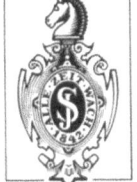

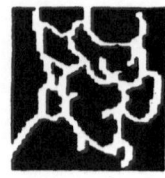

Editorial Board

R. Nakamura · R.L. Linscheid
T. Miura (Eds.)

Wrist Disorders

Current Concepts and Challenges

With 251 Figures, Including 8 in Color

Springer-Verlag
Tokyo Berlin Heidelberg
New York London Paris
Hong Kong Barcelona
Budapest

Ryogo Nakamura, m.d.
Associate Professor, Chief of Orthopaedic Surgery, Branch Hospital of Nagoya
University School of Medicine, 1-1-20 Daikominami, Higashi-ku, Nagoya, Aichi,
461 Japan

Ronald L. Linscheid, m.d.
Professor of Orthopedic Surgery, Department of Orthopedic Surgery, Mayo
Clinic, 200 First Street SW, Rochester, MN 55905, USA

Takayuki Miura, m.d.
Professor, Department of Orthopaedic Surgery, Nagoya University School of
Medicine, 65 Tsurumai-cho, Syowa-ku, Nagoya, Aichi, 466 Japan

On the front cover: Ulnar aspect, see Fig. 10/p. 20, and Scaphoid fracture evaluation, see
Fig. 6/p. 33.

ISBN 978-4-431-65876-4   ISBN 978-4-431-65874-0 (eBook)
DOI 10.1007/978-4-431-65874-0

Library of Congress Cataloging-in-Publication Data
Wrist disorders: current concepts and challenges/R. Nakamura, R.L. Linscheid, T. Miura
(eds.). p. cm. Includes bibliographical references and index.

Pathophysiology — Congresses. 3. Wrist Injuries — surgery — congresses. I. Nakamura, R.
(Ryogo), 1941– . II. Linscheid, R.L. (Ronald Lee), 1929– . III. Miura, Takayuki,
1930– . [DNLM: 1. Wrist — pathology — congresses. 2. Wrist — surgery — congresses.
WE 830 W9552] RD559.W753 1992 617.5′74059 — dc20, DNLM/DLC, for Library of
Congress. 92-49763

© Springer-Verlag Tokyo 1992
Softcover reprint of the hardcover 1st edition 1992

Typesetting, printing, and binding: Best-set Typesetter Ltd., Hong Kong

Preface

In recent years wrist problems have increasingly attracted the attention of orthopaedic and hand surgeons. Numerous advances have been achieved in functional anatomy, biomechanics, diagnosis, and treatment. There are, however, many controversial aspects to these problems.

Many clinical and associated investigators from around the world have attempted to increase our knowledge of the wrist with enthusiastic and devoted studies. An international symposium was held at the Nagoya Castle Hotel, Nagoya, Japan from March 6th through March 8th, 1991 to further understanding and promote discussion of wrist problems among a representative international group. Approximately 300 participants from 16 different countries assembled for these discussions.

This monograph consists of 40 selected papers based on presentations given at the international symposium. The topics are divided into six chapters: Functional Anatomy, Diagnosis and Basic Studies; Kienböck's Disease; Scaphoid Fracture, Distal Radius Fracture; Carpal Instability and Wrist Pain; and Wrist Arthroplasty. A number of unique observations as well as detailed surgical techniques were presented. These include topics such as the vascularity of the triangular fibrocartilage, radial wedge osteotomy and vascular bundle implantation into the lunate for Kienböck's disease, Herbert screw insertion though a minimal exposure for acute scaphoid fracture, and closing wedge oseotomy of the radial styloid for the early stage of the SLAC wrist.

It is hoped that this monograph will be of benefit to surgeons interested in not only achieving more satisfactory clinical outcomes, but also in stimulating further contemplation and research about these difficult wrist problems.

On behalf of the Organizing Committee of the International Symposium on the Wrist, we wish to express our gratitude to the authors who have generously taken time to prepare papers for publication.

RYOGO NAKAMURA
RONALD L. LINSCHEID
TAKAYUKI MIURA

Contents

Part III.   Scaphoid Fractures

Contributors

MUNEAKI ABE
Associate Professor, Osaka Medical College

A. HERBERT ALEXANDER
Chairman, Naval Hospital, Oakland

NICHOLAS BARTON
Consultant Hand Surgeon, Nottingham University Hospital

VAUGHAN BOWEN
Associate Professor, University of Toronto

ALESSANDRO CAROLI
Associate Professor, Modena University School of Medicine

JAMES H. DOBYNS
Professor (Emeritus), Mayo Graduate School

DIEGO L. FERNANDEZ
Associate Professor, University of Berne

TOSHIRO FUTAMI
Associate Professor, Kitazato University East Hospital

MOTONORI GOTO
Orthopaedic Surgeon, Fukuoka Orthopaedic Hospital

LOUIS A. GILULA
Professor, Mallinckrodt Institute of Radiology

YUICHI HIRASÉ
Assistant Professor, Jikei University School of Medicine

KOTARO IMAMURA
Assistant Professor, Nagasaki University School of Medicine

ADALBERT I. KAPANDJI
Clinique de l'Yvette

YASUKAZU KATSUMI
Professor, Meiji College of Oriental Medicine

JOHN M.G. KAUER
Professor, University of Nijimegen

IN KIM
Professor, Catholic University Medical College

YOSHIRO KIYOSHIGE
Chief, Saiseikai Yamagata Hospital

RONALD L. LINSCHEID
  Professor, Mayo Medical School

AKIO MINAMI
  Associate Professor, Hokkaido University School of Medicine

TAKAYA MIZUSEKI
  Chief, Hiroshima Prefectural Rehabilitation Center

YU MOCHIZUKI
  Hiroshima University School of Medicine

SHIN MUNESADA
  Tokai University

YOSHIFUMI NAGATANI
  Nagasaki University School of Medicine

RYOGO NAKAMURA
  Associate Professor, Nagoya University School of Medicine

TOSHIHIKO OGINO
  Professor, Sapporo Medical College

NOBUKI OHNISHI
  Associate Chairman, Oji General Hospital

TAKATOSHI OHNO
  Gifu University School of Medicine

HIROSHI ONO
  Nara Medical University

SEUNG-KOO RHEE
  Associate Professor, Catholic University Medical College

J. PAUL RYLEY
  Consultant Psychiatrist, Ashford Mental Health Center

MINORU SHIBATA
  Assistant Professor, Niigata University School of Medicine

KATSUMI SUZUKI
  Clinical Professor, University of Occupational and Environmental
  Health

SATOSHI TAKAHATA
  Hokkaido University School of Medicine

SATOSHI TOH
  Associate Professor, Hirosaki University School of Medicine

H. KIRK WATSON
  Associate Clinical Professor, University of Connecticut Medical School

HIROSHI YAJIMA
  Assistant Professor, Nara Medical University

KYU H. YANG
  Assistant Professor, Yonesei University College of Medicine

STEFANO ZANASI
  Senior Registrar, Modena University School of Medicine

Part I. Functional Anatomy, Diagnosis, and Basic Studies

The Wrist Joint: Functional Analysis and Experimental Approach

JOHN M.G. KAUER, ANTHONY de LANGE, HANS H.C.M. SAVELBERG, and
JAN G.M. KOOLOOS[1]

Abstract. The wrist allows the hand to combine dorsopalmar flexion and radioulnar deviation, a unique combination of functions that is made possible by a highly complex system of joints. The morphologic features of the carpal bones and of the radiocarpal and intercarpal contacts can be functionally interpreted by the mechanism that underlies the movements of the hand to the forearm. Displacements of the carpals take place in longitudinal articulation chains, with the proximal carpals having the position of an intercalated bone. The three articulation chains, radial, central, and ulnar, have interdependent movements at the radiocarpal and midcarpal levels. The linkage of movements in the longitudinal direction is associated to a transverse linkage by mutual joint contacts and by specific ligamentous interconnections. Kinematic analyses of the carpal joint motions have provided convincing evidence that each motion of the hand to the forearm demonstrates a specific motion pattern of the carpal bones. The stability of the carpus essentially depends on the integrity of the ligamentous system which consists of interwoven fiber bundles that differ in length, direction, and mechanical properties. Distinct separations into morphologic entities are difficult to make. From a functional point of view, the ligamentous interconnections can be regarded as a system that passively restricts movements of the carpals on one another and on the radius, but in a very differentiated way. The ligamentous system controls the linkage of the movements of the carpals, with the geometries of the bones and of the joint surfaces being, first of all, responsible for the kinematic behavior of the carpal joint.

Keywords: Wrist joint — Carpal mechanism — Articulation chains — Ligament behaviour — Ligament forces — Motion simulation

Introduction

Recognition and analysis of carpal joint disturbances require detailed insight into the normal function of the carpus. The understanding of the mechanism that underlies carpal function has been dominated for a long time by functional concepts developed in the second half of the 19th and the first half of the 20th centuries. These concepts are based on the principle that the hand moves in relation to the forearm at two joint levels in the wrist, the radiocarpal and the midcarpal joints. In these joints, two rigid transverse carpal rows are thought to move with respect to each other in the midcarpal joint, with the proximal transverse row moving to the radius in the radiocarpal joint. The two degrees of freedom of the hand with respect to the forearm, i.e., dorsopalmar flexion and radioulnar deviation, come about by differently directed movements at these two joints of the wrist. Different combinations of movements at the two joint levels establish the various positions of the hand relative to the forearm [1–9]. In this view, the movements take place around one or more fixed motion axes valid for the wrist as a whole. The functional importance of intercarpal mobility was recognized after discovery of the roentgenogram as a tool for the study of carpal bone displacements [10–12].

Destot [13] offered an important contribution to the understanding of the carpal mechanism, emphasizing the relations between carpal bone geometry, the shape of carpal bone contacts, and the mutual displacements of carpal bones in flexion and in deviation of the hand. He stressed the role of specific ligamentous interconnections

[1] Department of Anatomy and Embryology, University of Nijmegen, POB 9101, 6500 HB Nijmegen, The Netherlands

in carpal stability and specific mutual displacements of the carpals. However, the already accepted theory of the "fixed rows" had precluded a proper evaluation of these mutual displacements during motions of the hand to the forearm, as they did not fit the concept.

It has become apparent that functional concepts regarding the wrist joint, wherein specific morphologic features are omitted, are inadequate to explain the mechanism of action of the joint [14–21]. Moreover, they have been found to be useless in cases where intercarpal mobility assessment and the evaluation and classification of a disturbed carpal equilibrium are under discussion [14, 21–29].

The understanding of carpal disturbances has fundamentally increased the insight into normal wrist function. Classifications of instabilities of the carpal joint and the evaluation of clinical procedures show the necessity for detailed descriptions of the structures taking part in the joint system [3, 6, 16, 30–33] and of qualitative and quantitative data concerning the kinematics of the wrist [16, 34–42]. A close review of the literature shows that these data are not always interpreted in the same way.

The Carpal Link: A Model of Carpal Function

Gilford et al. [15] proposed a functional concept for the carpus in which they postulated that the joint functions as a system of three longitudinal articulation chains. In this system, proposed in

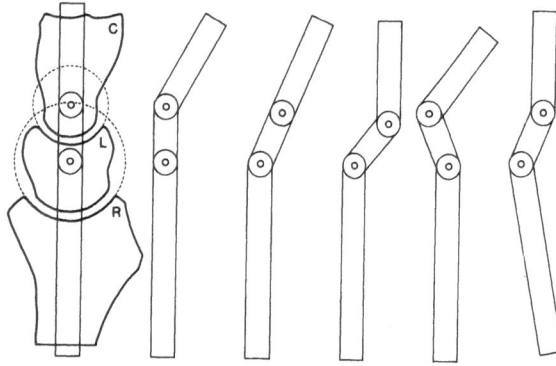

Fig. 1. The central chain, radius (R), lunate (L), capitate (C) modeled as a three-bar linkage, according to Gilford et al. [15]. The two joints — simple hinges — can move independently; the deformity of the link is unpredictible. (From [20] with permission)

order to give an explanation for the disturbed carpal equilibrium in some cases, they focused on the radiolunocapitate chain as the central part. Unaware of the concept of Navarro [43] that originated from the same principles, the central chain was modelled as a double trochlea: the mechanical equivalent of both the radiolunate and the radiocapitate joints is a simple pivot located at the "center of rotation" of each of the two joints. Figure 1 shows the central chain, modelled as a three-bar linkage. The model matches the approach of Reuleaux [44] which demonstrates that the direction in which the chain — on its own — will be deformed is unpredictible. The variety of mutual positions at the two joint levels, the result of the independence of the movements of the joints, offers an ever-changing shape of the central chain. In other words, the absence of a mutual attuning of the radiocarpal and midcarpal displacements creates the opportunity to move in every possible direction at both joint levels (Fig. 1).

The Intercalated Segments

The proximal carpals hold the position of intercalated bones without any muscular attachments. In the central chain, the lunate acts as the intercalated bone. The tendency of the lunate to move with respect to the radius and the capitate is highly dominated by the specific geometry of the lunate. The lunate has a larger proximo-distal dimension at the palmar aspect than at the dorsal aspect, being wedge-shaped in the dorsopalmar direction (Fig. 2). As a result, the lunate has an ever-present tendency to move into a dorsal rotation [17]. This moving tendency is independent from the position of the capitate to the radius. Another outcome of the specific geometry of the lunate is a simultaneous movement at both joint levels: the lunate tends to move with respect to the radius as well as with respect to the capitate.

It becomes obvious that the central chain can not function on its own. The lunate would become dislocated palmarly, so it would have to be stabilized. To explain the mechanism of stabilization of the central chain, mechanical models are proposed in which the scaphoid plays an essential role [14, 21]. In the radial chain (radius, scaphoid, trapezium, and trapezoid) the scaphoid is the intercalated bone. The position of the scaphoid is complicated in the functional sense since the scaphoid contacts the distal carpal row at two

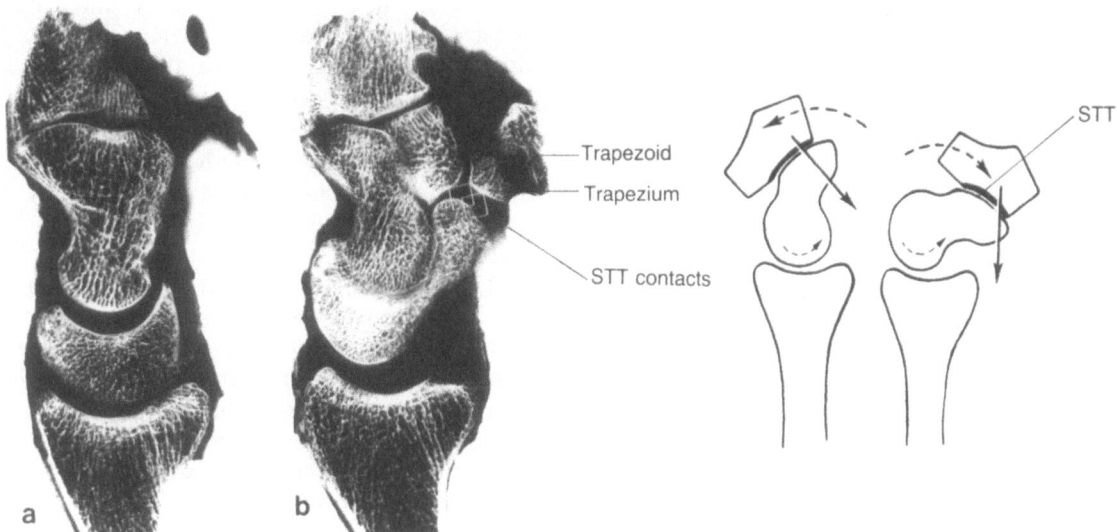

Fig. 2. Radiographed sagittal sections **a** through the lunate and **b** through the scaphoid. The dorsopalmar wedge shape of the lunate and the proximal part of the scaphoid suggests the tendency to rotate dorsally. The tendency to rotate dorsally of the scaphoid is counteracted by the scaphoid-trapezium-trapezoid (STT) contacts (*diagram*)

different levels, being interposed between trapezium, trapezoid, and radius and between the capitate and radius. The proximal part of the scaphoid, interposed between the capitate and radius, is wedge-shaped in the same direction as the lunate (Fig. 2). Therefore, this part of the scaphoid has the same tendency to move as the lunate, i.e., in a dorsal rotation. However, this moving tendency will be counteracted by the contact of the scaphoid with the trapezium and trapezoid (STT) (Fig. 2). The scaphoid will be forced into a palmar rotation together with the lunate and against the tendency to move when the hand is flexed palmarly or deviated radially. In dorsal flexion of the hand and in ulnar deviation, the scaphoid will come into the erect position with the dorsal rotation, a result of the wedge shape of the proximal part of the scaphoid and of the lunate, but only as far as is permitted by the STT contacts. The antagonism of the trapezium-trapezoid and capitate actions at the scaphoid makes the bone easily subject to trauma.

Scapholunate Interaction

Another point in the geometry of the scaphoid and the lunate should be mentioned. If, as is illustrated in Fig. 3, the radiocarpal surfaces of the scaphoid and lunate would be equally

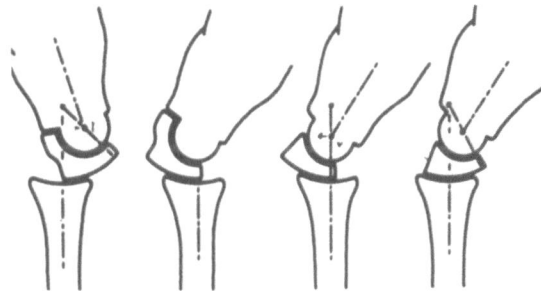

Fig. 3. Wedge-shaped scaphoid and lunate. In these models, both bones have equally curved contacts with the radius. The scaphoid and lunate will move together without mutual displacements

curved, both bones would move together, with the scaphoid slipping into a fixed end-position with respect to the trapezium and trapezoid. In fact, there would be no movement of the proximal carpals with respect to the distal carpals.

Lateral X-rays of the hand in the end-positions of flexion and of deviation show mutual displacements of the proximal carpals during their dorsopalmar rotation (Fig. 4). These displacements are based on differences in curvature at the radiocarpal joint contacts. The scaphoid, having a stronger curved proximal facet, will rotate faster

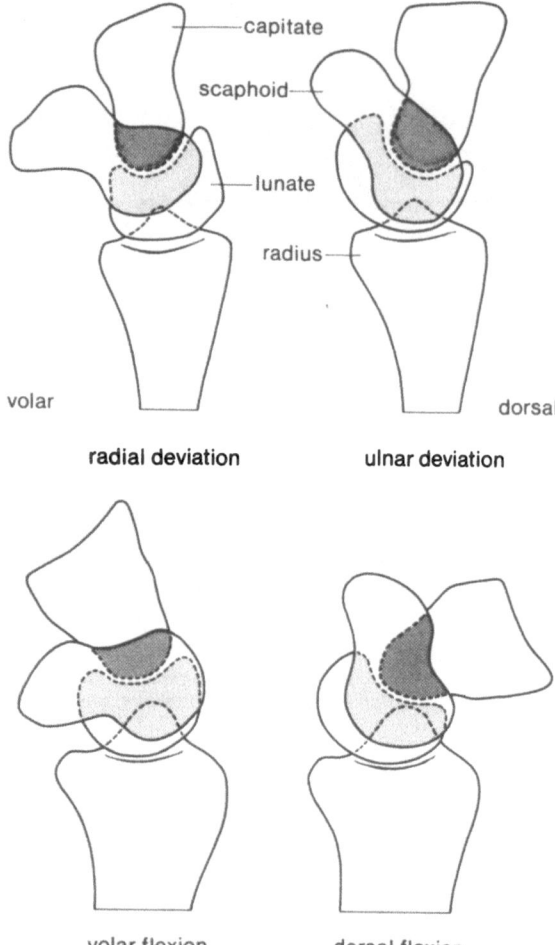

Fig. 4. The lateral projections of the radio-scapholunocapitate complex in the four end-positions of the hand. The overprojections of scaphoid, lunate and capitate are *shaded*. Note the unequally curved facets of the scaphoid and lunate in relation to the radius. (From [18] with permission)

in the palmar and dorsal directions in comparison with the lunate. As a result, the scaphoid shifts proximally relative to the lunate and relative to

the capitate when rotating palmarly, and will shift in the distal direction to these bones when rotating dorsally. The shift between the scaphoid and lunate will lead to differences in the angulations of the radial and central chains associated with dorsopalmar rotation of both bones.

The scapholunate shift is influenced by the scapholunate interosseous ligament. This ligament has a short dorsal part and a longer palmar part, thus making the mobility of the scaphoid to the lunate greatest at the palmar aspects of the bones. The shorter dorsal part serves as a turning point while the palmar part can bridge the cleft between the two bones which is present in the dorsiflexed hand. When the scaphoid and lunate come into the palmar rotated position, the palmar part has to bridge an increasing difference of level between the palmar parts of the scaphoid and lunate. As a result, the palmar cleft will close (Fig. 5). This mechanism includes the fact that the scaphoid and lunate move in the transverse plane, making pronation-supination movements along longitudinal axes while rotating in the dorsopalmar direction. These "out of plane" movements restrict the use of bony landmarks on conventional X-rays for making detailed comparisons of rotation angles [25].

Midcarpal Displacements

Displacements at the radiocarpal level will be followed immediately by displacements at the midcarpal level. The inequality of the curvature of the joints of the scaphoid and lunate to the radius will lead to different angulations of the central and radial chains during flexon and deviation of the hand. This includes midcarpal displacements as well. Radiocarpal and midcarpal displacements are interdependent. It is important to note the direction of the midcarpal displacement (Fig. 6). In the central chain, the four end-

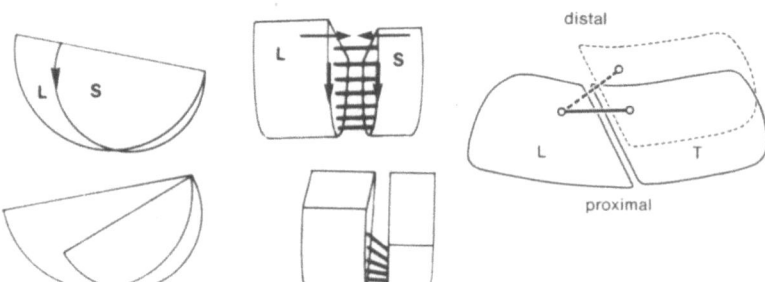

Fig. 5. Intercarpal mobility of the proximal carpal bones. Intercarpal displacements depend on differently curved joint facets and differently shaped interosseous connections. (From [16, 18] with permission)

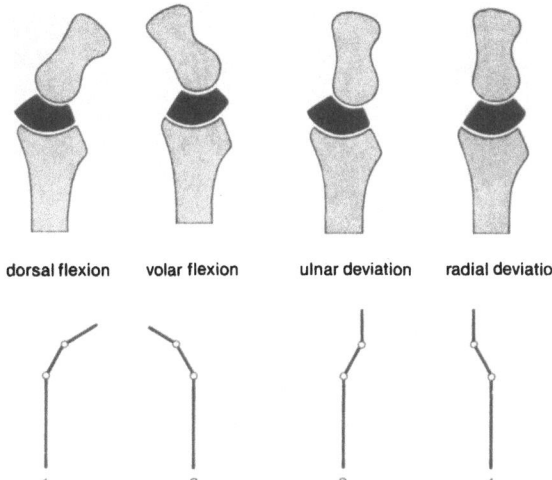

dorsal flexion   volar flexion   ulnar deviation   radial deviation

1   2   3   4

Fig. 6. Positions of the intercalated lunate in relation to the capitate and the radius in the four end-positions of flexion and deviation. *1,* The lunate shifts to the radius palmarly and to the capitate dorsally; *2,* the lunate shifts to the radius dorsally and to the capitate palmarly; *3,* the lunate shifts to the radius and to the capitate palmarly; *4,* the lunate shifts to the radius and to the capitate dorsally. (From [18] with permission)

positions of the lunate to the capitate and to the radius show that the intercalated lunate can move at the radiocarpal and midcarpal levels in the same as well as the opposite directions. Radiocarpally, the positions of the lunate in dorsal flexion and ulnar deviation are very similar, i.e., dorsally rotated, while, in palmar flexion, the position of the lunate resembles that in radial deviation. Midcarpally, the dorsal flexion end-position corresponds with the end-position in radial deviation and the palmar flexion end-position with the position in ulnar deviation. It becomes clear that the same phenomena can be observed in the radial and ulnar chains. At the midcarpal level, the proximal facets of the distal carpals have very irregularly curved and very specifically oriented joint contacts with the proximal carpals [45]. A midcarpal shift in either the palmar or dorsal direction of the proximal carpals to the distal carpals will change the orientation of the proximal carpals in the transverse plane. The direction of the "out of plane" motion associated with the dorsopalmar rotation is dependent on the direction of the midcarpal shift. Therefore, it can be assumed that the palmar-rotated proximal carpals in palmar flexion and in radial deviation show differences in their special positions. The same applies to the positions of the dorsal-rotated

proximal carpals in dorsal flexion and in ulnar deviation [18]. As a result of this mechanism, we can find very specific mutual positions of the carpals in every position of the hand in relation to the forearm.

The role of the triquetrum also has to be considered in this respect. The triquetrum moves with the lunate to the distal carpal row showing only a proximodistal shift to the lunate of 1 or 2 mm (Fig. 5). The lunotriquetrum interface is obliquely directed and is connected by only a short interosseous ligament. The triquetrum bridges the gap between the hamate and the lunate. The hamate-triquetrum joint can be described as a saddle joint with facets that have concave as well as convex parts. The saddle is irregularly curved, with a dorsopalmar groove on the hamate surface that is wound in a spiral fashion [45]. The spiral groove gives the triquetrum a swerving motion in the transverse plane when moving dorsopalmarly to the hamate. The dorsal rotation of the hamate to the triquetrum (in dorsal flexion and in radial deviation) will bring the triquetrum more radially with respect to the hamate and more ulnarly in the palmar rotation of the hamate to the triquetrum (in palmar flexion and in ulnar deviation). These movements of the triquetrum with respect to the hamate are in concert with the movements of the lunate with respect to the capitate. Capitolunate and hamate-triquetrum movements support each other.

In addition, the functional position of the triquetrum is dominated by the fact that all major ligaments, radiocarpal and ulnocarpal, have insertions into the bones of the ulnar carpal chain. This chain supports not only the movements in the central chain but anchors the wrist to the radius. In this way, the triquetrum plays the role of a keystone in the stability of the carpal joint.

Carpal Motion Axes

Analysis of the movements of the carpal bones during flexion and deviation of the hand gives the strong impression of specific motion patterns for each change in position of the hand to the forearm. A kinematic study of the human wrist joint based on roentgen-stereophotogrammetric experimentation [46] has offered precise data concerning the individual carpal bone motions in flexion and deviation of the hand [37, 39]. It can be concluded that the carpals move in re-

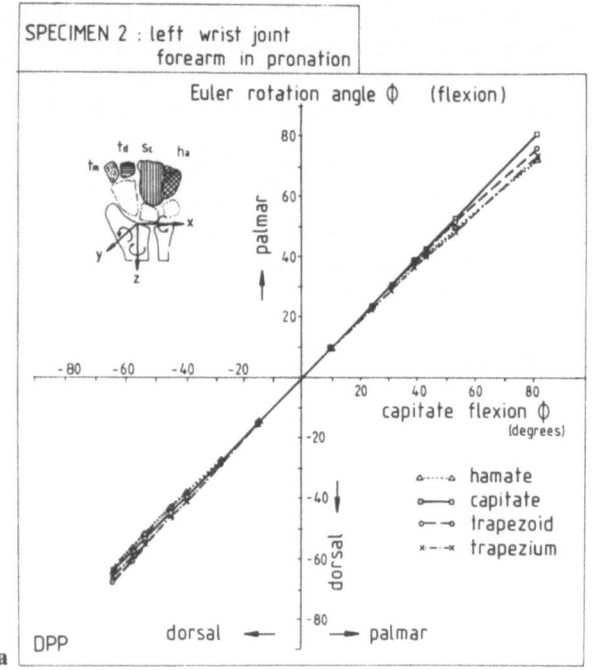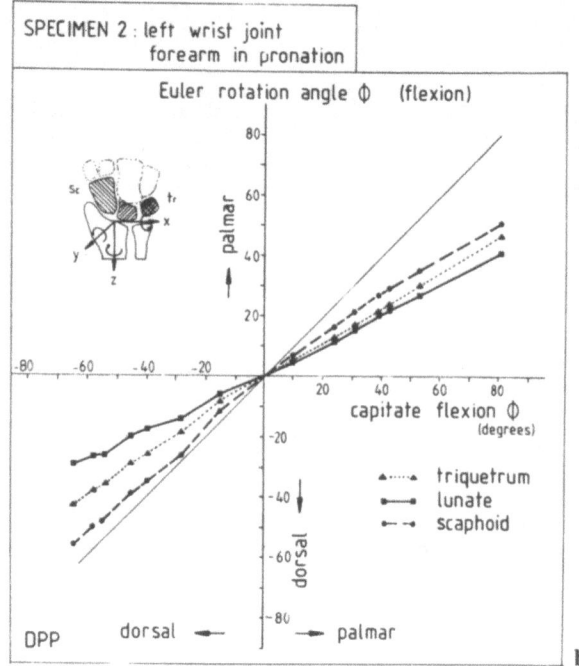

Fig. 7. Flexion angles (in degrees) **a** of the distal carpal bones and **b** of the proximal carpal bones as functions of the capitate flexion in dorsopalmar flexion of the pronated hand

producible patterns. In these patterns, the distal row moves as a solid block while the proximal carpals show differences in their rotational angles (Fig. 7). It can also be observed that the proximal carpals move simultaneously at the proximal and distal carpal joint levels.

The representation of spacial movements of the carpal bones can be approximated by a sequence of finite displacements. For each displacement, the helical axis can be calculated from measurements on the displacements of a number of anatomical or artificial landmarks in the carpal bone under consideration. The axis is the representation of a combination of translation along and a rotation about a line. The collection of these lines represents the motion of the carpal in relation to a fixed coordinate system. Each motion's step has its own motion axis, so the movement from end-position to end-position is characteristic and can be described by a bundle of axes for each carpal bone. It should be noted that there is no point of intersection of all axes of one bundle. The points of nearest approximation of the axes of one bundle (the pivot points) are all located within the carpus, around the capitolunate joint (Fig. 8). These experiments demonstrate that there is no point that functions as a center of

rotation for the carpus as a whole [37]. Additionally, it must be emphasized that the pivot points in flexion and deviation of the hand are located in different sites, data that concur with the concept that includes the effects of radiocarpal and midcarpal displacements in the same and in the opposite directions during flexion and deviation, respectively.

In this way, the carpal mechanism will generate specific motion patterns for each movement of the hand. The specificity of the motion patterns, primarily based on the specific carpal bone geometry, is a major factor in the stability of the carpal joint. The quantitative kinematic data have offered validation for this concept.

Ligament Function

The ligament system of the wrist joint consists of interwoven fiber bundles that differ in length, direction, texture, and mechanical properties [32, 47–50]. These properties are not always interpreted in the same manner [30, 32, 36, 47, 51, 52]. Therefore, it is not surprising that we encounter different classifications and different interpretations of the function of parts of the system,

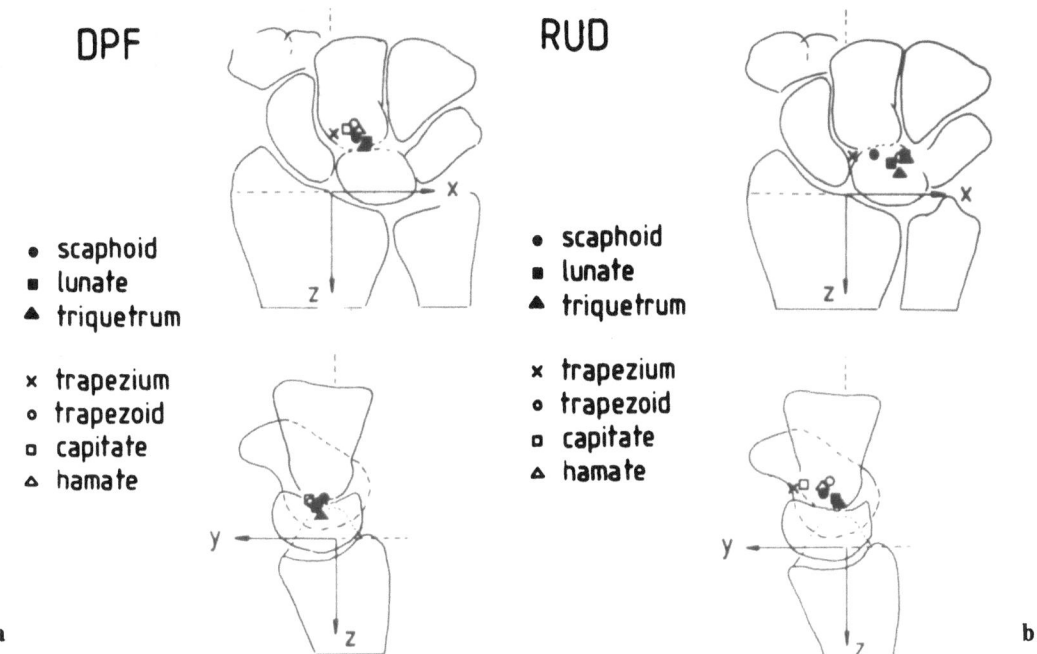

Fig. 8. The positions of the carpal pivot points relative to the coordinate system in the same carpus. **a** Dorsopalmar flexion (DPF) **b** Radioulnar deviation (RUD)

especially if we also take into consideration that it is quite difficult to make distinct separations in the morphologic sense. In general, the ligaments of the carpal joint are regarded as a system that passively restricts the mutual movements of the carpal bones and with respect to the radius and the ulna. For some intrinsic ligaments, i.e., the scapholunate and lunotriquetrum interosseous, a role as controls in the linkage of the movements of the proximal carpals could be demonstrated, a role that is consistent with the specific geometries of the carpal bones. The radiocarpal and ulnocarpal ligaments counteract the tendency of axial rotation of the hand with respect to the radius, but, at the same time, it can be established that the stability of the carpal joint depends on the integrity of the ligamentous system as a whole. Therefore, experimental procedures in which the

Fig. 9. Elastic moduli of some (parts of) carpal ligaments *RCP*, Palmar radiocapitate; *RLPp* and *RLPd*, proximal and distal part of the palmar radiolunate; *TCP*, palmar triquetrocapitate; *RTD*, dorsal radiocapitate; *RTD*, dorsal radiotriquetral; *TTD*, dorsal triquetrotrapezium. *RCP* and *RTD* are significantly stiffer than the other parts

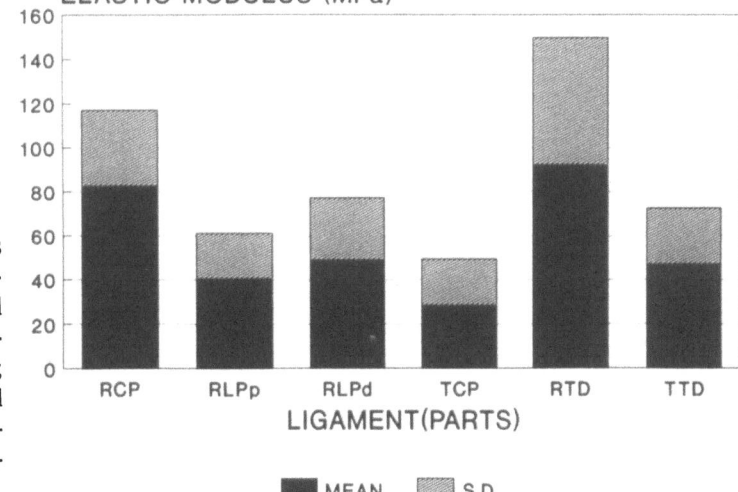

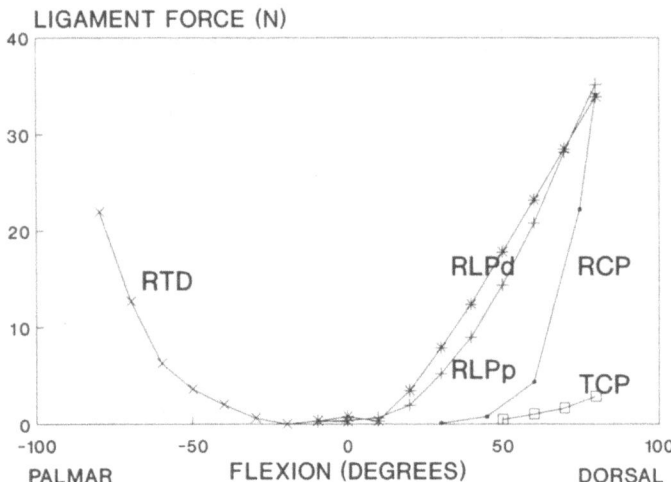

Fig. 10. The calculated ligament forces in the flexion of the hand. The forces are relatively low. The ligaments are strained in the endpositions. Abbreviations as in Fig. 9

role of selected ligaments is investigated, i.e., by cutting these ligaments sequentially, will not render significant information for evaluating trauma to ligaments.

In order to understand ligament function and the mechanism of ligament injury, more detailed knowledge is needed about the mechanical properties of ligaments [36, 50–52]. In recognizing that the carpal ligamentous system consists of only poorly stretchable material, functional concepts of the carpus in which ligaments function under the condition of a substantial elongation do not give justice to the mechanical properties of these structures [30, 32, 33]. In vitro assessment of carpal ligament behavior shows differences in stiffness between parts of the ligamentous system (Fig. 9). The palmar radiocapitate and dorsal radiotriquetrum ligaments have the highest elastic moduli, while the other parts show significantly lower values. However, in order to establish the function of ligaments as constraints in the motion pattern of the carpal bones, data are needed about the forces that are generated in the ligaments during movements of flexion and deviation.

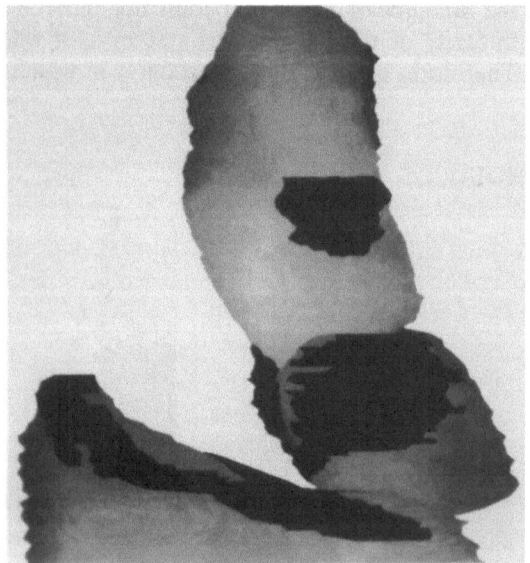
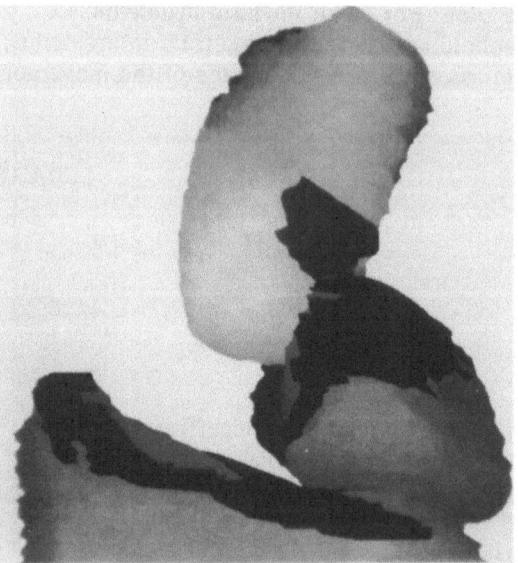

Fig. 11. The reconstructed positions **a** of the radiolunocapitate in the neutral position and **b** in the ulnar deviation position, palmar view. The changes in the spacial positions of some of the ligament insertion sites can be noted

These data can be obtained by combining the experimental data on ligament length changes and force-elongation relationships. Ligament forces have been calculated for some ligaments (Fig. 10). It can be suggested that, under normal conditions, the loading of the ligamentous system is relatively low, while some ligaments become strained only at the end-positions of the hand with respect to the forearm. To what extent these in vitro experiments, in which only small parts of the ligaments are under consideration, offer reliable quantitative data has to be further investigated [53]. Data concerning the changes in the mutual positions of ligament insertion sites can be collected by simulation of the kinematics in computer-reconstructions of serial-sectioned carpal joints (Fig. 11). The kinematics of the joint and the function of the ligaments can thus be assessed in conjunction.

It has been established that muscles which cross the carpal joint are an essential part of the stabilizing system of the wrist [17]. Within this framework, the absence of true collateral ligaments should be noted. True collaterals would support the flexion movement of the hand but, at the same time, would affect the range of radioulnar deviation. Experimental data have offered the suggestion that the extensor carpi ulnaris, abductor pollicis longus, and extensor pollicis brevis tendons can function as a dynamic collateral system, being able to adjust both their length and their strain. To what extent the tendons crossing the wrist will influence the behavior of the ligaments which are closely interwoven with their tendon sheaths is yet unknown.

The function of the carpal ligamentous system has to be regarded as the support of the motion patterns based upon mutually attuned carpal bone geometries, which are essential linkages in the interdependency of the carpal articulation chains.

References

1. Bonin von G (1929) A note on the kinematics of the wrist joint. J Anat 63:259–262
2. Cyriax EF (1926) On the rotary movements of the wrist. J Anat 60:199–201
3. Fick R (1904, 1910, 1911) Handbuch der Anatomie und Mechanik der Gelenke. In: von Bardeleben K (ed) Handbuch der Anatomie des Menschen. I. Anatomie der Gelenke; II. Allgemeine Gelenk- und Muskelmechanik; III. Spezielle Gelenk- und Muskelmechanik. Gustav Fischer, Jena
4. Fischer O (1897) Über Gelenke von zwei Graden der Freiheit. Arch Anat Entwickelungsgesch Suppl Bd, pp 242–272
5. Fischer O (1907) Kinematik organischer Gelenke. Vieweg, Braunschweig
6. Günther GB (1850) Das Handgelenk in mechanischer, anatomischer und chirurgischer Beziehung. Meissner, Hamburg
7. Henke W (1859) Die Bewegungen der Handwurzel. Z Rat Med 7:27–42
8. Strasser H (1917) Lehrbuch der Muskel- und Gelenkmechanik. IV. Spezieller Teil: Die obere Extremität. Springer, Berlin
9. Wright RD (1935) A detailed study of movement of the wrist joint. J Anat 70:137–142
10. Forssel G (1902) Über die Bewegungen im Handgelenke des Menschen. Scand Arch Physiol 12:168–258
11. Virchow H (1902) Die Weiterdrehung des Naviculare carpi bei Dorsalflexion, und die Beziehungen der Handbänder. Anat Anz 21:111–126
12. Virchow H (1902) Über Einzelmechanismen am Handgelenk. Anat Anz 21:369–388
13. Destot E (1923) Anatomie et physiologie du poignet. In: Destot E (ed) Traumatismes du poignet et rayons X. Masson, Paris
14. Fisk GR (1970) Carpal instability and the fractured scaphoid (Hunterian lecture). Ann R Coll Surg Engl 46:63–76
15. Gilford WW, Bolton RH, Lambrinudi C (1943) The mechanism of the wrist joint with special reference to fractures of the scaphoid. Guys Hosp Rep 92:52–59
16. Kauer JMG (1974) The interdependence of carpal articulation chains. Acta Anat 88:481–501
17. Kauer JMG (1980) Functional anatomy of the wrist. Clin Orthop 149:9–20
18. Kauer JMG (1986) The mechanism of the carpal joint. Clin Orthop 202:16–26
19. Kauer JMG (1988) The longitudinal carpal chain, a model of carpal function. Ann R Coll Surg Engl 70:166
20. Kauer JMG, Lange de A (1987) The carpal joint. In: Taleisnik J (ed) Management of wrist problems. Hand Clin 3(1):23–29
21. Linscheid RL, Dobyns JH, Beabout JW, Bryan RS (1972) Traumatic instability of the wrist. J Bone Joint Surg [Am] 54:1612–1632
22. Bellinghausen HW, Gilula LA, Young LV, Weeks PM (1983) Posttraumatic palmar carpal subluxation. J Bone Joint Surg [Am] 65:998–1006
23. Fisk GR (1980) An overview of injuries of the wrist. Clin Orthop 149:137–144

24. Fisk GR (1988) Malalignment of the scaphoid after lunate dislocation. In: Razemon JP, Fisk GR (eds) The wrist. Churchill Livingstone, Edinburgh, pp 135–137

25. Gilula LA (1979) Carpal injuries: Analytic approach and case exercises. Am J Roentgenol 133:503–517

26. Gilula LA, Weeks PM (1978) Posttraumatic ligamentous instability of the wrist. Radiology 129:641–651

27. Green DP (1988) Carpal dislocations and instabilities. In: Green DP (ed) Operative hand surgery. Churchill Livingstone, New York, pp 875–938

28. Johnson RP (1980) The acutely injured wrist and its residuals. Clin Orthop 149:33–44

29. Lichtman DM, Martin RA (1988) Introduction to the carpal instabilities. In: Lichtman DM (ed) The wrist and its disorders. Saunders, Philadelphia, pp 244–250

30. Mayfield JK, Johnson RP, Kilcoyne RG (1976) The ligaments of the human wrist and their functional significance. Anat Rec 186:417–428

31. Reicher MA, Kellerhouse LE (1990) Carpal instability. In: Reicher MA, Kellerhouse LE (eds) MRI of the wrist and hand. Raven, New York, pp 69–85

32. Taleisnik J (1976) The ligaments of the wrist. J Hand Surg [Am] 1:110–118

33. Taleisnik J (1984) Current concepts of the anatomy of the wrist. In: Spinner M (ed) Kaplan's functional and surgical anatomy of the hand. Lippincott, Philadelphia, pp 179–201

34. Berger RA (1980) Analysis of carpal bone kinematics. Thesis, University of Iowa, Iowa

35. Berger RA, Crowninshield RD, Flatt AE (1982) The three-dimensional rotational behavior of the carpal bones. Clin Orthop 167:303–310

36. Lange de A, Huiskes R, Kauer JMG (1990) Wrist joint ligament length changes in flexion and deviation of the hand: An experimental study. J Orthop Res 8:722–730

37. Lange de A, Huiskes R, Kauer JMG (1990) Effects of data smoothing on the reconstruction of helical axis parameters in human joint kinematics. J Biomech Eng 112:107–113

38. Lange de A, Huiskes R, Kauer JMG (1990) Measurement errors in roentgen-stereophotogrammetric joint-motion analysis. J Biomech 23:259–269

39. Lange de A, Kauer JMG, Huiskes R (1985) Kinematic behavior of the human wrist joint: A roentgen-stereophotogrammetric analysis. J Orthop Res 3:56–64

40. Rozing PM, Kauer JMG (1984) Partial arthrodesis of the wrist. Acta Orthop Scand 55:66–68

41. Youm Y, Flatt AE (1980) Kinematics of the wrist. Clin Orthop 149:21–32

42. Youm Y, McMurthy RY, Flatt AE, Gillespie TE (1978) Kinematics of the wrist. 1: An experimental study of radio-ulnar deviation and flexion-extension. J Bone Joint Surg [Am] 60:423–432

43. Navarro A (1921) Luxaciones del carpo. Cited by Taleisnik J (1985) The bones of the wrist. In: Taleisnik J (ed) The wrist. Churchill Livingstone, New York, pp 1–12

44. Reuleaux F (1878) Theoretische Kinematik, Grundzüge einer Theorie der Maschinenwegens. Vieweg, Braunschweig

45. Johnston HM (1907) Varying positions of the carpal bones in the different movements at the wrist. J Anat Phys 41:109–222; 280–292

46. Selvik G (1974) A roentgen-stereophotogrammetric method for the study of the kinematics of the skeletal system. Thesis, University of Lund, Lund

47. Bonjean P, Houton JL, Linarte R, Vignes J (1981) Anatomical bases for the dynamic exploration of the wrist joint. Anatomia Clinica 3:73–85

48. Logan SE, Nowak MD, Gould Ph L, Weeks PM (1986) Biomechanical behavior of the scapholunate ligament. Biomed Sci Instrum 22:81–85

49. Mayfield JK (1980) Mechanism of carpal injuries. Clin Orthop 149:45–54

50. Nowak MD, Logan SE (1991) Distinguishing biomechanical properties of instrinsic and extrinsic human wrist ligaments. J Biomech Eng 113:85–93

51. Savelberg HHCM, Kooloos JGM, Kauer JMG (1989) Kinematics of the human carpal bone-ligament complex. Ann Soc R Zool Belg 119:65

52. Savelberg HHCM, Kooloos JGM, Lange de A, Kauer JMG, Huiskes R (1991) Human carpal ligament recruitment and three-dimensional carpal motion. J Orthop Res 9:693–704

53. Kooloos JGM (1991) The insertion sites of selected human carpal ligaments. A quantitative morphological study using three-dimensional computer reconstructions. Eur J Morphol 29(2):77–87

Examination of the Wrist

RONALD L. LINSCHEID[1]

Keywords: Wrist — Examination — Tendinitis — Sprains — Fractures — Instabilities

Introduction

The wrist is a very complicated joint which is susceptible to a number of diseases, injuries, and arthritic changes. Because there is very little subcutaneous fat and the skin is closely applied to the various structures of the wrist, physical examination is enhanced. Obviously, a very through knowledge of the anatomy of the region is required, especially that of the surface representation of the various bony landmarks. Since many of these are palpable, the best teaching aid is examination of one's own wrist, especially in conjunction with a skeletal specimen for referral.

The actual examination of the wrist is dependent on a thorough case history which elicits the site of pain, the motions that elicit discomfort, and the characteristics of the pain. These results and the physical examination then help to determine what further imaging techniques or laboratory tests may be indicated. While there are a number of ways of discussing the examination of the wirst, representative diagnoses that occur in various aspects of the wrist may be instructive in presenting the differential diagnoses of the various areas as well as point out some of the characteristic findings of each aspect. Comparison with the opposite normal wrist should be routine.

Radial Aspect of the Wrist

On the radial aspect of the wrist, one may palpate the radial styloid process, the trapezium and trapezoid, and the tendons of the anatomic snuff box including the abductor pollicis longus and extensor pollicis brevis palmarly and the extensor pollicis longus dorsally. The radial artery may be palpated within the snuff box.

Intersection Syndrome

The intersection syndrome is associated with post-traumatic inflammation between the "outcropping" muscles of the abductor pollicis longus and the underlying extensor tendons of the wrist [1]. This is often brought on by acute repetitive exertion. Besides a positive Finkelstein's test, there is tenderness over the taut muscle bellies. Crepitus associated with either flexion extension of the wrist or motion of the thumb is often felt under the abductor pollicis longus muscle belly. This condition is usually self-limiting but in some instances may become chronic (Fig. 1.a).

DeQuervain's Disease

DeQuervain's disease, or stenosing tenosynovitis, is associated with tenderness directly over the radial styloid aggravated by resisted extension and by pain elicited by the Finkelstein's test [2, 3]. This test is performed by clasping the thumb under the fingers and acutely deviating the wrist ulnarly. There is often a prominence over the radial styloid associated with hypertrophy of the dorsal retinaculum that overlies the first dorsal compartment. A ganglion sometimes arises from the area (Fig. 1.b).

Wartenberg's Cheiralgia

This is discomfort due to the irritation of the superficial sensory branch of the radial nerve over the radial styloid which is usually brought on by

[1] Department of Orthopedic Surgery, Mayo Clinic, 200 First Street SW, Rochester, MN 55905, USA

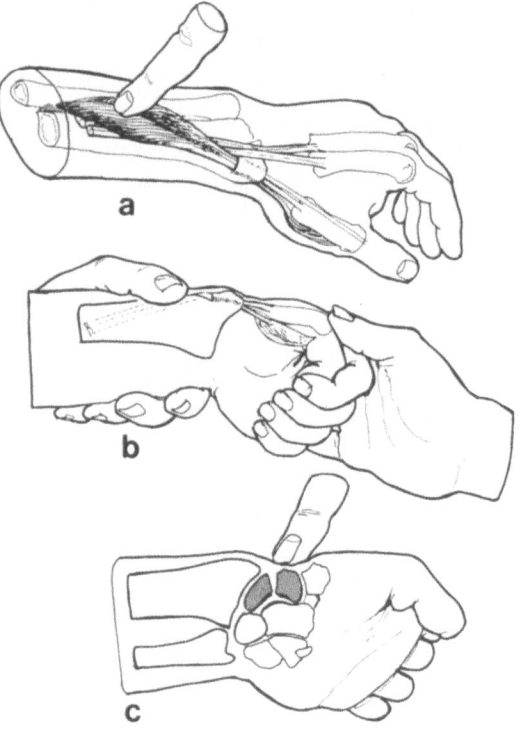

Fig. 1. Radial aspect. **a** "Intersection syndrome", peritendinitis, crepitans of "outcropping" muscles. Tenderness is elicited with direct pressure. Crepitus beneath the abductor pollicis brevis is noted on thumb or wrist extension while palpating the muscle. **b** Finkelstein's test for DeQuervain's disease. Stenosing tenosynovitis of the first dorsal compartment is painful with a forced ulnar deviation of the thumb and wrist. There is often swelling and tenderness over the radial styloid. **c** Tenderness in the anatomic snuff box may be due to scaphoid fracture, radioscaphoid degenerative disease, and calcific capsulitis

mechanical irritation of the nerve from direct blows or compressive objects about the wrist such as casts, splints, or bracelets. The nerve is often readily palpable just beneath the cephalic vein. When the fingers are rubbed over the nerve pain or paresthesias may be elicited into the thumb or first web space. The Tinel's test is usually positive.

Scaphoid Fracture and Radioscaphoid Degenerative Disease

Tenderness in the snuff box is well known as a sign for scaphoid fracture, particularly of the scaphoid waist. It may also be positive with

scaphotrapezial degenerative disease and radioscaphoid degenerative change (Fig. 1.c).

Dorsoradial Aspect of the Wrist

The dorsoradial aspect of the wrist includes that area between the extensor carpi radialis longus and the extensors of the fingers and from Lister's tubercle to the carpometacarpal joints. The bony landmarks are Lister's tubercle, the dorsal rim of the scaphoid, trapezoid, and capitate.

Occult Ganglion

An occult ganglion, as differentiated from the usual dorsoradial ganglion, implies that the occult variety arising from a defect in the dorsal aspect of the scapholunate ligament has not penetrated the dorsal capsule of the wrist and, therefore, is not as obvious to observation or palpation. These ganglia are most commonly seen in young women, and tenderness may be elicited by direct pressure over the scapholunate junction with the

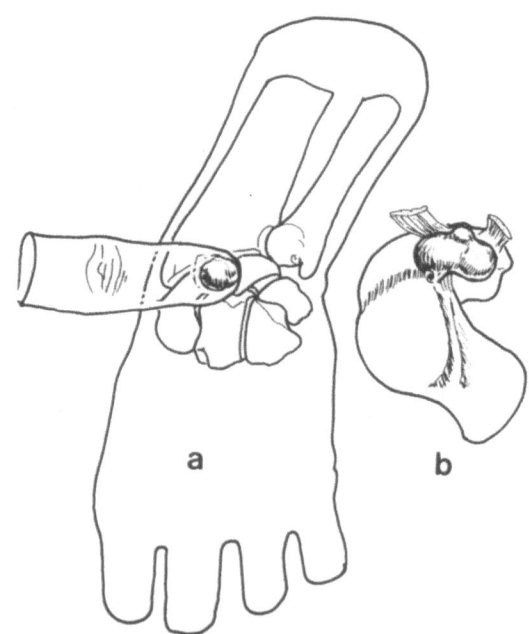

Fig. 2. Dorsal aspect. **a** Occult ganglion is suspected in younger women with point tenderness over the dorsal aspect of the scapholunate ligament. **b** A small sessile mass may be palpated with mild palmar flexion of the wrist

wrist in slight palmar flexion. A small sessile mass may be palpated in some individuals [4] (Fig. 2).

Radioscaphoid Impingement

This condition, as the name implies, usually occurs with repetitive dorsiflexion stress such as that which afflicts gymnasts or physical development enthusiasts. Localized tenderness directly over the scaphoid rim just radial to the site of the tenderness in the previous example can be elicited by direct pressure. Forced extension in radial deviation is painful. Standard X-rays are usually negative and help to exclude scaphoid fracture. Sclerosis or a small loose body may occasionally be seen on tomography [5] (Fig. 3.b).

Proximal Pole Instability or Dynamic Rotary Subluxation of the Scaphoid

This diagnosis, popularized by Watson, has pain and tenderness in the same area. Its presence is best determined by dorsally pressuring the

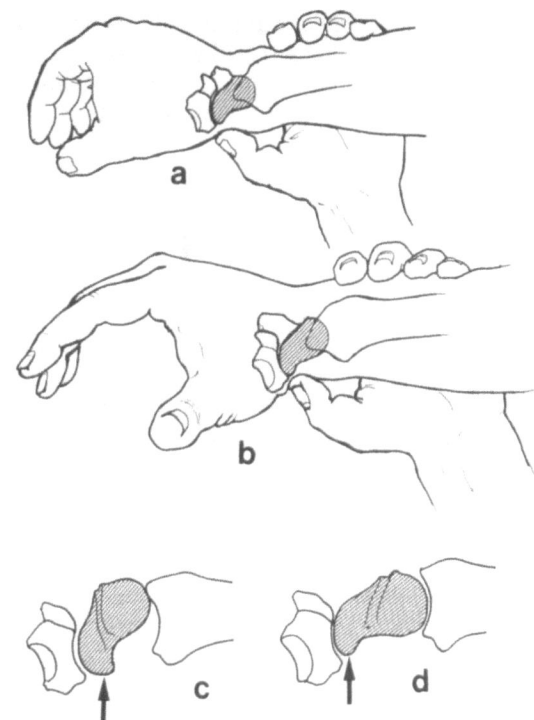

Fig. 4. Palmar aspect. Displacement of the scaphoid tuberosity dorsally as the hand is swung from ulnar (**a**) to radial (**b**) deviation may elicit pain from dorsal subluxation of the proximal scaphoid pole (Watson test) (**c**) or impingement of degenerative articular surfaces of the scapho-trapezio-trapezoidal (STT) joint (**d**). *Arrows*, direction of applied force

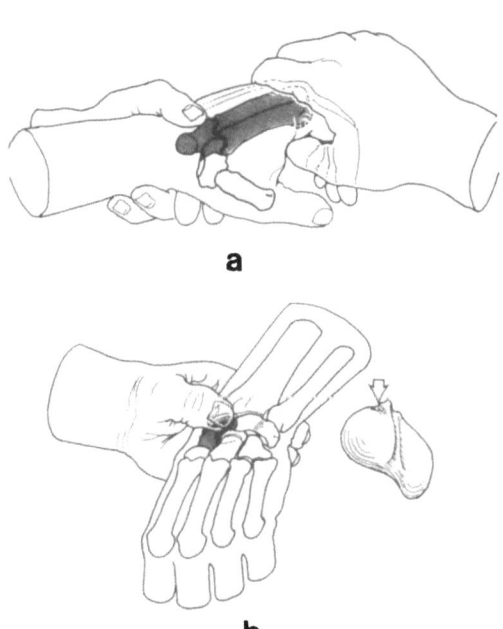

Fig. 3. a Chronic sprains of the second, third, and fourth carpometacarpal joints are easy to overlook. Manipulation of the respective metacarpal and its proximal carpal and elicitation of pain by direct pressure are suggestive signs. **b** Scaphoid impaction syndrome is suggested by point tenderness to palpation over the scaphoid ridge, especially in gymnasts, weight lifters, etc., where chronic impaction of the scaphoid against the radial rim occurs

scaphoid tuberosity while the wrist is in ulnar deviation and then passively deviating the wrist radially. Elicitation of pain or a snap as the scaphoid dorsally subluxes is thought to be diagnostic (note also scaphotrapezial degenerative joint disease) [6] (Fig. 4a–c).

Posterior Interosseous Nerve Syndrome

This is a diagnosis even more difficult to make. The posterior interosseous nerve does supply the dorsal capsule after branching profusely just proximal to the scapholunate junction. Whether or not it conveys pain impulses is not firmly established, but neuromata in this nerve, especially following ganglion excisions or surgical approaches to the dorsum of the wrist, are not uncommon. Excision of a segment of this nerve at the time of exploration is considered by many to be a worthwhile adjunct to exploration of the dorsum of the wrist. Injection of a small amount of lidocaine subperiosteally just ulnar to Lister's tubercle may be helpful in evaluating this problem.

Occult Fractures of the Wrist

Occult fractures in the dorsoradial aspect of the wrist are easily missed. This includes lunate fractures, Kienböck's disease, capitate fractures, and fractures of the scaphoid not readily seen on standard X-rays. These are best detected by eliciting point tenderness over the bone by the physical examination and confirmed with Tc_{99} scans or tomography. Kienböck's disease may have only minimal tenderness in its early stages and may at times be preceded by occult fractures. Pain is usually best elicited by direct pressure over the dorsal pole of the lunate with the wrist slightly flexed (Fig. 1).

Dorsal Aspect of the Wrist

The dorsal aspect of the wrist overlies the previous area in part but also includes the carpometacarpal joints and a great many underlying structures. Most superficially, one can occasionally see swelling over the dorsum of the wrist not associated with any known systemic disease.

Isolated Tenosynovial Effusion

Isolated tenosynovial effusion in the fourth dorsal compartment may be a harbinger of early rheumatoid arthritis but may also occur as part of a stenosing tenosynovitis. The most important diagnostic sign is the scalloped, demarcated edge of the tenosynovial sheath that moves proximally and distally as the fingers are flexed and extended. This is prolonged slightly further on the ulnar aspect than on the radial and ends roughly at the carpometacarpal joint level. Occasionally, a small ganglion arising from the extensor tendons may also be seen to move with tendon excursion.

Vestigial Manus Brevis Muscles

A vestigial manus brevis muscle is usually an indicis or medius and also presents a mass that is more evident on extension of the fingers.

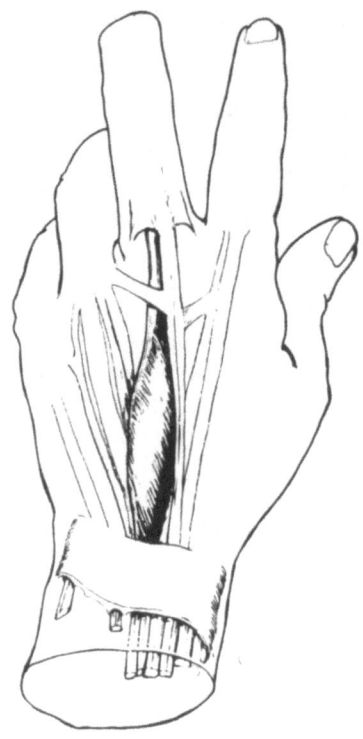

Fig. 5. Manus brevis muscles may simulate tumors of the dorsum of the hand and are occasionally painful. Increased turgor with isolated finger extension is diagnostic

These are occasionally of a size sufficient to elicit anxiety in the patient. They may also occasionally be uncomfortable due to impingement against the distal rim of the dorsal retinaculum during extension of the wrist [7]. They are also easily mistaken for ganglia of the wrist. The diagnosis can usually be made by eliciting the difference in turgor associated with the mass when the finger is first extended and then relaxed (Fig. 5).

Secretan's Disease

Secretan's disease of the wrist area usually extends onto the metacarpals. It is also known as hard dorsal edema of the hand. It often is first seen after an impaction injury to the dorsum of the hand, but the persistence of swelling and induration may also be associated with factitious aggravation. Involvement of the subaponeurotic fascia may lead to significant limitation of excursion of the extensor tendons. The indurated area may be several centimeters in diameter but usually has a relative demarcation on palpation.

Carpometacarpal Sprains

Chronic sprains of the carpometacarpal joints are far more frequent than usually considered. These may, when acute, give rise to marked dorsal edema as well and may, in fact, precipitate the previous condition. This is a forme fruste of carpometacarpal dislocation or fracture-dislocation but usually presents with negative X-rays. The diagnosis is best established by well-localized tenderness at the carpometacarpal joints: the second and third are most commonly injured, but occasionally the fourth may also be sprained alone or in combination. This injury to the fifth carpometacarpal joint is considerably less frequent in contradistinction to the fracture-dislocation that may occur. Manipulation of the joint by securing the trapezoid, capitate, or hamate between the thumb and forefinger of one hand while manipulating the respective metacarpals with the other will often elicit moderately severe discomfort. Occasionally, a click or crepitant snap may be elicited which the patient identifies with the pain. An injection of a small amount of lidocaine into the joints may help to confirm the diagnosis. Standard X-rays are usually negative although a Tc$_{99}$ scan is occasionally positive, and tomography may show osteopenia extending from the dorsal contact areas of these joints [8] (Fig. 3.a).

Carpe Bossu

This is a dorsal swelling usually of the third, or occasionally the second, carpometacarpal joint and is sometimes painful and probably represents a reactive stage to a chronic sprain of this joint which induces hypertrophic bone formation [9].

Triquetrohamate Impaction

This injury is probably an analog of the triquetral rim fracture and is associated with rather specific tenderness over the dorsal rim of the triquetrum exaggerated by dorsiflexion and ulnar deviation of the hamate on the triquetrum. The distal dorsal rim of the triquetrum is tender to palpation. X-rays are seldom diagnostic and even exploration infrequently demonstrates any recognizable impaction pattern [4] (see Dorsal Subfluxion below).

Palmar Aspect of the Wrist

The radiovolar aspect of the wrist includes the area between the abductor pollicis longus and flexor carpi radialis including the scaphotrapezial joint and radial styloid area. The radial artery is palpable just before it passes under the abductor pollicis longus towards the dorsum of the first web space. The artery in older individuals often becomes tortuous, but this is seldom of consequence.

Radiovolar Ganglion

A multinodular lump in the same area is often associated with a radiovolar ganglion. These are only occasionally uncomfortable but often provoke some anxiety. The protuberance is usually noted just proximal to the thickened portion of the deep antebrachial fascia which extends approximately 2 cm proximal to the proximal edge of the transverse carpal ligament. The ganglion may travel down the tendon sheath of the flexor carpi radialis to present in this location and may arise from either the scapho-trapezial joint or from the radiocarpal joint capsule. A history of fluctuation in size with joint activity can usually be elicited from the patient. There is a characteristic smooth, turgid feel to the mass [10].

Scaphotrapeziotrapezoidal Degenerative Joint Disease

Isolated degenerative arthritis of this joint has become increasingly recognized but it also may occur as part of a pantrapezial arthritis. Tenderness can be elicited by displacing the scaphoid tuberosity on the trapezium. It is also painful to apply the same test described above for dynamic subluxation of the proximal pole of the scaphoid. When pressure is applied directly over the tuberosity, it prevents the scaphoid from translating volarly on the trapezium during radial deviation. This aggravates a site of degenerative change eliciting a sharp pain. The diagnosis can be confirmed by X-ray [10] (Fig. 4a,b,d).

Flexor Carpi Radialis Tenosynovitis

This is similar to the other stenosing tenosynovitities and is usually seen in middle-aged industrial workers who have highly repetitive flexion-extension requirements in their occupation. Tenderness may be elicited over the scaphoid

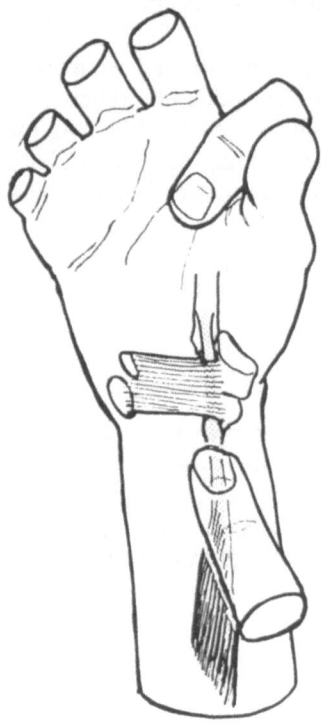

Fig. 6. Stenosing tenosynovitis of the flexor carpi radialis is tested by resisting strong active flexion of the wrist with one hand and palpating the FCR tendon as it passes adjacent to the scaphoid tuberosity

tuberosital area but can also be aggravated by asking the patient to flex the wrist against resistance while intermittent pressure is applied to the tendon by palpation. Less commonly, there is a palpable swelling over the tendon sheath. Diagnostic and therapeutic injection of a mixture of lidocaine and steroid may aid in making the diagnosis [4] (Fig. 6).

Trapezial Ridge Fracture

Fracture of the trapezial ridge, although uncommon, may occur from a fall on the outstretched hand and result in specific tenderness along the insertion of the flexor retinaculum into the rim of the trapezium. The area of tenderness is specific on palpation. X-ray confirmation usually requires a carpal tunnel view. If this is negative, one may consider a sprain of this insertion as an equally valid explanation for the discomfort [4]. Similar tenderness after a carpal tunnel release is indicative of a "pillar" syndrome. A fibrotic response at the site of ligamentous section is often evident. The course is usually self-limited. (Figs. 5, 7.a)

Linburg's Syndrome

This syndrome is an unusual cause of pain in the wrist in a small percentage of people with an anomalous interconnecting tendon or musculotendinous unit between the flexor pollicis longus and index profundus. Repetitive use may cause a mechanical irritation and a tenosynovial reaction which elicits pain and occasionally median nerve irritation with carpal tunnel symptoms. The condition is suspected if the patient is asked to flex the tip of the thumb into the palm and simultaneously extend the index finger. Passive extension of the index finger at this time may cause rather intense pain, the residual of which simulates the pain of which the patient complains. There are a few patients in whom this test is

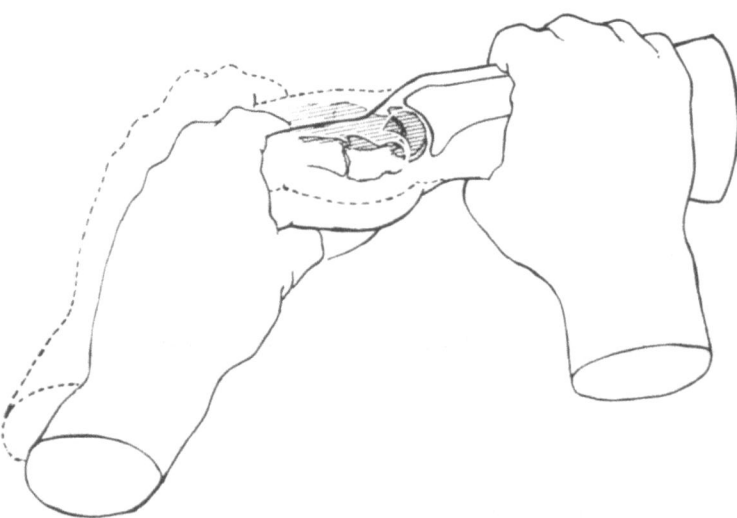

Fig. 7. Midcarpal laxity is seen to varying degress in normal individuals. In the symptomatic patient, the ability to sublux the mid carpal joint with a forceful passive motion may be indicative of ligamentous laxity or attenuated ligamentous support. Comparison with the contralateral side is imperative in judging the significance of the subluxation. Study under video fluoroscopy is often the helpful in analyzing the significance of the findings

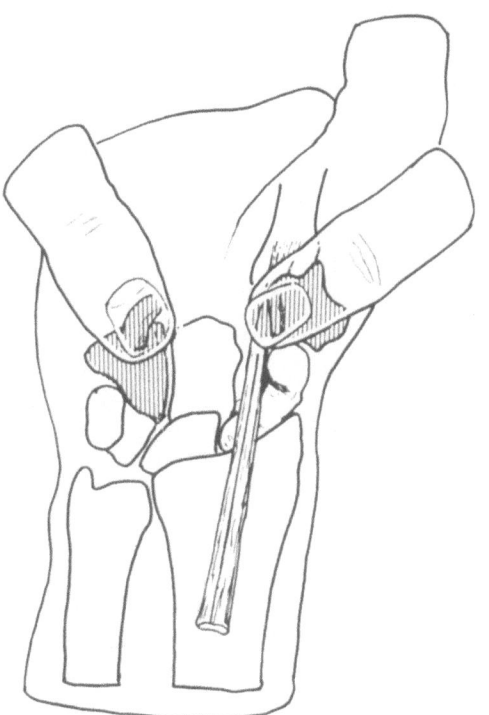

Fig. 8. Fracture of the hamate hook or trapezial ridge is suggested by eliciting point tenderness over either structure by direct palpation

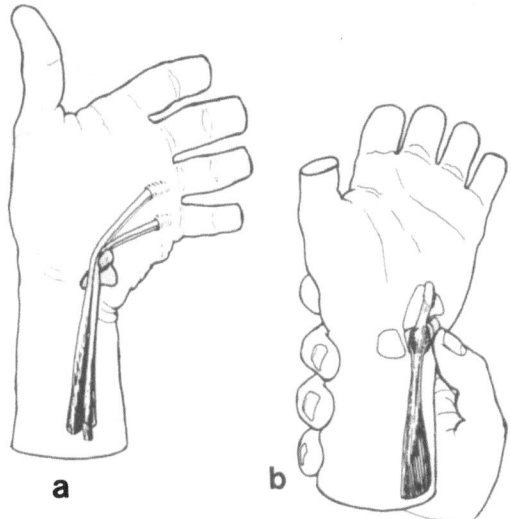

Fig. 9. a Fracture of the hamate hook may also be confirmed by resisting forceful ulnar deviation of the fourth and fifth fingers as the taut bowstringing deflects the hamulus. **b** Pisotriquetral degenerative changes are aggravated by displacement of the pisiform over the triquetral articular surface. Several positions of the wrist should be tried to alter the contact areas

positive and in which subsequent exploration reveals no interconnecting structure. Thus, the results of the test must be carefully evaluated [11].

Hook of the Hamate Fracture

Fracture of the hamulus is often missed on both examination and X-ray study. It may be a result of direct injury but often occurs as a stress fracture in golfers, ball players, and racqueteers (tennis, badminton, etc.) where there is direct abutment of a handle. Pain may be appreciated dorsally over the fourth and fifth carpometacarpal joints, but point tenderness is usually maximal at 1 cm distal and radial to the pisiform. Another reliable test is to resist little finger flexion first in radial and then ulnar deviation. Bowstringing of the finger flexors against the hamulus during the latter manuever elicits diagnostic pain [12, 13] (Figs. 8, 9.a).

Pisotriquetral Degenerative Arthritis

Pain on the ulnar aspect of the wrist brought on by motions of the wrist while clenching the fingers or rotating the forearm suggest the possibility of

degenerative change at the pisotriquetral joint. This most often occurs in older individuals but occasionally a young adult or even an adolescent will develop a chondromalacic area on this joint from a fall, injury, or racquet sport. In the more advanced case, crepitus is readily elicited by manipulation of the pisiform on the triquetrum but, in some instances, a specific configuration of the joint must be obtained before pain is produced by the manipulation since only a small portion of the articular surface may be involved. Therefore, when checking for this suspected condition, the wrist should be extended, flexed, and ulnarly and radially deviated during the grinding process. (Fig. 9.b)

Flexor Carpi Ulnaris Tendinitis

This condition usually begins with exquisite tenderness and pain over the proximal aspect of the pisiform and at its insertion with the tendon of the flexor carpi ulnaris. The area may be swollen and red. A localized infection may be suspected, but an X-ray will usually show amorphous calcification at the insertion of the tendon.

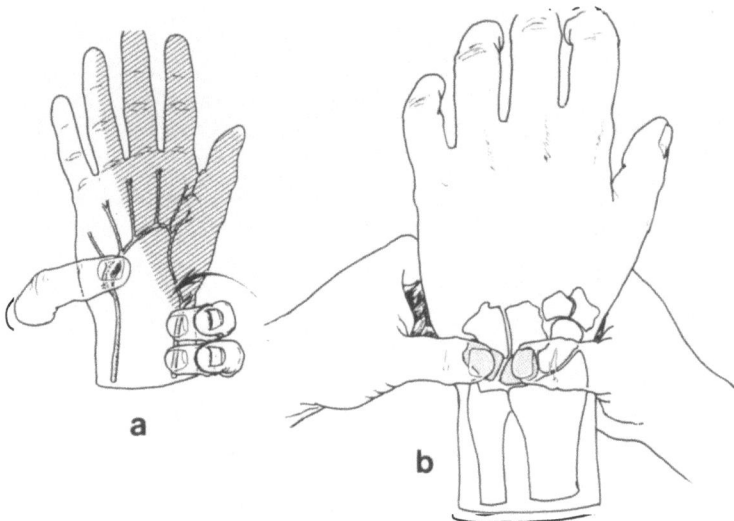

Fig. 10. Ulnar aspect. **a** A thrombosed ulnar artery aneurysm is readily palpable and painful to direct pressure in Guyon's canal. Vascular compromise of the ulnar digits may be obvious. Allen's sign tests the patency of the radial and ulnar arteries by alternately releasing one artery and then the other after exsanguinating the hand by three rapid and complete grasping exercises with the arteries manually occluded. A rapid return of color is seen on the intact side within 30 seconds when the hand is relaxed. **b** A tear of the lunotriquetral ligament or injury to the lunotriquetral joint is aggravated by ballottment motions of the lunate on the triquetrum. If the joint is destabilized, as with lunotriquetral dissociation, excessive motion is observable and especially noteworthy if the opposite wrist is uninvolved. *Arrow*, direction of applied force

Ulnar Artery Thrombosis

Ulnar artery thrombosis may also elicit pain in the proximal hypothenar area. The onset is usually subacute with persistent aching and induration present in the hypothenar area. There is often a history of recurrent trauma, such as using the butt of the hand to hammer an object. It is also more common in smokers and is often accompanied with coldness and numbness particularly of the little and ring finger. An additional classic finding is a positive Allen's sign [14] which consists of exsanguinating the hand by three rapid firm clenched first maneuvers. On the last clenching, both the radial and ulnar arteries are occluded by the examiner's fingers at the distal forearm, first one and then the other arteries are loosened, and the rapidity of color return into the fingers is noted. The hand must be held relaxed during this maneuver and the fingers not extended fully since this may retard arterial filling even in the normal individual. Capillary filling should occur in 10 seconds or less, but comparison with the opposite hand is the best gauge. The portable Doppler unit, when available, also makes this examination quick and reliable. (Fig. 10.a)

Carpal Instabilities

Carpal instabilities require consideration of the wrist area as a whole [15].

Scapholunate Dissociation

This is the best known of the carpal instabilities and occurs more frequently in males than in females. There is usually a history of injury in younger individuals. The symptoms include weakness, pain, limitation of motion, and, occasionally, a snapping sound or feeling within the wrist. Tenderness is usually well centered over the scapholunate junction. The proximal pole of the scaphoid may be ballottable either by displacement from pressure over the tuberosity from the volar aspect or, if dorsally subluxed, by direct pressure over the proximal pole of the scaphoid. A click may be elicited during radial ulnar deviation. The diagnosis is usually confirmed by X-ray examination which shows a gap developing between the proximal pole of the scaphoid and the lunate as well as an increased scapholunate angle on the sagittal view [15] (Fig. 4a–c).

Lunotriquetral Dissociation

This problem is significantly less common than the preceding instability. It also presents with limited motion and weakness. The site of primary tenderness is over the lunotriquetral joint, and a positive ballottement test may be elicited between the lunate and triquetrum if the lunate is stabilized by a thumb and forefinger of one hand and the triquetrum ballotted dorsovolarly with the thumb and forefinger of the other hand. This may be checked against the opposite normal wrist. In the more severe cases, the wrist also has a fork-like deformity since the distal carpal row sags volarly relative to the proximal row. This also leads the ulnar head to have a very prominent appearance. This is often easily correctable by simultaneously pressing down on the ulnar head and pressing up on the pisiform, giving the sensation of a reduction of a subluxation. Tenderness may also be elicited by direct pressure on the ulnar aspect of the triquetrum, exerting a grinding effect on the lunate. X-rays changes are usually more subtle. In the full-blown case, there is a disruption of the arcs of the line drawn alongside the proximal carpal row such that the triquetrum appears to be displaced proximally relative to the lunate. A similar disruption of the distal arcs may occur in the mid-carpal joint. On the sagittal view, there is usually a palmar angulation of the proximal carpal row relative to the distal carpal row and a palmar displacement of the distal carpal row (Fig. 10.b).

A variant of this condition is a lunotriquetral tear in which the interosseous membrane between the lunate and triquetrum is only partially torn. The same tenderness is usually elicited but the ballottement test is negative and displacement is not seen. This condition may occur not as an extension injury to the wrist, as are most full lunotriquetral dissociations, but rather as an impingement with the distal radioulnar joint. It may occur concomitantly with ulnocarpal impingement or triangular fibrocartilage tear [16] and will be covered more thoroughly below, under the heading of the distal radioulnar joint.

Carpal Instability Non-Dissociative (CIND)

This is a term implying that the ligaments that bind the lunate to the scaphoid and to the triquetrum are intact but there is mechanical instability between the carpal rows. This is more often seen in people with lax ligamentous habitus although it may be accentuated after unusual stress or injury. Pain, weakness, and limited motion are often associated with mild to marked deformity of the wrist, similar to that seen in lunotriquetal dissociation with palmar angulation of the proximal carpal row. In a few instances, the deformity is reversed, with the proximal carpal row dorsiflexed. Most patients complain of a snapping of the wrist, particularly in going from radial to ulnar deviation. A rather marked and prominent alteration in contour of the wrist is sometimes seen while observing it from the sagittal aspect. A definitive click may be heard or felt. This click and sudden change in position of the proximal carpal row from a dorsiflexed to a palmar-flexed position is an exaggerated instantaneous expression of the conjunct rotation of the proximal carpal row which occurs normally during radial ulnar deviation as a smooth synchronous movement. Another feature of this which is occasionally seen under the image intensifier is a so-called "catch-up clunk", where the lunate trails behind the scaphoid during ulnar deviation as it is forced up the inclined plane of the distal radius. The lunate suddenly traverses radially and rotates from a palmar to a dorsiflexed position. The distal carpal row translates from a palmar to a dorsal position in following the concavity of the lunate. This movement may at times be rendered normal by displacing the proximal carpal row radially with moderate thumb pressure on the ulnar aspect of the triquetrum. This would appear to help relax the palmar radiocarpal ligaments and allow the smoother kinematic rotation to resume. In these lax wrists, it is also often possible to sublux the distal row on the proximal row by manual displacement dorsopalmarly with the forearm fixed. The classic tests for lax ligamentous habitus are usually positive in this group of patients [17, 18] (Fig. 7).

Ulnar Translation of the Wrist

This condition is quite common in rheumatoid arthritis where capsular distention and erosion of ligamentous attachments allows the carpus to slide down the inclined plane of the radius. In late stages, this usually results in erosion of the palmar rim of the radius, dorsal displacement of the ulnar head, and translation of the lunate out of the lunate fossa to lie volarly to the ulnar head. The condition is markedly less common as a traumatic entity but may be recognized both clinically and radiographically by displacement of the entire carpus in an ulnar direction. It is usually possible to redisplace the carpus into a normal position by radially directed pressure on the hand. Early recognition is especially important since the condition is very difficult to correct in the later stages [19].

Post-Fracture Instability

This condition is most commonly seen following a fracture of the distal radius with dorsal angulation and proximal displacement. As the palmar inclination is lost, there is a tendency for the lunate to slide up the now dorsally inclined plane of the articular surface of the radius. It maintains its normal relationship with the articular surface but appears to be dorsiflexed relative to the longitudinal axis of the forearm. The distal carpal row, however, flexes palmarly. In this situation, the proximal row can no longer undergo its normal synergistic angulation with the distal row during flexion extension and has great difficulty in adjusting to the conjunct rotation that occurs on radial ulnar deviation. This markedly limits the range of motion of the wrist, particularly in dorsiflexion, and results in weakness and discomfort. The condition is suspected from the dorsal prominence of the carpus and is readily confirmed by standard X-rays. Carpal tunnel symptoms and ulnar impingement symptoms are often recognized in the same patient.

Distal Radioulnar Joint

Dorsal Subluxation

Dorsal subluxation of the ulna is a misnomer, since this is a condition in which the radius and carpus are subluxed on the ulnar head. The prominence of the ulna is usually seen most readily with the forearm pronated, and supination may be restricted since the ulnar head cannot displace into the palmar aspect of the sigmoid notch of the radius during attempted supination. This is often painful and occasionally crepitant. Diagnosis is best made by the above findings and comparison with the opposite wrist. Subluxation of the ulnar head can usually be corrected by displacing the ulnar head palmarly while displacing the carpus dorsally with firm pressure under the pisotriquetral area. If supination is obtained with passive motion, the instability

is corrected until pronation again occurs. The condition may be associated with rupture of the triangular fibrocartilage, particularly the volar limb, ulnar styloid fractures, or a variety of fractures of the distal forearm. Chondromalacia of the articular surface of the ulnar head may occur due to the dorsal subluxation against the sigmoid notch of the radius. The so-called "piano key" sign is elicited by displacing the prominent ulnar head palmarly and watching it spring back when pressure is released. Standard X-rays are often unreliable in making this diagnosis but cross-section CAT scans or MRIs are helpful [20] (Fig. 11.b).

Palmar Subluxation

Palmar subluxation of the distal ulna is much less common and may result in a frank dislocation in which the ulnar head becomes locked under the palmar rim of the sigmoid notch. There is a distinct narrowing of the forearm in the AP plane and a widening in the sagittal plane. Ulnar nerve symptoms are occasionally present and pronation is usually severely restricted. Surprisingly, this condition may be overlooked both by clinical examination and by X-ray unless sought for specifically [5] (Fig. 12.b).

Triangular Fibrocartilage Injuries

The triangular fibrocartilage may be disrupted as a result of acute injuries or as a result of compressive stress which generally results in central perforations and degenerative changes. The above instabilities are commensurate with traumatic disruptions of the triangular fibrocartilage at either the radial or the ulnar styloid attachment. The latter condition is more often seen in patients with a so-called positive ulnar variance in which a combination of compression and torque between the ulnar head and proximal carpal row result in degeneration of the cartilage. This may be associated with a click or crepitus during wrist motions, and the pain can often be increased by depressing the ulnar head while raising the ulnar carpus and then having the patient deviate the wrist ulnarly. This acts to compress the whole area and may, therefore, be indicative of a lunotriquetral tear, a triangular fibrocartilage tear, or an ulnocarpal impingement. An arthrogram is usually a reliable method of making the diagnosis but must be interpreted cautiously on the basis of the clinical examination and other findings (Figs. 11.b, 13).

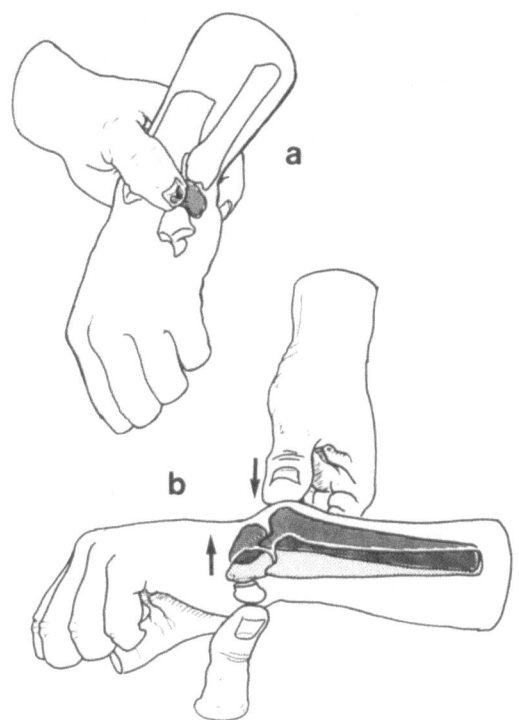

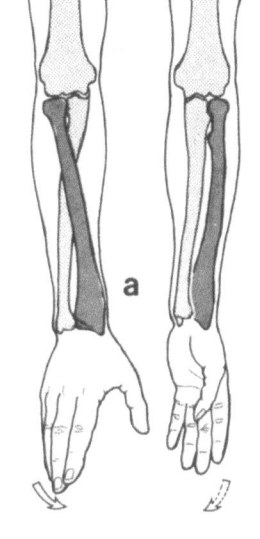

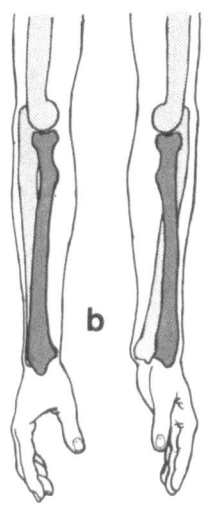

Fig. 12. a Palmar dislocation of the ulnar head is suggested by inability to pronate the left forearm, and **b** a narrowing of the AP and widening of the lateral aspect of the distal forearm. *Arrows*, direction of attempted angulation

Fig. 11. a A dorsal triquetral rim avulsion fracture may be easily missed on standard X-rays. Point tenderness over this area readily identified by a bony landmark is easily confirmed. **b** Distal radioulnar. The "piano key sign" is shown by depressing the ulnar head while the pisiform is supported and the forearm is pronated. The ulnar head springs back into position like a piano key. This may be present in females with lax ligaments and must be compared to the contralateral wrist. It may signify dorsal subluxation of the ulnar head. *Arrows*, direction of applied force

Subluxation of Extensor Carpi Ulnaris

Subluxation of the extensor carpi ulnaris is an uncommon problem which also elicits pain and discomfort particularly with pronosupination motions of the wrist during stressful use. The condition may come on after a vigorous and forceful movement and is usually seen in patients with a lax ligamentous habitus. The diagnosis is most easily confirmed by having the patient fully

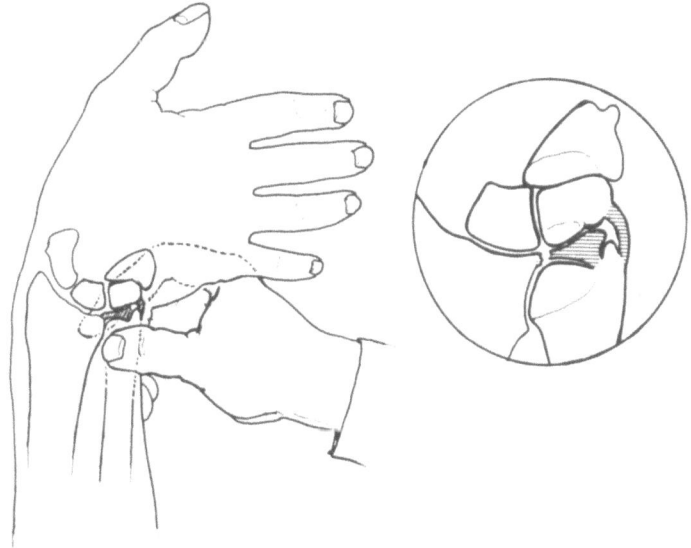

Fig. 13. Triangular fibrocartilage injuries and ulnocarpal impaction are suggested by pain elicited with the ulnar head depressed while the pisiform is supported and the wrist deviated ulnarly. This compresses the triangular fibrocartilage between the ulnar head and triquetrum

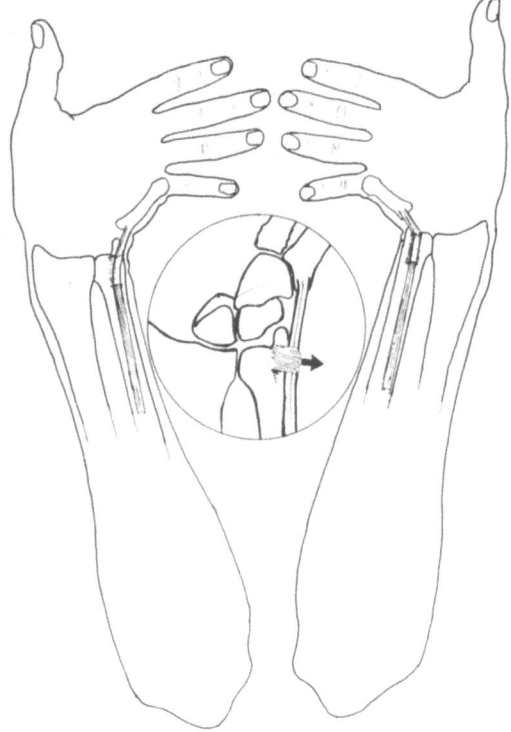

Fig. 14. Subluxation of the extensor carpi ulnaris is best demonstrated when the patient supinates both forearms before their face and strongly ulnarly deviate. The tendon slides out of the sixth dorsal compartment and over the ulnar styloid with a snap. It may be held in place with direct thumb pressure. *Arrow*, direction of tendon subluxation

supinate both forearms and then deviate the hands from the radial to the ulnarly deviated position. The extensor tendon which has occupied a dorsal position adjacent to the dorsal rim of the radius will slip out of its groove over the ulnar styloid process with an audible and palpable snap [21] (Fig. 14).

Instability of Ulnar Stump Following Excision of Distal Ulna

This postoperative condition is associated with impingement of the ulnar stump against the ulnar aspect of the radius, particularly during forceful motions and pronosupination. It may result in a snapping of the ulna and induces pain and giving way in the distal forearm. The diagnosis is easily confirmed by manipulating the ulnar stump against the radius and by X-rays which show scalloping at the site of impingement [22].

Miscellaneous

There are a number of other conditions of the wrist which are not covered in this short chapter. Inflammatory conditions which may cause pain and effusion in the wrist include septic arthritis, gout, and pseudogout. The latter may closely simulate an acute septic arthritis when calcium pyrophosphate crystals are released from the triangular fibrocartilage or ligaments of the wrist in older patients. There are many subtle injuries to the wrist which also cannot be covered in detail, as well as the effects of systemic diseases, such as rheumatoid arthritis.

When in doubt, it is often better to re-examine the patient's wrist on two or more occasions at distinct intervals, since generalized tenderness sometimes encouraged by apprehension may mask more specific point tenderness. The use of differential injections into the wrist may also be helpful, particularly if there is a negative arthrogram, thereby implying integrity of the intercarpal, radiocarpal, and distal radioulnar joints. This may make it possible to isolate the area of injury.

Lastly, there may be secondary gain factors which may make a definitive diagnosis difficult. This is not an infrequent occurrence in patients who have suffered injuries which they deem to be another's fault and in those patients who are in a compensable situation. While newer imaging and diagnostic modalities, such as arthroscopy, have markedly increased our diagnostic capabilities, they have also added substantially to the cost of medical work-ups. Therefore, a careful history and physical examination should continue to remain the most important part of our diagnostic evaluation. Substituting an expensive battery of tests and procedures for the examination is ultimately deleterious to the patient, our medical systems, and the economy.

References

1. Wood MB, Linscheid RL (1973) Abductor pollicis longus bursitis. Clin Orthop 93:293–296
2. deQuervain F (1913) Clinical surgical diagnosis for students and practitioners (translated from the 4th edn by J Snowman). William Wood, New York
3. Finkelstein H (1930) Stenosing tenovaginitis at the radial styloid process. J Bone Joint Surg [Am] 12:509–540
4. Linscheid RL, Dobyns JH (1987) Physical examination of the wrist. In: Post M (ed) Physical

examination of the musculoskeletal system. Year Book, Chicago, pp 80–94

5. Linscheid RL, Dobyns JH (1985) Wrist sprains. In: Tubiana R (ed) The hand, vol 2. Saunders, Philadelphia, pp 970–985

6. Watson HK, Goodman ML, Johnson TR (1981) Limited wrist arthrodesis. Part II. Intercarpal and radiocarpal combinations. J Hand Surg 6:223–233

7. Fernandez-Vazquez JM, Linscheid RL (1972) Anomalous extensor muscles simulating dorsal wrist ganglion. Clin Orthop 83:84–86

8. Joseph RB, Linscheid RL, Dobyns JH, Bryan RS (1981) Chronic sprains of the carpometacarpal joints. J Hand Surg [Am] 6:172–180

9. Fiolle J (1931) le "Carpe Bossu." Bull Mem Soc Nat Chir 57:1687–1690

10. Crosby EB, Linscheid RL, Dobyns JH (1978) Scaphotrapezial trapezoidal arthrosis. J Hand Surg [Am] 3:223–234

11. Linburg RM, Comstock BE (1979) Anomalous tendon slips from the flexor pollicis longus to the flexor digitorum Profundus. J Hand Surg [Am] 4:79–83

12. Bishop AT, Beckenbaugh RD (1988) Fracture of the hamate hook. J Hand Surg [Am] 13:135–139

13. Crosby EB, Linscheid RL (1974) Rupture of the flexor profundus tendon of the ring finger secondary to ancient fracture of the hook of the hamate: Review of the literature and report of two cases. J Bone Joint Surg [Am] 56:1076

14. Allen EV (1929) Thromboangiitis obliterans: Methods of diagnosis of chronic occlusive arterial lesions distal to the wrist with illustrative cases. Am J Med Sci 178:237–244

15. Linscheid RL, Dobyns JH, Beabout JW, Bryan RS (1972) Traumatic instability of the wrist: Diagnosis, classification and pathomechanics. J Bone Joint Surg [Am] 54:1612–1632

16. Reagan DS, Linscheid RL, Dobyns JH (1984) Lunotriquetral sprains. J Hand Surg [Am] 9:502–514

17. Schernberg F (1984) Static and dynamic radio-anatomy of the wrist. Ann Chir Main 4:301–312

18. Wright TW, Dobyns JH, Linscheid RL (to be published) Carpal instability nondissociative. J Hand Surg [Am]

19. Rayhack JM, Linscheid RL, Dobyns JH, Smith JH (1987) Posstraumatic ulnar translation of the carpus. J Hand Surg [Am] 12:180–189

20. Darrow JC, Linscheid RL, Dobyns JH, Mann JM, Wood MB, Beckenbaugh RD (1985) Distal ulnar recession for disorders of the distal radioulnar joint. J Hand Surg [Am] 10:482–491

21. Burkhart SS, Wood MB, Linscheid RL (1982) Posttraumatic recurrent subluxation of the extensor carpi ulnaris tendon. J Hand Surg [Am] 7:1–3

22. Bieber EJ, Linscheid RL, Dobyns JH, Beckenbaugh RD (1988) Failed distal ulna resections. J Hand Surg [Am] 13:193–200

Imaging of the Painful Wrist

Louis A. Gilula and Neal R. Stewart[1]

In this presentation we will cover a few topics relating to imaging approaches to the painful wrist which we believe are very important to surgeons in this field. Due to the lack of time and space; only a few major areas can be presented, including some newer, current concepts of computed tomography (CT) that have evolved in our own practice [1]. Next some major aspects of magnetic resonance imaging (MRI) of the wrist will be presented which are quite pertinent to those interested in the wrist. Finally a few summary remarks about wrist arthrography will be made.

General Approach to Wrist Pain

Wrist pain is currently a major problem area, and it is obviously quite important for the patient to get a good history and physical. If radiographic examination is indicated, we believe routine examination of the wrist should have four views: (1) a posteroanterior (PA) view which describes an X-ray beam entering the posterior and exiting the anterior (palmar) aspect of the wrist, (2) a PA ulnar deviation view or an angled view which will show the scaphoid waist better, (3) a 45° oblique view which is the best for looking at the scaphotrapeziotrapezoidal joint, and (4) a lateral view, which is mandatory for every wrist and hand problem. If examination of the hand or wrist is performed without a lateral view, some major errors can be made. Fractures off the dorsal and/or palmar surfaces of hand and wrist bones can be entirely missed without these views. In addition, with more and more interest being paid to ulnar variance (the relative length of the ulna

with respect to the adjacent radius), we should insist on a standardized PA view of the wrist. To our knowledge, the standardized position that most people accept when we talk about ulnar variance is the PA view taken with the elbow at the same level as the shoulder. A true lateral view at right angles to this standardized PA view can be taken either as a cross-table lateral or with the elbow fully adducted to the patient's side. Unless a technologist is instructed to do this routinely, the surgeon will not know if the views are standardized or not. When choosing a procedure based on the relative length of an ulna, where there are differences of only a few millimeters, having standard views is very important. One quick and easy way to see if the PA and lateral views are taken at right angles to each other is to look at the ulnar styloid. The ulnar styloid should not be centered on the distal end of the ulna in the same way on both of these views if they are at right angles to each other.

A routine radiographic wrist examination providing an obvious diagnosis can lead to a further work-up of choice based on physical examination and the favored method of treatment. If the four views are completely normal and examination does not warrant further investigative imaging studies, then no further imaging studies should be ordered. If the four radiographic views are normal, or if it is uncertain if they are abnormal and clinical findings warrant further investigation, bone scintigraphy can be very helpful. When bone scintigraphy is abnormal, especially if the bone scintigraphy is not just subtly but very abnormal, and if the abnormality confirms physical examination findings the work-up should be continued until the abnormality on the scan can be explained. If bone scintigraphy is normal, usually the radiographic work-up for an osteochondral abnormality can be stopped. With a normal bone scan and

[1] Mallinckrodt Institute of Radiology, 510 South Kingshighway Boulevard, St. Louis, MO 63110, USA

with a suspect intercarpal ligament injury, the arthrogram can be of value to demonstrate the abnormal intrinsic ligaments or show some other abnormal capsular or ligament structure. If a bone scan is diffusely abnormal, a diffuse synovitis and a systemic arthritis work-up should be considered. If the bone scan is focally very hot, a bone or osteochondral abnormality should be considered and further work-up with CT or MRI may be necessary. Sometimes an arthrogram may be indicated depending on the questions that need answering. In the following sections, an approach to CT, MRI, and arthrography will be presented.

Tailored Approach to Wrist CT

Currently we believe that CT of the wrist should be a "tailored" examination [1]. In other words, the CT examination should be made to fit the patient's problem. We prefer CT to routine thin section tomography because there is not as much blur of the bone structures and sharper bone edges can be seen. To obtain the desired CT results, the best position necessary to obtain the referring physician's desired answer should be used. A basic principle of CT is that sections at right angles to the surface of interest are required. Scanners can do a very good job of reproducing anatomic details if the area of interest lies in a plane at right angles to the plane of section. If a CT examination is performed in an incorrect manner or plane, an obvious fracture or abnormality can be missed. Therefore radiologists, or whoever is performing the CT examination must know the specific reason for the examination to get the best result.

There are several different methods to examine the wrist [1]. Different positions will be valuable is different situations.

Axial Position (Fig. 1)

The axial or transaxial position is excellent to look at the hamate hook, carpal tunnel, distal radial fractures, and dorsal and/or palmar cortical detail. This position can be used in patients with questionable distal radioulnar subluxation, where the hands and the wrists are first positioned so that that patient is comfortable, usually in the prone position (Fig. 1a). Then the hands and wrists are placed in the position that causes the patient pain, usually the supine (Fig. 1b), over-supinated or even over-pronated position

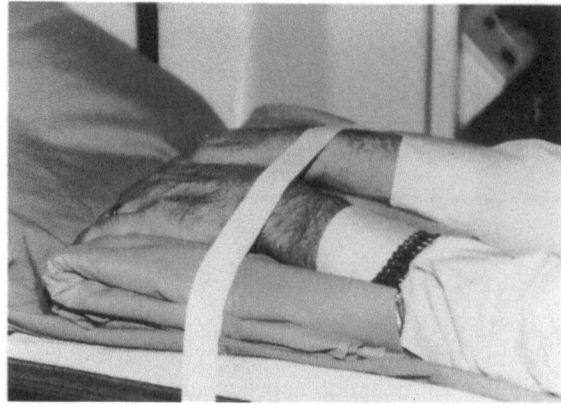

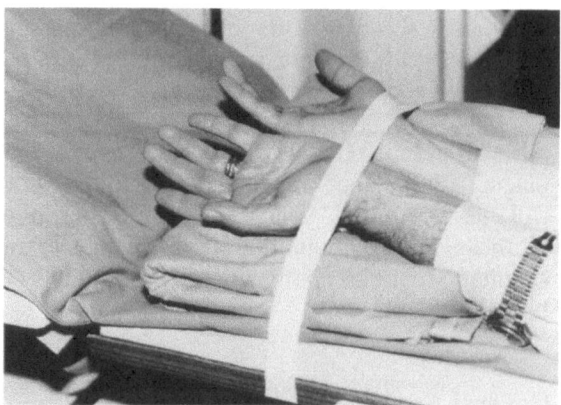

Fig. 1a,b. Positions for axial CT. **a** Prone. **b** Supine

(Fig. 2c). This second position must be designed to hold the wrists in the painful position to see if the ulna is subluxed. Currently the hands and wrists are taped together in the second position to fix them symmetrically, and the wrists are then taped to the table. In the axial position, both wrists can be imaged simultaneously. In the patient shown in Fig. 2 who had distal radioulnar joint pain, in the prone position with the opposite wrist for comparison there was some asymmetry but nothing that could be called definitely abnormal (Fig. 2a,b). In the over-pronated position (the major position that produced the patient's pain) there was left distal radioulnar joint diastasis as compared to the opposite side (Fig. 2c,d). Rarely is there the need to use CT to show the hook of hamate fractures, but if there is a question, CT performed in the axial or sagittal plane is a valuable example of an application of CT to look at this specific problem.

Fig. 2a–d. Distal radioulnar joint (DRUJ) diastasis. Prone topogram (**a**), and CT section (**b**). No definite DRUJ abnormality is identified. With over-pronation to point of patient pain on topogram (**c**), and CT section (**d**), diastasis of the left DRUJ is present (*arrowheads*)

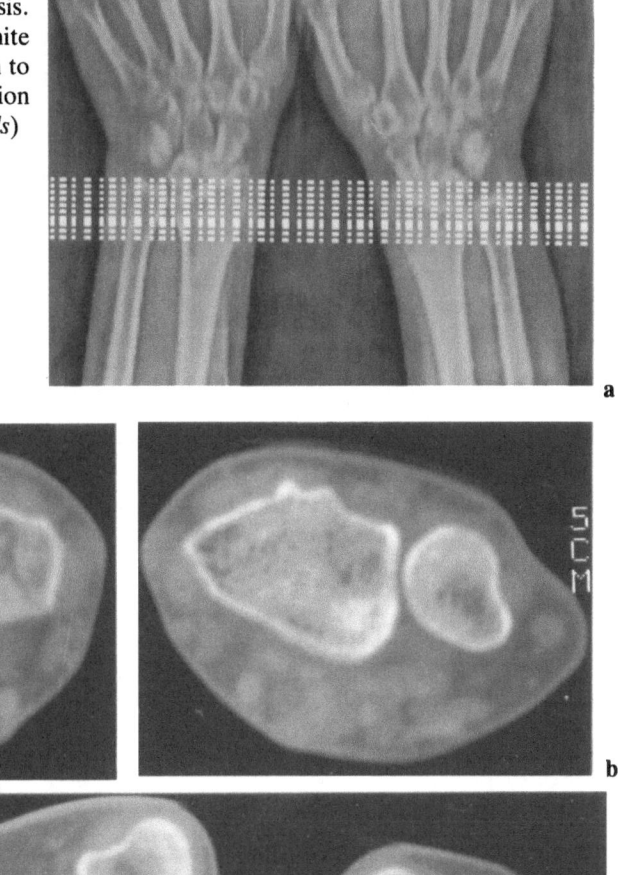

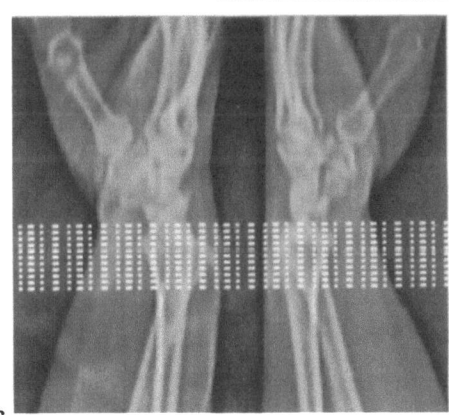

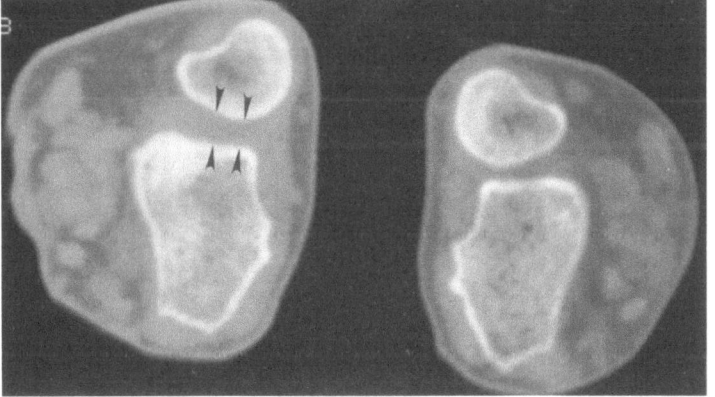

Coronal Plane

We perform coronal CT by two methods [1]. One method, described by Pennes et al. [2], uses a flexed wrist placed above the head (Fig. 3a). A second method is to place the wrist in an extended position or on a wrist holder (Fig. 3b) [1, 3] or in some manner to simulate this holder. In our opinion, this plane provides the easiest way to survey the entire wrist and to understand the wrist anatomy. This position can provide information about intercarpal and radiocarpal arthrodeses, and the status of the radiocarpal articulation. For instance, it can be determined whether there is degenerative joint disease as evidenced by osseous changes or joint space narrowing in a deep portion of the joint that cannot be recognized on routine radiographs. This position can also display the pattern of fracture lines of carpal bone fractures much more accurately than plain films [1] (Pruitt D.L., Gilula L.A., Manske P.R., Vannier M.W., CT distal radial fractures, in preparation).

CT can be very helpful to evaluate the status or extent of bone fusion in patients with intercarpal

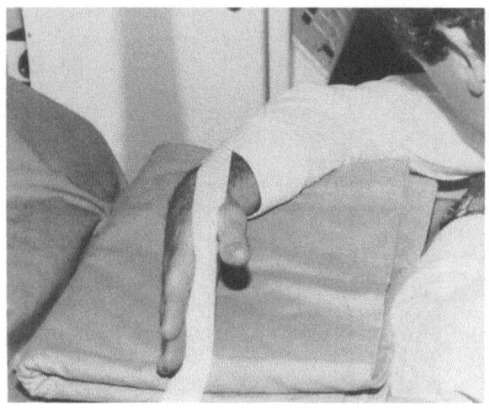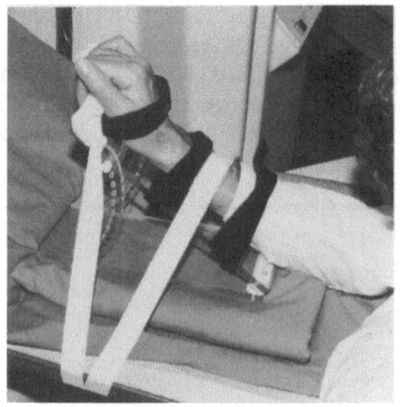

Fig. 3a,b. Positions for coronal CT. **a** "Pennes" position for coronal CT. The hand is flexed slightly with ulnar side of the hand and wrist on the CT table [1]. **b** "Vannier" position for coronal CT. The hand is held in an extended position on a wrist holder. The gantry of the CT machine is angled (not shown in this figure) during scanning to nearly tangent or parallel the dorsum of the carpus [1]

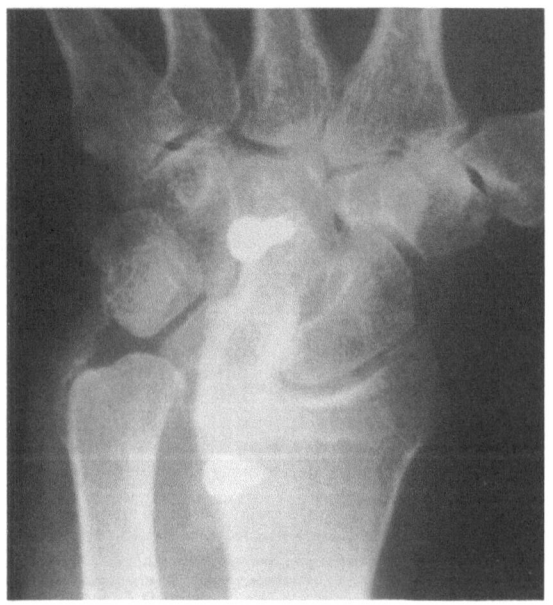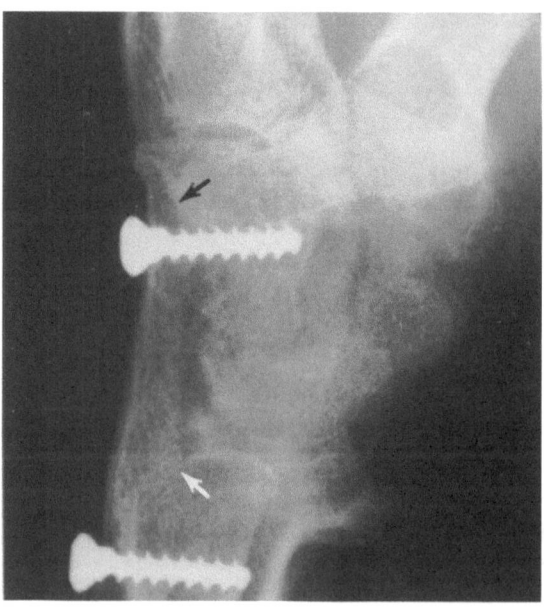

Fig. 4a–e. Coronal CT sections to evaluate status of wrist fusion in patient with pain post-arthrodesis. **a** Posteroanterio-view. **b** Lateral views show fusion between graft and radius (*white arrow*) and graft and capitate (*black arrow*). **c, d** Coronal CT sections with **c** dorsal to **d**. Solid bone fusion is evident between the radius and graft (*black arrow*), palmar aspect of the graft to lunate (*between arrowheads*), and at the capitolunate and scapholunate joints. Although the screws create some metal artifact, the CT examination is still adequate. **e** The patient's pain was subsequently proven to be due to a separate fragment of bone ulnar to the fusion mass (*arrow*) (*see p. 32*)

and/or radiocarpal arthrodeses. One example (Fig. 4) is of a patient that had pain after a radiocarpal arthrodesis procedure. There was a question as to whether the intercarpal fusion was solid and indeed, one hand surgeon told the patient that the fusion would have to be taken down and reperformed. It can be very difficult to establish the amount of solid radiocarpal and intercarpal bone bridging present unless the specific joint in question is clearly profiled on plain radiographs. Fluoroscopic spots of specific joints can be performed as a second step to

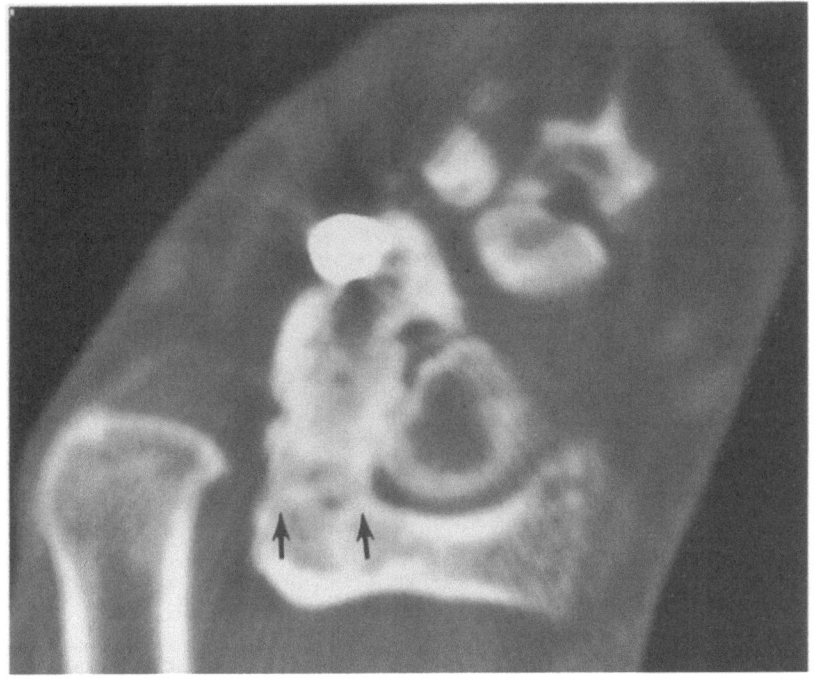

c

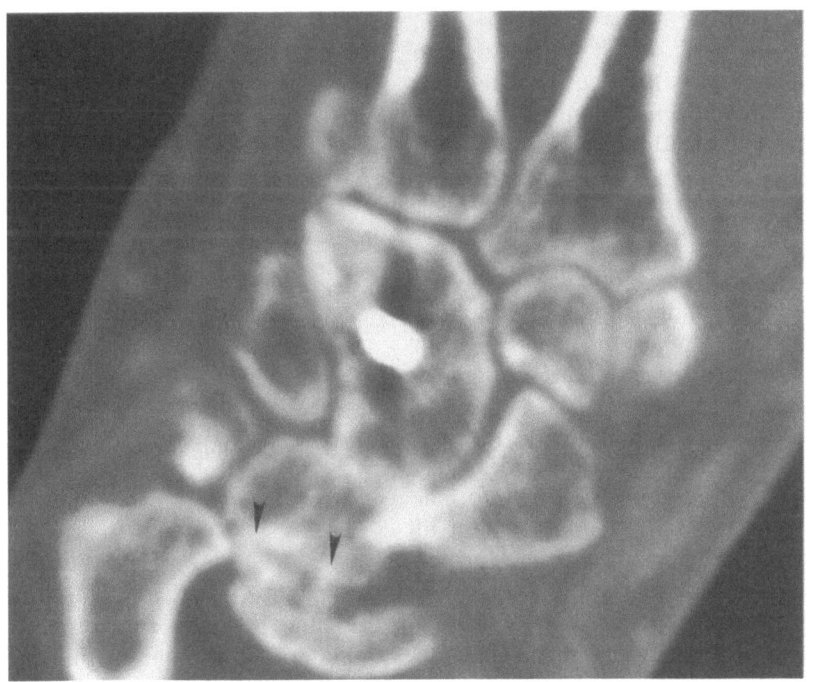

d

evaluate an arthrodesis prior to CT. If decisions about healing are made without profiling an arthrodesed joint, mistakes can be made because of curved overlapping anatomic structures [4]. Also, central portions of articulations may not be clearly evaluated because of overlapping bone structures. For the patient shown in Fig. 4, in the coronal CT plane the intercarpal and radiocarpal anatomy were easily seen. There was solid bone fusion between the graft to radius and lunate, capitate and lunate, and scaphoid and lunate. A separate bone fragment was present along the

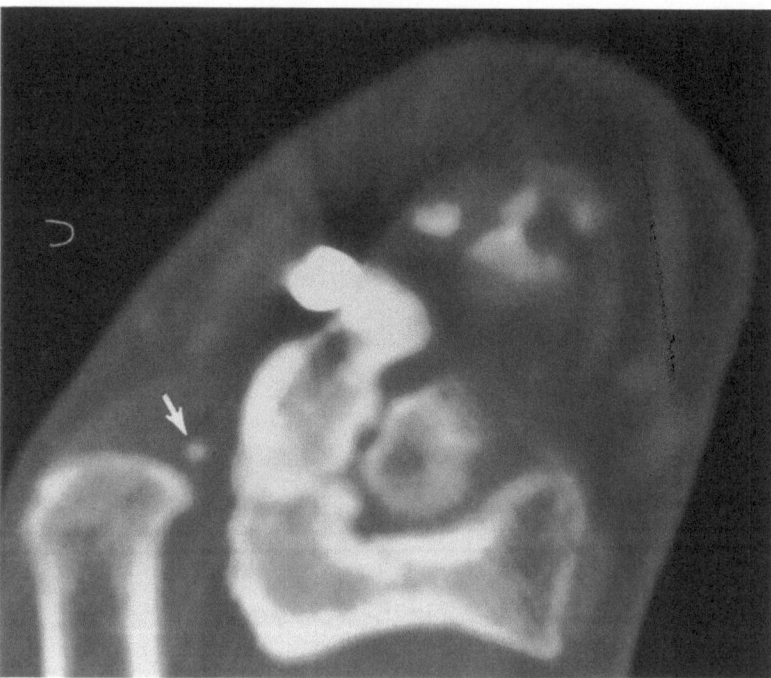

Fig. 4e

ulnar aspect of the graft which was related to the patient's pain (Fig. 4e). Once realizing this, the patient elected to accept the minor pain and left the fragment alone without further surgery.

Oblique Sagittal or "Long Axis of Scaphoid" Plane

This position provides a very good way to look at the long axis of the scaphoid to look for scaphoid fracture fragment alignment and healing. Some patients may have a scaphoid graft not easily evident on plain radiographs, such as a graft on the dorsal surface of the fracture, and the residual palmar gap of the fracture can be called a non-union. CT can provide us with very good information to see if there is union or displacement of fracture fragments. This method is performed by aligning the scan along the long axis of the scaphoid or by aligning the scan along the long axis of an intrascaphoid screw or wires if they are in place [1] with the hand at an oblique position above the head (Fig. 5). To evaluate the position of the scaphoid fracture fragments more fully, it is ideal to use both the coronal plane, which shows the scaphoid articulation with the capitate and radial ulnar displacement of fracture fragments, and the oblique sagittal plane, which shows dorsal and palmar displacement and/or rotation of fracture fragments. In one patient with a scaphoid waist fracture, on one coronal plane there was at

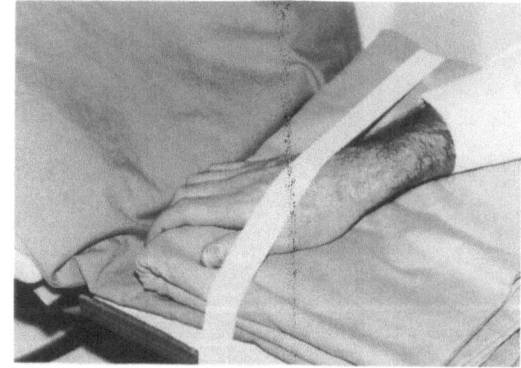

Fig. 5. Positioning of hand and wrist for oblique sagittal or long axis of the scaphoid plane

least 3- to 4-mm offset or displacement between the fracture fragments with no evidence of bony bridging (Fig. 6a). In a different patient, in the oblique sagittal plane or the true long axis plane of the scaphoid, the scaphoid showed some dorsal gapping at the fracture site (Fig. 6b). In a third patient a nonunion with a large dorsal exostosis was clearly demonstrated (Fig. 6c). Currently CT will show early bone bridging faster than any other imaging method.

In one patient with a Herbert screw, we used both thin section complex motion tomography and CT for comparison and preferred CT because it did not produce the blur as on polytomography.

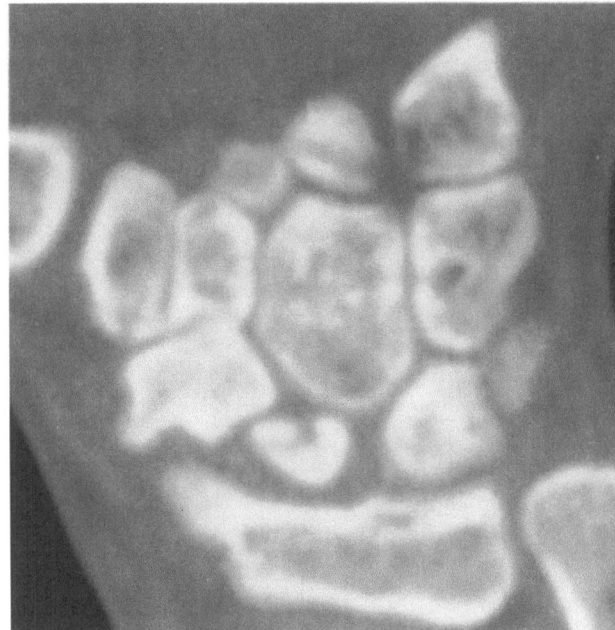

Fig. 6a–c. Scaphoid fracture evaluation. **a** Coronal plane. It can be seen that 3–4 mm of radial offset of the distal radial offset of the distal radial fracture fragment is present. **b** In a different patient, the oblique sagittal plane of the scaphoid shows dorsal gapping with no bone bridging. **c** In another patient with the oblique sagittal scaphoid plane, a nonunion of the scaphoid waist is present (*arrowheads*) with the dorsal exostosis (*arrow*) of the distal fragment

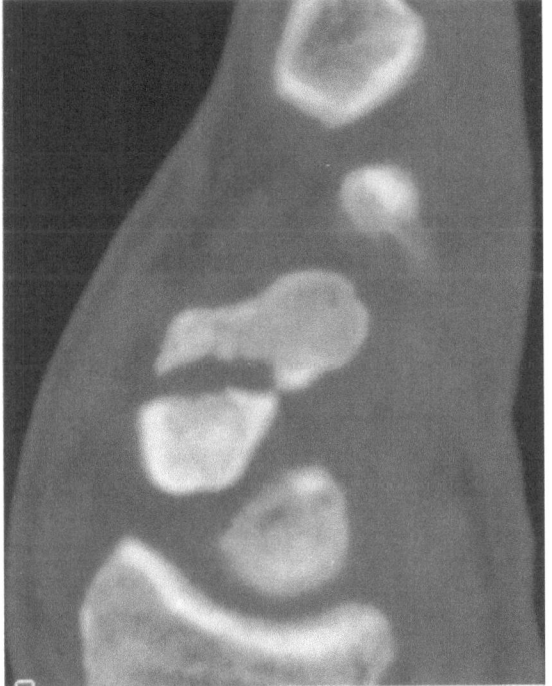

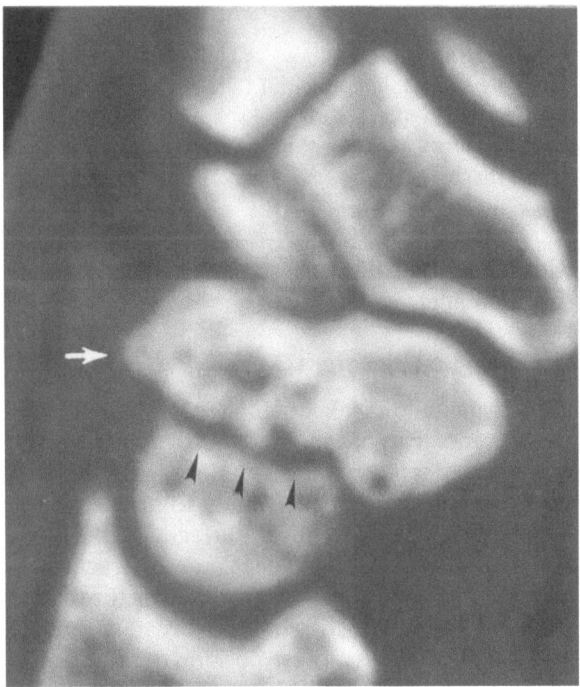

On some CT scanners there will be blur and streak artifacts from intrapatient metal, but the newer CT scanners do not have so many problems with metal. However when the CT section is passed along (parallel to) K-wires or the axis of the screw, metal artifacts are diminished (Fig. 7) (Wilson A.J. 1990, personal communication).

CT is valuable for the clinical questions as to the cause of block of motion of a healed scaphoid fracture and the status of the scaphoid fragments after healing. CT performed in the oblique sagittal plane parallel to the Herbert screw axis shows the screw very easily without much artifact, with an exostosis dorsally. Such an examination (Fig. 7) shows how CT can readily demonstrate a dorsal "humpback deformity" of the scaphoid, solid bone bridging of the scaphoid fracture fragments, and a long axis view of the scaphoid

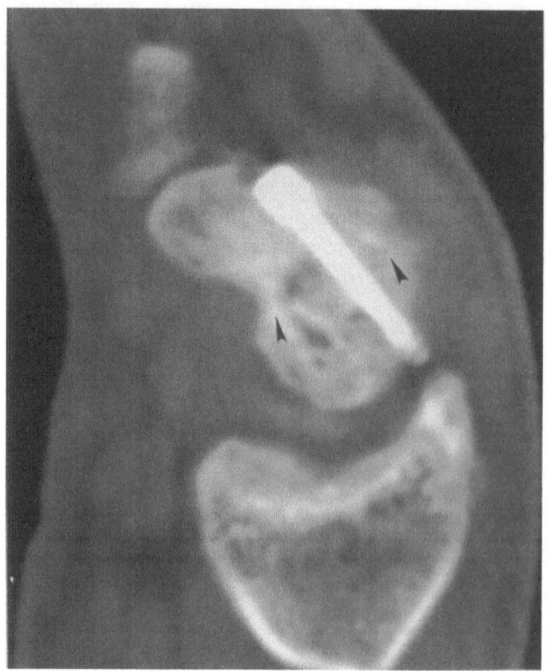

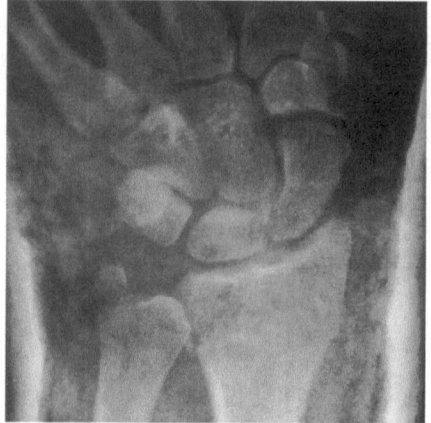

a

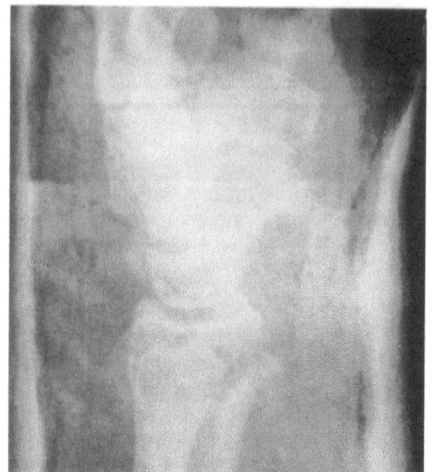

b

Fig. 7. Evaluation of the scaphoid with a Herbert screw by CT. Oblique sagittal CT section of scaphoid with screw in place shows a solid healed scaphoid fracture (*arrowheads*) without much artifact from the Herbert screw

which could enable measurement of an intra-scaphoid angle.

Direct Sagittal Plane for CT

This plane allows alignment evaluation of the third metacarpal-capitate-lunate-radius and other carpometacarpal axes in the sagittal plane. This plane is also a good method to demonstrate dorsal and palmar cortical surfaces. Offset of lunate (Kienböck's) and distal radius fractures, especially depression or pylon fractures of scaphoid and lunate fossae, can be readily shown in this plane. This is an easy position to assume, in or out of plaster, even if there is a long arm cast, by placing the hand straight above the head (Fig. 8d). One example of the value of this position can be illustrated by a distal radius fracture (Fig. 8). On the PA and lateral views of the casted and reduced distal radius fracture, the reduction appeared acceptable (Figs. 8a,b) as the distal radius articular surface was in a neutral position without any evident reason for operation. A direct axial scan was first performed in the patient with a right-angled cast. This showed the fracture

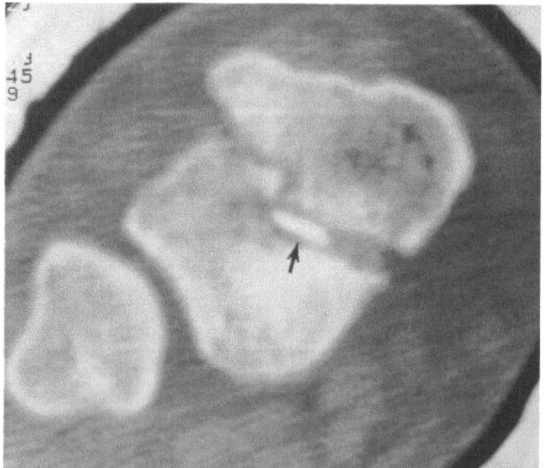

c

Fig. 8

in the sagittal plane going through the middle of the lunate and scaphoid fossa with a small amount of fragmentation along the scapholunate fossa junction (Fig. 8c).

The direct sagittal plane is the second position

Fig. 8a–e. Direct sagittal plane. **a** Distal radius fracture in PA. **b** Lateral views in cast. The distal articular surface of the distal radius after reduction is in a neutral position. No fracture fragment displacement is evident. **c** Transaxial plane CT. The fracture line in the sagittal plane is evident with the fracture fragment (*arrow*) in the fracture line. **d** Topogram of direct sagittal plane. **e** Direct sagittal plane CT shows fragment (*arrow*) inside the radiocarpal joint indicating need for surgical intervention. (From [1] with permission)

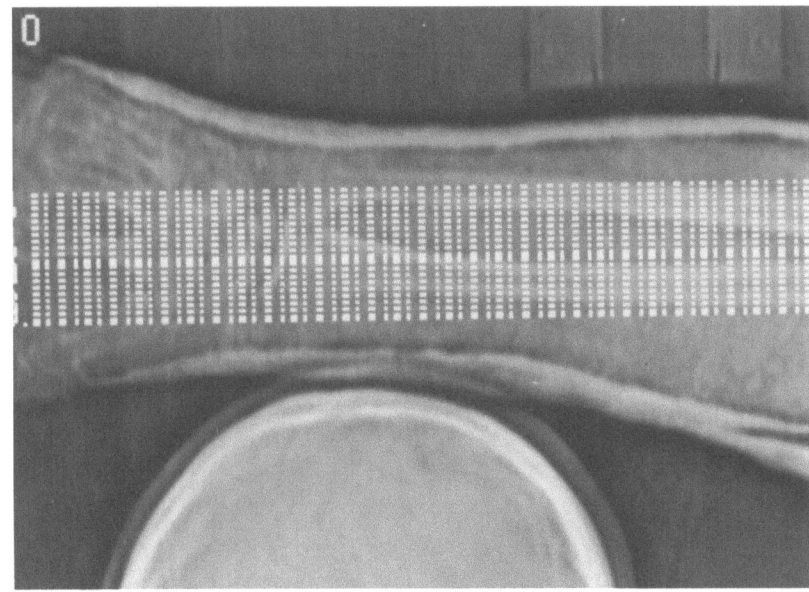

d

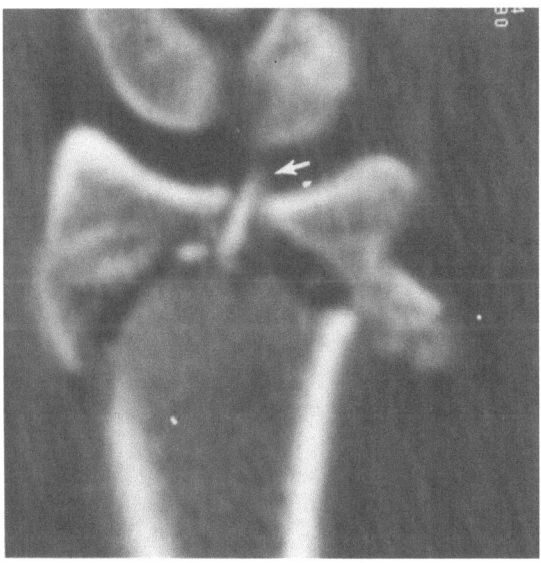

e

we prefer to use. In this case a fragment was sticking into the radiocarpal joint at least 2–3 mm and changed what was an apparent satisfactory reduction into an operative case (Fig. 8e). In other distal radius fractures, CT has shown pylon fractures in the middle of the scaphoid or lunate fossa that cannot be seen on plain films. We do not yet know how to apply CT in the overall patient population. Currently we believe that if a patient's treatment may be changed from conservative to surgical by further anatomic information, CT may provide a valuable method to gain this information. If the fracture plane is sagittal, a coronal plane CT may provide a second valuable exam to display depression or elevation of distal radius fracture fragments. A coronal plane CT can also be a valuable third position when more information is desired to understand unusual, very difficult fractures.

Parenthetically we have not yet found a patient on whom an axial CT could not be performed. A patient can lay on his side, can be placed supine on his elbows, or turned through 360° until an axial position is obtained. One patient with fractures of both legs and both arms was positioned flat on his back with one arm at a time above his head for a direct sagittal plane. This direct axial plane was performed, one wrist at a time with the hand in a somewhat saluting position, just to the side of the patient's face (thumb side down, small finger toward the ceiling). The head was in the scan plane, but was not included in the displayed scan sections.

Oblique View for STT Joint

A final position to present is an oblique view to look at the scaphotrapeziotrapezoidal joint. This was designed for one patient that needed the entire scaphotrapeziotrapezoidal joint profiled. To accomplish this, the wrist was positioned in a 30–45° reverse oblique position (ulnar side elevated) in order to profile those three bones as seen in a routine oblique wrist view (Fig. 9b). The resultant CT examination showed clearly the articulation between the trapezoid, trapezium, and scaphoid to verify some fusion between the graft and the scaphoid, but not between the graft, trapezium, and trapezoid (Fig. 9c). This position

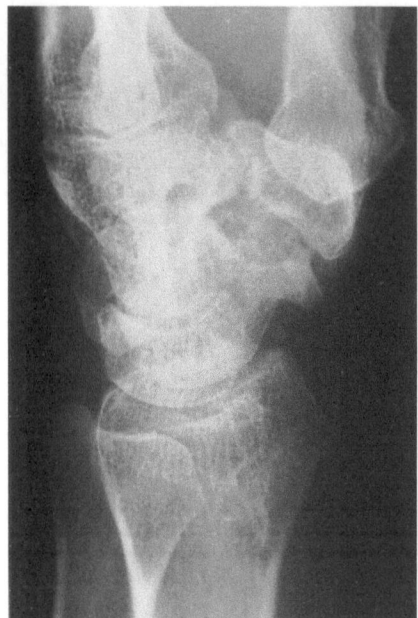

a

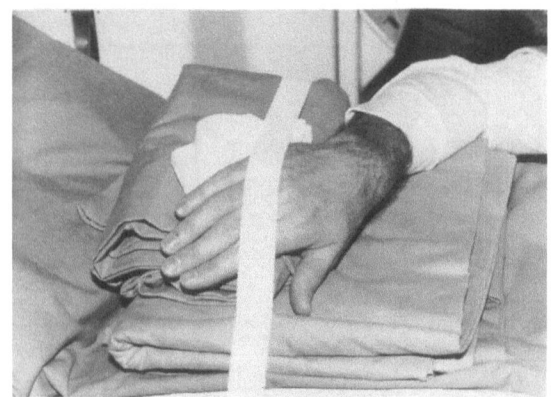

b

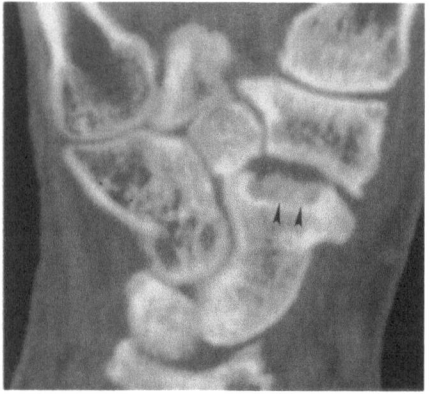

c

Fig. 9a–c. Scaphotrapeziotrapezoidal (STT) oblique view. **a** Lateral plain film (fusion procedure). The graft is in the STT space. **b** Hand position. **c** CT section of STT joint shows graft attached to scaphoid (*arrowheads*) but not to the trapezoid or trapezium

provides a very easy way to display the scapho-trapeziotrapezoidal joint and the adjacent articulation with the capitate. As this oblique view was designed to show a specific anatomic site, similarly, other positions could be designed to demonstrate other anatomic areas.

CT Reconstruction

CT reconstructions can be performed in many different ways. A reconstruction can be performed in different planes or can be reconstructed into a three-dimensional image. One example of three-dimensional reconstruction is that of a child with a "rosebud" hand (Fig. 10a). The clinical question concerned the status of the bone fusion or articulation distally for possible operative revision of the anomalous hand. A CT was performed in a routine transaxial plane (Fig. 10b) and then a three-dimensional reconstruction was performed. This showed the areas of fusion at the metacarpal bases. The hand was turned in multiple different directions to demonstrate how the distal tips of the fingers, metacarpals, and phalanges come together. The three-dimensional image allowed for ease of understanding and clarification of the anatomic abnormality. The major problem in the mature carpus for three-dimensional imaging is that for best carpal bone detail, each bone one wishes to examine may have to be separated or extracted.

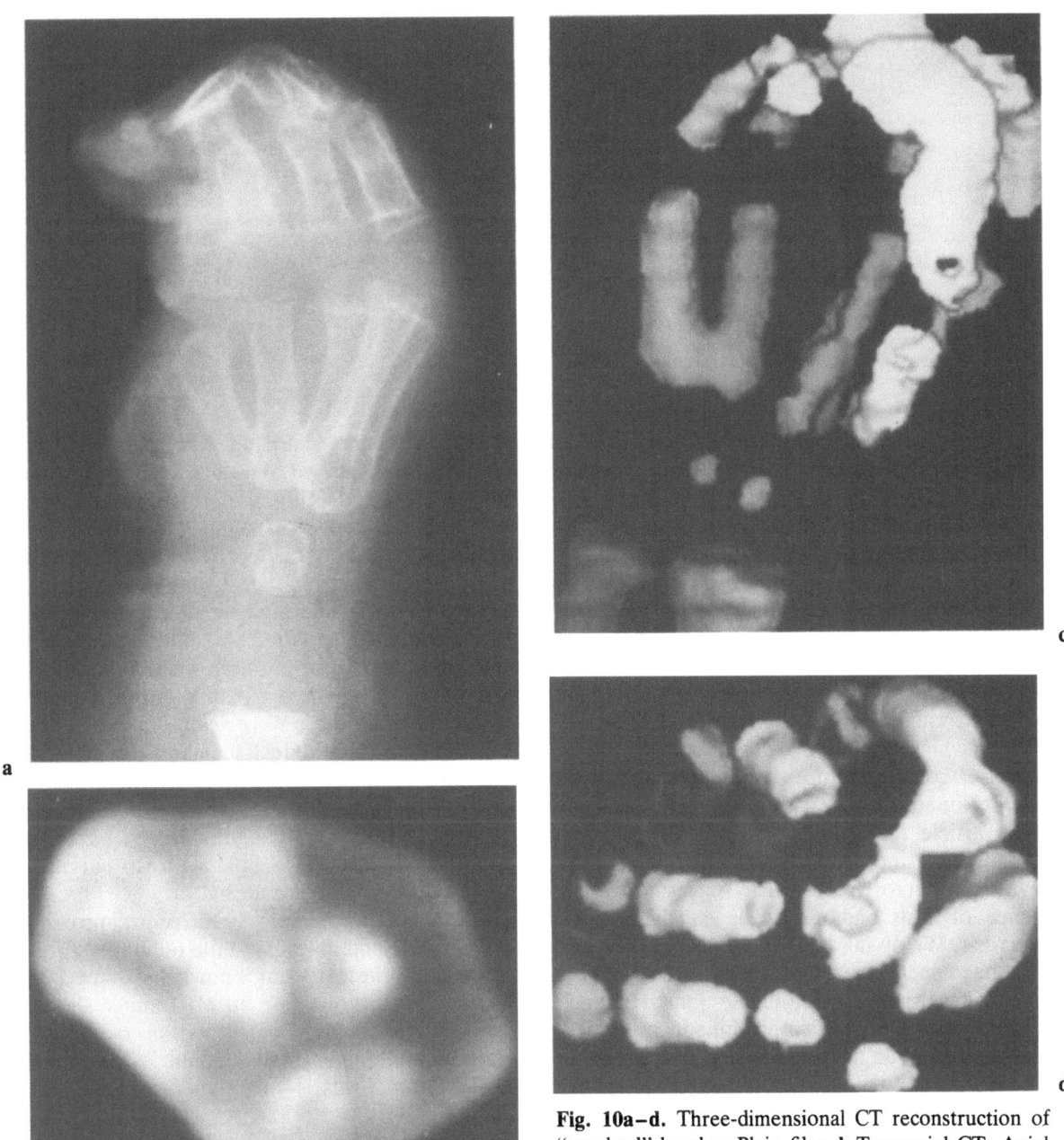

Fig. 10a–d. Three-dimensional CT reconstruction of "rosebud" hand. **a** Plain film. **b** Transaxial CT. Axial image through distal bone mass. **c, d** 3-D CT sections

Magnetic Resonance Imaging

MRI has some areas of definite current applications in the hand and the wrist, and other areas that are still developing. MRI is very sensitive to the presence of abnormal tissues, but is not tissue specific. The findings must be correlated with clinical evaluation and other imaging modalities. The purpose of this material is to provide an over-view of MRI use but not to present the basic physics background of MRI. Basically speaking, T_1-weighted images are very sensitive to bone marrow disorders and fat. T_2-weighted images are very sensitive to the presence of fluid. MRI can be very sensitive to the presence of marrow disorders including avascular necrosis, fractures, tumors, and infections. Cysts, ganglia, joint effusions, and

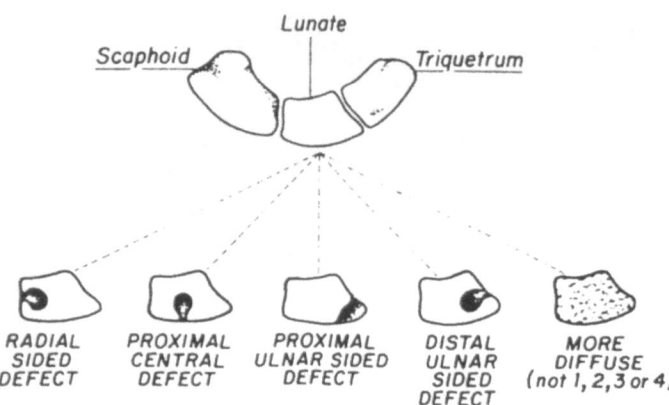

Fig. 11. Five patterns of lunate abnormalities

pus collections can be readily identified. The following is case material collected from the Mallinckrodt Institute of Radiology. Many of the examination were performed by fellow musculoskeletal radiologists Drs. William Totty, Tony Wilson, and William Murphy.

Mistakes have been encountered personally (LAG) and in the literature, and some can be avoided when dealing with the painful lunate. In our personal experience we have seen five different patterns of lunate abnormalities (Fig. 11), four of which we believe are not classic Kienböck's disease. Some literature suggests that any defect in the lunate may be Kienböck's disease [5, 6]. One article identified cysts and fibrosis in the lunate, and since both of these findings occur in avascular necrosis, the article suggested the presence of cysts and/or fibrosis equals avascular necrosis. We do not believe this to be true. What has been seen is a radial-sided defect that communicates to the scapholunate joint (Fig. 11). This commonly is corticated along its margin. Its contents may be fluid or fibrous, and no specific tissue may be found at operation. We have seen a similar unoperated ulnar-sided lucent defect communicating to the lunotriquetral joint not illustrated here. We have had two cases with a proximal central defect that connects to the radiolunate joint. Not uncommonly a proximal ulnar-sided defect occurs (Fig. 11) which may represent ulnar impaction syndrome changes or aging phenomena. These changes may be that of a lucent defect with cystic or fibrous material, or can be an area of solid sclerosis. A more diffuse pattern of MRI abnormality would be supportive of current or evolving Kienböck's disease. The following examples will help clarify these observations.

A patient with a painful lunate had a well-defined radial sided lucent defect (Fig. 12a) which

was hot on bone scan (Fig. 12b). An MRI was obtained which showed a well-defined in the radial side of the lunate (Fig. 12c,d). The dark signal area (black) along the rounded margins of the defect represented the corticated margin. The center had low signal intensity on the T_1-weighted image (Fig. 12c) and high signal intensity on the T_2-weighted images (Fig. 12d). This was an operated case of a cyst or intraosseous ganglia. In our experience the patient's pain disappeared after operation when these were symptomatic.

The radial-sided defect seems to usually communicate to the scapholunate joint when it is one of these "painful holes." Differential diagnosis includes intraosseous ganglia, fibrous tissue, or cyst. It may just be a hole with no surgically recognizable enclosed material.

We do not know what is in the central proximal defect that communicates to the radiolunate joint as none of these to our knowledge have been operated on. In one case an MRI image showed the lucency that connected to the radiolunate joint to contain a small amount of fluid, and we question if this is enlargement of a vascular channel.

⟶

Fig. 13a–e. Ulnar impaction syndrome. **a** Plain film demonstrates subtle increased density in the ulnar proximal aspect of the left lunate (*arrowheads*). **b** Bone scan shows prominent increased uptake over the left lunate or lunotriquetral area (*arrow*). **c** On CT examination, a sclerotic area (*arrow*) is verified in the proximal ulnar aspect of the lunate. An MRI examination with T1 weighting (**d**) and T2 weighting (**e**) confirms the abnormality ulnarly with low signal on both sequences (*arrows*) compatible with the area of bone sclerosis seen on plain films and CT. (Actually the MRI was performed first and the CT was later performed for anatomic clarification)

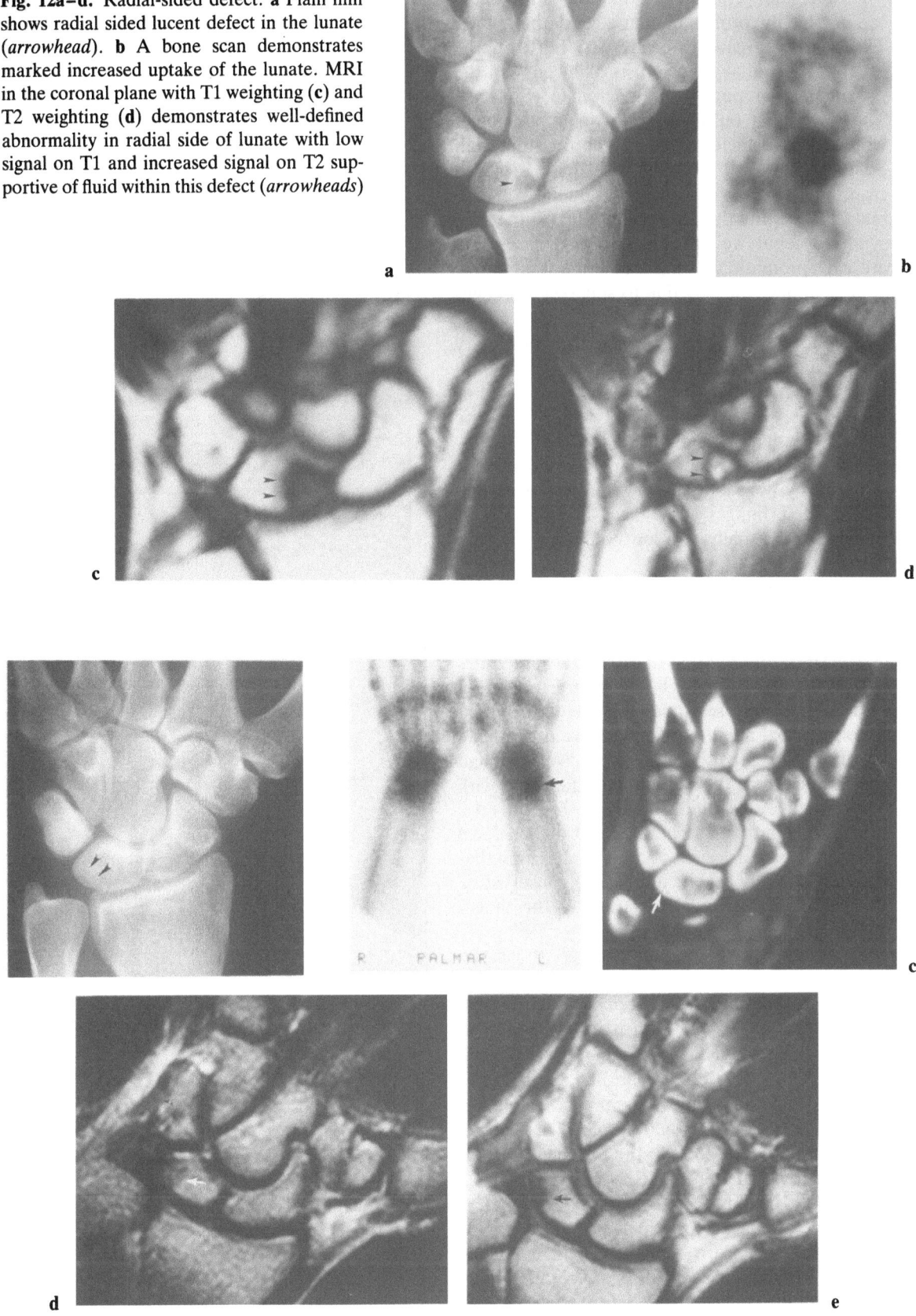

Fig. 12a–d. Radial-sided defect. **a** Plain film shows radial sided lucent defect in the lunate (*arrowhead*). **b** A bone scan demonstrates marked increased uptake of the lunate. MRI in the coronal plane with T1 weighting (**c**) and T2 weighting (**d**) demonstrates well-defined abnormality in radial side of lunate with low signal on T1 and increased signal on T2 supportive of fluid within this defect (*arrowheads*)

A fourth abnormal pattern in the painful lunate can involve the proximal ulnar edge of the lunate. The bone scan can be focally very hot over the lunate. There may be sclerosis or lucency in the proximal ulnar portion of the lunate (Fig. 13). The low signal on T_1- and T_2-weighted images would be satisfactory for just fibrous material. Some of these can be cysts with fluid, in which case they become a bright signal on T_2-weighted images. This fits the pattern for ulnar impaction syndrome, but we have encountered cases that are asymptomatic and some of these ulnar-sided abnormalities could be due to senescent changes [7].

The more diffuse patterns of signal abnormality in the lunate will probably represent osteonecrosis or Kienböck's disease. An obvious case of Kienböck's disease in a patient with a sclerotic collapsed lunate typically has a low signal on T_1-weighted images, which means the marrow is replaced by fibrous tissue or sclerotic bone. The T_2-weighted images may have a fairly bright signal, but is usually also low compared to other carpal bones.

When a *very* hot lunate is encountered is on a bone scan we should look further to explain the scan. We prefer next to go to CT; other people may wish to proceed first to MRI, and sometimes both CT and MRI may be necessary to explain the abnormal bone scan and the patient's problem.

Focal carpal abnormalities that are painful can involve other carpal bones as well. We have had operated cases of the capitate and trapezoid with fibrous and cystic fluid and tissue respectively. When a patient with a carpal lucent defect, focal tenderness, and a very hot bone scan has pain that does not go away despite all types of conservative therapy, then just focal curettage of the defect may relieve the pain.

MRI can be valuable for trauma. It can be especially helpful to detect a fracture not shown by other techniques. This can be suspected when a patient has persistent focal pain. With a bone scan that is focally hot in the area of tenderness, and plain films and CT are normal, both occult fractures and "bone bruise" may be found on MRI in such clinical situations. MRI is also an excellent method to look at the proximal portion of a scaphoid fracture to see if there are changes to support healing or avascularity. If on T_1-weighted images the proximal pole has low or normal signal marrow, and T_2-weighted images have the same signal as the distal pole, this change would support a vascularized proximal pole. If

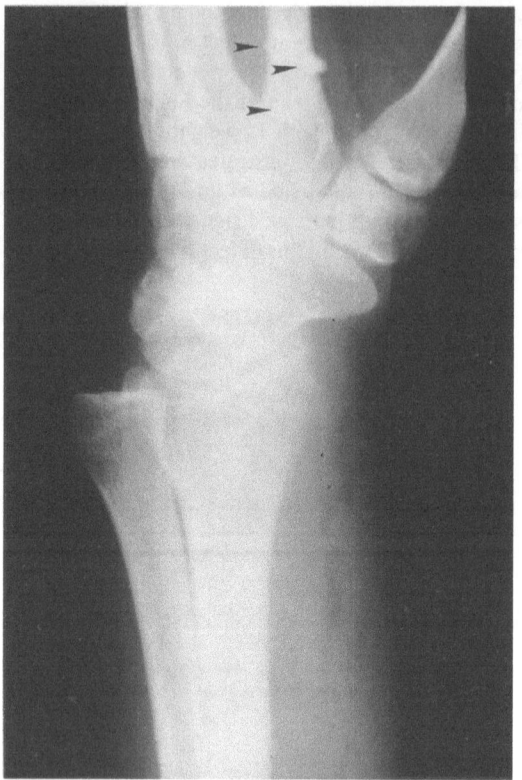

a

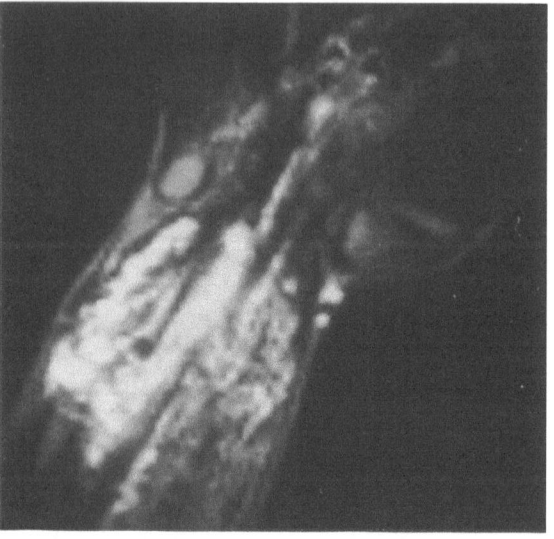

b

Fig. 14a,b. MRI of AV malformation of the forearm. **a** An oblique lateral view shows irregular soft tissue enlargement palmarly with calcifications (*arrowheads*) distally. **b** Coronal T2 weighted MRI shows a bright signal mass (*white areas*) involving palmar aspect of the distal forearm and extending into the wrist due to an anteriovenous malformation

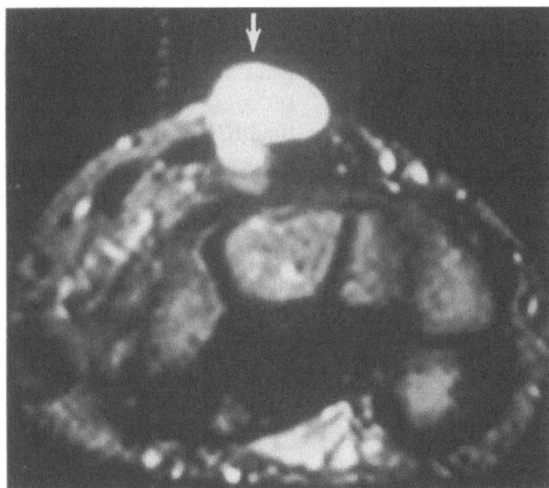

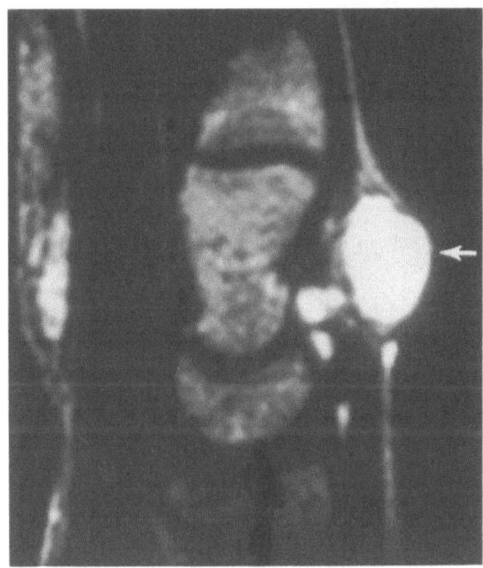

Fig. 15a,b. Dorsal ganglia. T2 weighted MRI in axial (**a**) and sagittal (**b**) planes demonstrate very bright focal signals (*white*) due to a dorsal ganglia (*arrows*) in the wrist

both T_1 and T_2 signals are decreased in the proximal scaphoid pole compared to the distal pole, this supports decreased vascularity of the proximal fragment.

MRI can readily show the soft tissue involvement of neoplastic processes, therefore if a potential or definite neoplastic process involves the wrist and/or the hand, MRI is the best way to demonstrate its extent. MRI can determine the extent of arteriovenous malformation in the forearm, wrist, and hand (Fig. 14).

Similarly, MRI typically shows ganglia with decreased signal on T_1-weighted images and in-

creased signal on T_2-weighted images typical of fluid composition (Fig. 15). MRI can be valuable to detect a subtle or occult ganglia or glomus tumor if it cannot be found clinically.

MRI has been described to show anatomic abnormalities in carpal tunnel syndrome. When clinically indicated it can be used to show abnormal changes of the median nerve such as swelling of the nerve, fluid around the nerve or an adjacent pathologic process.

Greenan and Zlatkin have described identifying defects in the scapholunate ligament, lunotriquetral ligament, and triangular fibrocartilage (TFC) [8]. Anecdotally, some people believe they can show the TFC fairly routinely, but most people in our experience have a difficult time looking at the scapholunate and lunotriquetral ligaments routinely. Normally the TFC is seen as a very dark signal without increased signal. Seeing an increased signal passing entirely through the TFC is the type of signal change we would see with a TFC defect. Recently we have been very impressed with the work of Dr. Saara Totterman, a radiologist doing specialized work in MRI, who has been producing advanced, state-of-the-art MRI images of the wrist, and who has been working with a hand surgeon, Dr. Richard Miller of Rochester, New York. With dedicated wrist coils and sequencing she has produced improved details of the TFC and scapholunate, lunotriquetral, and extrinsic ligaments (Fig. 16). As imaging continues to improve, the future use of MRI for ligament and capsular abnormalities should increase. When MRI is finally able to routinely demonstrate both intrinsic and extrinsic ligaments, capsule margins and their abnormalities, we believe wrist arthrography may be replaced.

The major advantages of MRI are that it shows high soft tissue contrast, it is very sensitive to fluid, and shows accurate anatomic location. The major disadvantages of MRI are its higher cost and unreliable detection of calcification, ossification or gas. Some patients cannot tolerate MRI examination because of claustrophobia.

Wrist Arthrography

Wrist arthrography has received a lot of attention largely due to work that has been done by Levinsohn et al. [9] We have been performing wrist arthrography for many years and have personal experience (LAG) of over 1000 cases. The last 500–700 cases were performed using the triple joint arthrogram technique. Only a few points will be mentioned here. We prefer to use diluted

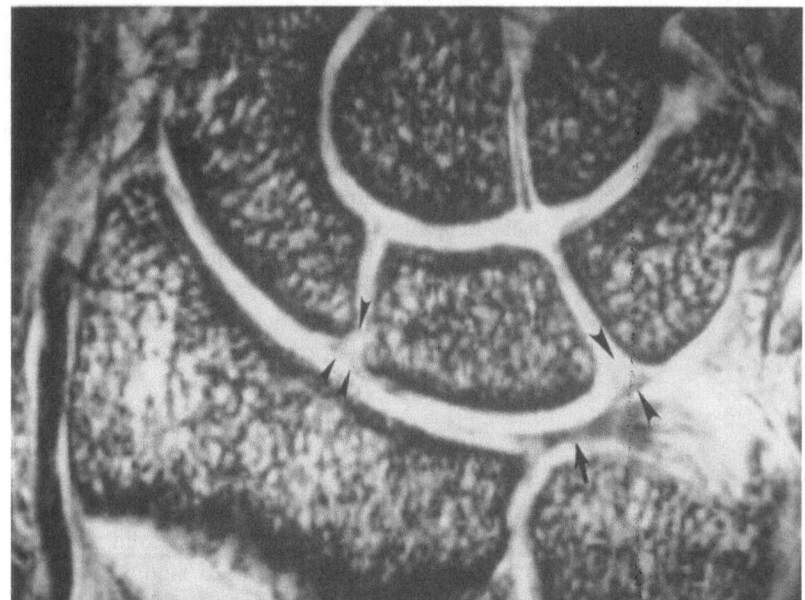

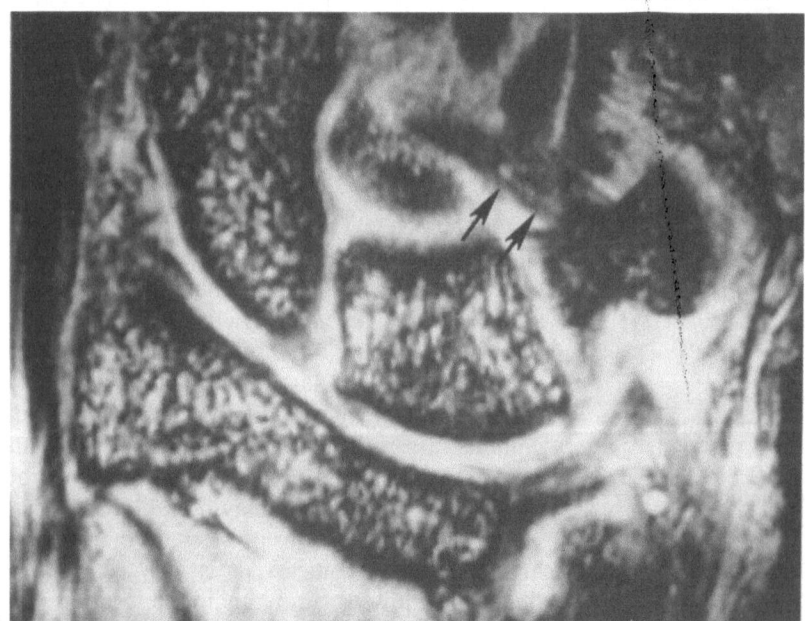

Fig. 16a,b. Dedicated wrist coil images. Coronal gradient echo images at 1-mm thick sections with **a** more dorsal than **b**. These show triangular fibrocartilage (*small arrow*), scapholunate (*between small arrowheads*), lunotriquetral (*between large arrowheads*) and extrinsic ligaments (*large arrows*). (Courtesy of Saara Totterman, Rochester, New York)

contrast, as a thick or denser contrast produces more synovitis. Contrast diluted with anesthetic tells if the compartment being bathed by contrast and anesthesia is the source of pain. We believe contrast should be injected until the joint is fully distended within the patient's comfort level. The needle should be placed away from the symptomatic site at the midcarpal level when there are ulnar-sided symptoms. In that situation, the needle can be placed at the distal ⅓–¼ of the scaphocapitate joint. With radial-sided symptoms, it is easy to put the needle on the ulnar side of the wrist between the capitate, hamate, triquetrum, and lunate. For the radiocarpal joint, for ulnar-sided symptoms, the needle can be placed between the radial styloid and scaphoid. In the midportion of the radiocarpal joint, a needle can be placed in the middle of the radiolunate joint. On the ulnar side of this joint the needle can be placed along the proximal ulnar surface of the triquetrum. Contrast injection must be followed and recorded by fluoroscopic spots, 105 mm filming, videotape or digital subtraction techniques.

There may be various sized holes (defects) in the scapholunate and lunotriquetral ligaments. There are smaller "pinholes" or large defects, and the size of ligament defects may be important to think about in the future. Concern about a flap-like defect of scapholunate, lunotriquetral ligament or TFC is one of the main reasons that triple joint arthrography to fill all three compartments is currently emphasized [9]. A small flap of one of these structures has been seen at operation, arthroscopy and anatomic dissection that could potentially block contrast from entering an adjacent wrist compartment from one side of a ligament but would allow contrast to enter from the other side of a ligament. Therefore, the claimed advantage of three compartment wrist arthrography is that it is capable of demonstrating unidirectional ("flap") ligament tears. These tears may be missed by injecting only one compartment, but the major question remains in the minds of many people that have personally contacted us is whether this is necessary, and whether the additional information contributes to patient managements. We examined 250 patients in one series where the midcarpal joint (MCJ) was injected first, the distal radioulnar joint (DRUJ) injected second, and the radiocarpal joint (RCJ), last [10]. This study showed that all one-way scapholunate and lunotriquetral defects were shown from the first joint injected, the midcarpal joint. We had two capsule defects communicating between RCJ and MCJ that showed only from the radiocarpal to midcarpal joint. There were a few one-way defects in the TFC that were seen from the radiocarpal and from the DRUJ injections. We did another study where we looked at 100 patients, injecting 50 patients randomly in the radiocarpal joint first and 50 patients in the midcarpal joint first [11]. This study showed all scapholunate and lunotriquetral ligament communicating defects that were unidirectional (filled from only one direction) filled from the first joint injected. Our feeling is that these two studies support the idea that when the midcarpal or radiocarpal joint is fully distended (comfortably) with contrast, all communicating scapholunate and lunotriquetral ligament defects (tears) are demonstrated. To show all capsular defects, all three compartments need to be injected separately. To verify the status of the TFC, both surfaces of the TFC must be outlined. However, the major point to bring out with wrist arthrography currently and in the future is that there is an increasing need to determine which arthrographic findings are significant. Many other questions remain to be answered, such as whether a defect found on one side of a TFC is important, what is the meaning of a defect (communicating to another compartment or noncommunicating, just focal extravasation) found in the capsule, and whether a capsular defect is a sign of an adjacent extrinsic ligament tear.

Regardless of the imaging procedure performed, careful wrist examination is the most important part of evaluating the "unexplained" painful wrist. A lot of work remains to be done. The diagnosing and treating physician needs to work closely with radiologists to find out which of the abnormalities are important and how we should best proceed to investigate the painful wrist.

References

1. Stewart NR, Gilula LA (1992) Tailored approach to wrist CT. Radiology 183:13–20
2. Pennes DR, Jonsson K, Buckwalter KA (1989) Direct coronal CT of the scaphoid bone. Radiology 171:870–871
3. Biondetti PF, Vannier MW, Gilula LA, Knapp R (1987) Wrist: Coronal and transaxial CT scanning. Radiology 163:149–151
4. Nelson DL, Pruitt DL, Martin RA, Manske PR, Gilula LA, Szerzinski JH (to be published) Lunotriquetral Arthrodesis. J Hand Surg [Am]
5. Sowa DT, Holder LE, Patt PG, Weiland AJ (1989) Application of magnetic resonance imaging to ischemic necrosis of the lunate. J Hand Surg [Am] 14:1008–1016
6. Reicher MA, Kellerhouse LE (1990) MRI of the wrist and hand. Raven Press, New York pp 108–111
7. Nakamura R, Tanaka Y, Imaeda T, Miura T (1991) The influence of age and sex on ulnar variance. J Hand Surg [Br] 16:84–88
8. Greenan T, Zlatkin MB (1990) Magnetic resonance imaging of the wrist. Semin Ultrasound CT MR 11:267–287
9. Levinsohn EM, Palmer AK, Coren AB, Zinberg E (1987) Wrist arthrography: The value of the three compartment injection technique. Skeletal Radiol 16:539–544
10. Wilson AJ, Gilula LA, Mann FA (1991) Unidirectional joint communications in wrist arthrography. An evaluation of 250 cases. AJR 157:105–109
11. Mann FA, Wilson AJ, Gilula LA (to be published) Triple joint wrist arthrographic prospective study of technical variations and their effect on unidirectional communication. J Hand Surg [Am]

Wrist Kinematics

Yu Mochizuki, Yoshikazu Ikuta, Akira Ikeda, and Tsuneji Murakami[1]

Abstract. Although many experimental and clinical studies have been reported in the past, the nature of kinematics of the wrist joint remains controversial, with wrist motion being notoriously difficult to measure on radiographs. Consequently, we have elected to use a technique for directly measuring carpal motion by means of a strain gauge attached to a unique measuring apparatus. To investigate intercarpal movement, we selected four carpal bones for measurement, the lunate, capitate, scaphoid, and triquetrum. We attached the measuring apparatus to each carpal bone by 1-mm diameter screws.

The intercarpal movement showed different kinematics in each directional motion of wrist joint. In extension, the movement increased over a 40° angle between the capitate and scaphoid and the triquetrum and capitate. In radial flexion, the movement increased over a 10° angle between the capitate and triquetrum and the triquetrum and lunate.

The measuring apparatus was very useful for analyzing the three-dimensional movements of wrist joints. This study offers fundamental data which can contribute to the understanding of the pathogenesis of wrist joint disorders.

Keywords: Intercarpal motion — Direct measurement — Measuring apparatus — Strain gauge — Normal movement

Introduction

In spite of the many experimental and clinical studies which have been reported on the subject, the nature of kinematics of the wrist joint remains controversial. The reasons for this are both anatomical and functional [1, 2]. The carpal bones are small, irregularly shaped structures, without obvious longitudinal axes or prominent, easily identifiable landmarks. In addition, their motion is primarily rotational and often in more than one axis. This type of movement is notoriously difficult to measure on radiographs. It is also difficult to detect rotation if only a small portion of the bone is visible, as is the case during dissection or surgical exposure. Furthermore, most relative motion is quite small, which increases the possibility of error in radiographic readings.

For these reasons, recent investigators have labeled the carpal bones and have used sophisticated, accurate, and minimally invasive techniques to measure three-dimensional motion, such as light-emmitting diodes and sonic pulsation markers. However, these techniques of carpal bone marking have specific limitations: (1) they can only be used in vitro, (2) they require exposure of the carpals and the implantation of markers, and (3) they have the potential for disturbing normal intercarpal motion by injuring normal structures.

We carried out an experimental study in order to analyze the intercarpal movement of wrist joints. We used a technique of direct measurement of carpal motions with a unique apparatus.

Materials and Methods

We used 36 wrist joints from 30 cadavers which were preserved by an arterial embalming technique.

The measuring apparatus which we used was comprised of a 20 × 6 × 1mm polyethylene bar with a dome-shaped center portion, 5mm in diameter. The strain gauges were attached to

[1] Department of Orthopaedic Surgery, Hiroshima University School of Medicine, Kasumi, 1-2-3, Minami-ku, Hiroshima 734, Japan

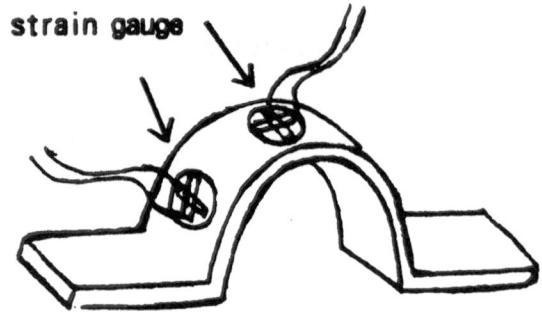

strain gauge

Fig. 1. The measuring apparatus which was comprised of a 20 × 6 × 1 mm polyethylene bar with a dome-shaped center portion, 5 mm in diameter. The strain gauges (*arrows*) were attached to the top and sides of the center portion along the center line of the long axis

the top and sides of the center portion along the center line of the long axis (Fig. 1). In a preliminary study, we found that the amount of strain indicated a visible change in the angle between the 2 points. The strain gauge on the top portion showed a larger amount of strain than did the sides. This fact suggested that the strain gauge on the top portion had a higher sensitivity than that of the sides. Therefore, we decided to use the data of the strain gauge on the top portion.

To investigate intercarpal movement, we selected four carpal bones for measurement, the lunate, capitate, scaphoid, and triquetrum. The dorsal side of the cadaver wrist joint was exposed, keeping the ligaments and capsule intact. We decided upon the screw insertion point by using two-directional roentgenography and attached the measuring apparatus to each carpal bone by

1-mm diameter screws. The forearm of each specimen was rigidly mounted onto a holding device in a neutral position. All movements were powered by the operator's hand. Measurements were performed 5 times at each measuring site and in each direction. The data were analyzed statistically by regression analysis.

Results

In extension, the capitolunate site showed the largest change of strain. The scaphocapitate and triquetrocapitate sites showed sudden increases of strain of over a 40° angle. The scapholunate and triquetrolunate sites did not show any increases in change of strain (Fig. 2). The data demonstrated each site to be significantly different from the others. In flexion movement, all measured sites showed an increase of strain, with the triquetrocapitate site showing the largest change of strain and the scapholunate site showing the smallest change of strain. In addition, each measured site indicated a significant difference from the others.

In radial flexion movement, the scaphocapitate site showed the largest change of strain, and the triquetrolunate and triquetrocapitate sites evidenced a sudden increase of strain of over 10°. The scapholunate site showed the smallest change of strain, and each measured site was significantly different from the others (Fig. 3).

In ulnar flexion movement, all measured sites showed an increase of strain. In particular, the triquetrocapitate site showed the largest change of strain, and the triquetrolunate site showed the

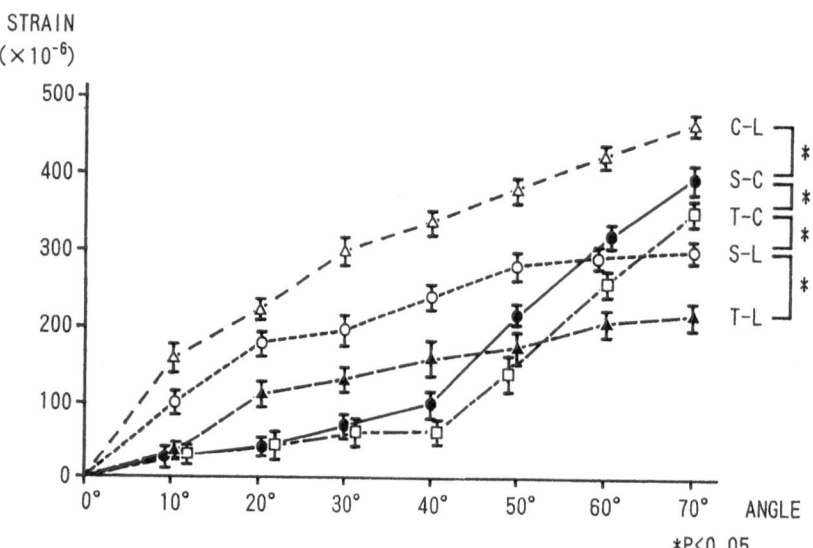

Fig. 2. The strain change at each measured site during extension movement. *Open circle*, scapholunate motion; *closed circle*, scaphocapitate motion; *open triangle*, capitolunate motion; *closed triangle*, triquetrolunate motion; *square*, triquetrolunate motion. *C*, Capitate; *L*, lunate; *S*, scaphoid; *T*, triquetrum

Fig. 3. The strain change at each measured site during radial flexion movement. *Open circle*, scapholunate motion; *closed circle*, scaphocapitate motion; *open triangle*, capitolunate motion; *closed triangle*, triquetrolunate motion; *square*, triquetrolunate motion. *C*, Capitate; *L*, lunate; *S*, scaphoid; *T*, triquetrum

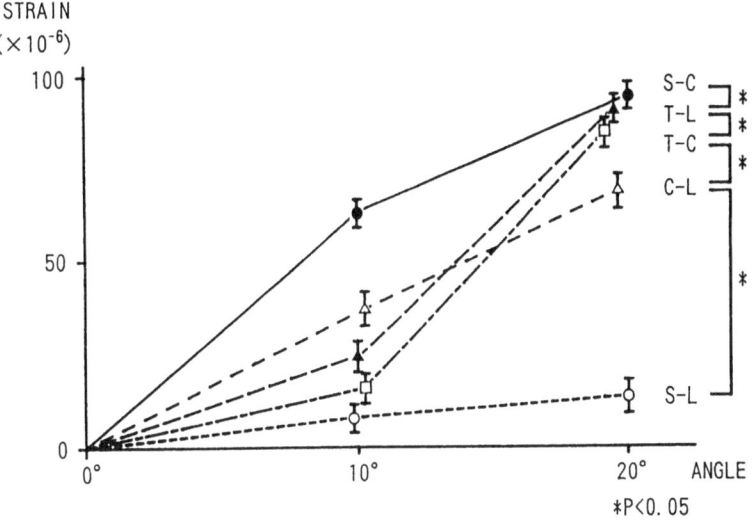

smallest change of strain. We could not find any significant difference between the scaphocapitate and the scapholunate sites. The other measured sites were significantly different from the others.

Discussion

We hypothesized that any statistical difference would reflect a difference in kinematics of the movements. In the extension movement, each carpal bone showed a different movement, with the largest being between the capitate and lunate. The movement increased over a 40° angle between the capitate and scaphoid and the triquetrum and capitate, while between the scaphoid and lunate and the triquetrum and lunate the increase in movement was slight.

Each carpal bone showed different movement in flexion, with the largest movement being observed between the triquetrum and capitate and the smallest between the scaphoid and lunate.

Each carpal bone showed different movement in radial flexion, with the largest being between the scaphoid and capitate and the smallest between the scaphoid and lunate. The movement increased over a 10° angle between the capitate and triquetrum and the triquetrum and lunate.

In ulnar flexion, each carpal bone showed a different movement except at the scaphocapitate

and scapholunate sites. During ulnar flexion, the scaphoid, capitate, and lunate showed almost the same amount of movement, with the largest being between the capitate and triquetrum and the smallest between the triquetrum and lunate.

Conclusions

The intercarpal movement had different kinematics in each directional motion of the wrist joint. In extension, the movement increased over a 40° angle between the capitate and scaphoid and the triquetrum and capitate. In radial flexion, the movement increased over a 10° angle between the capitate and triquetrum and the triquetrum and lunate.

The measuring apparatus was very useful for analyzing the three-dimensional movements of wrist joints. This study offers some fundamental data which can contribute to the understanding of the pathogenesis of wrist joint disorders.

References

1. Linscheid RL (1972) Traumatic Instability of the wrist. J Bone Joint Surgery [Am] 54:1612–1632
2. Volz RG (1980) Biomechanics of the wrist. Clin Orthop 149:112–117

Analysis of Wrist Motion During Basketball Shooting*

Nobuki Ohnishi[1], Jaiyoung Ryu, In-Seol Chung, Richard Colbaugh, and Bruce Rowen[2]

Abstract. The purposes of this study were to establish the efficacy of a custom-designed electrogoniometer (biaxial) in monitoring wrist motion and to analyze the function of the wrist in basketball shooting. Six NCAA basketball players participated and a total of 578 shots (free-throws) were recorded and analyzed with the custom-designed electrogoniometer attached to both wrists of each player.

The dominant wrist motion was divided into 3 phases, acceleration, constant velocity, and deceleration. For the dominant wrist, the average range of motion was 120° (extension 50°, flexion 70°) in the flexion-extension movement (FEM), and 23° (radial deviation 12°, ulnar deviation 11°) in radioulnar deviation (RUD). The non-dominant side showed a smaller range of motion, 32° in FEM and 16° in RUD. The velocity of motion of the dominant wrist at the constant velocity phase ranged from 2500° to 3100° per second in FEM and 150°–750° in RUD. No statistically significant difference was found in the range or velocity of the wrist motion between good shots and those which were too short or too long. The players with smaller deviations in their range of wrist motion, however, were the more accurate shooters. This study has established the efficacy of the electrogoniometer in monitoring wrist motion.

Keywords: Wrist — Basketball — Electrogoniometer — Motion analysis

Introduction

Throwing is a crucial element in many sports. However, differences exist in throwing techniques across the broad spectrum of sports with each sport needing specific extremity movements to achieve the desired style. While extensive investigations in other sports, such as baseball, have been performed [1–5], there is, to our knowledge, no study explaining the wrist kinematics in basketball shooting. Most studies of the throwing mechanism have been focusing on the shoulder, and, to a lesser degree, on the elbow. Journals of sport medicine have expressed concern with the wrist only in relation to injury [6–9]. In the same way, basketball has been of interest only in relation to injuries in this field [10–12]. Even with three-dimensional cinematography, it is difficult to monitor the rapid motions of small joints, such as those in the wrist. This may contribute to the lack of biomechanical information on the wrist in sport activities. Since the shoulder and the elbow seem to be more vulnerable to injuries with greater frequency and severity than are other joints in the act of throwing, the wrist has not received much attention by researchers.

In order to thoroughly understand the mechanics of throwing activities, one must understand the kinematics of the wrist as well as those of other joints. The purposes of this study are to analyze (1) the range of flexion-extension movement (FEM) and radioulnar deviation (RUD) undergone by the wrist in shooting a basketball, (2) the angular velocity of the wrist motion when shooting the ball, and (3) correlation of the wrist motions and quality of the shooting action.

Subjects Methods and Materials

Six male NCAA basketball players from the University of Texas at El Paso (UTEP) participated in this study. Subject information is shown in

* No benefits in any form have been or will be received from a commercial party related directly or indirectly to the subjects of this article
[1] Department of Orthopaedics, Ohji General Hospital, Omotemachi-4, Tomakomai 053, Japan
[2] Orthopaedic Biomechanics Research Laboratory, Texas Tech University — Health Science Center, El Paso, Texas, USA

Table 1. Subject information

Player	Age (years)	Height (feet)	Weight (pounds)	Position (on team)	FT (%)[a]	FG (%)
1 (J.T)	21	6.2	155	Guard	80	53
2 (B.G)	30	6.5	180	Guard	79	55
3 (T.B)	24	6.3	240	Forward	85	56
4 (M.P)	25	6.4	200	Forward	90	55
5 (C.B)	24	6.5	205	Guard	83	51
6 (F.E)	23	6.8	215	Forward	50	36

FT, Free-throwing; *FG*, field goal
[a] Percentage for both FT and FG means the rate of successful shootings in official games during 1 year

Table 1. None had a history of a major injury or of wrist disorders. Physical examination showed no abnormality in the upper extremities. All were right-hand dominant. They understood the purposes, methods, and materials comprising this study, and cooperated willingly. The experiment was performed in indoor basketball courts. The players were given enough time to warm up.

Custom-designed biaxial electrogoniometers (goniometers) (Fig. 1) were attached to both wrists of the players to simultaneously monitor angular movement of the wrist in two planes, FEM, and RUD. The goniometer was attached so that its two potentiometers were colinear with the axes of FEM and RUD. It was then calibrated at 0° in both planes while the wrist was kept in a

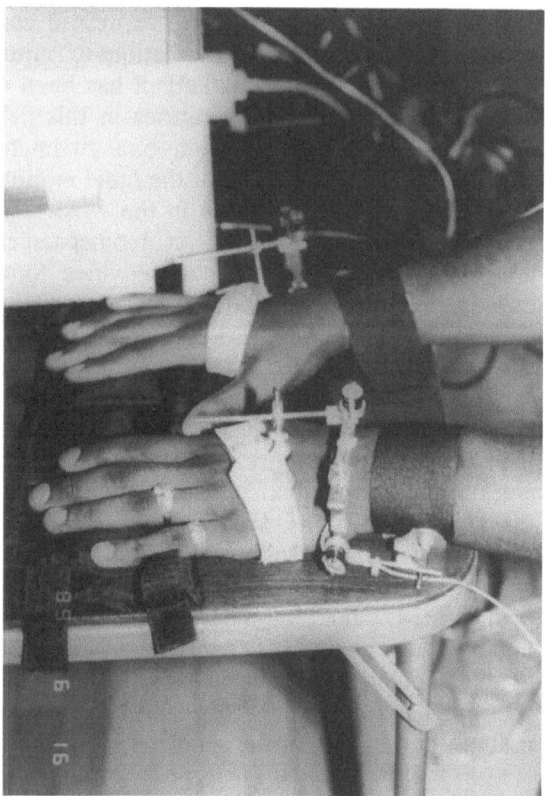
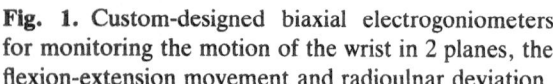

Fig. 1. Custom-designed biaxial electrogoniometers for monitoring the motion of the wrist in 2 planes, the flexion-extension movement and radioulnar deviation

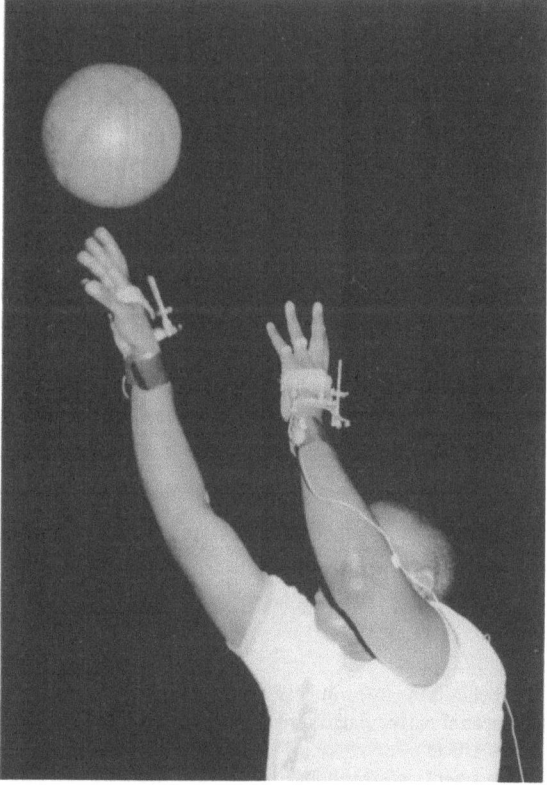

Fig. 2. Players were requested to shoot free-throws with the goniometers attached to their wrists

neutral position. Tracking of the goniometer and its 0° calibration were rechecked and adjusted after every 10 shots. All data from the goniometer were converted into analogue modes and recorded with a strip-chart recorder. After each player felt that he was adequately prepared and familiarized with the devices and their settings, he was requested to shoot 100 free-throws just as he would do in actual games (Fig. 2). In order to analyze the correlation of the wrist motions and shot quality, the shots were divided into 3 categories: good (through the hoop without backboard rebound), short (hitting the anterior part of rim of the hoop and bounding out), and long (hitting the posterior part of the rim or backboard and bounding out). The players were also filmed with a high-speed 16-mm motor-driven video camera throughout the entire shot sequence to capture movements of the upper extremities, including the wrist, and to compare and contrast these movements with the data from the goniometers. For statistical analysis, a standard PC software package was used.

Results

A total of 578 shots were recorded and analyzed. Successful shooting rates for each player ranged from 60% to 87% (average 80%). Of the missed shots, 14% were too short and 6% too long. While the players themselves showed highly consistent patterns of motion in both wrists during shooting, shot form was quite different among the players.

According to the characteristics of the slope on the graph and direction of the movement of the wrist in RUD, the motion of the dominant wrist from maximum extension to maximum flexion in the FEM plane was divided into 3 phases, acceleration, constant velocity, and deceleration (Fig. 3). The acceleration phase began at the maximally extended position and continued to the point where acceleration was lost. In this phase, wrist flexion was not accompanied by RUD wrist motion in 2 of the players, ulnar deviation in 2, and radial deviation in 2. In the constant velocity phase, flexion movement was at a constant speed,

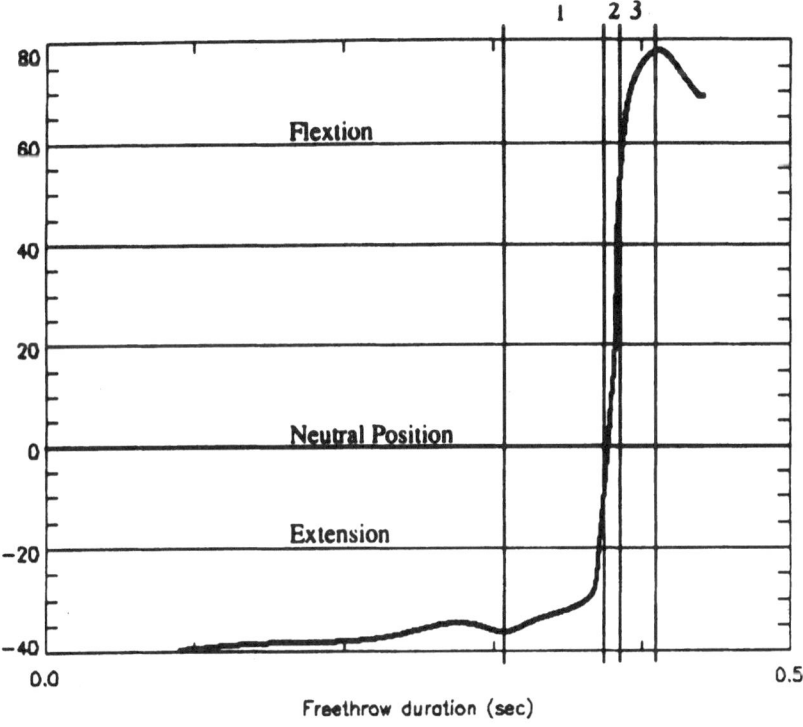

Fig. 3. Motion of the dominant wrist from maximum extension to maximum flexion was divided into 3 phases, *1* acceleration, *2* constant velocity, and *3* deceleration

so the relationship of time and angular motion of the wrist was shown on the graph by a straight line. In this phase, wrist flexion motion was accompanied by ulnar deviation in all players. In the deceleration phase, the speed of flexion motion of the wrist decreased, until it stopped flexing at the end point. In this phase, the wrist flexed with radial deviation in 4 players, ulnar deviation in 1, and no RUD movement in 1. Just after termination of the deceleration phase, the wrist began to extend acutely from the maximally flexed position, resembling a rebound phenomenon, so this phase may be called the recovery phase. The video recording showed that the basketballs were released between the late stage of acceleration phase and the early stage of the constant velocity phase.

Non-dominant wrists began to move in flexion and ulnar direction 0.08–0.12 seconds earlier than dominant wrists, and showed slower movement over a longer period.

The range of wrist motion during shooting is shown in Table 2. For the dominant side, the wrist extension ranged from 40.2° to 56.5°, the group average being 50°. Wrist flexion for each player ranged from 48° to 84°, the average for the 6 players being 70°. The average of the total range in FEM for each player ranged from 102° to 138°, with the average for the 6 players being 120°. The average of radial deviation for the 6 players was 12° (ranging from −3° to 20°). The average of ulnar deviation for the 6 players was 10° (ranging from 3° to 21°). The range of motion in RUD for each player ranged from 12° to 35°, and the average for the 6 players was 23°. For the non-dominant side, the average of range of motion in FEM was 32°, nearly one-fourth of that of the dominant side. In RUD, it was 16°.

Each player showed some degrees of variation in the range of wrist motion. Table 3 shows comparisons of shooting results with the standard deviation (SD) of the dominant wrist motion in FEM for each player. A player with a 61% success rate (lowest in this series) showed an SD

Table 2. Range of motion of the dominant wrist in basketball shooting (in degrees)

Direction	Average	Range
Extension	50	40–56
Flexion	70	48–84
Radial deviation	12	−3–20
Ulnar deviation	10	3–21

Table 3. The relationship of standard deviation (SD) of the range of motion of the dominant wrist in flexion-extension and the rates of successful shots (G.S.)

Player	Average (°)	SD	G.S. (%)
M.P.	122	3.1	87
C.B.	123	7.1	87
J.T.	132	4.2	86
B.G.	138	6.8	81
T.B.	107	7.0	81
F.E.	102	18.3	60

of 18.3, while players with 87% success rates showed SDs of 3.1 and 7.1. There was a tendency for players with better success rates to show more constant wrist motion, i.e., these players had smaller deviations in the range of motion of the wrist among their shots.

The velocity of the dominant wrist motion at constant velocity phase ranged from 2500° to 3100° per second in FEM, and from 150° to 750° per second in RUD. The velocity of the non-dominant wrist in FEM ranged from 250° to 800° per second.

Comparisons of wrist motions among the types of shots, good, short, and long, are shown in Table 4. There was no statistically significant difference among these 3 groups in the range of wrist motion in any direction. No significant difference was found in the velocity of wrist motion among these groups.

Discussion

Numerous investigations have been done on biomechanics of the wrist in clinical and basic research fields, but the field of sport medicine has largely bypassed the topic. Difficulty in monitoring rapid, highly coordinated, and complex motion of the wrist may have contributed to this lack of studies.

Three-dimensional analysis using high-speed cinematography with computer processing has proven useful in assessing motions of the upper extremities in baseball, tennis, water polo, and boxing [13, 14]. While this method excels in analyzing the movements of relatively large joints, such as the shoulder and the elbow, close-up viewing is required for digitization of the wrist. Should the wrist move in a wide range, it would be difficult to keep an orthogonally located camera focused. Such cinematography is further

Table 4. Correlation of the wrist motions in both planes and quality of shots. Shots were divided into 3 categories, good, short, and long

| | ROM in Shooting: dominant side | | | | | | | ROM in Shooting: non-dominant side | | | | | |
| | FEM | | | RUD | | | | FEM | | | RUD | | |
Player no.	Good	Short	Long	Good	Short	Long	Player no.	Good	Short	Long	Good	Short	Long
1	131.8	133.7	132.3	38.8	38.0	36.8	1	18.9	18.0	20.6	35.7	35.8	36.0
2	122.6	124.0	122.3	35.6	35.7	37.5	2	44.4	44.4	47.0	14.4	14.0	14.3
3	138.0	133.3	134.9	18.4	18.0	19.7	3	23.7	22.7	23.7	16.0	14.7	14.8
4	107.0	106.3	108.0	11.4	11.2	12.0	4	16.1	15.9	16.0	4.0	3.9	4.0
5	102.2	102.0	106.0	35.9	35.6	38.8	5	34.7	36.8	27.1	17.7	18.1	18.3
6	123.8	123.4	122.0	32.8	39.4	28.6	6	51.4	50.0	54.0	24.3	25.5	23.7

ROM, Range of motion; *FEM*, flexion-extension movement; *RUD*, radioulnar deviation

complicated by the fact that the marker points on the hand which need to be targetted are often hidden by the basketball and the player's own body during motion.

Electromyographic techniques have been used to quantify activities of muscles involved in motion [15–21]. This technique has been applied mainly to muscles around the shoulder and the elbow during activity, especially in throwing baseballs. This method provides important information in analyzing muscle activity, but it is inadequate for studies of joint kinematics by itself.

In order to monitor the motion of small joints, a new technique needed to be developed. By comparing the data from a high-speed video camera, the way in which players actually do the shooting, and the consistency of the data for each player, the results of this study have established the efficacy of the electrogoniometer in monitoring wrist motion in basketball shooting. The players who participated in this study reported that the devices did not hamper wrist motion, nor did they alter the pattern of their shooting. However, some points of the devices need to be revised. Velcro straps were used to attach the devices to the wrists of the players. Should slipping occur between the bones and the covering skin, the resulting measurement may be inaccurate. A more reliable method of application needs to be developed. In this study, data was converted into an analog mode and recorded on a strip-chart recorder. For increased accuracy and convenience, data should be directly fed into a computer and digitized. This revised method is currently being used on other projects.

Motion analysis in this study revealed consistency and individuality of wrist motion during each player's shooting. Dominant wrist motion, when divided into 3 phases, moved uniformly in an ulnar direction when the wrist was flexed acutely at constant velocity phase, while there was variety in RUD wrist motion among the players in the acceleration and deceleration phases.

A large amount of range of wrist motion (120° in FEM) was required for basketball shooting, a fact which should be taken into account by hand surgeons treating the dominant wrists of basketball players, as this is much more than the reported functional range of motion for the activities of daily living [22, 23]. Any disorder restricting the range of wrist motion less than reported in this study may easily decrease the shooting ability of a basketball player. Interestingly, the range of wrist motion needed for basketball shooting is near that reported as the retained range of motion following triscaphe arthrodesis [24] (Table 5).

The results also showed that the dominant wrist moved at high speeds (2500°–3100° per second). These values are lower than those required for the shoulder and the elbow in baseball pitching (at acceleration phase, 6180° and 4595° per second, respectively) [2], but much higher than

Table 5. ROM of the dominant wrist in basketball shooting compared with ROM after triscaphe athrodesis. (From [24])

Range of motion	Shooting	STT-FUSION
Extension	50°	55°
Flexion	70°	68°
Radial deviation	12°	12°
Ulnar deviation	11°	28°

STT, Scaphoid-trapezium-trapezoid

the average peak angular velocity of the elbow needed for throwing in water polo (1137°) [13]. This means that basketball shooting demands high wrist performance in both speed and range of motion.

One of the purposes of this study was to investigate how motions of the wrist affected the vector or accuracy of shots. There was no statistically significant difference in the wrist motion (range or velocity) among the 3 groups, good, too short, and too long shots. It is suggested that constant, accurate movements of the wrist are needed for good shots, since the data showed that players with higher accuracy (success rate) had less variation in the range of wrist motion among the shots. Shooting, just like pitching in baseball, seems to result from integrated motions of whole body [25], and the wrist plays an important role in the terminal movement of sequential body activation through a link system. The results of this study will provide fundamental understanding of wrist function in basketball players, and also provide a kinematic data base for further studies of the wrist during high-speed activities.

Conclusions

This study has established the efficacy of custom-designed biaxial electrogoniometers in monitoring wrist motion in basketball shooting. The function of the wrist in basketball shooting was analyzed and the results were described. No statistically significant difference was found in range or velocity of wrist motion between good shots and those which were too short or too long. However, those players with the more constant range of wrist motion achieved greater accuracy.

Acknowledgements. The authors thank coach Don Haskin, assistant coach Greg Lackey, and the participating players of University of Texas at El Paso, Miner, for their generous cooperation in this study. The authors also acknowledge that the goniometer used in this study was originally designed by the staffs of Biomechanics Laboratories of the Mayo Clinic/Mayo Foundation (Rochester, Minn.).

References

1. Tullos HS, King JW (1973) Throwing mechanism in sprots. Orthop Clin North Am 4:709–720

2. Papas AM, Zawacki RM, Sullivan TJ (1985) Biomechanics of baseball pitching. A preliminary report. Am J Sports Med 13:216–222

3. Perry J (1983) Anatomy and biomechanics of the shoulder in throwing, swimming, gymnastics, and tennis. Clin Sports Med 2:247–270

4. Albright JA, Jokl P, Shaw R, Albright JP (1978) Clinical study of baseball pitchers: Correlation of injury to the throwing arm with method of delivery. Am J Sports Med 6:15–21

5. Barnes DA, Tullos HS (1978) An analysis of 100 symptomatic baseball players. Am J Sports Med 6:72–67

6. Bergfeld JA, Weiker GG, Andrish JT, Hall R (1982) Soft playing splint for protection of significant hand wrist injuries in sports. Am J Sports Med 10:293–296

7. McCleland SJ, Fithan DC (1988) Ipsilateral carpal, metacarpal, and ankle fractures resulting from an attempted basketball slam-dunk. Am J Sports Med 16:544–545

8. Roy S, Caine D, Singer KM (1985) Stress changes of the distal radial epiphysis in young gymnasts. A report of twenty-one cases and review of the literature. Am J Sports Med 13:301–308

9. Tehranzadeh J, Labosky DA (1984) Detection of intraarticular loose osteochondral fragments by double-contrast wrist arthography. A case report of basketball injury. Am J Sports Med 12:77–79

10. Henry JH, Lareau B, Neigut D (1982) The injury rate in professional basketball. Am J Sports Med 10:16–18

11. Sane J (1988) Comparison of maxillofacial and dental injuries in four contact team sports: American football, bandy, basketball, and handball. Am J Sports Med 16:647–652

12. Zelisko JO, Noble B, Porter M (1982) A comparison of men's and women's professional basketball injuries. Am J Sports Med 10:297–299

13. Whiting WC, Puffer JC, Finerman GA, Gregor RJ, Maletis GB (1985) Three-dimensional cinematographic analysis of water polo throwing in elite performers. Am J Sports Med 13:95–98

14. Whiting WC, Gregor RJ, Finerman GA (1988) Kinematic analysis of human upper extremity movements in boxing. Am J Sports Med 16:130–136

15. Groppel JL, Nirschl RP (1986) A mechanical and electromyographical analysis of the effects of various joint counterforce braces on the tennis player. Am J Sports Med 14:195–200

16. Mann RA, Moran GT, Dougherty SE (1986) Comparative electromyography of the lower extremity in jogging, running, and sprinting. Am J Sports Med 14:501–510

17. Ryu RKN, McCormick J, Jobe FW, Moynes DR, Antonelli DJ (1988) An electromyographic analy-

sis of shoulder function in tennis players. Am J Sports Med 16:481–485

18. Sisto DJ, Jobe FW, Moynes DR, Antonelli DJ (1987) An electromyographic analysis of the elbow in pitching. Am J Sports Med 15:260–263

19. Jobe FW, Tibone JE, Perry J, Moynes DR (1983) An EMG analysis of the shoulder in throwing and pitching. Am J Sports Med 11:3–5

20. Jobe FW, Moynes DR, Tibone JE, Perry J (1984) An EMG analysis of the shoulder in pitching. AM J Sports Med 12:218–221

21. Gowan ID, Jobe FW, Tibone JE, Perry J, Moynes DR (1987) A comparative electromyographic analysis of the shoulder during pitching. Professional versus amateur pitchers. Am J Sports Med 15: 586–590

22. Palmer AK, Welner FW, Murphy D, Glisson R (1985) Functional wrist motion: A biomechanical study. J Hand Surg [Am] 10:39–46

23. Ryu J, Cooney WP III, Askew LJ, An KN, Chao ESY (1991) Functional ranges of motion of the wrist joint. J Hand Surg [Am] 16:409–419

24. Watson HK, Ryu J, Akelman E (1986) Limited intercarpal arthrodesis for rotatory subluxation of the scaphoid. J Bone Joint Surg [Am] 68:345–349

25. Toyoshima S, Hoshikawa T, Miyashita M, Oguri T (1974) Contribution of the body parts to throwing performance. In: Nelson RC, Morehouse CA (eds) Biomechanics 4. University Park Press, Baltimore, pp 169–174

Aging and Ulnar Variance: Features of the Elbow Joint Affecting Positive Variance

Motonori Goto and Akira Kobayashi[1]

Abstract. Although asymptomatic increase in the incidence of ulnar positive variance with aging has been reported, the cause of this phenomenon is not yet known. The purpose of this study was to clarify whether it is due to narrowing of the humeroradial joint with aging. Bilateral roentgenograms in 50 normal males and 50 normal females, ranging in age from 20 to 89 years, were randomly selected and evaluated in order to determine ulnar variance, humeroradial distance, and ratio of radial to ulnar length.

The results showed that the mean ulnar variance became positive and the mean humeroradial distance narrowed after 50 years of age. There was no correlation between the ratio of radial to ulnar length and age.

On the basis of these results, we concluded that the proximal shift of the radius associated with the narrowing of the humeroradial joint observed during aging is one of the causes of ulnar positive variance.

Keywords: Aging — Ulnar variance — Elbow joint — Humeroradial distance — Positive variance

Introduction

Since Hultén first called attention to the frequent association of negative ulnar variance and Kienböck's disease [1], ulnar lengthening or radial shortening procedures have been recommended for the treatment of this disease. The accurate measurement of ulnar variance is also an important factor in various surgical procedures.

In 1982, Palmer introduced an accurate method of measuring ulnar variance [2]. He showed that the relative lengths of the radius and ulna were dependent on the position of the antebrachium. To attain an accurate value for ulnar variance, Palmer suggested a standard posterior-anterior (PA) X-ray of the wrist with the arm abducted to 90°, the elbow flexed to 90°, and the arm, forearm, and hand placed flat on the X-ray table. A transparent template with concentric semicircles at 1-mm intervals was used for accurate measurement of distances.

In 1988, using the template designed by Palmer, Tanaka showed that the ulnar variance of the elderly in both males and females is more positive than that in younger subjects, and that the ulnar variance of males is more negative than that of females [3].

In the present study, we measured ulnar variance by Palmer's method as well as humeroradial distance and radial and ulnar length on bilateral X-ray films in 100 randomly selected normal individuals.

Materials and Methods

One hundred normal randomly selected subjects (50 males and 50 females), ranging in age from 20 to 89 years, were studied. The number of subjects by sex in each age group is shown in Table 1.

Ulnar variance, humeroradial distance, and radial and ulnar length were measured on bilateral X-ray films as follows:

1. Measurement of ulnar variance was done by Palmer's method, using a template with concentric semicircles. The patient was positioned for a PA radiograph of the wrist with neutral forearm rotation, the elbow flexed to 90°, and the shoulder abducted to 90°.

[1] Fukuoka Orthopaedic Hospital, Yanagouchi 2-10-50, Minami-ku, Fukuoka, 815 Japan

Table 1. Subjects

Age (years)	Male (n)	Female (n)	Total
20~29	5	5	10
30~39	5	5	10
40~49	5	5	10
50~59	10	10	20
60~69	10	10	20
70~79	10	10	20
80~89	5	5	10
Total	50	50	100

Table 2. Results according to age

Age (years)	Mean ulnar variance (mm)	Mean humeroradial distance (mm)	Mean ratio of radial to ulnar length (%)
20~29	0.35 ± 0.74	2.43 ± 0.43	89.3 ± 1.3
30~39	0.28 ± 0.73	2.38 ± 0.41	88.7 ± 1.2
40~49	0.38 ± 0.54	2.35 ± 0.39	89.2 ± 1.6
50~59	1.0 ± 1.19	2.14 ± 0.27	88.6 ± 1.1
60~69	1.01 ± 1.11	2.14 ± 0.33	88.7 ± 1.4
70~79	1.01 ± 1.32	2.09 ± 0.39	88.4 ± 1.3
80~89	1.03 ± 1.44	2.0 ± 0.16	88.9 ± 1.9

2. Humeroradial distance was measured between points A and B as shown on Fig. 1. The patient was positioned for an AP radiograph with the elbow joint extended to 0°.
3. The lengths of the radius and ulna were measured with the distance between points B and C being the radial length and that between Points D and E being the ulnar length (Fig. 1).

The ratio of radial to ulnar length was expressed in percentages.

Results

Mean ulnar variance, humeroradial distance, and ratio of radial to ulnar length for each age group are shown in Table 2. There was a significant difference between subjects under 50 years of age and those 50 years or more in ulnar variance, which was significantly more positive in the latter. Mean ulnar variance was 0.68 mm in males and

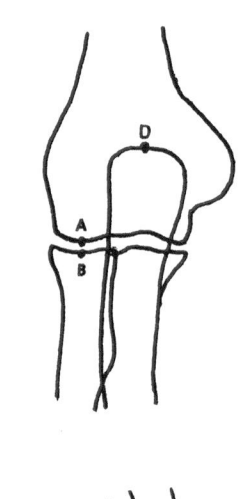

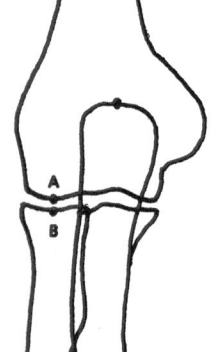

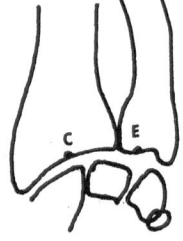

Humero-Radial Distance A-B

Length of Radius and Ulna
Radial Length B-C
Ulnar Length D-E

Fig. 1. Methods of measurement. Point **A** is the point of greatest convexity on this facet of the humerus, **B** is the center of the joint surface of the radial head, **C** is the center of the distal radial joint surface, **D** is the most proximal point of the olecranon, and **E** is the center of the horizontal ulnar joint surface

0.96 mm in females, the difference not being significant. There was no significant difference between the right and left sides in ulnar variance.

There was a significant difference between subjects younger than 50 years and those who were older, in humero-radial distance, which was significantly more narrow in the latter. The mean humeroradial distance in males (2.29 mm) was significantly greater than that in females (2.11 mm). No significant difference in humeroradial distance was found between the right and left sides.

No significant differences among the age groups in ratio of radial to ulnar length were found.

Discussion

We have previously reported that the triangular fibrocartilage complex in the wrist joint shows degeneration in aged persons and in subjects with positive variance [4]. In addition, it has been reported that ulnar variance becomes more positive during aging and, in 1988, Sadahiro reported that the distal radial joint surface moves more proximally during aging [5]. In 1977, Minami found that the humeroradial distance decreased during aging and that there was a high correlation between humeroradial distance and age [6].

However, few studies on the relationship between features of the elbow joint and ulnar positive variance have been conducted. We had postulated that the ulnar positive variance would be influenced by conditions in the elbow and the wrist joints. On the basis of the present findings, we conclude that ulnar variance is related to aging and to narrowing of the humeroradial distance, and that proximal shift of the radius is, therefore, one of the causes of ulnar positive variance.

References

1. Hultén O (1928) Über anatomische Variationen der Hand Gelenkknochen. Acta Radiol 9:155–172
2. Palmer AK (1982) Ulnar variance determination. J Hand Surg [Am] 7:376–379
3. Tanaka Y (1988) Study of ulnar variance (second report). J Jpn Soc Surg Hand 5:505–508
4. Kobayashi A (1985) Carpal lunate lesion in ulna-plus variant. J Jpn Soc Surg Hand 2:426–429
5. Sadahiro T (1988) Radiological studies on aging process of the distal radio-ulnar joint. J Jpn Soc Surg Hand 5:501–504
6. Minami M (1977) Roentogenological studies of osteoarthritis of the elbow joint. J Jpn Orthop Assoc 51:1223–1236

Microvasculature of the Triangular Fibrocartilage Complex of the Wrist

Yasukazu Katsumi,[1] Yasusuke Hirasawa,[2] Satoshi Hitomi,[2] Jun Seri,[2] Yoshikuni Ohta,[3] Hitoshi Okuda,[3] and Takao Tokioka[4]

Abstract. The microvascular anatomy of the triangular fibrocartilage complex (TFCC) of the human wrist was investigated by the acrylic plastic and India ink injection method in 16 cadaver specimens, whose ages had ranged from 24-weeks (stillborn) to 84 years. It was found that the TFCC was supplied by the branches of the ulnar artery and of the anterior interosseous artery. The microvascular supply of the articular disc was basically the same as that of the meniscus of the knee joint. In the TFCC of the adult, the articular disc was avascular, with the exception of the border to the meniscus homologue and the radioulnar ligaments. A capillary plexus originating in the meniscus homologue and the radioulnar ligaments supplied the peripheral 10%–15% of the articular disc. The prestyloid recess was coverd with layers of vascular synovial tissue. In the TFCC of the fetus and the infant, capillaries were observed at the surface of the TFC and the attachment to the radius. Avascular areas of articular discs in the fetus and the infant were relatively smaller than that in the adult. Cellularity was more prominent in the fetus and the infant.

Keywords: Triangular fibrocartilage complex — Microvascular system — Histological study — Aging

[1] Department of Orthopaedic Surgery, Meiji College of Oriental Medicine, Hiyoshi-cho, Funai-gun, Kyoto 629-03, Japan
[2] Department of Orthopaedic Surgery, Kyoto Prefectural University of Medicine, Kamigyou-Ku, Kyoto, 602 Japan
[3] Department of Anatomy, Osaka Dental University, Chuo-Ku, Osaka, 540 Japan
[4] Second Department of Oral Anatomy, School of Dentistry, Meikai University, Sakado, Saitama, 350-02 Japan

Introduction

Tears of the triangular fibrocartilage (articular disc, TFC) are one of the recognized causes of ulnar wrist pain [1, 2]. A recent study reported that the triangular fibrocartilage complex (TFCC) functions as a cushion for the ulnar carpus and as a major stabilizer of the distal ulnar joint [3]. Excision of the TFC would lead to unsatisfactory long-term results, thus primary repair should be considered in a traumatically torn TFC.

The vascularity of the TFCC is one of important factors needing repair in wrist surgery. The vascularity of the TFC was reported to be in the outer 15%–20% of the TFC [4]. Detailed knowledge of the internal vascularity of the TFC, however, is not clear because studies were done by standard histological examinations. It is also unknown what are the differences in the microvascular anatomy of the TFCC with regard to age.

The purpose of this study was to evaluate the microvascular system of the TFCC and the effects of aging, using the resin and India ink injection method.

Materials and Methods

Sixteen cadaver wrists were used in evaluating the blood supply of the TFCC. All upper extremities were obtained from fresh and old cadavers with an age range from 24-weeks (stillborn) to 84 years. The 16 specimens were divided into 3 groups.

In the first group, two upper extremities of a fresh specimen (age 62 years) were injected with 500 cc red acrylic resin through the brachial artery, using the Taniguchi-Ohta plastic injection method [5]. One of the limbs was dissected and observed under a stereoscopic microscope. The other specimen was fixed on a band saw and 5 mm-thick

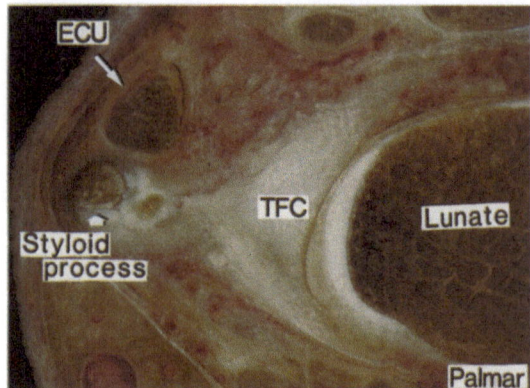

Fig. 1. The triangular fibrocartilage complex (TFCC) viewed from its carpal side in the transverse section after injection of red acrylic resin. The red resin was abundantly observed in the dorsal and palmar radio-ulnar ligaments, but was absent in the body of the *TFC*, with the exception of the border to the radioulnar ligaments. *ECU*, Tendon of the extensor carpi ulnaris

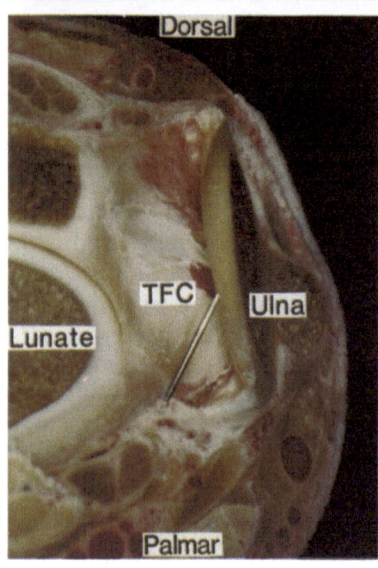
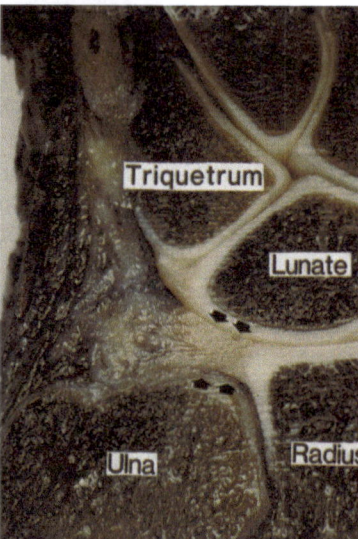
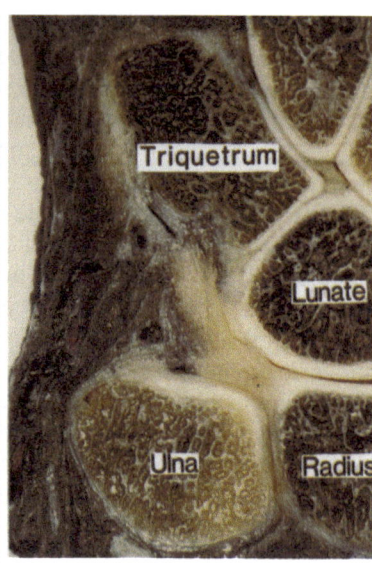

Fig. 2

Fig. 3

Fig. 4

Fig. 2. TFCC viewed from its ulnar side in a transverse section after injection of red acrylic resin. The ulnar head is lifted by a pin in order to observe the TFC. Red resin was seen locally on the surface of the TFC. Partial separation of the TFC was observed in this specimen

Fig. 3. A 5-mm coronal section of TFC at the level of the dorsal third after vascular perfusion with red acrylic resin and India ink. India ink was clearly observed on the meniscus homologue and ulnar collateral ligament, but it was absent in the area of the TFC which was under mechanical pressure from the lunate and ulna (*arrows*)

Fig. 4. A 5-mm coronal section of the TFC at the level of the palmar third after vascular perfusion with red acrylic resin and India ink. No prestyloid recess was seen at this level. India ink was clearly observed on the meniscus homologue and ulnar collateral ligament

sections were cut in a transverse plane and observed under a light microscope.

In the second group, two upper extremities of a fresh specimen (age 40 years) were injected with 500 cc India ink followed by 200 cc red acrylic resin. In addition to injections of the adult specimen, two upper extremities of a fresh specimen of a full-term infant were injected with 50 cc India ink through the aorta. They were fixed on a band saw and 5 mm-thick sections were cut in a sagittal plane. After decalcification with 10% nitric acid, the specimens were each sectioned serially (200 μ

in thickness) in a sagittal plane and observed under a light microscope.

In the third group, ten wrists of old specimens were examined histologically. They included four wrists from cadavers with an age range from 66 to 84 years, and six wrists from those of full-term infants and from 24 to 32-week-old stillborns. They were each sectioned serially (5 μ in thickness) in sagittal and frontal planes after decalcification. The sections were stained with hematoxylin and eosin (HE), elastica van Gieson, toluidin blue, and safranin-0 stains.

Results

Observation of the Specimens after Vascular Perfusion with Red Acrylic Resin

The vascular supply of the TFCC originated predominantly from the two radiocarpal branches (palmar and dorsal) of the ulnar artery. They anastomosed the palmar and dorsal branches of the anterior interosseous artery to each other. The palmar and dorsal branches gave rise to a capillary plexus in the capsular-ligamentous tissue.

On the TFCC viewed from its carpal side in the transverse section, the red resin was observed abundantly in the dorsal and palmar radioulnar ligaments, but was absent in the TFC, with the exception of the border of the radioulnar ligaments (Fig. 1). On the TFCC viewed from its ulnar side, the red resin was seen locally on the surface of the TFC (Fig. 2). Partial separation of the TFC was observed on the same specimen.

Observation of the Specimens after Vascular Perfusion with Red Acrylic Resin and India Ink

On the 5 mm-thick coronal sections before decalcification, India ink was clearly observed on the meniscus homologue, prestyloid recess, and ulnar collateral ligament. However, it was not seen in the area of the TFC which was under mechanical pressure from the lunate and ulna (Figs. 3, 4). A prestyloid recess was seen on the dorsal third of the section (Fig. 3), but was absent on the palmar third (Fig. 4).

A decalcified 200-micron coronal section revealed the vascularity of the TFC more clearly. On the section of the dorsal third, India ink was well observed on the meniscus homologue, prestyloid recess, and ulnar collateral ligament (Fig. 5), but no India ink was seen on most areas of the TFC. Vessels in the meniscus homologue penetrated the TFC tissue for a short distance and ended in terminal capillary loops. The capillary plexus was an arboraceous network of vessels that supplied the peripheral border of the TFC throughout their attachments to the radioulnar ligament. The prestyloid recess was covered with layers of vascular synovial tissue (Fig. 6). The synovial membranes had many capillary loops well-stained with India ink.

No prestyloid recess was detected on the section of the palmar third (Fig. 7). The microvascular anatomy of the TFC at the level of the palmar third was similar to that observed at the level of dorsal third. The TFC was not stained with India ink with the exception of the border of the meniscus homologue. Vessels in the meniscus homologue penetrated the TFC tissue for a short distance and ended in the terminal capillary loops.

The extensor carpi ulnaris tendon and its tendon sheath were observed on the dorsal side (Fig. 8) and capillary loops were observed on them. The tendon sheath had good vascularity.

The radiotriquetral ligament, which was well stained with India ink, was observed on the the palmar side (Fig. 9).

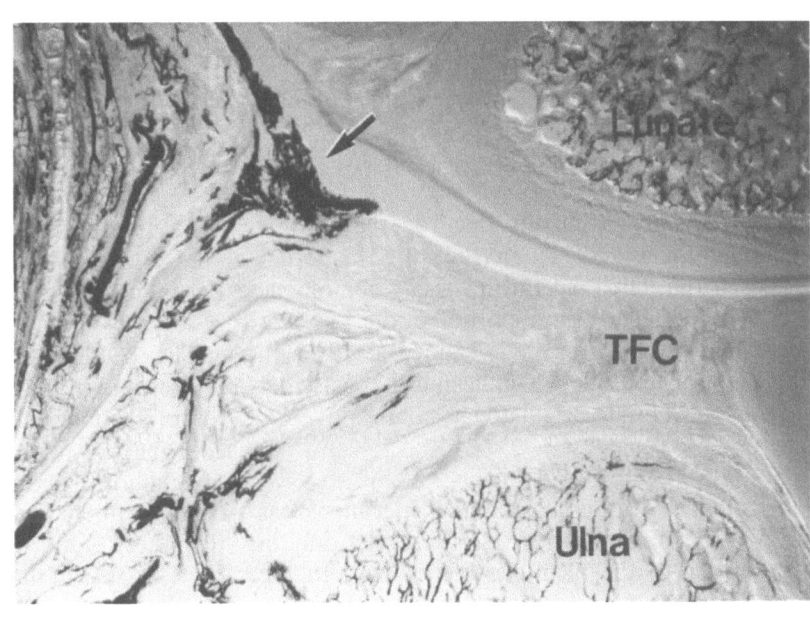

Fig. 5. A 200μ coronal section of the TFC at the level of the dorsal third after vascular perfusion with red acrylic resin and India ink. India ink was clearly observed on the meniscus homologue, the prestyloid recess (*arrow*), and on the ulnar collateral ligament. Vessels in the meniscus homologue penetrated the TFC tissue for a short distance and ended in terminal capillary loops

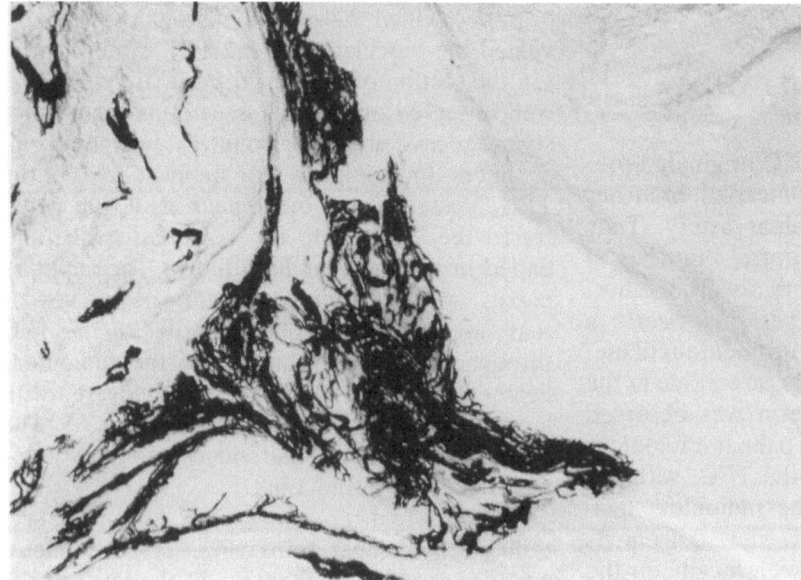

Fig. 6. The prestyloid recess was covered with layers of vascular synovial tissue. The synovial membranes had many capillary loops well-stained with India ink

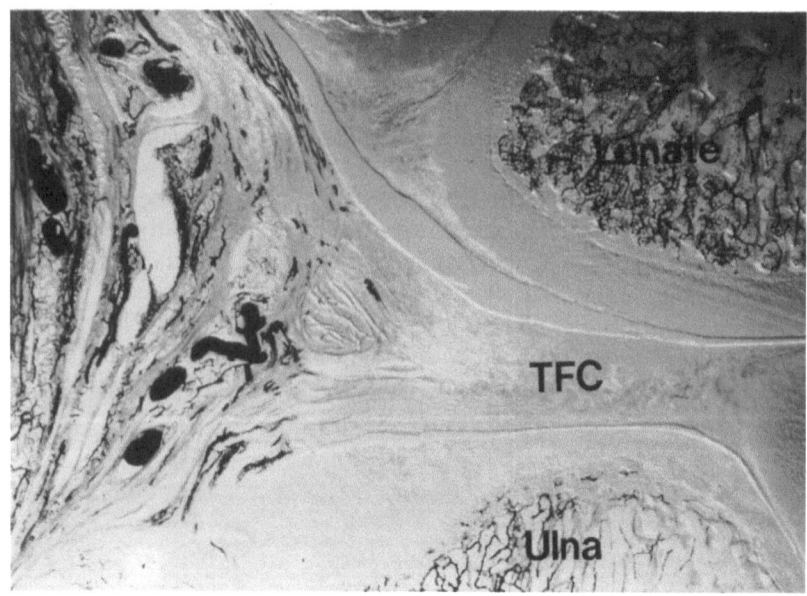

Fig. 7. A $200\,\mu$ coronal section of the TFC at the level of the palmar third after vascular perfusion with red acrylic resin and India ink. The microvascular anatomy of the TFC at this level was similar to that observed in the dorsal side

The TFC was relatively thick on the coronal section of the fetal specimen (Fig. 10). The border between the TFC and the meniscus homologue was not clear. The central portion of the TFC was avascular but its surface was stained locally with India ink. These findings indicated the avascular area of the TFC to be relatively small.

Histological Examination

The cellularity of the TFC of adult specimens was low (Fig. 11). Capillaries were observed only in the border to the meniscus homologue. In the central area of the TFC, collagen fibers proliferated and its structure was arranged randomly. Partial hyaline and mucoid degeneration was also observed.

The cellularity was more prominent in the fetuses and in the infant, with the cells appearing to be fibroblastic (Fig. 12). The production of collagen was poor in the specimen of a 24-week-old stillborn. The production and structure of the collagen fibers in the full-term infant were richer than those of the 24-week-old stillborn. The vascularity of TFC in the infant was slightly higher than

Fig. 8. A 200μ coronal section of the TFC at the dorsal side after vascular perfusion with red acrylic resin and India ink. The extensor carpi ulnaris tendon and its tendon sheath were observed. Capillary loops were also observed on it. The tendon sheath had good vascularity. *ECU*, Tendon of the extensor carpi ulnaris

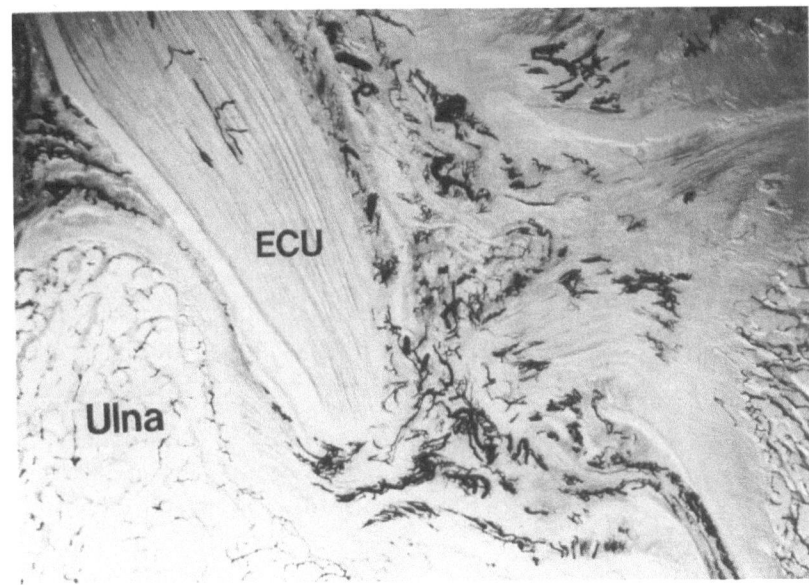

Fig. 9. A 200μ coronal section of the TFC at the palmar side after vascular perfusion with red acrylic resin and India ink. The radiotriquetral ligament was observed to be well stained with India ink

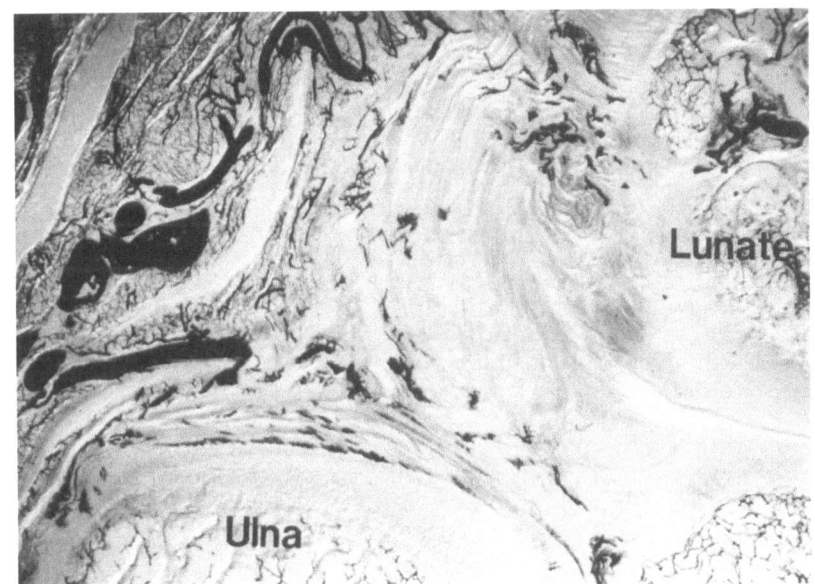

that in the stillborn. Capillaries were observed at the surface of the TFC and the attachment to the radius.

Discussion

In 1989, Palmar classified lesions of the TFCC as traumatic or degenerative [6]. Degeneration of the TFC is seen from the third decade of life and is a less common cause of ulnar wrist pain [7–9].

Whereas traumatic lesions are far less common than degenerative ones, they cause more painful wrists and thus are more important clinically. Repair of the vascularity of the TFCC is one of the major aims of wrist surgery.

The body of the adult TFC is avascular, whereas its peripheral ligamentous portion is highly vascularized. The capillary plexus in the ligamentous tissue is an arboraceous network of vessels that supply the peripheral border of the TFC throughout their attachment to the radioulnar ligament.

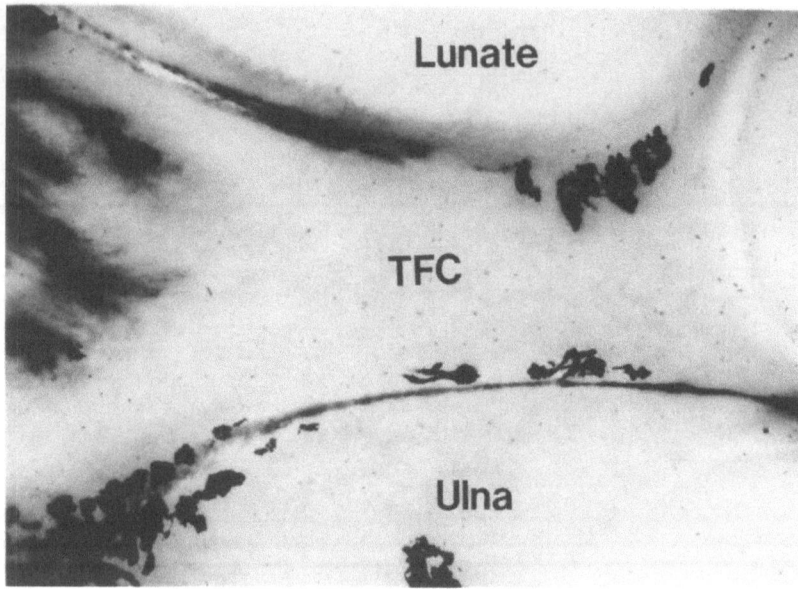

Fig. 10. A 200μ coronal section of an infant TFC at the palmar side after vascular perfusion with red acrylic resin and India ink. The TFC was relatively thick. The border between the TFC and the meniscus homologue was not clear. The central portion of the TFC was avascular, but its surface was stained with India ink. These findings indicated that the avascular area of the articular disc is relatively small

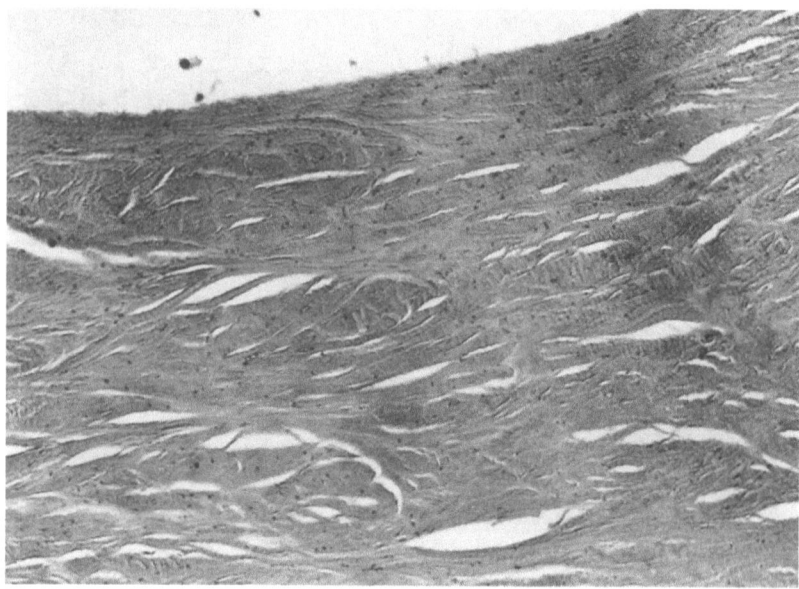

Fig. 11. Section of the adult TFC. The cellularity was low and capillaries were observed only in the border to the meniscus homologue. Collagen fibers proliferated it and its structure was arranged at random in the central area of the TFC. Partial hyaline and mucoid degeneration was observed. Hematoxylin and eosin, $\times 100$

In a 40-year-old specimen, the degree of vascular penetration into the periphery of the TFC ranged from 10% to 15% of TFC width. In a specimen older than 60 years of age, the degree was less than 10%. The results of this study agree with a previous report on the limited peripheral blood supply of the TFC [4]. The basic vascular supply of the TFCC is similar to that of the meniscus of the knee joint [10]. It appears that capillaries cannot exist under pressure.

The structure of the TFCC in the fetus and infant was different from that in the adult. The components of the TFCC were not clearly distinguished histologically, but the cellularity was more prominent in the fetus and infant. The blood supply of the TFC, even in the fetus, was fundamentally avascular, although the avascular areas in the TFC of the fetus and infant were relatively small. With aging, the cellularity of the TFC decreased significantly and the vascularity

Fig. 12. Section of a 24-week-old stillborn TFC. The cellularity was more prominent than in the adult. The cells appeared to be fibroblastic. Capillaries were observed at the surface of the TFC and at the attachment to the radius. Hematoxylin and eosin, × 100

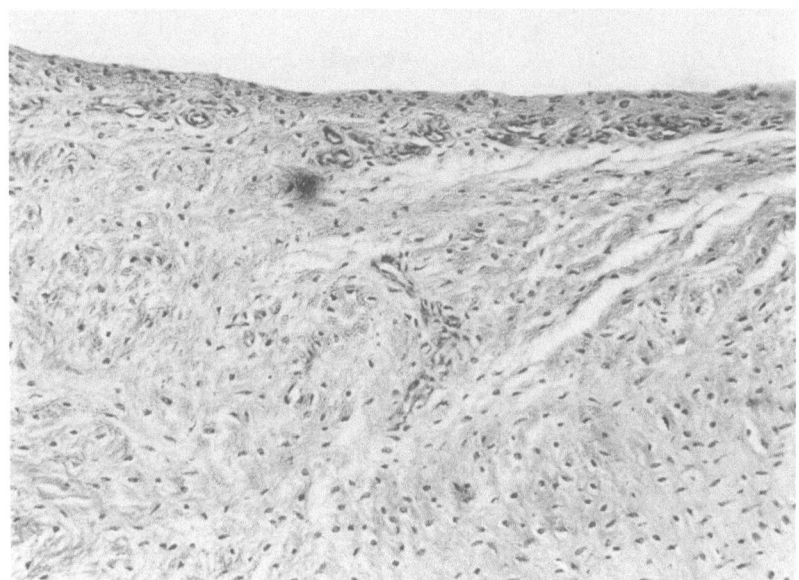

decreased as well. These findings indicate that the potential for healing torn TFC is greater in the young adult.

It is not certain whether lesions in the avascular portion of the TFC can heal. Arnoczky and Warren suggested that lesions in the avascular portion of the meniscus can heal by the creation of a vascular access channel that joins the avascular lesions to the peripheral blood supply [11]. Similarly, the peripheral blood supply in the TFC may provide the possibility of healing a small torn TFC in young adults.

Conclusions

In an investigation carried out on 16 cadaver specimens, the blood supply to the TFCC was found to be maintained by the branches of the ulnar artery and of the anterior interosseous artery. The prestyloid recess of the adult TFCC was covered with layers of vascular synovial tissue.

In the adult TFCC, the TFC was avascular with the exception of the border to the meniscus homologue and radioulnar ligaments. A capillary plexus originating in the meniscus homologue and radioulnar ligaments supplied the peripheral 5%–10% of the TFC. Capillaries were observed at the surface of the TFC and the attachment to the radius in the TFCC of the fetus and infant. Avascular areas of articular discs in the fetus and infant were found to be smaller than those in the adult.

References

1. Coleman HM (1960) Injuries to the articular disc at the wrist. J Bone Joint Surg [Br] 42:522–529
2. Linden AJ (1986) Disc lesion of the wrist joint. J Hand Surg [Am] 11:490–497
3. Palmar AK, Werner FW, Eng MM (1981) The triangular fibrocartilage complex of the wrist — anatomy and function. J Hand Surg [Am] 6:153–162
4. Thiru-Pathi RG, Ferlic DC, Clayton ML, McClure DC (1986) Arterial anatomy of the triangular fibrocartilage of the wrist and its surgical significance. J Hand Surg [Am] 11:258–263
5. Taniguchi Y, Ohta Y, Tajiri S, Okano H, Hanai H (1953) New improved method for injection of acrylic resin. Okajimas Folia Anat Jpn 24:259–267
6. Palmar AK (1989) Triangular fibrocartilage complex lesion: A classification. J Hand Surg [Am] 14(4):594–606
7. Weigl K, Spira E (1969) The triangular fibrocartilage of the wrist joint. Reconstr Surg Traumatol 11:139–153
8. Lewis OJ, Hamshere RJ, Bucknill TM (1970) The anatomy of the wrist joint. J Anat 106:539–552
9. Mikic JDJ (1978) Age changes in the triangular fibrocartilage of the wrist. J Anat 126:367–384
10. Arnoczky SP, Warren RF (1982) Microvasculature of the human meniscus. Am J Sports Med 10:90–95
11. Arnoczky SP, Warren RF (1983) The microvasculature of the meniscus and its response to injury. Am J Sports Med 9:131–141

Three-Dimensional Reconstruction of the Carpal Bones

Kyu H. Yang,[1] Eung S. Kang,[1] Hui W. Park,[1] Sang S. Chung,[2] Sun H. Kim,[2] and Sun K. Yoo[3]

Abstract. Three-dimensional reconstruction of the carpal bones was performed by using GE CT/T 9800, IBM PC/AT, and three-dimensional reconstruction software of hierarchical representation which was developed in our colleges. Four carpal reconstructions were performed: one normal wrist (elbow disarticulation specimen), one lunate volar dislocation with carpal tunnel syndrome (preoperative and postoperative evaluations), and one naviculocapitate syndrome which was associated with trans-scaphoid dorsal perilunate dislocation and carpal tunnel syndrome. After reconstruction, we observed the carpus from the dorsal and volar sides and from the radiocarpal and carpometacarpal joints. We then seperated the proximal and distal carpal rows, observed the midcarpal joint surface of both carpal rows, and removed the three ulnar-sided carpal bones (triangular, pisiform, and hamate) to evaluate the radiolunocapitate-third metacarpal axis.

Three dimensional reconstruction of the carpal bones and separation of the carpal rows offered extremely valuable information on the general configuration of the traumatized carpal bones as well as on displacement and rotation of each carpal bone individually.

Keywords: Three-dimensional reconstruction — Carpal bones

Introduction

The carpus consists of eight small carpal bones and is traditionally divided into the proximal and distal carpal rows (PCR and DCR). There are many other concepts of how to describe the functional anatomy of the carpus, e.g., the columnar, oval ring, and longitudinal columns theories, but that of PCR and DCR prevails and facilitates the understanding of the complex anatomy of the carpus. In the PCR, the scaphoid, lunate, and triquetral bones articulate proximally at the radiocarpal joint and the pisiform bone articulates directly only with the articular surface of the triquetral bone. The DCR consists of the trapezium (greater multangular), trapezoid (lesser multangular), capitate, and hamate. Some authors divide the scaphoid into proximal and distal segments and assign them PCR and DCR, respectively. Because of the complexity of the carpus, the ordinary roentgenogram, arthrogram, and tomogram cannot depict the precise spatial relationship of each component of the carpal row in the normal and injured carpus [1–3].

Introduction of computerized axial tomography (CT scan) in 1972 by Hounsfied had a major impact on musculoskeletal imaging. However, while the conventional CT scan and multiplanar reconstruction add significant information on carpal abnormalities, difficulties can still arise in the interpretation of these images. Because these are all two-dimensional images, both a radiologist and hand surgeon are needed to construct a three-dimensional (3-D) mental image. The mental image is not retainable, and that is one of the causes of misinterpretation, especially in small complex structures such as a carpus. Rotation and seperation of these structures are even more difficult in mental images. The reconstruction of a 3-D image from serial slice data (CT and MRI scans) has been accomplished since the late 1970s

[1] Department of Orthopedic Surgery and
[2] Department of Neurosurgery Yonsei University College of Medicine, 134 Shinchon-Dong, Seodaemun-ku, Seoul, Korea.
[3] Department of Electrical Engineering, College of Engineering, Soonchunhyang University, 657 Hannam-Dong, Yongsan-ku, Seoul, Korea

in many institutes in order to overcome these drawbacks [4–21].

Our research team has developed a new software algorithm by using a hierarchical representation method which was applicable to a small IBM personal computer. We reconstructed the normal carpus and complicated carpal injuries and evaluated the various viewpoints for attaining the best observation.

Materials and Methods

Four carpal reconstructions were performed: one normal wrist, one neglected lunate volar dislocation with carpal tunnel syndrome (preoperative and postoperative reconstructions) and one naviculocapitate syndrome which was associated with trans-scaphoid perilunate dislocation. CT scans of the carpus were taken by GE CT/T 9800 scanner (slice thickness 1.5 mm, slice interval 1.5 mm, 120 KV, 100 mA, level 250, window 1000) from the distal radius to the base of the third

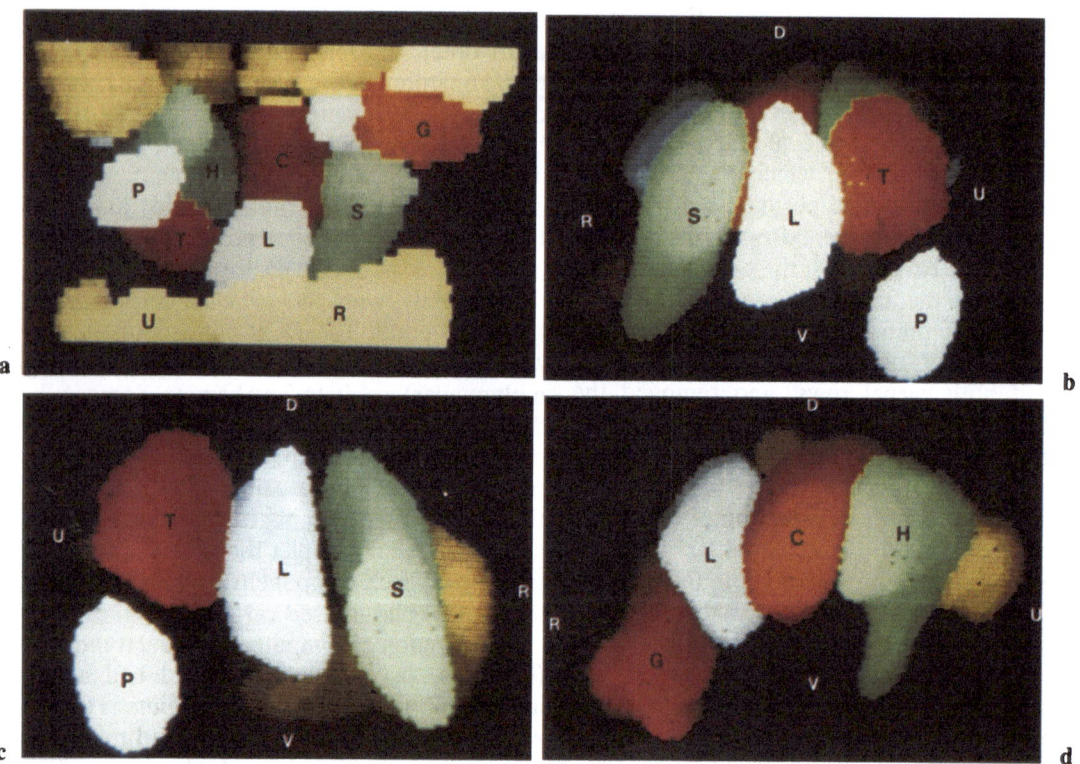

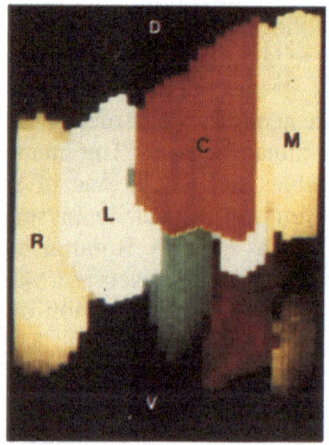

Fig. 1. a Volar aspect of the normal carpus. **b** Observation of the carpus from the radiocarpal joint revealed general configuration of each carpal bone and articular surface of the proximal carpal row. **c** Observation of the proximal carpal row from the midcarpal joint revealed the precise contour of the four carpal bones. The upper and lower borders of the scaphoid, lunate, and triquetral bones are straight and could be used as reference lines. **d** Observation of the distal carpal row from the midcarpal joint. The articular surface and transverse carpal arch were clearly visible. **e** The triangular, pisiform, hamate, and fourth and fifth metacarpal bone were removed and the carpus was observed from the ulnar side after three-dimensional reconstruction. The Radiolunocapitate-third metacarpal axis and longitudinal alignment of the carpus were clearly displayed. *R*, Radius or radial side; *U*, ulnar or ulnar side; *S*, scaphoid; *L*, lunate; *T*, triangular; *P*, pisiform; *G*, greater multangular (trapezium); *L*, lesser multangular (trapezoid); *C*, capitate; *H*, hamate; *M*, metacarpal bone; *F*, fragment; *D*, dorsal side; *V*, volar side

metacarpal bone in full pronation, neutral deviation, and flexion.

After reconstruction, we first observed the carpus from the dorsal and volar sides for acquiring a general configuration. Next, we separated the radius from the PCR and the metacarpal bones from the DCR for evaluation of the proximal articular surface of the PCR and distal articular surface of the DCR. Following this, we separated the PCR and DCR at the midcarpal joint to observe the midcarpal joint surfaces of the two carpal rows. We then removed the ulnar, triquetral, pisiform, hamate, and fourth and fifth metacarpal bones to observe the carpus from the ulnar side in order to evaluate the radio-lunocapitate-third metacarpal bone axis (RLCMA).

Results

Three-Dimensional Reconstruction of the Normal Carpus

The dorsal and volar view of the carpus revealed a clear general configuration of the eight carpal bones and adjacent bony structures (Fig. 1.a). Observation of the carpus from the radiocarpal joint showed spatial orientation of the scaphoid, lunate, triquetral, and pisiform bones. The upper and lower borders of the first three bones were straight, indicating a normal alignment. The relationship of the triquetral and pisiform bones was

well delineated (Fig. 1.b). Observation of the carpus from the carpometacarpal joint provided a clear view of the distal four carpal bones, transverse carpal arch, humulus, and pisiform bone. The views of the PCR and DCR from the midcarpal joint were striking and depicted far clearer and more detailed anatomy and spatial orientation of the eight carpal bones than could be achieved previously (Fig. 1.c,d). Once again, the upper and lower borders of the scaphoid, lunate, and triquetral bones were straight and could be used as reference lines. Removal of the ulnar-sided carpal bones and observation of the capus from the ulnar side depicted a normal RLCMA (Fig. 1.e).

Three-Dimensional Reconstruction of the Neglected Lunovolar Dislocation

A CT scan of this case confirmed the lunate volar dislocation. However, more information on the spatial orientation of the lunate and adjacent carpal bones seemed to be very helpful for the reduction of a long-standing dislocation. Therefore, we performed a 3-D reconstruction and observed the PCR from the mid-carpal joint. It provided a clear image of volar dislocation and rotation (palmar and 90° clockwise rotation) of the lunate. Upper and lower reference lines were disrupted (Fig. 2.a). Observation from the ulnar side depicted the disruption of the RLCMA and the amount of volar displacement of the lunate, suspected as being a chief offender of carpal tunnel syndrome (Fig. 2.b).

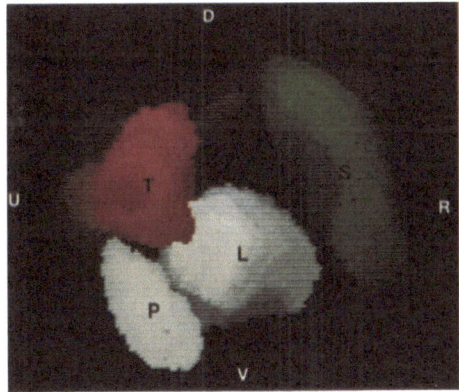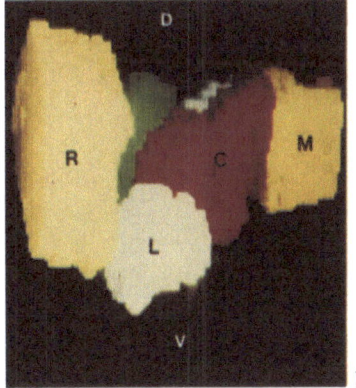

Fig. 2. a The proximal carpal row was observed from the midcarpal joint after reconstruction of the neglected volar lunate dislocation. Dislocation and rotation (about 90° clockwise) of the lunate into the carpal tunnel were clearly visible. Two reference lines of the upper and lower borders of the scaphoid, lunate, and triangular bones were disrupted. b Observation from the ulnar side revealed disruption of the radiolunocapitometacarpal axis and volar displacement and rotation of the lunate into the carpal tunnel in a neglected lunate volar dislocation

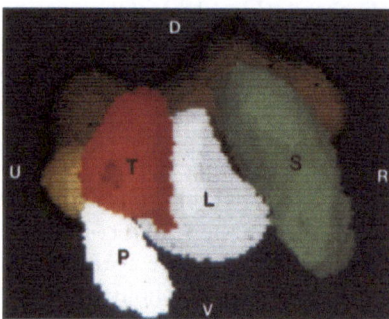

Fig. 3. Observation of the proximal carpal row from the midcarpal joint after open reduction and internal fixation of the neglected volar lunate dislocation revealed incomplete reduction of the lunate. The reference line of the upper border of the scaphoid, lunate, and triangular bones was not completely restored

Post-Operative 3-D Reconstruction of the Lunovolar Dislocation

Open reduction and internal fixation of the above case was performed through volar and dorsal approaches. The lunate was dislocated into the carpal tunnel, pressing the median nerve tightly to the volar side. The lunate was reduced and fixed with multiple Kirschner wires. After removal of the wires, a postoperative CT scan and 3-D reconstruction were performed. Observation of the PCR from the midcarpal joint revealed incomplete reduction of the lunate. The most sensitive indicator of the dislocation and its reduction was the reference line of the upper border of the scaphoid, lunate, and triquetrum (Fig. 3).

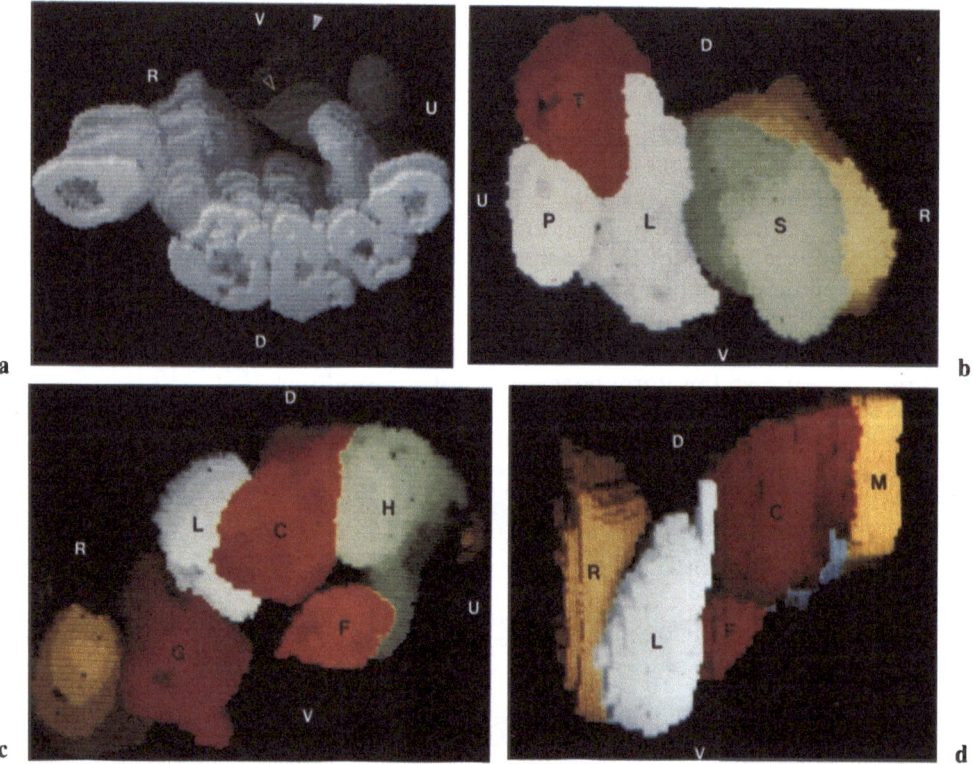

Fig. 4. a Preliminary 3-D reconstruction revealed two bony shadows at the volar aspect of the carpus indicating lunate (*closed arrow*) and head fragment of the capitate (*open arrow*). **b** The proximal carpal row was observed from the midcarpal joint after reconstruction of naviculocapitate syndrome which was associated with trans-scaphoid perilunate dislocation. Horizontal orientation of the mal-united scaphoid and dorsal displacement of the triangular and pisiform bone were noted. **c** The distal carpal row was observed from the midcarpal joint after reconstruction of naviculocapitate syndrome which was associated with trans-scaphoid perilunate dislocation. The capitate head fragment seemed to be seperated from the body of the capitate and displaced into the carpal tunnel. **d** Observation of the radiolunocapitometacarpal axis revealed dorsal displacement of the distal carpal row. No fragment of the head of the capitate was displaced to the carpal tunnel

Three-Dimensional Reconstruction of Naviculocapitate Syndrome

There was evidence of a malunited scaphoid fracture and perilunate dislocation of the DCR on the anteroposterior and lateral views in the reontgenograms. Preliminary 3-D reconstruction revealed two bony shadows at the volar aspect of the carpus, indicating lunate and head fragmentation of the capitate (Fig. 4.a). Observation of the PCR from the midcarpal joint revealed horizontal malalignment of the scaphoid and dorsal displacement of the triquetrum and pisiform bone over the lunate (Fig. 4.b). Observation of the DCR from the midcarpal joint showed seperation of the head fragment from the body of the capitate. After analysis of the CT scan (not shown) and the above conformation, we confirmed that the head fragment of the capitate was rotated about 90° to the dorsal side (Fig. 4.c). Observation from the ulnar side depicted disruption of the lunocapitate relationships and seperation of the head and body of the capitate (Fig. 4.d).

Discussion

Development of the CT scan and multiplanar reconstruction technique made it possible to understand the complex pathoanatomy of the carpal body. However, the inherent limitation of the two-dimensional image was a major impetus for the development of a more realistic image. In the 2-D image the surgeons can not see the transverse or sagittal sections of the structure but only the outer surface of the bone and joint [9–11]. This means that a precise, high quality CT scan is useful chiefly for purposes of diagnosis, because it is more accurate for evaluating the small changes in details. Three-dimensional reconstruction is better for preoperative planning because it can provide a realistic view of the pathoanatomy from the side from which the surgeon wants to approach. Due to that reason, it was first applied to craniofacial surgery [16, 19] and evaluation of the pelvic bone and acetabular fractures [7, 18]. Three-dimensional reconstruction of the bony structure from CT and MRI images is a major advance in the orthopedic field. Reversal surgery of congenital dislocations of the hip, revision of total hip arthroplasty, and osteotomy has now been made possible [11, 21].

In medical 3-D imaging, the main objectives are to visualize, manipulate, and analyze human internal structures [22]. When we construct a 3-D system, we put emphasis on reducing computation time and memory requirement in addition to the above-mentioned three features of performance. The octree representation method [23] was adapted to compactly represent the large amount of volumic data and to allow the time-efficient implementation of many graphical and image-processing operations. This system consists of an automatic two-dimensional pre-processing and three-dimensional reconstruction by a hierarchical representation method, and three-dimensional image processing by a tree-traversal operation. In 2-D processing, organs are segmented by combining the histogram separation and boundary tracer with curvature information [24]. These segmented images are converted to a quadtree [25] with a 1-to-4 data structure [26]. Because system memory is limited, the 1-to-8 structure [26] is adapted to represent the octree and the octree is built in a bottom-up fashion by recursively merging each of the adjacent quadtrees. This hierarchical structure enables many 3-D procedures, such as hidden surface removal, artificial shading, transparent display, rotation, organ removal, and image modification. In image modification, user-defined sections are extracted from the octree by partially traversing the octree in pre-order. Using a graphics input device, such as a mouse, the clinician draws the model in an arbitrary shape on the screen. The modified organ is created by carrying out the intersection of the octree of the original organ and recreated an octree of that model. All the above procedures are programmed by "C" language and the 3-D system is thus developed with a personal computer.

Since the mid-1980s Weeks et al. [20], Belsole et al. [1], Biondetti et al. [5], and Nakamura et al. [14] reported their experiences in various articles concerning the value of the preoperative and biomechanical evaluation of 3-D reconstruction in the carpus. Weeks et al. [20] varied the orientation of the CT scanner planes with respect to the carpus in order to optimize the best image after the 3-D reconstruction, and selected an oblique plane of the section for the best overall images. However, a CT scan of the carpus alone gives us much important information and is better for evaluation of changes in the small structures. In the oblique slice, identification of the individual bones and fragments and processing for color application are much more difficult. Biondetti et al. [5] compared the transaxial and coronal techniques in CT scanning for the 3-D reconstruction of the wrist. They obtained more detailed 3-D images of the wrist from the coronal than from the transaxial CT scans because the resolution of the articular surface is limited by the small pixel size (about 0.15–0.2 mm) in the former and by the slice thickness (1.5 mm–2.0 mm) in the latter. This is true in the evaluation of the carpus as a whole, but has some limitation for the evaluation of the PCR and DCR when they are seperated and observed from the logitudinal axis for the evaluation of displacement and rotation of the traumatized carpal bones; i.e., its limitation is reversed by the change of the viewpoint.

Conclusions

In this study, we attempted to create a standard method for the evaluation of the carpus. Specifically, this included observation from the dorsal and volar sides, from the radiocarpal, carpometacarpal and midcarpal joints, and finally from the ulnar side. To achieve this purpose, we took CT scans in a transaxial manner in all cases because the most accurate information is obtained when the stacked sections are viewed perpendicular to the plane observed. As a result, the most accurate imaging was obtained when we observed the region of interest from the radiocarpal, carpometacarpal, and midcarpal joints. The most inaccurate coarse image was obtained when we conducted the observations from the dorsal, volar, and ulnar sides (parallel to the scanner plane). Fortunately, the ordinary anteroposterior roentgenogram shows minimal overlapping of the carpal bones, so that the dorsal and volar inspections are not so important. Observation of the carpus from the ulnar side is chiefly for the evaluation of the radioulnocapitate metacarpal bone axis (RUCMA), so coarse images do not limit preoperative diagnosis and planning.

The drawbacks of our system are limitation of available random access memory (RAM) and central processing unit (CPU) of the small personal computer. They limit the number of the slices which are to be reconstructed and require much time due to slow data-processing ability. We hope that the step-up of the image observed from the ulnar side will be reduced if we increase the available CT slices by partial overlapping of the slices and interpolation.

Three-dimensional reconstruction of the carpus is not necessary in all carpal injuries, but is selec-

tively applicable to the complicated and unusual ones in order to evaluate the movement of each carpal bone for preoperative planning as well as for general education. Transaxial CT scanning and observation of the carpus from the radiocarpal, carpometacarpal, and midcarpal joints provided us valuable information on the changes of individual carpal bones, PCR, and DCR.

References

1. Belsole RT, Hilbelink D, Llewellyn JA, Dale M, Stenzler S, Rayhark JM (1986) Scaphoid orientation and location from computed three-dimensional carpal model. Orthop Clin North Am 17:505–510
2. Green DP, O'Brien EF (1980) Classification and management of carpal dislocation. Clin Orthop 149:55–72
3. O'Brien ET (1984) Acute fractures and dislocation of the carpus. Orthop Clin North Am 15:237–258
4. Belsole RT, Hilbelink DR, Llewellyn JA, Stezsler S, Greene TL, Dale M (1988) Mathematical analysis of computed carpal models. J Orthop Res 6: 116–122
5. Biondetti PR, Vannier MW, Gilula LA, Knapp RH (1988) Three-dimensional surface reconstruction of the carpal bones from CT scans. Trans-axial versus coronal technique. Comput Med Imag Graphics 12:67–73
6. Bresina ST, Vannier MW, Logan SE, Weeks PM (1986) Three-dimensional wrist imaging. Evaluation of functional and pathological anatomy by computation. Clin Plast Surg 13:389–405
7. Burk DL, Mears DC, Kennedy WH, Cooperstein LA, Herbert DL (1985) Three-dimensional computed tomography of acetabular fractures. Radiology 155:183–186
8. Engel J, Salai M, Yaffe B, Tadmor R (1987) The role of three-dimension computerized imaging in hand surgery. J Hand Surg [Br] 12:349–352
9. Fishman EK, Magid D, Ney DR, Drebin RA, Kuhlman JE (1988) Three-dimensional imaging and display of musculoskeletal anatomy. J Comput Assist Tomogr 12:465–467
10. Herman GT, Vose WF, Gomoru JM, Gegter WB (1985) Stereoscopic computed three-dimensional surface displays. Radiographics 5:825–852
11. Lobregt S, Schaars HWGK (1987) Three-dimensional imaging and manipulation of CT data. Medica mundi 32:92–98
12. Moutet F, Chapel A, Cinquin P, Rose-Pitet L (1990) Three-dimensional imaging of the carpus. Ann Chir Main 9:32–37

13. Murphy SB, Kijewski P, Millis MB, Hall JE, Simon SR, Chandler HP (1988) The planning of orthopedic reconstructive surgery using computer-aided simulation and design. Comput Med Imag Graphics 12:33–45

14. Nakamura R, Horii E, Tanaka Y, Imaeda T, Hayakawa N (1989) Three-dimensional CT imaging for wrist disorders. J Hand Surg [Br] 14:53–58

15. Quinn SF, Belsole RJ, Greene TL, Rayhack JM (1989) CT of the wrist for the evaluation of traumatic injuries. Crit Rev Diagn Imaging 129:357–380

16. Roberts D, Pettigrew J, Udupa J, Carol R (1984) Three-dimensional imaging and display of the temporo-mandibular joint. Oral Surg Oral Med Oral Pathol 58:461–474

17. Sundberg SB, Clark BR, Foster BK (1986) Three-dimensional reformation of skeletal abnormalities using computed tomography. J Pediatr Orthop 6:426–420

18. Totty WG, Vannier MW (1984) Complex musculoskeletal anatomy: Analysis using three-dimensional surface reconstruction. Radiology 150:173–177

19. Vannier MW, Marsh JL, Warren JO (1984) Three-dimensional CT reconstruction images for craniofacial surgical planning and evaluation. Radiology 150:179–184

20. Weeks PM, Vannier MW, Stevens WG, Gayou D, Gilula LA (1985) Three-dimensional imaging of the wrist. J Hand Surg [Am] 10:32–39

21. Woolson ST, Parvati DEV, Fellingham LL, Vassiiadis A (1986) Three-dimensional imaging of bone from computerized tomography. Clin Orthop 202:239–248

22. Udupa JK (1986) Computerized surgical planning: Current capabilities and medical needs. SPIE 626:474–482

23. Samet H (1988) Hierachical data structures and algorithms for computer graphica. IEFE CG and A:48–68

24. Seitz P, Ruegsegger P (1983) Fast contour detection algorithm for high precision quantitative CT. IEFE Med Imag MI-2, 3:136–141

25. Yau MM, Srihari SN (1983) A hierarchical data structures for multi-dimensional digital images. Commun ACM 26:504–515

26. Oliver MA (1985) Display algorithms for quadtrees and octrees and their hardware realization. Eurographics Netherlands: 9–37

Part II. Kienböck's Disease

The Kienböck's Dilemma — How to Cope

A. Herbert Alexander[1] and David M. Lichtman[2]

Abstract. Etiology, blood supply, early diagnosis, staging, and treatment in Kienböck's disease are the subjects of numerous manuscripts in the literature. We present an insight into Kienböck's disease as we understand it and a rationale for approaching the Kienböck's dilemma. Kienböck's disease is an isolated disorder of the lunate manifested by radiodensity changes and often accompanied by fracture lines, fragmentation, and progressive collapse. Ultimately, its etiology is vascular insufficiency, but contributing factors that put the lunate at risk include negative ulnar variance, limited extraosseous blood supply, limited intraosseous blood supply and repeated "microtrauma." Though there are numerous treatment modalities, we recommend several methods based on staging and ulnar variance. For Stage I, immobilization is helpful to establish the diagnosis with certainty and theoretically may allow the lunate to revascularize. In patients with Stage II or IIIA and ulnar negative variance, radial shortening is recommended. If there is positive ulnar variance, a revascularization procedure is preferred (DML) but radial shortening (AHA) also has been successful. In Stage IIIB, there being fixed deformity of the lunate and carpus, scapho-trapezio-trapezoid fusion or scaphocapitate fusion is utilized. If there is significant synovitis, then the lunate is excised as well. In Stage IV (pan-carpal arthrosis), proximal row carpectomy or wrist arthrodesis is indicated.

[1] Department of Orthopaedic Surgery, Naval Hospital, Oakland, California, USA; Uniformed Services University of the Health Sciences, Bethesda, Maryland, USA
[2] Naval Hospital and Uniformed Services University of the Health Sciences, Bethesda, Maryland, USA

The opinions or assertions expressed herein are those of the authors and are not to be construed as official or as necessarily reflecting the views of the Department of the Navy or of the Naval service at large.

Keywords: Kienböck's disease — Lunate avascular necrosis

Introduction

Between the years 1843 and 1985, a span of 143 years, approximately 85 articles appeared in the literature on Kienböck's disease. Over the next 5 years (1986–1990), another 43 were published. Despite an information explosion and volumes of material published on this entity, we still do not know all the answers. Issues of etiology, blood supply, early diagnosis, staging, and treatment remain controversial. That is why we have called this chapter the Kienböck's *dilemma.* Consequently, the purpose of this discussion is to provide some insight on Kienböck's disease as the authors understand it, and to provide a mechanism to cope with the dilemma. We will highlight the various proposed etiologies and treatments from a historical perspective. This will be followed by a discussion of the necessary "tools" and information (clinical presentation, X-ray findings, MRI, ulnar variance, staging, patient desires, and response to immobilization) required in formulating a treatment algorithm. Finally, based on these latter concepts, we will present our preference of treatment.

Etiology

Kienböck's disease is an isolated disorder of the lunate manifested by radiodensity changes and often accompanied by fracture lines, fragmentation, and progressive collapse. Recently, there has been some discussion whether or not Kienböck's disease represents an acute compression fracture or whether it may be due to chronic trauma. In 1980, Beckenbaugh and associates pointed out that 82% of the patients

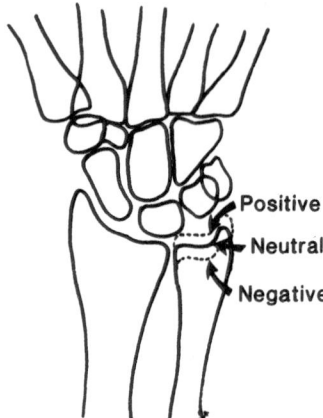

Fig. 1. Schematic representation of the radiographic appearance of *ulnar variance*. Neutral variance occurs when the distal articular surfaces of the radius and ulna are equal. If the ulna is "shorter" relative to the radius, *negative* ulnar variance exists; if the ulnar is "longer" than the radius, then *positive* variance exists

have evidence of fracture lines [1]. He was not the first to implicate trauma. In 1843, before the advent of X-ray, Peste described collapse of the lunate and ascribed its cause to trauma [2]. Others have also implicated trauma [3–5], including Kienböck [6] (in 1910), who believed that repeated sprains and contusions lead to ligamentous injury and vascular compromise. This was followed by avascular necrosis and collapse of the bone.

In 1928, Hultén noted that 78% of his patients with Kienböck's disease had a short ulna, or *negative* ulnar variance whereas 23% of normal patients have a short ulna [7] (Fig. 1). Generally, this concept of negative ulnar variance being etiological is well supported in the literature [8–15]. With a short ulna, radiocarpal pressure is shifted to the radiolunate fossa, resulting in increased shear on the lunate which apparently increases the risk of avascular necrosis.

Ultimately, however, it is the lack of tissue perfusion which is the critical event in Kienböck's disease. Thus, there have been several discussions of the lunate's tenuous blood supply [4, 5, 9, 16]. Lee found three vascular patterns in cadaver lunates: a single vessel, either volar or dorsal, supplying the whole bone (26%); several vessels at either the dorsal or volar surface without central anastomosis (8%); and several vessels at volar and dorsal surfaces with central anastomosis (66%) [4]. According to Lee, the first two patterns of vascularity are more likely

to put the lunate in jeopardy. However, it is unlikely that injury to a single vessel (as in the first pattern) is a likely cause, since one would expect entire involvement of the lunate clinically, when, in fact, we find that the proximal surface becomes avascular first.

Seemingly, injection studies of Panagis, Gelberman, and colleagues [16] support Lee's contention. In 20% of fresh lunate specimens, they found a single palmar nutrient vessel. In Gelberman and associates' other study, however, the incidence of a single volar vessel was only 7% [9]. Theoretically, it follows that a single traumatic event, such as a fracture or dislocation of the carpus, would result in avascular necrosis. But seldom is this history present in a patient with Kienböck's disease. Additionally, they found 3 intraosseous vascular patterns: *Y* in 59%, *I* in 31%, and *X* in 10%. Evaluation of the terminal vessels showed that the proximal subchondral bone, adjacent to the radial articular surface, was least vascular. Because of the relatively rich extraosseous blood supply, Gelberman and associates concluded that it was disruption of intraosseous vascularity, due to repeated trauma with compression fracture, that causes Kienböck's disease.

The problem with all these studies is that none of the specimens actually had Kienböck's disease. Therefore, we still do not know if there is some entirely different vascular pattern, currently unrecognized, that predisposes a patient to lunate avascular necrosis.

To summarize, our current feeling is that Kienböck's disease is the result of multiple factors. The patient usually has a lunate "at risk". The lunate "at risk" is one in which there is a short ulna that causes increased shear stress and/or has a tenuous blood supply. The tenuous blood supply may be due to a single nutrient vessel, a limited intraosseous blood supply, blood dyscrasia, septic embolism, or even vasculitis. By adding either an acute fracture or repeated "microtrauma" to a lunate "at risk", Kienböck's disease results.

Treatment Methods

There are over 20 treatment modalities for Kienböck's disease. Each surgeon has his/her favorite, and, upon seeing a patient with Kienböck's disease, is likely to choose that procedure, operate on the patient, and then report on the results of that procedure. This leads to the current dilemma and confusion. Generally, published reports do not specifically cover what was characteristic of a patient's wrist or why the surgeon chose the particular operation performed.

Immobilization

Immobilization has been tried in all stages of Kienböck's disease. Stahl [5] advocated prolonged immobilization of up to 2 months and showed 80% good results. Similarly, Evans et al. tried immobilization and had poor results in 38%, implying that at least 62% did well [17]. Generally, however, most clinicians have had poor experience with immobilization [18–21], except in specific instances. Our own experience [13] with 22 cases of Kienböck's disease immobilized over 2 months showed no improvement in lunate architecture, while it deteriorated in 17. Thus, we concluded that immobilization was not worthwhile. At the time, however, these 22 cases were not really staged as to the degree of involvement. Presently, we consider immobilization to be useful in stage I Kienböck's disease for two reasons: (1) it may keep the vascular insult at a minimum and give the lunate a chance to heal, and (2) if the diagnosis remains in question, a trial period of immobilization may be therapeutic or it may result in the characteristic radiographic changes that establish the diagnosis.

Radial Shortening and Ulnar Lengthening

Radial shortening and ulnar lengthening, along with capitate shortening, scapho-trapezio-trapezoid fusion, scaphocapitate fusion and capitohamate fusion fall into the category of decompressive procedures. That is to say, they all are intended to decompress the forces on the lunate and theoretically allow the lunate to revascularize. The basic science supporting this concept will be discussed later.

Radial shortening has had an excellent track record in the literature. Almquist [18] reported good results in 11 out of 12 of his group's patients followed for 5 years. In 1987, at the time of this literature review, he noted 69 out of 79 patients reported in the literature as having good results, without even taking staging into consideration. More recently, Nakamura et al. reported satisfactory results in 19 out of 23 patients in all stages of Kienböck's disease [22]. He got a few poor results only in those with the ulnar positive

variant where he also shortened the radius more than 4 mm.

Ulnar lengthening does essentially the same thing as radial shortening, except in ulnar lengthening one must insert a segment of bone in the osteotomy site before applying the compression plate. Sundberg and Linscheid reported 18 out of 19 cases to be successful with this technique and with no non-unions [14]. Generally, one should try for 1–2 mm positive variance whether doing radial shortening or ulnar lengthening. The advantage of radial shortening is that a second surgical incision is not required for obtaining bone graft. A potential problem with both procedures is the possibility of non-union, while being small, is a little higher for ulnar lengthening. Also, eventual plate removal in some symptomatic patients may be required.

Capitate Shortening

Almquist also described capitate shortening done in conjunction with capitohamate fusion. From 3 to 5 mm of the midportion of the capitate are removed through a dorsal approach. In 17 patients seen over a 7-year period, results were "encouraging" [18].

Scapho-trapezio-trapezoid Fusion (STT)

Triscaphe fusion or STT fusion, as described by Watson et al. [15], is designed to decompress the lunate by shifting radiocarpal forces to the scaphoid fossa. The procedure may be done with or without silicone replacement arthroplasty, as described in their original article. However, Watson recently indicated that one may leave the lunate in place or simply excise it if found to be very fragmented and necrotic. Scaphocapitate fusion achieves the same kinematic result as STT fusion and is a little easier to do.

Capitohamate Fusion

Chuinard and Zeman [23] proposed capitohamate fusion to prevent proximal capitate migration in the face of a collapsing lunate. Since the capitate is already bound to the hamate by stout ligaments, the two act as a unit. Thus, it seems unlikely that capitohamate fusion alone can decompress the lunate and prevent proximal migration of the distal carpal row. This is borne out in the biomechanical studies discussed below. For this reason, we do not recommend it.

Excisional Arthroplasty

Historically, lunate excision is second only to immobilization as a popular form of treatment for Kienböck's disease. Some investigators have reported very good results [24–27]. The rationale for simple excision is that removal of sequestered bone will reduce the amount of synovitis and concomitant symptoms. The problem with simple excision is that the capitate then remains unsupported. Although the patient may have a good result in the short term because the synovitis has been "excised", theoretically, problems may result in the long term due to proximal migration of the capitate [5, 28, 29] with subsequent abnormal carpal kinematics. For that reason, many of the "interpositional" arthroplasties were developed to accompany lunate excision. Also, it should be mentioned that it seems a bit extreme to excise the lunate in stages I or II, when there still exists a chance for lunate revascularization and healing.

Biomechanics of Decompressive Procedures

Trumble and colleagues [30] studied the reduction in lunate compression in whole arm specimens after performing radial shortening, ulnar lengthening, capitohamate fusion, and STT fusion. Using electronic strain gauges, they found radial shortening, ulnar lengthening, and STT fusion successful in relieving lunate loading throughout wrist and forearm motion. Only the capitohamate fusion was ineffective. However, since the STT fusion was accompanied by a significant reduction in range of motion, radial shortening and/or ulnar lengthening were preferred.

Horii and associates [31] used a two-dimensional computer model to predict the total amount of force transmitted through the radiolunate joint after limited intercarpal fusion, capitate shortening, and ulnar lengthening/radial shortening of 4 mm. Limited intercarpal fusion reduced the radiolunate force by only 15% whereas shortening of the radius or lengthening of the ulna by 4 mm resulted in a 45% reduction in radiolunate force. Although capitate shortening reduced radiolunate loading, it dramatically overloaded the scaphotrapezial and triquetrohamate joints.

To summarize, based on these studies, the decompressive procedures generally do what they are supposed to do. Furthermore, radial shortening/ulnar lengthening appear to have distinct advantages over the intercarpal procedures.

Collagen Arthroplasty

The so-called collagen arthroplasties have also met with limited success [32–34]. In this operation, either a coiled tendon, such as the palmaris longus, or "epitendinous" tissue from the flexor tendons is used to fill the gap of the excised lunate. However, collagen arthroplasty in a young active patient is not likely to prevent late proximal migration of the capitate.

Silicone Replacement Arthroplasty (SRA)

The senior one of us (DML) began using SRA in the late 1960s. SRA is simply another method of preventing proximal migration of the capitate following lunate excision [35]. In our initial publication in 1977, it was concluded that early SRA was indicated in Kienböck's disease because of the poor results seen in stage III (late) of the disease: 4 (out of 10) unsatisfactory results for stage III at an average follow-up of 25 months [13]. In 1982, we expanded our indications for SRA after reviewing an additional 16 patients treated with the new Swanson high-performance (HP) silicone lunate prosthesis and obtaining satisfactory results in 12 out of 13 patients with stage III disease (average follow-up, 18 months) [12]. Unfortunately, long-term results did not substantiate our "1982 enthusiasm". In 1990, we .eported on a 5-year follow-up of SRA, noting only 50% satisfactory results [8]. As previously reported by others, [36–39], the presence of wear-particle synovitis was present in 3 out of 5 patients who returned for radiographs at an average of 57 months post-operatively. Consequently, we have abandoned SRA as a primary treatment modality for Kienböck's disease, as has Dr. Swanson.

Revascularization

Several methods for restoring blood supply to the lunate are available. It is important to remember, however, that once the lunate has reached an advanced stage of collapse, revascularization can do little to restore lunate architecture. Braun [40] (personal communication, 1989) described a method of taking a small piece of volar radial bone, still attached to the pronator quadratus muscle, which is then grafted to the avascular lunate (Fig. 2). A similar procedure, described

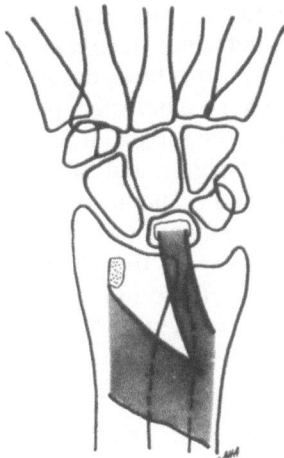

Fig. 2. The pronator quadratus muscle pedicle revascularization procedure. *Shaded area*, pronator quadratus; *dotted area*, donor site

by Erbs and Böhm [41], uses the pisiform on its vascular pedicle. They had uniformly good results at 5-years average follow-up. Hori et al. demonstrated that one need only perform direct transfer of a vascular bundle into the avascular lunate [42]. They successfully treated 8 out of 9 patients with Kienböck's disease in their original report. By personal communication, Hori (1991) recently noted that he has done this procedure successfully in over 25 patients. Uchida and Sugioka's experimental work seems to support the direct transplantation of vessels versus a vascularized bone pedicle [43]. Using a rabbit model, they found that the bone grafts were gradually resorbed and that the main function of the procedure was the provision of vessels.

In our own experimental study, we demonstrated that blood supply can be restored to avascular bone by direct vessel transfer [44]. Amputated and transplanted avascular rat femoral heads, isolated with silicone, were studied with technetium scans, latex injection, and tetracycline labeling after routing vessels through the bone. All specimens in which the anastomosed vessels remained patent demonstrated neovascularization and restoration of blood supply.

Salvage Procedures

In advanced Kienböck's disease, options include proximal row carpectomy and radiocarpal arthrodesis.

Staging

After having reviewed the available treatment modalities, the practitioner is left with a large variety of choices. These can be narrowed down and individualized for a particular patient after determining two additional factors — stage and ulnar variance.

We have modified Stahl's original staging largely because it was based on pathology and histology, information generally not available for the preoperative decision-making process. The following describes 4 stages of Kienböck's disease based on radiographic and clinical presentations (Fig. 3).

Stage I

Radiographs are normal except for the possibility of either a linear or a compression fracture.

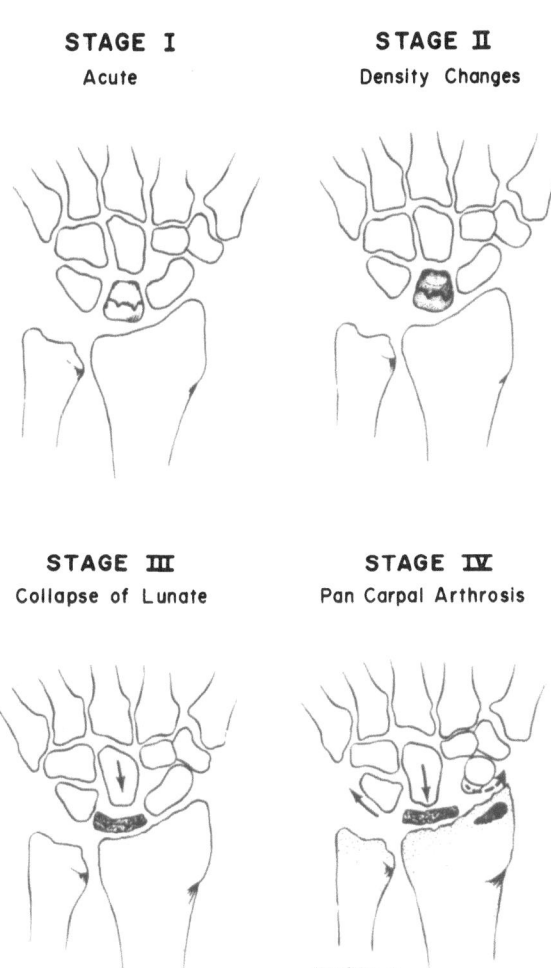

Fig. 3. Schematic representation of the radiographic appearance of stages I–IV of Kienböck's disease

Unless a compression fracture is visible, this stage is clinically indistinguishable from a wrist sprain. MRI is helpful in making the diagnosis, particularly when the MRI shows the entire lunate to be involved. One must be careful not to diagnose Kienböck's disease on MRI alone in the face of focal changes alone. Symptoms in the earliest stage are persistent pain, aggravated by use of the hand.

Stage II

There are definite density changes apparent in the lunate relative to the other carpal bones; however, the size, shape, and anatomic relationship of the bones are not significantly altered. Fracture lines may be noted. Later in this stage, anteroposterior radiographs show loss of height on the radial side of the lunate. The patient exhibits symptoms of recurrent pain, swelling, and tenderness in the wrist.

Stage III

The entire lunate has collapsed in the frontal plane and is elongated in the sagittal plane. The capitate migrates proximally. Scapholunate dis-

sociation, rotation of the scaphoid (the "ring" sign, Fig. 4), and ulnar deviation of the trique-trum may be seen on the anteroposterior radio-graph. Stage III is subdivided into stage IIIA, lunate collapse without fixed scaphoid rotation (negative "ring" sign), and stage IIIB, lunate collapse with fixed scaphoid rotation and other secondary derangements (positive "ring" sign). Clinically, patients in these stages have the same symptoms as those in stage II but with an increased level of wrist stiffness.

Stage IV

All the radiographic findings characteristic of stage III are present as well as generalized degenerative changes in the carpus. The symptoms are those of degenerative arthritis of the carpus. Long periods of quiescence may be intermixed with acute flare-ups of synovitis and pain.

Ulnar Variance

There are basically 2 ways of measuring ulnar variance. The first is easier and the one which we utilize. As described by Gelberman and associates [10], a line is extended from the distal radial articular surface toward the ulna and the distance between this line and the carpal surface of the ulna is measured (Fig. 5). We routinely take this measurement on a posteroanterior radiograph of the wrist with the patient's shoulder abducted 90°, the elbow flexed 90°, and the forearm in neutral rotation, a position advocated by Palmer and coworkers [45].

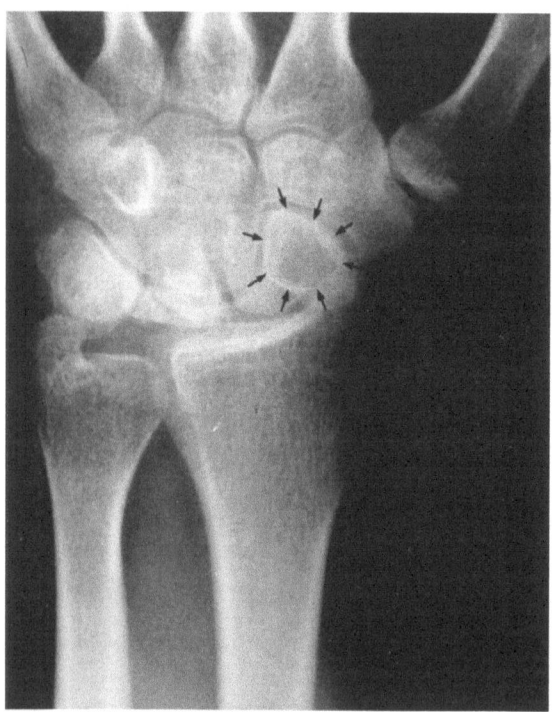

Fig. 4. Stage IIIB Kienböck's disease with scaphoid rotation demonstrating the "ring sign" (*arrows*) on an anteroposterior view

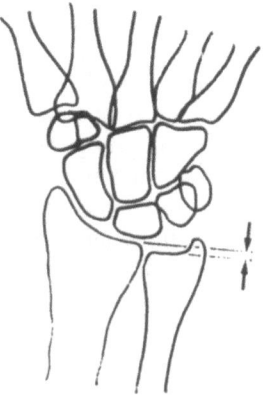

Fig. 5. Measurement of ulnar variance

In the second method [45], Palmer utilized a template of concentric circles (similar to the one used in establishing sphericity in Legg-Calvé-Perthes disease). The concentric circle that best approximates the distal radial surface is selected as a reference and compared in millimeters to the carpal surface of the ulna.

Rationale for Treatment

Stage I

Previously, in stage I, it was often difficult to make a diagnosis since lunate density change and collapse were absent. Sometimes a compression fracture might be present, but still the uncertainty of the diagnosis prevents the clinician from proceeding with abandon to a surgical solution. Even with the invention of the MRI, it is possible to over-diagnose Kienböck's disease. Consequently, we prefer a period of immobilization (up to 3 months) until the diagnosis is established with certainty. An external fixator in lieu of a simple cast is a reasonable alternative and may actually be preferable since a simple cast is unlikely to relieve axial compression. Over-distraction is to be avoided as carpal ligamentous instability may result.

The choice of treatment for stages II and IIIA of Kienböck's disease is dependent on ulnar variance; i.e. patients with the ulna positive variant are treated differently than patients with the ulna minus variant. Specifically, it would not make a lot of sense to shorten a radius or lengthen an ulna in a patient who already has profound ulnar positive variance. However, realizing that the literature is very convincing about the effectiveness of radial shortening and ulnar lengthening, even in those who have positive variance, we have recently been somewhat less strict in avoiding radial shortening/ulnar lengthening in patients with neutral variance or only minimal positive variance.

Stage II, Stage IIIA — Ulna *Positive* Variance

The senior one of us (DML) prefers a revascularization procedure as outlined below for stage II and stage IIIA when there is ulna positive variance. In addition, in cases of stage I not responding to conservative measures, and whose MRIs show total involvement of the lunate, revascularization is preferred.

A small piece of bone is harvested from the dorsum of the distal radius and a 2-mm hole is drilled through the middle of it. The second dorsal metacarpal artery and vein is then identified distally and mobilized so that the vessels can be drawn through the hole in the bone graft. In 15% of the patients, these vessels may be absent and an alternate vascular supply required. The ligated ends of the vessels are then anchored to the hole in the bone graft using the ligature. The lunate is exposed through a dorsal capsular flap and a hole is drilled in it to accommodate the bone graft and vessel transplantation. Alternatively, if lunate collapse is present, the lunate may be wedged open and the graft can be used to hold it open. At this point, release of the tourniquet should result in pulsation of the vessel. It must be insured that the vessels are not compressed by the extensor carpi radialis tendons; if they are, tendon lengthening is done. Postoperatively, the patient is immobilized with an external fixator for 10 weeks.

Stage II, Stage IIIA — Ulna *Minus* Variance

With little doubt, clinical reports support the use of equalization procedures (radial shortening or ulnar lengthening). Now, with biomechanical studies supporting their use, the rationale for radial shortening/ulnar lengthening appears irrefutable. We prefer radial shortening because an incision for bone graft is obviated and the likelihood of non-union is probably somewhat smaller. An oblique osteotomy (Fig. 6) is made

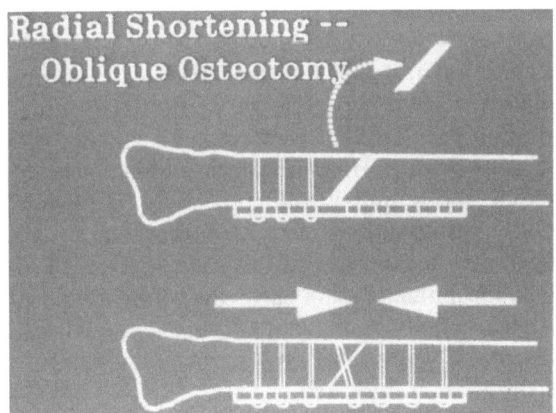

Fig. 6. Lateral schematic representation of the radial shortening type of osteotomy. Fixation is done with a 3.5 mm dynamic compression plate and an interfragmentary screw

through a volar approach. Using AO/ASIF technique, we apply either a 7- or 8-hole 3.5 mm dynamic compression plate with an interfragmentary screw through the osteotomy. Enough bone should be removed to leave the ulna in 1–2 mm ulnar positive variance. Plate removal is not usually necessary unless it becomes troublesome.

Stage IIIB

In stage IIIB, there are already fixed deformities of the lunate and carpus. Consequently, equalization procedures are less likely to be successful. This is because the equalization, though it may unload the lunate, is not likely to reestablish normal carpal architecture and mechanics. Therefore, for stage IIIB, STT fusion or scaphocapitate fusion is recommended. If there is significant synovitis, then the lunate should be excised as well.

Stage IV

Finally, in stage IV, we are virtually no longer dealing with Kienböck's disease per se. The disease process has progressed to involve the entire carpus, and the treatment must address more than just the lunate and its articular surfaces. Depending on patient desires and the condition of the proximal capitate and the radial articulation, proximal row carpectomy or wrist arthrodesis is our treatment of choice.

In summary, although Kienböck's disease is now less of an enigma, it still remains a dilemma. Using the stage of the disease and the ulnar variance, we have been able to deal with the maze of treatment options to our patients' satisfaction. We recommend immobilization in stage I. For stage II and for stage IIIA with *positive* ulnar variance, revascularization (DML) or radial shortening (AHA) is preferred. In patients with stage II or stage IIIA and *negative* ulnar variance, radial shortening is our procedure of choice. Once carpal architecture and mechanics have been affected permanently (stage IIIB), STT or scaphocapitate fusion are the treatments of choice. Finally, in the face of pan-carpal arthrosis (stage IV), proximal row carpectomy or wrist arthrodesis is indicated.

References

1. Beckenbaugh RD, Shives TC, Dobyns JH, Linscheid RL (1980) The natural history of Kienböck's disease and consideration of lunate fractures. Clin Orthop 149:98–106
2. Peste JL (1843) [Discussion] Bull Soc Anat Paris 18:169–170
3. Kashiwagi D, Fukiwara A, Inoue T, Liang FH, Imanoto Y (1977) An experimental and clinical study on lunatomalacia. Orthop Trans 1:7
4. Lee M (1963) The intraosseous arterial pattern of the carpal lunate bone and its relation to avascular necrosis. Acta Orthop Scand 33:43–55
5. Stahl F (1947) On lunatomalacia (Kienböck's disease), a clinical and roentgenological study, expecially on its pathogenesis and the late results of immobilization treatment. Acta Chir Scand [Suppl] 126:1–133
6. Kienböck R (1910) Über traumatische Malazie des Mondbeins und ihre Folgezustande: Entartungsformen und Kompressionsfrakturen. Fortschritte auf dem Gebiete der Roentgenstrahlen 16:78–103
7. Hùlten O (1928) Über anatomische Variationen der Handgelenkknochen. Acta Radiol Scand 9:155
8. Alexander AH, Turner MA, Alexander CE, Lichtman DM (1990) Lunate silicone replacement arthroplasty in Kienböck's disease — a long term follow-up. J Hand Surg [Am] 15:401–407
9. Gelberman RH, Bauman TD, Menon J, Akeson WH (1980) The vascularity of the lunate bone and Kienböck's disease. J Hand Surg 5:272–278
10. Gelberman RH, Salamon PB, Jurist JM, Posch JL (1975) Ulnar variance in Kienböck's disease. J Bone Joint Surg [Am] 57:674–676
11. Kawai H, Yamamoto K, Yamamoto T, Tada K, Kaga K (1988) Excision of the lunate in Kienböck's disease. Results after long-term follow-up. J Bone Joint Surg [Br] 70:287–292
12. Lichtman DM, Alexander AH, Mack GR, Gunther SF (1982) Kienböck's disease — update on silicone replacement arthroplasty. J Hand Surg [Am] 7:343–347
13. Lichtman DM, Mack GR, MacDonald RI, Gunther SF, Wilson JN (1977) Kienböck's disease: The role of silicone replacement arthroplasty. J Bone Joint Surg [Am] 59:899–908
14. Sundberg SB, Linscheid RL (1984) Kienböck's disease — results of treatment with ulnar lengthening. Clin Orthop 187:43–51
15. Watson HK, Ryu J, DiBella A (1985) An approach to Kienböck's disease: Triscaphe arthrodesis. J Hand Surg [Am] 10:179–187
16. Panagis JS, Gelberman RH, Taleisnik J, Baumgaertner M (1983) The arterial anatomy of the human carpus. Part II: the intraosseous vascularity. J Hand Surg 8:375–382
17. Evans G, Burke FD, Barton NJ (1986) A comparison of conservative treatment and silicone replacement arthroplasty in Kienböck's disease. J Hand Surg [Br] 11:98–102

18. Almquist EE (1987) Kienböck's disease. Hand Clin 3:141–148
19. Grassi G, Santoro D, Coli G, Cianciulli M (1978) The surgical treatment of Kienböck's disease. Ital J Orthop Traumatol 4:149–154
20. Kristensen SS, Thomassen E, Christensen F (1986) Kienböck's disease — late results by non-surgical treatment. A follow-up study. J Hand Surg [Br] 11:422–5
21. Viernstein K, Weigert M (1967) Die Radiusverkurzungsosteotomie bei der Lunatummalzie. Munch Med Wochenschr 109:1992
22. Nakamura R, Imaeda T, Miura T (1990) Radial shortening for Kienböck's disease: Factors affecting the operative result. J Hand Surg [Br] 15:40–45
23. Chuinard RG, Zeman SC (1980) Kienböck's disease: An analysis and rationale for treatment by capitate-hamate fusion. Orthop Trans 4:18
24. Cave EF (1939) Kienböck's disease of the lunate. J Bone Joint Surg 21:858–866
25. Dornan A (1949) The results of treatment in Kienböck's disease. J Bone Joint Surg [Br] 31:518–520
26. Gillespie HS (1961) Excision of the lunate bone in Kienböck's disease. J Bone Joint Surg [Br] 43:245–249
27. Marek RM (1957) Avascular necrosis of the carpal lunate. Clin Orthop 10:96–107
28. Blaine ES (1931) Lunate osteomalacia. JAMA 96:492
29. McMurtry RY, Youm Y, Flatt AE, Gillespie TE (1978) Kinematics of the wrist, II. Clinical applications. J Bone Joint Surg [Am] 60:955–961
30. Trumble TE, Glisson RR, Seaber AV, Urbaniak JR (1986) A biomechanical comparison of the methods for treating Kienböck's disease. J Hand Surg [Am] 11:88–93
31. Horii E, Garcia-Elias M, Bishop AT, Cooney WP, Linscheid RL (1990) Effect on force transmission across the carpus in procedures used to treat Kienböck's disease. J Hand Surg [Am] 15:393–400
32. Ishiguro T (1984) Experimental and clinical studies of Kienböck's disease — excision of the lunate followed by packing of the free tendon. J Jpn Orthop Assoc 58:509–522
33. Kato H, Usui M, Minami A (1986) The long-term results of Kienböck's disease treated by excisional arthroplasty using a silicone implant or a coiled palmaris longus tendon. J Hand Surg [Am] 11:645–653
34. Schmitt E, Hassinger M, Mittelmeier (1984) Die lunatummalazie und ihre Behandlung mit Lunatumexstirpation. Z Orthop 122:643–650
35. Swanson AB (1970) Silicone rubber implants for the replacement of the carpal scaphoid and lunate bones. Orthop Clin North Am 1:299–309
36. Atkinson RE, Smith RJ, Jupiter JB (Jan 1985) Silicone synovitis of the wrist. 40th annual meeting of the American Society for Surgery of the Hand, January 21–23, Las Vegas, NV
37. Carter PR, Benton LJ (Jan 1985) Late osseous complications of carpal silastic implants. 40th annual meeting of the American Society for Surgery of the Hand, January 21–23, Las Vegas, NV
38. Peimer CA, Medige J, Eckert BS, Wright JR, Howard BS (1986) Reactive synovitis after arthroplasty. J Hand Surg [Am] 11:624–638
39. Swanson AB, Wilson KM, Mayhew DE, Page BJ II, Swanson GG, Maupin BK (Jan 1985) Long-term bone response around carpal bone implants. 40th annual meeting of the American Society for Surgery of the Hand, January 21–23, Las Vegas, NV
40. Braun R (March 1983) The pronator pedicle bone grafting in the forearm and proximal carpal row. 38th annual meeting of the American Society for Surgery of the Hand, May 7–9, Anaheim, CA
41. Erbs G, Böhm E (1984) Langezeitergebnisse der os pisiforme-verlagerung bei Mondbeinnekrose. Handchirurgie 16:85–89
42. Hori Y, Tamai S, Okuda II, Sakamoto II, Takita T, Masuhara K (1979) Blood vessel transplantation to bone. J Hand Surg [Am] 4:23–33
43. Uchida Y, Sugioka Y (1990) Effects of vascularized bone graft on surrounding necrotic bone: An experimental study. J Reconstruct Microsurg 6:101–7
44. Saldana MJ, Niebauer JJ, Brown R, McCarroll R, Lichtman DM (1990) Microsurgical revascularization of ischemic rat femoral heads. J Hand Surg [Am] 15:309–15
45. Palmer AK, Glisson RR, Werner FW (1982) Ulnar variance determination. J Hand Surg [Am] 7:376–379

Kienböck's Disease and Ulnar Variance

RYOGO NAKAMURA, SATOSHI TSUGE, KENTARO WATANABE, KENJI TSUNODA,[1] and TAKAYUKI MIURA[2]

Abstract. Although positive ulnar variance in Kienböck's disease is rare in Europe and the USA, it occurs frequently in Japan. To clarify whether Kienböck's disease with positive ulnar variance in Japan is different clinically than Kienböck's with zero or negative ulnar variance, 39 patients with positive ulnar variance were compared to 81 patients with zero or negative variance. The sex and age distribution, roentgenographic findings, and the results of 99mTc scintigraphy and MRI in patients with positive ulnar variance were found to be identical to those in patients with zero or negative variance. Therefore, Kienböck's disease with positive variance appears to be the same clinical entity as Kienböck's disease with zero or negative variance. These results indicate that negative ulnar variance is not a dominant predisposing factor for this disease.

Keywords: Kienböck's disease — Ulnar variance — Bone scintigraphy — Magnetic resonance imaging — Negative ulnar variance — Positive ulnar variance — Lunatum malacia

Introduction

Since Kienböck's description in 1910 [1], lunatomalacia has been called Kienböck's disease. Over the 80 years since, its etiology and treatment have been discussed extensively, but remain controversial. Extrinsic etiological factors implicated in Kienböck's disease are a single acute episode which results in lunate fracture and repeated minimal trauma to the wrist. However, Hultén (1928) found a high incidence of negative ulnar variance among patients with Kienböck's disease and postulated that negative ulnar variance predisposes patients to Kienböck's disease [2]. Hultén's theory has been supported by a number of clinical [3–12] as well as biomechanical studies [13, 14], although other authors have questioned the soundness of this theory [15–19].

Unlike Europe and the United States, where most patients with Kienböck's disease show negative ulnar variance, Kienböck's disease with positive ulnar variance is observed frequently in Japan, with the incidence of positive ulnar variance being at least equal to that of negative ulnar variance. If it is true that negative variance plays a major role in the development of Kienböck's disease, the pathogenesis, symptons, and clinical finding in patients with positive ulnar variance should be different from those with negative variance. Furthermore, it has been hypothesized that Kienböck's disease with positive variance may be a distinct clinical entity, as is ulnocarpal abutment syndrome. To elucidate these questions, sex and age distribution, occupation, symptoms, roentgenographic findings, and results of bone scan and magnetic resonance imaging (MRI) of patients with positive ulnar variance were compared to those of patients with zero and negative variance.

Patients and Methods

The diagnosis of Kienböck's disease was made in 136 patients on the basis of roentgenographic findings at Nagoya University Hospital from 1973 to 1989 by either of two of the authors (R. N. and T. M.). At the time the patients were first seen, a

[1] Department of Orthopaedic Surgery, Branch Hospital of Nagoya University School of Medicine 1-1-20 Daikominami, Higashiku, Nagoya 461, Japan
[2] Department of Orthopaedic Surgery, Nagoya University: School of Medicine, 65 Tsurumaicho, Syowa-Ku, Nagoya, 466 Japan

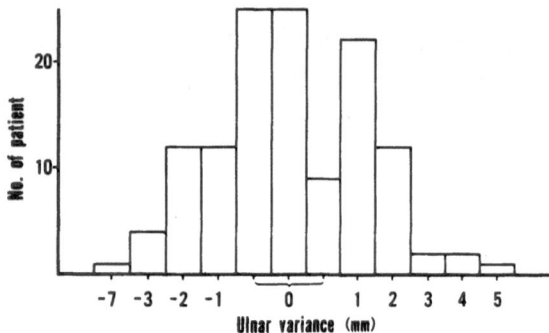

Fig. 1. Ulnar variance distribution in patients with Kienböck's disease

relevant history regarding type and duration of manual labor, sports activity, history of trauma, and duration of symptoms was obtained. The study included 120 patients whose roentgenograms of both wrists (affected and contralateral, unaffected wrists) were available for evaluation. The ulnar variance of the affected wrist was measured in millimeters on the PA wrist roentgenograms using Palmer's template of concentric circles [20]. The patients were divided into 3 groups according to the ulnar variance: group A consisted of 39 patients (33%) with a positive ulnar variance (ulnar variance of 1 mm or more), group B of 51 patients (43%) with zero variance, and group C of 30 patients (25%) with negative variance (ulnar variance of −1 mm or less) (Fig. 1).

Demographies and Roentgenographic Studies

Averages of age, sex distribution, and the percentage of manual workers in each group were determined and compared between the 3 groups. Patients were considered as manual laborers if they had engaged in hard physical work for more than 1 year before the onset of symptoms.

The range of wrist flexion-extension and the grip strength of the affected side were expressed as a percentage of the unaffected side and compared between the 3 groups in order to determine any difference in the severity of clinical symptoms.

The ratio of the lunate height to width as measured on lateral roentgenograph and expressed as a percentage (Ståhl's index) [21], and the carpal height index (the ratio of the affected to the unaffected carpal height) [22, 23] also were measured and compared.

To increase objectivity, the severity of the disease was staged according to both Ståhl's index

and the carpal height ratio: stage I was defined as corresponding to a Ståhl's index of 45 or more, stage II to 30–44, and stage III less than 30. Cases in which the carpal height ratio on the affected side was 0.03 less than the unaffected side were considered as carpal collapse and were graded as stage IV, regardless of Ståhl's index [24]. Cases in which arthritic changes were present throughout the wrist were defined as stage V. Distribution of stages by group was examined and compared.

Bone Scintigraphy and MRI Study

In order to investigate any difference at the site of the bone lesions in the 3 groups, 99mTc scintigraphy was performed in 24 patients (9 in group A, 7 in group B, and 8 in group C). Two hours after the intravenous injection of 15～20 mCi 99mTc pyrophosphate, bone scintigraphy was performed using a gamma camera.

MRI was performed in 16 patients (6 each in groups A and B, and 4 in group C) to detect any differences at the site of the bony avascular change [25]. A 1.5 tesla superconductive MRI scanner (Sigma MR system) and an accompanying surface coil for wrist imaging were used for this study. T_1-weighted coronal images at a slice interval of 3 mm were obtained.

Results

Clinical Demographic and Roentgenographic Findings (Table 1)

The majority of patients were male in all groups (82% in group A, 75% in group B, and 70% in group C), while the distribution of patients' age was similar in the 3 groups. No significant difference in the percentage of males or the mean age between groups existed (X^2-test and t-test respectively; $0.1 < P < 0.5$).

Eighty-three patients had engaged in manual labor in which the wrist suffered repeated impacts. The most common type of manual work was hammering (23 cases; carpentry or sheet metal), followed by using an impact wrench (14), lifting heavy objects (9), and electric installation (7). The remaining 30 manual laborers were engaged in 12 different occupations, such as spot welding and farming. Thirteen patients had a history of trauma to the wrist, and ten patients had participated in sports activities in which the wrist suffered repeated impact. The remaining 14 of the 120 patients were housewives, office

Table 1. Clinical demographics and roentgenographic findings in patients with Kienböck's disease

Ulnar variance	Cases (n)	Sex Male	Sex Female	Age distribution mean ± SD range:years	Related etiological factor Manual work	Wrist trauma	Sports activity	None	Range of wrist flexion-extension mean ± SD (degree)	Grip strength (percent of contralateral wrist mean ± SD%)	Ståhl's[a] index (mean ± SD%)	Carpal[b] height index (mean ± SD%)	Stage of illness I	II	III	IV	V
Positive	39	32	7	38 ± 15 (17 ~ 70)	27	5	2	5	83 ± 20	61 ± 27	31 ± 9	0.95 ± 0.04	1	14	5	19	0
Zero	51	38	13	35 ± 14 (16 ~ 68)	38	4	3	6	82 ± 22	62 ± 22	33 ± 10	0.95 ± 0.04	8	19	6	17	1
Negative	30	21	9	31 ± 15 (10 ~ 75)	16	4	5	3	86 ± 22	65 ± 25	30 ± 9	0.95 ± 0.04	1	7	5	17	0
Total	120	83	38	35 ± 13 (10 ~ 75)	83	13	10	14	83 ± 21	62 ± 24	31 ± 9	0.95 ± 0.04	10	40	16	53	1

[a] Ståhl's index: the ratio of the lunate height to width as measured on lateral radiography, expressed as a percentage
[b] Carpal height index: the ratio of the carpal height ratio of affected wrist to contralateral non-affected wrist

workers, and others without a history of wrist trauma and in whom external force was not believed to have been an etiological factor. Manual workers accounted for 69%, 75%, and 60% of cases in groups A, B, and C, respectively. The percentage of manual workers in group A was not significantly different than that in groups B or C (X^2-test; $P > 0.5$).

Average range of motion and grip strength were similar in the 3 groups. Patients in each group presented most commonly with stage IV of the disease followed by stage II.

Bone Scintigraphy and MRI Results

The results of 99mTc bone scintigraphy revealed high uptake areas confined to the lunate and surrounding carpal bones in all 24 patients regardless of group. MRI demonstrated more clearly on T_1-weighted images that the affected area was confined to the lunate (Figs. 2, 3). The avascular area of the lunate appeared as low signal intensity and involved either the radial half or the whole lunate. No case presented with low-signal intensity confined to the ulnar lunate, which would have been diagnostic of ulnocarpal abutment syndrome. No difference in MRI findings among the 3 groups was detected.

Discussion

The incidence of Kienböck's disease with positive ulnar variance is low in Europe and the United States. Hultén [2], Wette [12], and Persson [8], using the criterion of 2 mm or more for positive ulnar variance, stated that the incidence of positive variance in Kienböck's disease is null. According to Persson, only 3 cases with positive variance had been reported in the literature at that time (1950), and these were considered to be exceptional cases. Using the criterion for positive variance of 1 mm or more, Viernstein et al. [26] reported that 3 out of 108 (3%) patients with Kienböck's disease had positive variance, and Beckenbaugh et al. [4] reported positive variance in only one (2%) out of 42 patients. A relatively high incidence of positive variance has been reported by Joeck [6] and Kristensen, et al. [17] Joeck had previously reported (1937) that 6 out of 36 patients (17%) had a positive ulnar variance of 2 mm or more. In 1986, Kristensen, et al. reported that 6 out of 47 patients (13%) had a positive variance of 1 mm or more. In contrast,

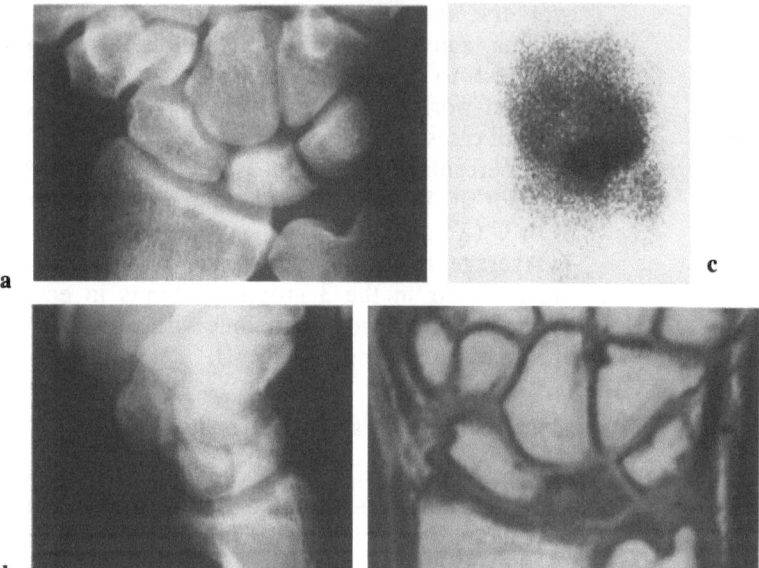

Fig. 2. Kienböck's disease with positive ulnar variance in a 38-year-old male who experienced right wrist pain for 3 months and had engaged in lifting heavy objects for 6 years. **a** PA Roentgenography showing positive ulnar variance (2 mm) and sclerosis of the lunate. **b** Lateral roentgenograph showing flattening and the fracture line of the lunate. **c** A 99mTc bone scan revealing increased uptake of isotope in by the lunate. **d** T_1-Weighted MRI showing evident low signal confined to and involving the entire lunate

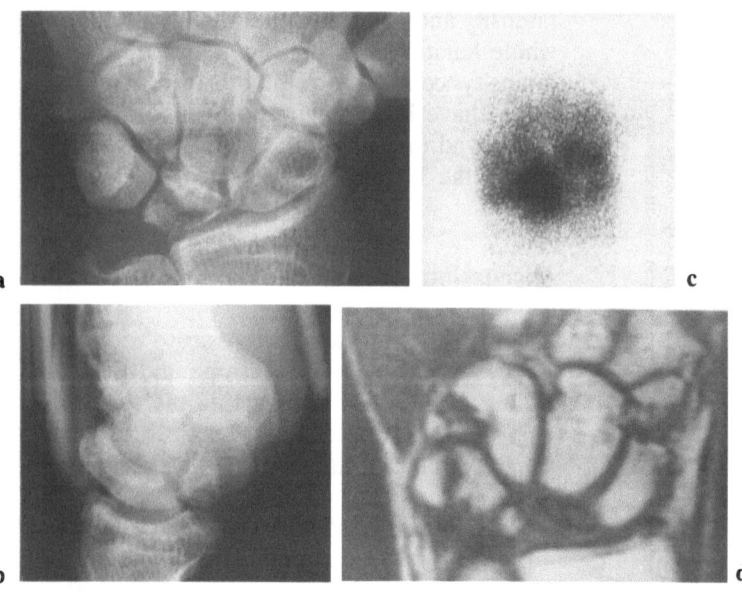

Fig. 3. Kienböck's disease with negative ulnar variance in a 28-year-old male who experienced left wrist pain for 2 years and had operated an impact wrench for 7 years. **a** PA Roentgenogrphy showing negative ulnar variance (−2 mm), flattening of the radial side of the lunate, and fracture. **b** Lateral roentgenography showing flattening and the fracture line of the lunate. **c** 99mTc bone scan revealing high uptake of the lunate and surrounding carpal bone. **d** T_1-Weighted MRI showing low-signal density confined to the lunate

the incidence of patients with Kienböck's disease with positive ulnar variance is higher in Japan. Takada [27] found that 27 out of 146 cases (18%) had positive variance of 1 mm or more, 83 (57%) had zero variance, and 36 (25%) had negative variance of −1 mm or less. Hu [28] studied 204 patients with Kienböck's disease and reported that 45 (22%) had positive variance greater than 2 mm, 122 (59%) had zero variance, and only 37 (19%) had negative variance of more than −2 mm. However, these authors concluded that

the incidence of negative ulnar variance was high in Kienböck's disease because the incidence of negative variance among healthy wrists of the Japanese is lower (Takada, 6%; Hu, 1%). Contrary to these two reports, Okutsu et al. [29] have concluded that the incidence of negative ulnar variance among Japanese is not increased significantly, based on a study comparing 198 wrists with Kienböck's disease to 150 normal wrists. Additionally, in our studies [30], 108 out of 325 (32.2%) normal wrists had positive ulnar variance of more than 1 mm, 128 (39.3%) had zero variance, and 89 (27.4%) had negative variance of more than 1 mm. Therefore, we agree with Okutsu et al., and believe that the incidence of negative ulnar variance is not significantly different between wrists with Kienböck's disease and normal wrists.

An important question which arises from these controversies is whether Kienböck's disease with positive ulnar variance is the same entity as that with negative or zero variance. If it is different, then what has been called "Kienböck's disease with positive ulnar variance" is actually a "Kienböck-like" disease which is frequent among the Japanese. If the clinical entity is the same, Hultén's proposition — that negative ulnar variance is a predisposing factor of Kienböck's disease — must be questioned.

Our investigation has demonstrated that demographic factors, such as age and sex distribution and type of labor, and clinical manifestations, such as restricted wrist motion, weakness of grip, and roentgenographic and radiological findings on bone scan and MRI, show no difference between Kienböck's disease with positive ulnar variance and that with zero or negative variance. These results demonstrate, at least, that negative ulnar variance is not a predominant predisposing factor to Kienböck's disease, if it is a predisposing factor at all. We are concerned that undue emphasis on negative ulnar variance as a predisposing factor to Kienböck's disease may delay the investigation of other more important etiological factors, such as the influence of external force on the wrist.

Conclusion

Kienböck's disease with positive ulnar variance, occurring frequently among the Japanese, has the same clinical manifestation as Kienböck's disease with zero or negative variance and is believed to be the same clinical entity. Therefore, negative ulnar variance cannot be considered a predominant predisposing factor of Kienböck's disease.

References

1. Kienböck R (1910) Über traumatische Malazie des Mondbeins und ihre Folgezustände: Entartugsformen und Kompressionfracturen. Fortschr Röntgenstr 16:77–103
2. Hultén O (1928) Über anatomische Variationen der Handgelenkknochen. Acta Radiol 9:155–69
3. Axelsson R (1973) Niveauoperationen bei Mondbeinnekrose. Handchirurgie 5:187–196
4. Beckenbaugh RD, Shives TC, Dobyns JH, Linscheid RL (1980) Kienböck's disease: The natural history of Kienböck's disease and consideration of lunate fracture. Clin Orthop 149:98–106
5. Gelberman RH, Salamon PB, Jurist JM, Posch JL (1975) Ulnar variance in Kienböck's disease. J Bone Joint Surg [Am] 57:674–676
6. Joeck H (1937) Der Einfluß der minus Variante Hulténs auf die Entstehung der Lunatummalazie, zugleich Einversuch einer einheilichen Deutung. Arch Orthop Unfall-Chir 37:618–640
7. Mirabello SC, Rosenthal DI, Smith RJ (1987) Correlation of clinical and radiographic findings in Kienböck's disease. J Hand Surg [Am] 12:1049–1054
8. Persson M (1950) Causal treatment of lunatomalacia. Further experiences of operative ulnar lengthening. Acta Chir Scand 100:531–544
9. Stahl S, Reis ND (1986) Traumatic ulnar variance in Kienböck's disease. J Hand Surg [Am] 11:95–97
10. Steinhäuser J, Posival H (1982) Doppelseitige Mondbeinnekrose; Ein Beitrag zur Pathogenese. Zeitshrift für Othopadie und Ihre Grenzgebiete 120:151–157
11. Watson HK, Ryu J, Dibella A (1985) An approach to Kienböck's disease. Triscaphe arthrodesis. J Hand Surg [Am] 10:179–187
12. Wette W (1936) Die Bedeutung der "Minusvariante" (Hultén) für die Ätiologie der Lunatumnekrose. Arch Orthop Unfall-Chir 36:41–46
13. Palmer AK, Werner FW (1984) Biomechanics of the distal radioulnar joint. Clin Orthop 187:26–35
14. Trumble T, Glisson RR, Seaber AV, Urbaniak JR (1986) A biomechanical comparison of the methods for treating Kienböck's disease. J Hand Surg [Am] 11:1:88–93
15. Chan KP, Huang P (1971) Anatomic variations in radial and ulnar length in the wrists of Chinese. Clin Orthop 80:17–20
16. Fisk GR (1984) The wrist. J Bone Joint Surg [Br] 66:396–407
17. Kristensen SS, Thomassen E, Christensen F (1986) Ulnar variance in Kienböck's disease. J Hand Surg [Br] 11:258–260
18. Kristensen SS, Søballe K (1987) Kienböck's disease — the influence of arthrosis on ulnar variance measurements. J Hand Surg [Br] 12:301–305
19. Nathan PA, Meadows KD (1987) Ulna-minus variance and Kienböck's disease. J Hand Surg [Am] 12:777–778

20. Palmer AK, Glisson RR, Werner FW (1982) Ulnar variance determination. J Hand Surg 7(4):376–379
21. Ståhl F (1947) On lunatomalacia (Kienböck's disease): A clinical and roentgenological study, especially on its pathogenesis and late results of immobilization treatment. Acta Chir Scand 126:1–133
22. Youm Y, McMurtry RY, Flatt AE, Gillespie TE (1978) Kinematics of the wrist. I. An experimental study of radio-ulnar deviation and flexion-extension. J Bone Joint Surg [Am] 60:423–431
23. Kato H, Usui M, Minami K (1986) Long-term results of Kienböck's disease treated by excisional arthroplasty with a silicone implant or coiled palmaris longus tendon. J Hand Surg [Am] 11:645–653
24. Nakamura R, Imaeda T, Miura T (1990) Radial shortening for Kienböck's disease: Factors affecting the operative results. J Hand Surg [Br] 15:40–45

25. Sowa DT, Holder LE, Patt PG, Weiland AJ (1989) Application of magnetic resonance imaging to ischemic necrosis of the lunate. J Hand Surg [Am] 14:1008–1016
26. Viernstein K, Weigert M (1967) Die Radiusverkursungsosteotomy bei der Lunatummalazi. Münch Med Wochenschr 109:1992–1994
27. Takada S (1972) Lunatomalacia — A clinical observation and experimental study by tetracycline marking method. J Jpn Orthop Assoc 46:661–674
28. Hu ST (1977) The relationship between "variant", relative, length of distal ulna and radius, and Kienböck's disease. J Jpn Orthop Assoc 51:15–26
29. Okutsu S, Ninimiya S, Iwaya T, Iwao T, Takami H, Miyaji N, Abe I, Azuma A, Okai K, Shiba M (1977) Clinical study of Kienböck's disease. Orthop Surg (Jpn): 28:1549–1552
30. Nakamura R, Tanaka Y, Imaeda T, Miura T (1991) The influence of age and sex on ulnar variance. J Hand Surg [Br] 16:84–88

The Incidence of Kienböck's Disease Among Adults with Cerebral Palsy

Takaya Mizuseki,[1] Shigeo Jyoji,[1] Shotaro Katayama,[1] Kenya Tsuge,[1] and Yoshikazu Ikuta[2]

Abstract. The incidence the Kienböck's disease among adults with cerebral palsy (CP) was studied. The 202 wrists of 101 subjects who lived mainly in homes for the physically disabled were evaluated regardless of complaints or type of CP. The survey revealed six wrists of five patients (3%) to be affected by Kienböck's disease. The type of CP was of the mixed (athetospastic) type in all the cases. Wrist position was neutral at rest, but was either volarly or ulnovolarly flexed for firm gripping. None of the subjects remembered undergoing any trauma to the wrist and nor having done any strenuous manual labor in the past. The mean ulnar variance of the wrists in this survey was $+0.27$ mm in the males and -0.15 mm in the females, while that of the wrists with Kienböck's disease was -1.25 mm. It was postulated that repeated high pressure at the wrist joint created by abnormal pull of the forearm flexors and extensors, together with negative ulnar variance can cause repeated trauma to the lunate, eventually leading to Kienböck's disease.

Keywords: Kienböck's disease — Cerebral palsy — Ulnar variance — Incidence — Spasticity

Introduction

The real cause of lunatomalacia, Kienböck's disease, remains unknown, although several factors such as negative ulnar variance [1, 2], acute fracture [3], repeated trauma [4], or prejudiced blood supply [3, 5] are reported to be highly related. We cannot delineate any single factor to be the prime cause because racial, social, and occupational backgrounds of these patients vary from one to another. While it is very difficult to make an *in situ* model of repeated high pressure in the wrist joint, the wrists of the subjects with cerebral palsy (CP), especially of the spastic, athetotic, or mixed (athetospastic) type, are characteristically prone to repeated high pressure since voluntary control of the hand and forearm muscles is difficult. Our first encounter with Kienböck's disease in CP raised the question if this long-standing spasticity of the limbs can have any effect on the carpal bone, i.e., causing a higher incidence of aseptic necrosis of the lunate. An epidemiological survey was conducted on those adults with CP who lived mainly in homes for the physically disabled in Hiroshima Prefecture, in order to see if repeated high pressure can cause Kienböck's disease among this population.

Patients

The adult subjects with CP were interviewed and, in those who gave consent, bilateral wrist radiographs were taken whether or not they had complaints concerning the wrist. A history of past or present wrist pain was taken.

There were 101 people with CP in this survey, 46 males and 55 females. Their ages ranged from 17 to 60 years with an average of 35.1 years (males 36.4, females 34.0) years. The types of CP included in this study were either spastic quadriplegia, athetosis, or a combination of athetosis and spasticity. Occupationally, none had been exposed to strenuous manual work, although all had been using their hands for light manual work or activities of daily living (ADL).

[1] Hiroshima Prefectural Rehabilitation Center, Taguchi, Saijyo, Higashi-Hiroshima City, 724-05 Japan
[2] Department of Orthopedic Surgery, Hiroshima University, Hiroshima, 734 Japan

95

Table 1. Data of the subjects with cerebral palsy (CP) and Kienböck's disease

Case	Age (years)	Sex	Type of CP	Affected wrist	Age at onset of pain (years)	Stage[a]	Ulnar variance[b]	Hand dominancy	Wrist position in grasping
1	24	M	Mixed	Bilateral	Right: 21	II	−0.5 mm	Right	Ulnovolar flexion
					Left: none	II	+1.5 mm		Ulnovolar flexion
2	36	F	Mixed	Left	30	IV	−4.0 mm	Right	Volar flexion
3	36	M	Mixed	Right	22[c]	IIIB	−3.0 mm	Right	Slight ulnar deviation
4	32	F	Mixed	Left	20[c]	IIIB	0.0 mm	Right	Ulnar deviation
5	36	F	Mixed	Right	36	I	−1.5 mm	Right	Ulnar deviation

[a] Lichtman's radiological stage classification [7, 8]
[b] Project-a-line method was employed for ulnar variance determination [1]
[c] Pain had been present in the past but was absent at the time of investigation

Table 2. Comparison of the mean ulnar variance

	All the patients with CP	Patients with CP and Kienböck's disease	Normal population[a]
Males	+0.27 mm	−1.25 mm	+0.67 mm (Average, 36.4 years of age)
Females	−0.15 mm		+0.81 mm (Average, 34.0 years of age)

[a] Calculated according to the equation of Sadahiro et al. [11]
CP, Cerebral palsy

Methods

Bilateral radiographs of the wrists were taken regardless of the presence or absence of wrist symptoms. The patients were asked to maintain a so-called standard position of the wrist [6], with the elbow flexed at 90°, the forearm neutral in prono-supination, and the wrist neutral in extension-flexion. However, this position was difficult for some because of their spasticity, and a compromise wrist position was accepted. The radiographs were studied for abnormality of the lunate and for determining ulnar variance. For those whose lunates were sclerotic or collapsed, Lichtman's radiological classification [7, 8] was employed to determine the degree of collapse. The project-a-line method [1] was used for deciding ulnar variance. At this time, the subjects were questioned about past or present wrist pain.

Results

Kienböck's disease was diagnosed in six wrists of five patients. One patient had bilateral wrist involvement and another was diagnosed as having

stage I Kienböck's disease with slightly increased density and localized pain on the lunate. (Table 1). The over-all incidence rate, therefore, was 3.0%. The CP in all the subjects with affected wrists was of the mixed (atheto-spastic) type. The affected sides of the wrist were evenly distributed although all the patients were right-handed. There was a tendency toward either ulnovolar flexion or ulnar deviation of the wrist during firm gripping. The resting position, however, was neutral in all cases. For the subjective symptoms, two wrists which had been symptomatic in the past were no longer so at the time of investigation, three were symptomatic, and the remaining one had never been symptomatic. The onset of symptoms was at around 20 years of age in 3 cases, and after 30 years of age in the other 2 (Table 1). None of the five patients remembered any history of trauma to their wrists.

According to Lichtman's radiological stage classification [7, 8], one-half of the wrists were in the advanced stages III and IV, and the other half were in stages I and II. The average ulnar variance of the 202 wrists of the 101 subjects was +0.27 mm in the males and −0.15 mm in the females. On the other hand, the mean ulnar variance of all the affected wrists was −1.25 mm (Table 2).

Treatment

For those patients who were found to have Kienböck's disease, treatment by surgery was necessary for only one. Four other patients did not seek surgical treatment for the condition since their symptoms were either no longer present, periodic, or tolerable. The other case (case #2) had required a carpal tunnel release operation in the past since a fragmented lunate migrated into the volar carpal tunnel, causing carpal tunnel syndrome of the affected wrist (Fig. 1). The only patient (case #1) who underwent surgery of the lunate had severe wrist pain after work and sought relief of the pain.

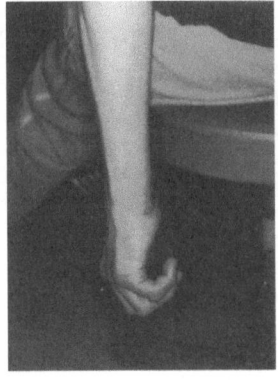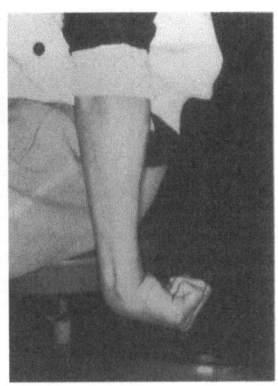

Fig. 2. Case 1. A 24-year-old male whose grasping posture was characteristic of an athetospastic hand. During firm gripping, the wrist was flexed ulnovolarly with simultaneous contraction of the extensor and flexor muscles (*right*). However, the resting posture of the wrist was neutral, not distorted (*left*)

Clinical Case

This 24-year-old male (case 1) with severe mixed CP had been working at making woolen gloves in a home for the physically disabled for the past 5 years. His manual grasping posture was characteristic of an athetospastic hand. During firm gripping, he showed an ulnovolarly flexed wrist with simultaneous contraction of the extensor and flexor muscles. However, the resting posture of the wrist was neutral and not distorted (Fig. 2). He started to feel slight pain over his right dorsal wrist at the age of 21 years. Two years after neglecting to receive medical care, he consulted our office and bilateral wrist X-rays were taken (Fig. 3). Bilateral involvement with the Kienböck's disease was revealed, although the left wrist had never been symptomatic. For the right symptomatic wrist, conservative treatments such as local steroid injections and a wrist splint failed to provide any relief. The anchovy procedure was chosen and the surgery was carried out in January, 1990. One year postoperatively, the severity of his complaint diminished, he is back to his former work, and is satisfied with the results although there was no change in the spasticity.

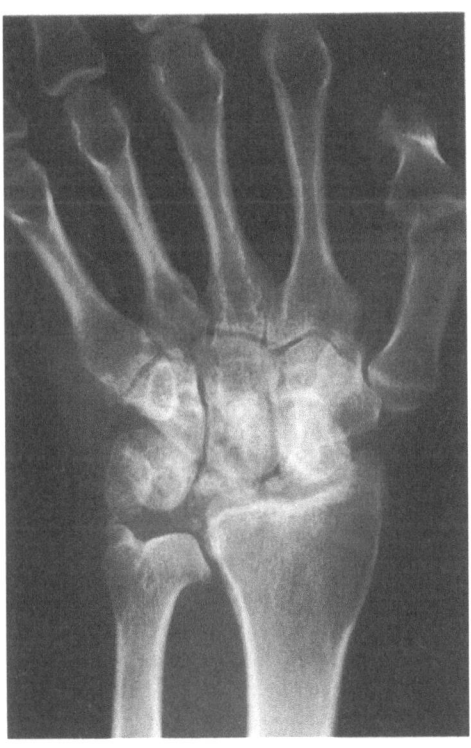

Fig. 1. Case 2. A 36-year-old female with severe mixed CP and stage IV of Kienböck's disease of the left wrist. The lunate is fragmented and the proximal pole of the scaphoid is absorbed. Although she did not seek surgical treatment for lunate pain, she suffered from carpal tunnel syndrome. Carpal tunnel release of the affected left wrist was carried out at the age of 34 years

Discussion

Our study revealed that the incidence rate of Kienböck's disease was 3% among the adult subjects with CP. Although there are no reports

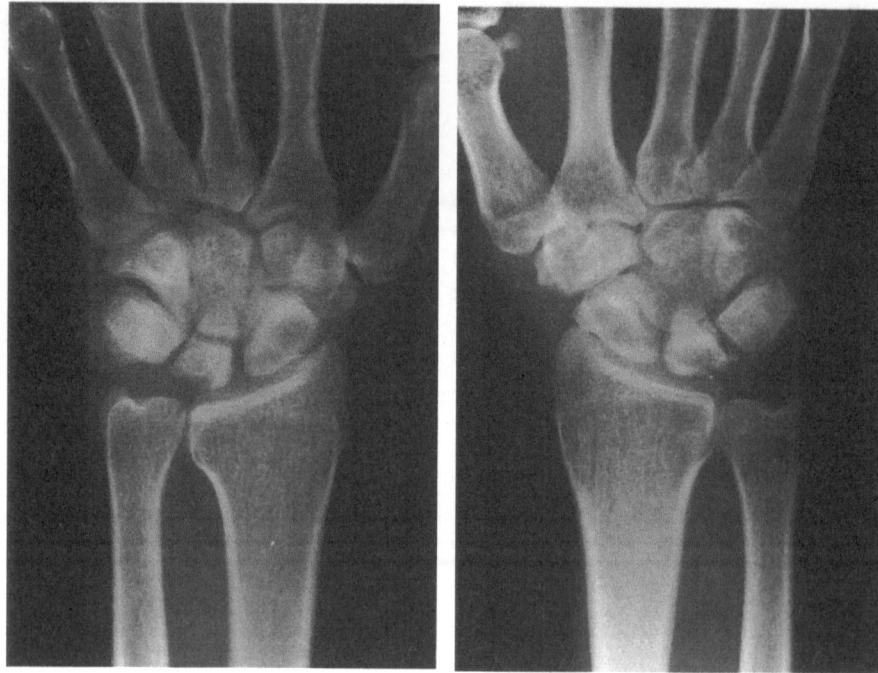

Fig. 3. Case 1. Onset of right wrist pain was at the age of 21 years. He had bilateral involvement of the wrists. Right wrist *right* and left wrist *left*. The Ulnar side of the proximal pole is collapsed

in the literature on the incidence of Kienböck's disease in the normal population, it was the impression of Alexander et al. [8] that the average orthopedist, not the hand specialist, encounters 1 case of Kienböck's disease every 1 or 2 years. As for the incidence of Kienböck's disease among adults with CP, the only report to date has been by Rooker and Goodfellow [5], who reported five wrists of Kienböck's disease out of 53 (4.7%) persons with cerebral palsy in residential homes. When we take these and our figures into account, even though our rate is not as high as that reported by Roocker and Goodfellow's [5], we can deduce that the incidence of Kienböck's disease among this population is higher than in the normal one.

Why, then, should people with CP have a higher incidence of Kienböck's disease? According to Rooker and Goodfellow [5], the resting posture of the affected wrists were all flexed, and this compromised the blood supply to the lunate. Additionally, in 4 out of 5 of their cases, the radiographs demonstrated definite negative ulnar variance, although the authors did not mention this specifically. Our results differ from their observations in that the resting position of the wrists was not necessarily in volar flexion.

Although Rooker and Goodfellow believed that volar flexion of the wrist jeopardizes blood supply to the lunate, the position of the wrist is usually neutral when the individual is at rest or asleep, and in this neutral position, the blood flow should be restored barring any vasospastic condition. Marek [9] claimed that severe hyperextension of the wrist endangers blood supply as it enters the lunate. From our observation, we cannot agree to the hypothesis that vascular prejudice caused by constant wrist flexion causes Kienböck's disease among the patients with CP.

In our series, all the Kienböck's cases were patients with the mixed type of CP. They somehow managed to use their hands in daily activities, and there was no preponderance of right or left hand dominancy. The resting position of their wrists was usually neutral. However, when they tried to grasp something, not only their finger flexors but also their wrist flexors and extensors contracted simultaneously because of the nature of the CP. Usually the strongest flexor carpi ulnaris tendon causes the wrist position to be in ulnovolar flexion. At this point, undue pressure is created in the wrist joint, and these patients always have to use their wrists under high intra-articular pressure. It is not difficult to imagine how repeated stress could cause multiple traumas to the lunate as long as the hands were being used. Negative ulnar variance makes the stress more harmful.

Although negative ulnar variance is a well-recognized predisposing factor of Kienböck's disease in Caucasians [1, 2], this is controversial among the Japanese. Tanaka [10], in his matched study of sex and age between the normal population and those with Kienböck's disease, concluded that there is no statistical difference in ulnar variance between the 2 groups. However, although ulnar variance among the subjects with CP in our study was, on the average, slightly lower than that in the normal Japanese population as reported by Sadahiro et al. [11], in Kienböck's disease it was lower by an additional 2 mm. Even though the number of cases in our series is too small to draw any statistic conclusion, we can say that this negative variance is contributing to the cause of the disease, at least among the population with CP. From the above observations, we can conclude that the characteristic features of Kienböck's disease in CP were involuntary simultaneous contraction of the wrist flexors and extensors and the negative ulnar variance of the affected wrists.

The cause of Kienböck's disease has long been controversial since the first report of osteonecrosis of the lunate by Kienböck [12]. Lee [13] studied the vascular anatomy of the lunate and found no anastomosis between the palmar and dorsal vessels in 7.5% of the lunates, with 26% of the lunates having a single volar or dorsal vessel supply. He postulated that a horizontal single fracture alone can cause proximal pole avascular necrosis, disrupting blood supply to the pole. Rooker and Goodfellow [5] supported this theory from their experience with CP. Gelberman et al. [4] questioned this theory, citing Ståhl's retrospective roentgenological study [14]. In his anatomical study, intraosseous anastomosis of the vessels was found to be abundant and he concluded that it would be rare for avascular necrosis to be caused by a single fracture. Therefore, he devised the theory of repeated trauma-compression fracture as the cause of segmental interruption of the intraosseous blood supply. Almquist [15] believes that either a single trauma or repeated stress can cause devascularization of the lunate. In our experience with Kienböck's disease in CP no subject remembered any major episode of trauma to the wrists but all the subjects were exposed to re-peated minor trauma as they used their hands, and this supports the theory of Gelberman et al. that repeated trauma to the lunate causes compression fracture and disrupts intraosseous blood supply, causing Kienböck's disease.

Conclusions

The subjects with CP, especially of the mixed (athethospastic) type, were found to have a higher incidence of Kienböck's disease compared to the normal population. This implies that repeated higher pressure at the wrist joint brought about by abnormal pull of the forearm flexors and extensors together with a negative ulnar variance can cause repeated trauma to the lunate, eventually leading to Kienböck's disease.

References

1. Gelberman RH, Salamon PB, Jurist JM (1975) Ulnar variance in Kienböck's disease. J Bone Joint Surg [Am] 57:674–676
2. Hulten O (1928) Über anatomische Variationen der Hand gelenkknochen. Acta Radiol 9:155–169
3. Lee MLH (1963) The intraosseous arterial pattern of the carpal lunate bone and its relation to avascular necrosis. Acta Orthop Scand 33:43–55
4. Gelberman RH, Bauman TD, Menon J (1980) The vascularity of the lunate bone and Kienböck's disease. J Hand Surg 5:272–278
5. Rooker GD, Goodfellow JW (1977) Kienböck's disease in cerebral palsy. J Bone Joint Surg [Br] 59:363–365
6. Palmer AK, Glisson RR, Werner FW (1982) Ulnar variance determination. J Hand Surg 7:376–379
7. Lichtman DM, Mack GR, MacDonald RI (1977) Kienböck's disease: The role of silicone replacement arthroplasty. J Bone Joint Surg [Am] 59:899–908
8. Alexander AH, Lichtman DM (1988) Kienböck's disease. In: Lichtman DM (ed) The wrist and its disorders, 1st edn. Saunders, Philadelphia, pp 329–343
9. Marek F (1957) Avascular necrosis of the carpal lunate. Clin Orthop 10:96–96
10. Tanaka Y (1989) Study of ulnar variance. J Jpn Soc Surg Hand 6:120–130
11. Sadahiro T, Morisawa Y, Yamamoto H (1988) Radiological studies on aging process of the distal radio-ulnar joint. J Jpn Soc Surg Hand 5:501–504
12. Kienböck R (1980) The classic — Concerning traumatic malacia of the lunate and its conse-

quences: Degeneration and compression fractures. Clin Orthop 149:4–8

13. Lee MLH (1963) The interosseous arterial pattern of the carpal lunate bone and its relation to avascular necrosis. Acta Orthop Scand 33:43–55

14. Stahl F (1947) On lunatomalacia (Kienböck's disease). A clinical and roentgenological study, especially on its pathogenesis and the late results of immobilization treatment. Acta Chir Scand 95:Suppl 126

15. Almquist EE (1986) Kienböck's disease. Clin Orthop 202:68–78

Treatment of Kienböck's Disease with Vascular Bundle Implantation and Triscaphe Arthrodesis

Hiroshi Yajima, Susumu Tamai, Shigeru Mizumoto, Hiroshi Ono, and Yuji Inada[1]

Abstract. Since 1986, 21 patients with advanced Kienböck's disease have been treated with vascular bundle implantation into the lunate and with triscaphe arthrodesis. The former is a biological approach for Kienböck's disease and the latter is a biomechanical approach, both of which decrease the longitudinal stress on the diseased lunate as well as treat the accompanying rotary subluxation of the scaphoid. The 18 cases which were followed-up for more than 1 year were analyzed.

Fifteen of the subjects were males and 3 were females. The right hand was involved in 9 cases and the left in 9, 11 of which occurred in the dominant hand. The age at operation ranged from 20 to 54 years (average 39 years). Four patients were categorized according to Lichtman's criteria as being in stage IIIA, thirteen in stage IIIB, and one in stage IV. The follow-up periods ranged from 12 to 58 months (average 31 months). Triscaphe arthrodesis was performed in 16 patients and the temporary triscaphe arthrodesis procedure using C-wire percutaneous pinning was performed in 2 patients in stage IIIA.

Postoperative wrist pain disappeared in 11 patients and decreased in 7. The postoperative range of motion of the wrist was slightly increased, from 71 to 75 in average. The grip power improved in all patients, from 19.4 to 30.0 kg in average. Roentgenologically, the vertical height increased in 4 patients, decreased in 3, and was unchanged in 11. Radial styloid impingement was noted in three patients, and styloidectomy was performed in one of them 9 months after the first operation. In conclusion, vascular bundle implantation performed simultaneously with triscaphe arthrodesis is a useful surgical procedure in the treatment of Kienböck's disease with marked collapse of the lunate.

Keywords: Kienböck's disease — Vascular bundle implantation — Triscaphe arthrodesis — Lunate — Avascular necrosis

Introduction

Kienböck's disease was first reported in 1910 by R. Kienböck, an Australian radiologist [1]. Since then, numerous experimental and clinical studies on its etiology and pathophysiology have been performed, and various therapies have been attempted based on these studies.

Hori and his colleagues in our clinic [2] started canine experiments on vascular bundle implantation into bone in 1970, in order to revascularize and revitalize necrotized bone. The principle reason for a vascular bundle being used for implantation into bone was the fact that microcirculation exists abundantly in a vascular bundle, consisting of an artery and its concomitant vein. When a contrast media was injected from the artery of the isolated vascular bundle for performing microangiography, the injected media immediately flowed back from the vein and an intimate network between the artery and vein could be observed to be creating microcirculation. Hori experimentally demonstrated that vascular bundle implantation to isolated or necrotized bones resulted in intraosseous revascularization, leading to gradual activation of bone formation and remodeling. Since 1975, we have treated Kienböck's disease by promoting bone revitalization with vascular bundle implantation to the necrotized lunate, based on this experimental finding [3, 4]. Because some of the patients showed progression of lunate collapse or osteoarthritic changes after this procedure, we attempted to use

[1] Department of Orthopaedic Surgery, Nara Medical University, Kashihara, Nara 634, Japan

an external skeletal fixation device to apply a distraction force on the lunate in 8 cases, so as to increase or maintain its vertical height after the vascular bundle implantation with cancellous bone graft. This method improved the operative results in cases of advanced Kienböck's disease. However, some cases still showed decrease of the vertical height of the lunate (VH) after removal of the external skeletal fixation device. Increased postoperative VH compared to the preoperative VH was recorded in only 2 cases [4]. This unfavorable result may be explained by the facts that (1) a considerably long period may be necessary to produce bone formation by vascular bundle implantation, and (2) the application of an external fixation device can not correct the carpal malaligment permanently. In our experimental studies using rats, vascular proliferation from the implanted vascular bundle was recognized in a few weeks, but it took a long time for new bone formation occur [5]. Bearing this in mind, we recently attempted the combined use of vascular bundle implantation with triscaphe arthrodesis (fusion of the scaphoid, trapezium, and trapezoid) as reported by Watson and Ryu [6]. The combined surgical procedures were applied to 21 cases of Kienböck's disease (chiefly stage IIIB). Although the follow-up period for these cases is not long enough to draw valid conclusions, the results obtained so far are excellent. The following are the results in our 18 patients who were followed-up for more than 1 year.

Patients and Methods

Fifteen of the patients were males and 3 were females. The right hand was involved in 9 cases and the left in 9, 11 of which occurred in the dominant hand. The age of the patients at operation ranged from 20 to 54 years (average 39 years). The periods from onset to surgery varied from 4 months to 5 years (average 16 months). Four patients were categorized according to Lichtman's criteria [7] as being in stage IIIA, thirteen in IIIB, and one in IV. There was ulna minus variance in 1, zero in 13, and plus in 4. The follow-up periods ranged from 12 to 58 months (average 31 months) (Table 1).

Triscaphe arthrodesis according to the method of Watson and Ryu [6] was performed in 16 patients and the tentative triscaphe arthrodesis procedure using C-wire percutaneous pinning was performed in 2 patients in stage IIIA. Of the 18

Table 1. Patients and affected wrists

18 Patients (male: 15, female: 3)
Age: 20–54 years (average 39 years)
Right: 9, left: 9 (dominant: 11)
Interval from onset to surgery 4 months–5 years (average, 16 months)
Stage according to Lichtman (n, % of total) I (0, 0%)
II (0, 0%)
IIIA (4, 22%)
IIIB (13, 72%)
IV (1, 6%)
Ulnar variance (n, % of total) MINUS (1, 6%)
NULL (13, 72%)
PLUS (4, 22%)
Follow-up: 12–58 months (average, 31 months)

Table 2. Surgical results

Bone union[a]	15/16		(94%)
Pain (n, % of total) Disappeared			(11, 61%)
Relieved			(7, 39%)
Unchanged			(0, 0%)
Increased			(0, 0%)
	Preop.	Postop.	
ROM Flexion	32.2° →	32.2°	
Extension	38.9° →	42.8°	
	71.1°	75.0°	
Grip power	19.5 kg → 30.0 kg		

ROM, Range of motion; *Preop.*, preoperative; *Postop.*, postoperative
[a] Except for 2 cases treated with tentative triscaphe arthrodesis

patients, 8 underwent one-stage excision of the radial styloid process [8].

Results

Bone union was achieved in 15 out of 16 cases (94%). Pain disappeared completely in 11 cases. Four patients complained of wrist pain after hard work, but the degree of pain was not marked. Of these four patients, one had tenderness on the mid-wrist joint and the remaining three had tenderness on the styloid process. The postoperative range of motion of the wrist was slightly increased, from 71° to 75° on average. The grip power improved in all patients, from 19.4 to 30.0 kg on average (Table 2).

On X-ray evaluations, the vertical height of the lunate was seen to increase in 4 patients, decrease in 3, and was unchanged in 11. The mean carpal height ratio for all cases remained unchanged

Table 3. Postoperative X-ray findings (18 cases)

Vertical height Preop. (average)	36.4 (22–47)
Postop. (average)	35.7 (26–45)
Increased	4 (22%)
Unchanged	11 (61%)
decreased	3 (17%)
Carpal height ratio Preop. (average)	0.497
(according to Youm) Postop. (average)	0.494
Increased	3 (17%)
Unchanged	13 (72%)
Decreased	2 (11%)
Scapholunate angle Preop.	59.4° (48°–72°)
Postop.	51.2° (37°–58°)

Preop., Preoperative; *Postop.*, postoperative

(0.497 before the operation and 0.494 afterwards), although 3 cases showed an increase and another 2 showed a decrease in this parameter. The mean scapholunate angle improved from 59.4° to 51.2° (Table 3). Trabecular structures of the lunate improved in 12 cases (67%). In only 1 case was segmentation of the lunate accelerated post-operatively. Osteoarthritic changes between the radial styloid and the scaphoid were observed in three patients who did not undergo excision of the styloid process. Styloidectomy was performed in one of them 9 months after the initial operation and resulted in satisfactory relief of pain.

Representative Cases

Case 1

This 24-year-old male right-handed manual worker had been suffering from right wrist pain for 10 months before presenting to our clinic. Examination revealed swelling on the dorsum of the wrist and decrease of the range of motion (35° of flexion and 40° of extension). Grip power in the affected wrist was 30 kg compared to 42 kg for the normal one. On the preoperative roentgeno-grams, there was a marked collapse of the lunate

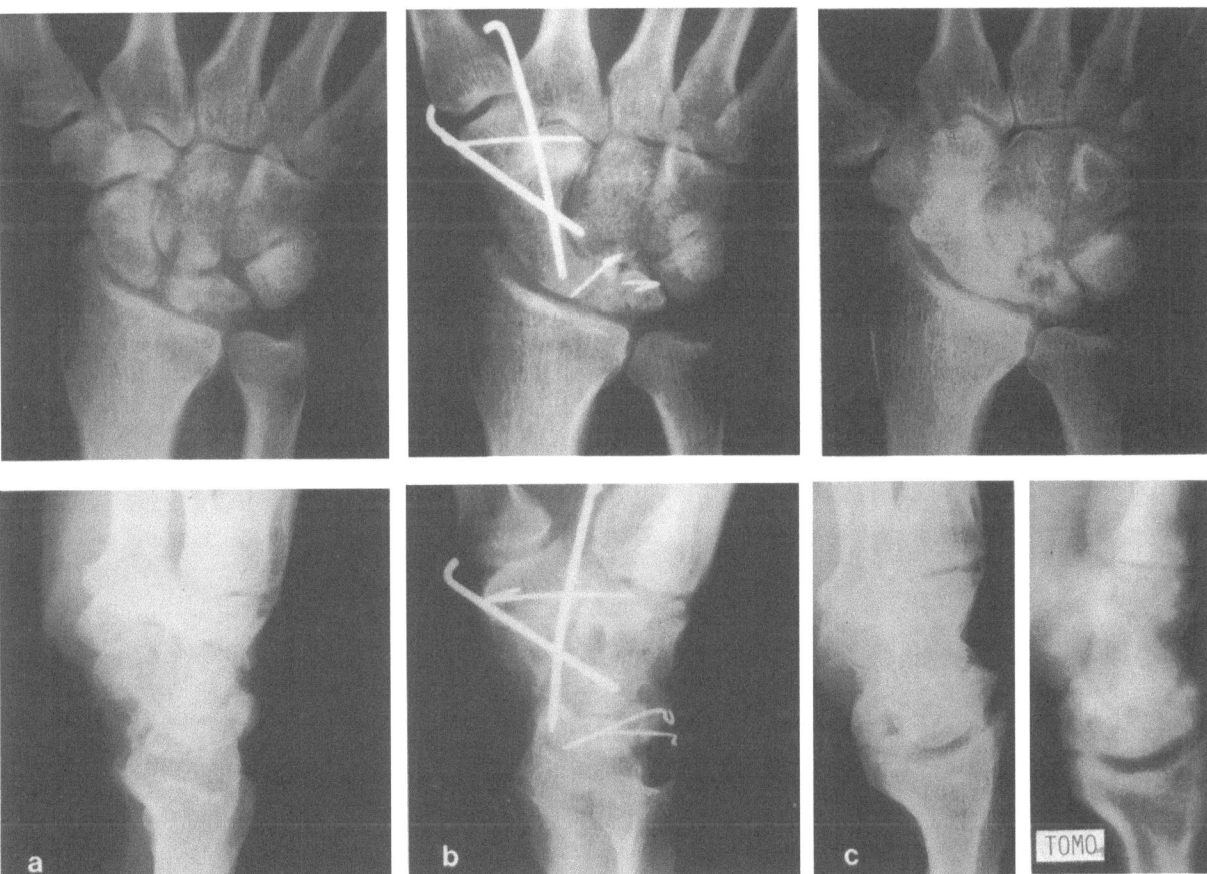

Fig. 1. Case 1, 24-year-old male, stage IIIB. **a** Preoperative view. **b** 2 Months after surgery. **c** 3 Years 6 months after surgery

with fragmentation, and the carpal height ratio was decreased to 0.491 (Fig. 1.a). Curettage of necrotized bone, cancellous bone graft from the ilium, vascular bundle implantation and triscaphe arthrodesis were performed on July 2, 1987 (Fig. 1.b). C-wires were removed 13 weeks postoperatively.

At 3 years 11 months postoperatively, the total wrist range of motion was 65° and the grip power was 40 kg. The patient was completely relieved from pain. The roentgenograms showed that the sclerosis had disappeared and that the trabecular architecture had improved; however an osteo-arthritic change was detected on the styloid process. The vertical height increased from 24 to 27 according to the Stähl index, and the carpal index increased from 0.491 to 0.524 (Fig. 1.c).

Case 2

This 45-year-old male right-handed public worker had been suffering from right wrist pain since January, 1987. He had received conservative treatment at another hospital, but the pain could

not be relieved. When he came to our clinic, he complained of severe motion pain at the right wrist joint and tenderness with slight swelling was present on the dorsum of the wrist. The flexion/extension of the wrist joint was 20°/20° and the grip power was decreased to 15 kg compared to that of 52 kg on the left. The roentgenograms revealed marked sclerosis and cystic changes of the lunate, with a slight fracture in the volar aspect of the lunate (Fig. 2.a).

At 2 years 6 months postoperatively, wrist motion increased to 45° in flexion and 45° in extension. The pain was entirely relieved. X-ray evaluations showed that the vertical height of the lunate had slightly increased (from 29 to 30), and that the scapholunate angle had also improved (from 70° to 43°) (Fig. 2.c).

Case 3

This 33-year-old male left-handed physical education teacher had complained of left wrist pain for 1 year 4 months. There was no history of trauma. On the first examination, left wrist

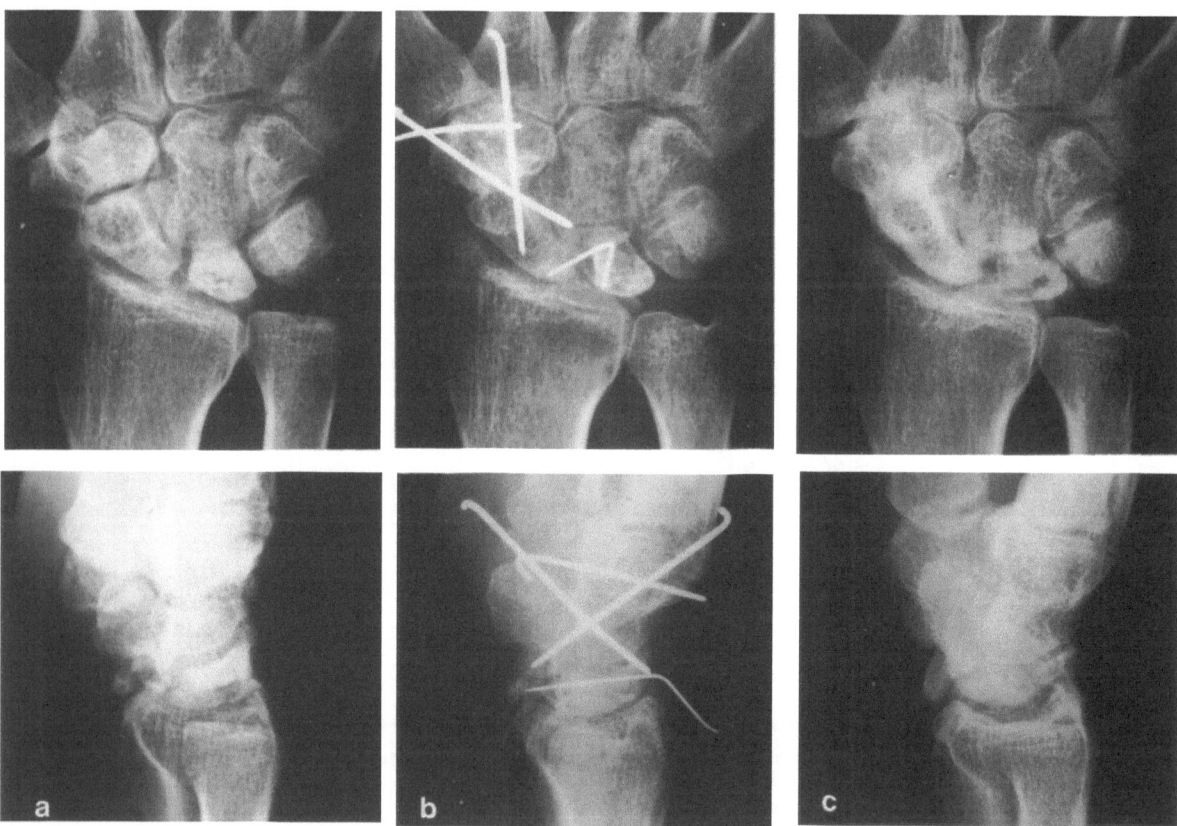

Fig. 2. Case 2, 45-year-old male, stage IIIB. **a** Preoperative view. **b** 2 Months after surgery. **c** 2 Years 6 months after surgery

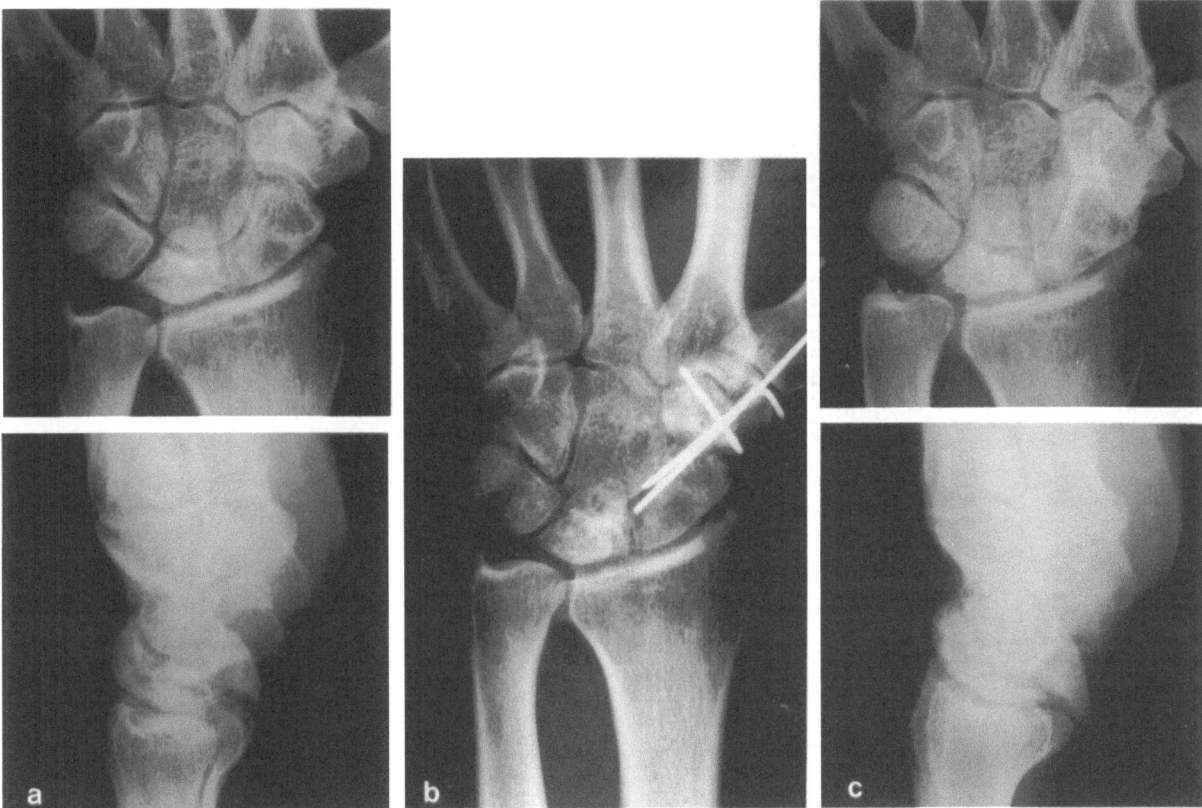

Fig. 3. Case 3, 35-year-old male, stage IIIB. **a** Preoperative view. **b** 2 Months after surgery. **c** 3 Years after surgery

motion had decreased to 30° in flexion and 45° in extension compared to the normal wrist. Conservative treatment was carried out for 2 months, but relief of pain could not be obtained. Vascular bundle implantation and triscaphe arthrodesis were performed on February 19, 1988 (Fig. 3.b).

At 3 years postoperatively, the total wrist range of motion was 75° (unchanged), and grip power was 28 kg (compared to 33 kg on the right side). He had no pain even after sports activities and returned to his original job. X-ray evaluation showed that bone union of the lunate had been obtained. The scapholunate angle improved from 52° to 40°, and carpal height was preserved at 0.50 (Fig. 3.c).

Case 4

This 49-year-old female right-handed factory worker had complained of right wrist pain for 1 month. Clinical examination revealed severe tenderness on the lunate. The total range of

motion of the wrist was 120° compared to that of 160°, on the left and grip power was 18 kg (the left being 20 kg). Preoperative roentgenograms showed a sclerotic change of the lunate without marked collapse (Fig. 4). MRI revealed that there was low signal intensity of the lunate on the T1- and T2-weighted images. A dorsal wrist splint had been applied for 2 months, but the wrist pain continued. Vascular bundle implantation and tentative triscaphe arthrodesis were performed on April 12, 1990. After curettage of the necrotized bone, cancellous bone graft and vascular bundle implantation were carried out, and tentative fixation of the trapezium, trapezoid, and scaphoid was performed with C-wire percutaneous pinning. The C-wires were removed 6 months postoperatively.

At 1 year 2 months postoperatively, the total wrist range of motion was 110° and grip power was 23 kg. She was relieved of pain and there was no residual tenderness. Postoperative roentgenograms showed that the trabecular structures of the lunate had improved, and the

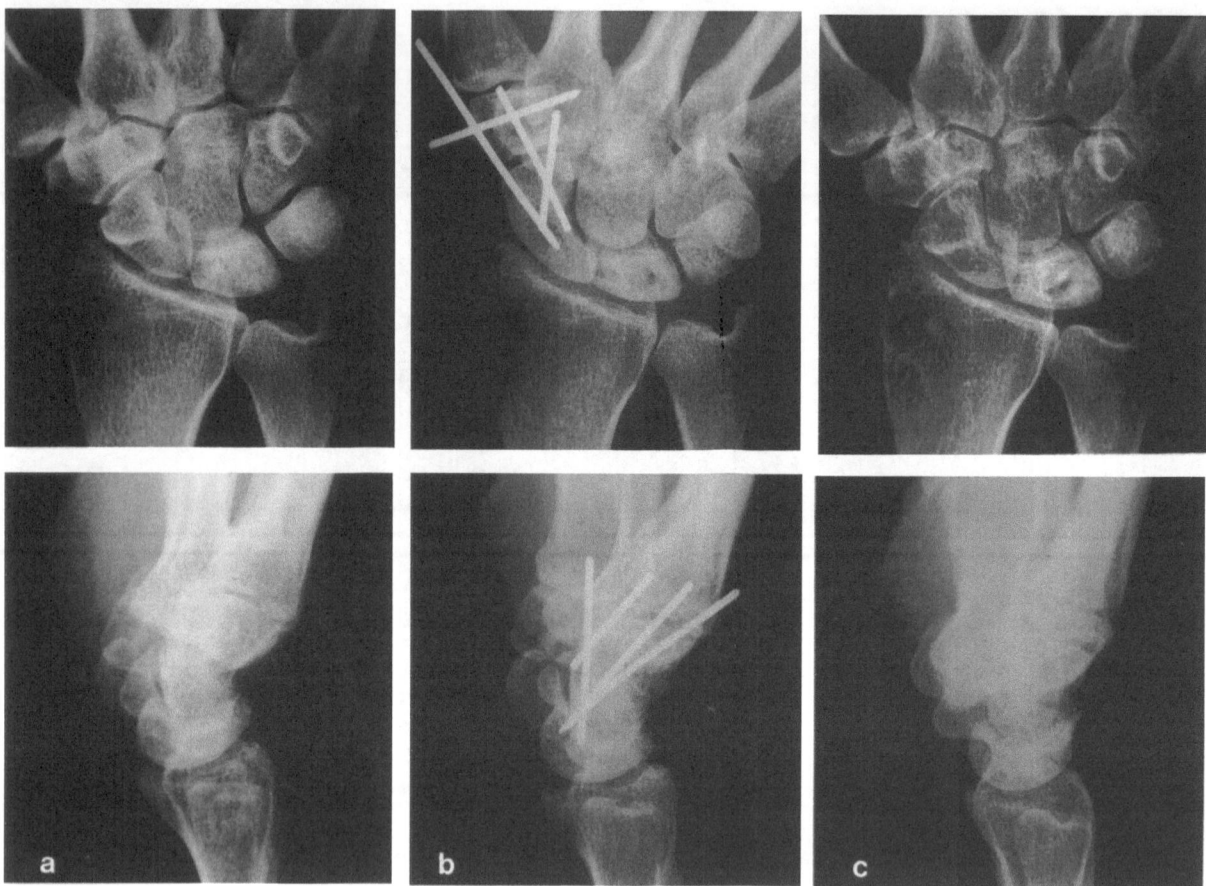

Fig. 4. Case 4, 46-year-old female, stage IIIA. **a** Preoperative view. **b** Percutaneous pinning of the triscaphe joint. **c** 1 Year after surgery

vertical height of the lunate was preserved even after removal of the wires.

Discussion

Various surgical procedures have been applied in treating Kienböck's disease. These procedures can be roughly divided into 4 groups (Table 4). The first group (biological approach) is represented by the vascular bundle implantation adopted by us [2–5]. Other methods in this group include implantation of a part of the radius together with the pronator quadratus muscle [9] and pedicle grafting of the dorsal metacarpal artery and vein. Many reports have indicated that these methods were effective at a relatively early stage of the disease. Gelberman et al. [10] and Lichtman [7] both limited the indication of vascular bundle implantation to stage I, II, and IIIA cases. In our previous investigations, the

Table 4. Groups of surgical procedures for Kienböcks disease

1. Biological approach
   Vascular bundle implantation
   Vascularized bone graft
   Muscle pedicled bone graft
2. Biomechanical approach
   Radial shortening
   Ulnar lengthening
   Radius wedged osteotomy
   Limited wrist arthrodesis
3. Replacement/resection arthroplasty
   Artificial lunate replacement
   Soft tissue replacement
   Proximal row carpectomy
4. Total wrist arthrodesis

results of this procedure were also excellent in cases of stage II, but some cases of stage IIIB or IV showed progression of osteoarthritic changes or collapse of the lunate postoperatively. After analysis of these previous results, we attempted to expand the lunate during implantation of cancellous bone and to apply a distraction force with an external skeletal fixation device after the operation. This attempt achieved excellent results in the clinical and X-ray evaluations for stages III and IV after the operation. The details of our method were presented at the 61st annual meeting of the Japanese Orthopedic Association (1988). However, a problem with this method is that the external skeletal fixation device cannot be applied for more than 2 months without disturbing wrist motion. One half of the cases developed lunate collapse after removal of the fixation device, although there was no case whose VH decreased more than that of preoperative results [11]. The high incidence of lunate collapse after removal of the fixation device suggests that the distraction apparatus could work on the carpal bones only temporarily for lessening the vertical pressure, and that it could not improve the malaligment of the carpal bones. This suggestion was borne out in our experiments using rats [4, 5]. In these experiments, vascularization from the implanted vascular bundle was seen soon after implantation, but a longer period of time was required for new bone formation. Based on these results, we believe that this method needs to be combined with some other biomechanical method in advanced Kienböck's disease. The

biomechanical approach categorized in the second group, such as radius shortening or ulnar lengthening, aims at decompressing the diseased lunate by rerouting the stress on the wrist joint to the ulnar side (Fig. 5, left) [12]. This approach came into use after Haltén [13] mentioned the negative ulnar variant as a possible cause for Kienböck's disease. However, the negative ulnar variant was found not to be common in Japanese patients, and ulnocarpal abutment syndrome can develop postoperatively with this approach. In the past, radiolunate or capitolunate fusion was used for partial fusion of the wrist joint, but these methods seem to be used only in special cases at present, and are rather indicated when arthrosis is present around the lunate (it seems more appropriate to allocate them to the third group of procedures). Triscaphe arthrodesis is a representative technique among partial wrist fusions. Its application to Kienböck's disease was probably first reported by Watson and Ryu [6]. This technique aims at decompressing the lunate by shifting the stress towards the radial carpal bones (Fig. 5, right). It can also prevent the radiocarpal arthrosis which is secondary to rotary subluxation of the scaphoid following lunate collapse. Rogers and Watson [8] reported on radial styloid impingement as a problem incurred with this technique. A similar change was also disclosed by X-ray evaluation in 3 of our cases. One of these

Fig. 5a,b. Schematic representation of **a** radial shortening. Advantages include good range of motion, but their is the disadvantage of osteoarthritis due to rotary subluxation of the scaphoid. **b** Schematic representation of triscaphe arthrodesis. This is an effective treatment for rotary subluxation of the scaphoid, but results in only limited range of motion and radial styloid impingement. *Arrows,* pathway for rerouting stress

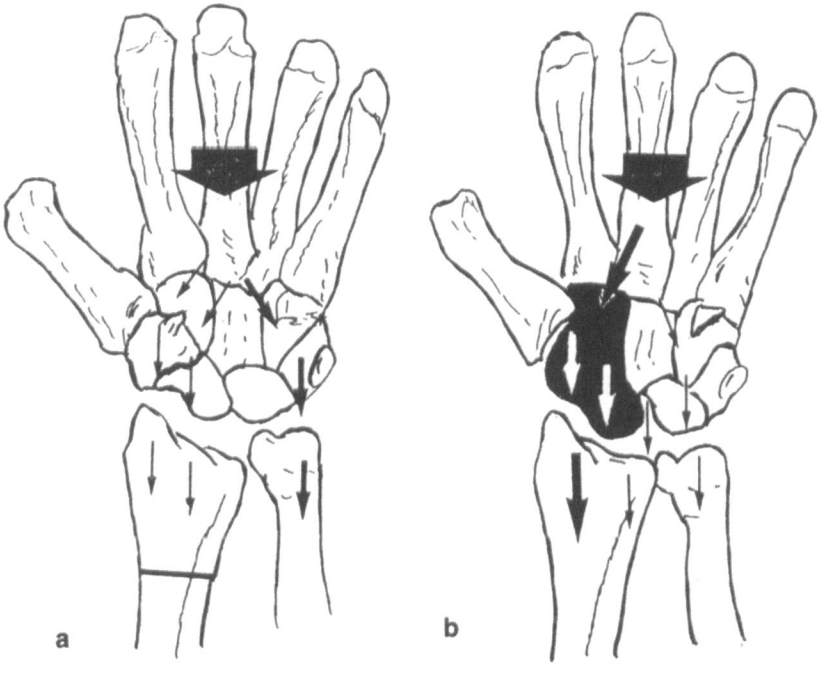

patients underwent excision of the radial styloid process after the initial operation and this led to the improvement of clinical symptoms. More recently, we have applied a one-stage excision of the styloid process to solve this problem. In any event, this problem should be studied more in depth through long-term follow-up of the surgically treated patients. As a new technique of triscaphe arthrodesis, we recently attempted tentative triscaphe arthrodesis with wire fixation in two cases of stage IIIA simultaneously with vascular bundle implantation. With this technique, the triscaphe joint was tentatively fixed with C-wires in the position of slight dorsiflexion of the scaphoid, in order to decompress the lunate. The wires were withdrawn 4–6 months later. This technique does not involve the risk of causing radial styloid impingement syndrome and can preserve wrist motion. Hence, this technique deserves trial application on stage IIIA cases. Other reported methods for limited wrist arthrodesis include capitoscaphoid fusion and capitohamate fusion. Of these two methods, the former seems to have a similar purpose and surgical effect as does triscaphe arthrodesis, because similar results were obtained in a dynamic study using amputated extremities [14]. The latter method aims at transferring the stress on the capitate to the hamate, triquetrum, and ulna. However, the results from dynamic experiments suggest that this method is almost ineffective [14].

The third group (excision and arthroplasty) seems to be indicated in cases of advanced Kienböck's disease. Finally, there is the fourth group which includes total wrist fusion techniques is selected in the most advanced cases. Each of these methods has been reported by many investigators and have both advantages and disadvantages.

We have been principally using vascular bundle implantation for the treatment of Kienböck's disease so that the lunate can be preserved, or rather revitalized, as far as possible. We extended our criteria for the indication of vascular bundle implantation, combining it with triscaphe arthrodesis. Although the follow-up period after the combined operation is still short, the results obtained thus far have been favorable. In recent years, artificial materials tend to be widely used not only in the field of hand surgery but also in other orthopedic fields. Pathological joints and bones are excised without careful consideration, and Swanson-type implants are frequently used for the treatment of Kienböck's disease. However, because the artificial materials currently available involve many problems, we should select the method that allows us to preserve the affected bone or joint as much as possible. It seems best to limit the use of artificial materials to cases for which there are no other possible therapeutic means.

Summary

Vascular bundle implantation with triscaphe arthrodesis was performed simultaneously in 18 cases of Kienböck's disease, staged from IIIA to IV, and clinically excellent results were obtained throughout, with an average follow-up period of 2 years 7 months.

X-ray evaluation showed that the vertical height of the lunate was maintained in 15 cases, and that the scapholunate angle improved in all cases.

Osteoarthritic changes between the radial styloid and the scaphoid after triscaphe arthrodesis were observed in 3 cases, and one-stage styloidectomy was considered to be effective for the prevention of osteoarthrosis.

References

1. Kienböck R (1910) Über traumatishe Malazie des Mondbeins und ihre Folgezustande: Entrtungsformen und Kompressions fracturen. Fortschr Rontgenstr 16:77–103
2. Hori Y, Tamai S, Okuda H, Sakamoto H, Takita T, Masuhara K (1979) Blood vessel transplantation to bone. J Hand Surg [Am] 4:23–33
3. Tamai S, Hori H, Fujiwara H (1987) Treatment of avascular necrosis of lunate and other bones by vascular bundle transplantation. In: Urbaniak JR (ed) Microsurgery for major limb reconstruction. Mosby, St Louis, pp 209–219
4. Yajima H, Tamai S, Mizumoto S, Nakata K, Hori Y (1987) Treatment of Kienböck's disease with vascular bundle implantation: Experimental and clinical studies. J Jpn Soc Surg Hand 4:332–336
5. Yajima H, Tamai S, Mizumoto S, Shono M, Masuhara (1989) Experimental study on secondary living bone graft: Method of creating new donor by vascular bundle implantation to isolated bone. J Jpn Orthop Assoc 63:539–548
6. Watson HK, Ryu J (1985) An approach to Kienböck's disease: Triscaphe arthrodesis. J Hand Surg [Am] 10:179–187

7. Lichtman DM (1988) The wrist and its disorders, 1st edn. Saunders, Philadelphia, pp 329–343

8. Rogers WD, Watson HK (1989) Radial styloid impingement after triscaphe arthrodesis. J Hand Surg [Am] 14:297–301

9. Braun RM (1984) Visible pedicle bone grafting in the wrist. In: Urbaniak JR (ed) Microsurgery for major limb reconstruction. Mosby, St Louis, pp 220–229

10. Gelberman RH, Szabo RM (1984) Kienböck's disease. Orthop Clin North Am 15:355–367

11. Yajima H, Tamai S (1988) Vascular bundle implantation for the treatment of Kienböck's disease. J Jpn Orthop Assoc 62:S973

12. Palmer AK, Werner FW (1984) Biomechanics of the distal radioulnar joint. Clin Orthop 187:26–35

13. Hultén O (1928) Über anatomische Variationen der Handgelenk-knochen. Acta Radiol 9:155–168

14. Trumble T, Glisson RR, Seaber AV, Urbaniak JR (1986) A biomechanical comparison of the methods for treating Kienböck's disease. J Hand Surg [Am] 11:88–93

Radial Shortening and Radial Wedge Osteotomy for Kienböck's Disease

Ryogo Nakamura, Satoshi Tsuge, Kentaro Watanabe, and Kenji Tsunoda[1]

Abstract. A radial wedge osteotomy with reduction of the inclination angle of the distal radius was performed in 27 patients with Kienböck's disease; radial shortening was performed in 23 patients. The results of the former are comparable, if not superior, to those of the latter. Radial wedge osteotomy yielded clinically satisfactory results in 25 out of 27 patients and radial shortening in 19 of 23 patients. Unlike radial shortening, radial wedge osteotomy unloaded the lunate by redistributing the axial load only to the radio-scaphoid joint without increasing the load on the ulnocarpal joint. Therefore, radial wedge osteotomy is believed to be preferable to radial shortening for Kienböck's disease with zero or positive ulnar variance.

Keywords: Kienböck's disease — Radial shortening — Radial wedge osteotomy — Ulnar variance — Radial inclination — Osteotomy

Introduction

Among the surgical methods currently used for treating Kienböck's disease, those best known for reducing the axial load on the lunate are radial shortening [1–7] and ulnar lengthening [8, 9]. The clinical results of these techniques have been reported by many authors, and lunate decompression has been confirmed by biomechanical analysis [11]. On the other hand, Tsumura et al. proposed radial wedge osteotomy as another surgical procedure which would reduce the axial load on the lunate [12]. They analyzed the biomechanics by using a rigid body spring model and demonstrated that the load through the lunate is reduced and the load through the scaphoid is increased by reducing the angle of radial inclination of the radius [13, 14].

Radial shortening has been the treatment of choice for Kienböck's disease at Nagoya University Hospital since 1975, and results have been favorable compared to Graner's method [15] and tendon replacement arthroplasty [16], which had been performed previously [17]. However, some patients have complained of postoperative ulnar wrist pain. As it was believed that ulnar wrist pain was caused by ulnocarpal abutment syndrome and disorders of the distal radioulnar joint secondary to a relative lengthening of the ulna, our surgical approach was modified in 1983 as follows: (1) radial shortening was limited to less than 3 mm, and (2) a radial wedge osteostomy was performed in patients with zero or positive ulnar variance at risk for postoperative ulnar wrist pain.

Recently, we have performed a radial wedge osteotomy together with radial shortening in this group of patients. This paper reports our results and discusses the effectiveness and usefulness of radial wedge osteotomy in comparison with radial shortening in terms of both symptoms and radiographic findings.

Patients and Methods

Osteotomy of the radius was performed from 1975 to 1988 in 51 cases of Kienböck's disease. This review includes 50 patients who were followed for at least 1 year. Radial wedge osteotomy was performed in 27 cases and radial shortening in 23 cases. Twenty-five males and two females, ranging in age from 14 to 54 years (average 32

[1] Department of Orthopaedic Surgery, Division of Hand Surgery, Branch Hospital of Nagoya University, School of Medicine, 1-1-20 Daikominami, Higashi-ku, Nagoya 461, Japan

Table 1. Patient data

Case no.	Sex	Age (years)	Ulnar variance (mm) (amount of shortening)	Amount of radial deviation of the distal radius (degrees)[a]	Stage	Wrist pain preop./postop.[b]	Range of motion: flexion-extension (degrees) preop./postop.	Grip strength (kg) preop./postop. (unaffected side)	Ståhl's index preop./postop.[c]	Carpal height ratio preop./postop. (unaffected side)	Results Lichtman's criteria	Results Outcome (score)	Follow-up (months)
A. Radial wedge osteotomy													
1	Male	24	0 (0)	7	IV	+/±	85/111	43/42 (55)	38/38	0.58/0.55 (0.58)	satisfactory	good (18)	28
2	Male	25	1 (1.5)	8	II	+/±	116/125	40/49 (49)	40/37	0.51/0.48 (0.52)	satisfactory	fair (15)	26
3	Male	34	1 (1)	10	II	+/±	82/130	35/41 (52)	38/38	0.50/0.50 (0.51)	satisfactory	good (19)	51
4	Male	34	0 (1)	8	II	+/±	80/85	19/38 (52)	33/32	0.55/0.54 (0.55)	satisfactory	fair (14)	47
5	Male	48	-1 (1)	6	II	++/±	97/95	15/31 (37)	35/30	0.57/0.54 (0.57)	satisfactory	fair (12)	36
6	Male	22	0 (1)	10	I	++/-	90/99	0/44 (45)	47/47	0.56/0.56 (0.56)	satisfactory	good (20)	25
7	Male	35	0 (0)	5	II	+/±	86/102	40/43 (54)	45/33	0.55/0.53 (0.55)	satisfactory	fair (16)	46
8	Male	21	-2 (2)	12	IV	+/±	82/112	14/31 (37)	41/33	0.52/0.52 (0.54)	satisfactory	good (18)	36
9	Male	23	-2 (2)	13	II	++/±	60/67	16/36 (54)	36/35	0.52/0.52 (0.57)	satisfactory	fair (15)	39
10	Female	42	1 (-2)	13	II	++/-	87/112	14/25 (34)	44/38	0.55/0.55 (0.57)	satisfactory	good (21)	61
11	Male	54	2 (0)	12	II	++/-	90/106	16/40 (42)	53/53	0.54/0.54 (0.54)	satisfactory	good (23)	38
12	Male	22	1 (0)	14	II	+/±	82/88	36/48 (57)	43/43	0.57/0.57 (0.57)	satisfactory	fair (16)	30
13	Male	22	0 (1)	15	II	++/-	75/112	24/36 (45)	45/45	0.52/0.53 (0.53)	satisfactory	excellent (27)	42
14	Male	22	1 (0)	11	III	+/-	94/128	45/50 (52)	35/22	0.57/0.57 (0.57)	satisfactory	excellent (24)	26
15	Male	40	2 (2)	7	II	++/±	60/88	36/48 (51)	27/27	0.51/0.49 (0.52)	satisfactory	good (19)	32
16	Male	24	0 (2)	14	IV	+/±	67/90	26/33 (47)	41/36	0.61/0.61 (0.63)	satisfactory	good (19)	25
17	Male	35	1 (2)	14	II	++/±	35/80	20/28 (34)	41/33	0.53/0.53 (0.56)	satisfactory	good (19)	27
18	Male	43	0 (2)	10	II	++/±	70/70	15/25 (40)	38/33	0.59/0.56 (0.59)	satisfactory	fair (12)	39
19	Female	14	-1 (0)	12	IV	+/±	52/93	25/27 (32)	13/15	0.48/0.48 (0.53)	unsatisfactory	good (23)	30
20	Male	46	3 (0)	8	IV	+/±	70/70	27/29 (38)	22/22	0.50/0.50 (0.54)	satisfactory	fair (12)	29
21	Male	24	2 (0)	6	II	+/±	85/98	39/38 (41)	38/38	0.51/0.51 (0.52)	satisfactory	good (19)	24
22	Male	38	2 (2)	9	II	++/±	95/98	31/28 (38)	38/38	0.57/0.55 (0.59)	unsatisfactory	fair (13)	28
23	Male	25	0 (1.5)	5	IV	+/±	100/110	34/40 (52)	43/36	0.56/0.55 (0.59)	satisfactory	fair (17)	26
24	Male	46	-1 (1)	8	III	++/-	76/83	33/34 (43)	24/24	0.52/0.52 (0.54)	satisfactory	fair (17)	26
25	Male	34	0 (2)	13	II	++/±	100/103	23/34 (43)	26/26	0.52/0.52 (0.53)	satisfactory	fair (13)	28
26	Male	40	1 (-1)	9	II	+/±	72/82	38/41 (52)	38/24	0.51/0.51 (0.52)	satisfactory	fair (16)	26
27	Male	33	5 (0)	10	II	+/±	113/120	31/42 (43)	40/30	0.50/0.50 (0.50)	satisfactory	good (18)	24
B. Radial shortening													
1	Male	35	2 (2)		II	+/-	100/110	20/37 (42)	36/36	0.54/0.52 (0.55)	Satisfactory	Good (20)	92
2	Male	37	1 (3)		II	+/±	65/63	20/25 (26)	38/33	0.50/0.50 (0.52)	Satisfactory	Fair (14)	21
3	Female	42	-2.5 (4.5)		IV	++/+	58/68	15/13 (27)	27/21	0.48/0.47 (0.51)	Unsatisfactory	Poor (10)	21
4	Female	25	0 (5)		I	+/±[d]	110/115	13/19 (29)	46/36	0.52/0.52 (0.53)	Satisfactory	Fair (15)	83
5	Male	23	2 (3)		IV	++/-	80/120	6/40 (43)	27/27	0.48/0.48 (0.53)	Satisfactory	Excellent (25)	77
6	Female	53	-1.5 (4.5)		IV	+/±	115/88	21/22 (16)	43/43	0.50/0.49 (0.53)	Unsatisfactory	Fair (14)	24
7	Male	21	1 (4.5)		IV	+/±[d]	75/68	21/34 (38)	25/32	0.50/0.49 (0.55)	Satisfactory	Fair (17)	127
8	Male	26	1 (5)		IV	+/±	75/86	30/31 (41)	43/41	0.53/0.55 (0.58)	Satisfactory	Good (18)	112

No.	Sex	Age		Stage	Pain[b]				CHR[c]			
9	Male	19	2 (1.5)	II	+/−	92/110	46/51 (57)	40/36	0.50/0.52 (0.52)	Satisfactory	Good (23)	81
10	Male	44	1 (8)	III	+/+[d]	107/75	20/29 (35)	12/21	0.53/0.52 (0.53)	Unsatisfactory	Fair (12)	102
11	Male	21	−1 (2)	IV	++/−	91/110	39/41 (47)	23/27	0.51/0.51 (0.54)	Satisfactory	Excellent (26)	94
12	Male	16	0 (2)	II	+/−	110/120	6/20 (22)	43/43	0.55/0.55 (0.55)	Satisfactory	Excellent (25)	12
13	Male	23	0 (1.5)	IV	+/±	73/85	25/29 (39)	23/26	0.47/0.50 (0.55)	Satisfactory	Excellent (24)	86
14	Male	27	−1 (2.5)	III	+/±	113/110	31/32 (40)	27/25	0.56/0.52 (0.55)	Satisfactory	Fair (13)	84
15	Female	37	0 (1)	IV	++/+	80/99	8/20 (26)	29/23	0.48/0.44 (0.54)	Unsatisfactory	Fair (12)	84
16	Male	21	0 (2.5)	II	++/−	55/132	16/47 (52)	36/36	0.51/0.51 (0.51)	Satisfactory	Excellent (24)	24
17	Male	29	0 (2.5)	IV	+/−	61/68	22/34 (32)	32/23	0.53/0.50 (0.57)	Satisfactory	Good (19)	75
18	Male	17	2 (1.5)	IV	+/−	78/108	42/49 (44)	29/33	0.50/0.55 (0.58)	Satisfactory	Excellent (30)	72
19	Male	26	−3 (3)	II	+/−	102/109	35/41 (49)	44/35	0.52/0.52 (0.54)	Satisfactory	Excellent (24)	72
20	Male	10	−3 (1.5)	IV	++/−	87/134	7/22 (21)	29/34	0.52/0.53 (0.56)	Satisfactory	Excellent (30)	54
21	Male	18	−2 (3)	II	+/±	85/128	31/38 (40)	42/40	0.52/0.52 (0.54)	Satisfactory	Excellent (30)	55
22	Female	16	−2.5 (2)	IV	++/±	84/146	7/26 (35)	24/22	0.50/0.50 (0.53)	Satisfactory	Fair (17)	47
23	Male	45	2 (3)	IV	+/±	82/88	43/42 (43)	30/30	0.56/0.56 (0.59)	Satisfactory	Good (19)	50

preop., Preoperative; *postop.*, postoperative
[a] Preoperative radial inclination angle minus postoperative radial inclination angle
[b] − No pain; ± mild pain with strenous activity; + mild pain with light work; ++ pain with daily use
[c] The ratio of the lunate height to width as measured on lateral radiograph
[d] Postoperative ulnar wrist pain

years), underwent radial wedge osteotomy. Eighteen males and five females, ranging in age from 10 to 53 years (average 27 years), underwent radial shortening (Table 1).

To avoid ambiguity regarding the disease stage, patients were classified according to Ståhl's index [18] and the carpal height ratio (CHR) [19]. Classification of patients according to Ståhl's index was: stage I, patients with an index of more than 45; stage II, an index from 30 to 44; and stage III, an index less than 30. Patients whose carpal height ratio (CHR) was less than 0.03, compared to the CHR of the normal side, were considered to have carpal collapse and classified as stage IV regardless of Ståhl's index. Patients with extensive osteoarthritic change of the wrist were defined as being in stage V. The 27 patients who underwent radial wedge osteotomy included stage I, 1 case; stage II, 18 cases; stage III, 2 cases, and stage IV, 6 cases. Twenty-three patients who underwent radial shortening included stage I, 1 case; stage II, 7 cases; stage III, 2 cases; and stage IV, 13 cases. Thus, many of the patients who underwent radial shortening had more advanced disease.

Surgical Procedure

An 8-cm longitudinal skin incision was made on the radial aspect of the forearm, centered on the distal one-fourth of the radius. The distal radius was exposed between the tendons of the brachioradialis and extensor carpi radialis, taking care to protect the sensory branch of the radial nerve. A step-cut osteotomy [20] was carried out in the distal one-fourth of the radius by the same surgical technique in both kinds of osteotomies. The long axis of the osteotomy was parallel to the anterior aspect of the forearm. The distal and proximal ends of the osteotomy were resected according to the amount of shortening or degree of angulation desired. Efforts were made to achieve 10°–15° of radial flexion of the radius during radial wedge osteotomy, and not to increase ulnar variance by resecting the trapezoidal bone segment with radial and ulnar heights of 5 and 2mm, respectively, instead of a wedge-shaped section of bone. When radial shortening was done, bone segments 3mm in height were resected from the both ends of the radius. The osteotomized radius was fixed internally with 2 or 3 screws (Figs. 1, 2), and the forearm and wrist were immobilized postoperatively with a plaster cast for about 8 weeks.

a   c   e

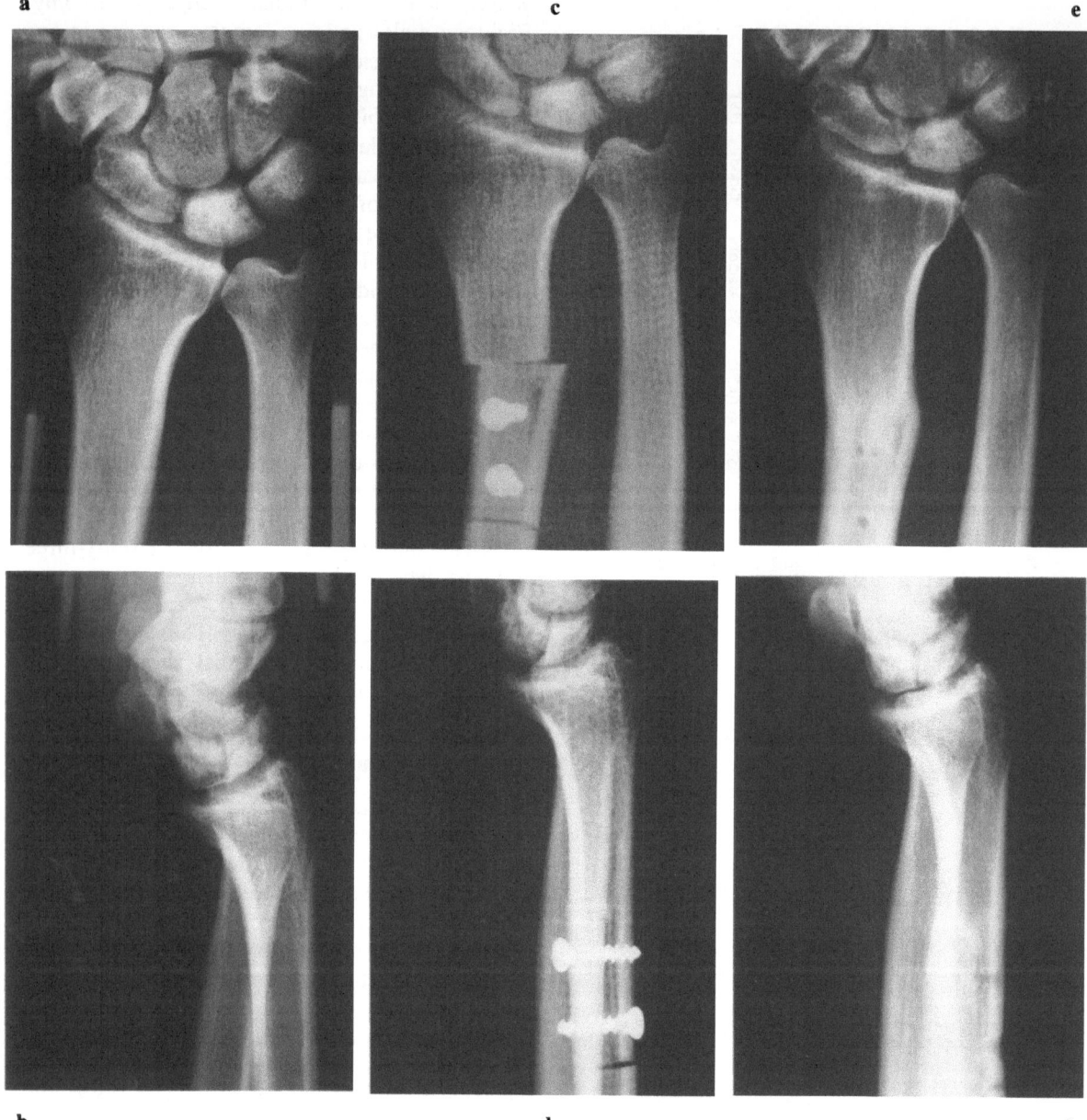

b   d   f

Fig. 1. Radial wedge osteotomy. A 22-year-old male employee in an automobile manufacturing plant complained of right wrist pain after operating a pneumatic impact wrench for 8 months. **a, b** Preoperative radiographs show sclerosis and cystic changes of the lunate. Flattening and fracture of the lunate can be seen in the lateral view. **c, d** Early postoperative radiographs taken with the wrist in a plaster cast show the operative procedure of radial wedge osteotomy utilizing a step-cut technique. **e, f** Postoperative radiographs taken 29 months after surgery demonstrate favorable remodeling of the lunate

The follow-up time was from 1 to 4 years (average 2 years 5 months) after radial wedge osteotomy and from 1 year to 10 years and 7 months (average 5 years 6 months) after radial shortening.

Wrist pain, range of motion for flexion and extension, and grip strength were assessed, and Lichtman's criteria [21] were used to evaluate the postoperative results. Post-operative radiographic findings of the lunate, including sclerotic changes, cystic changes, and fragmentation, were compared to the preoperative findings. Results were classified as "improved", "unchanged", or aggravated. Ståhl's index and the carpal height

a c e

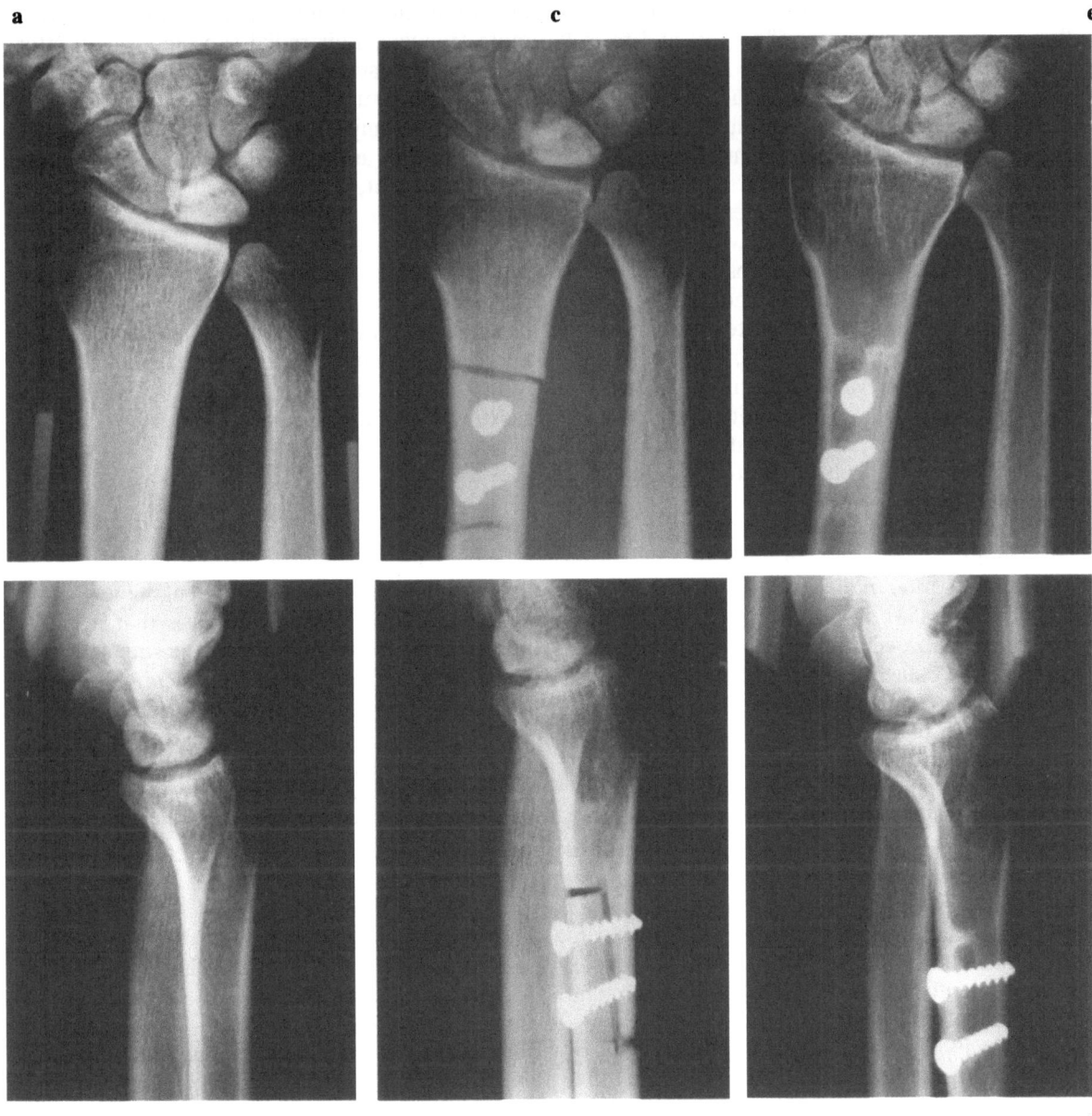

b d f

Fig. 2. Radial shortening. A 25-year-old male who had used a pneumatic wrench for 4 years. **a, b** Pre-operative radiographs showing sclerosis and flattening of the lunate. Cystic change of the lunate can be seen in the lateral view. **c, d** Early postoperative radiographs showing radial shortening by the step-cut osteotomy. **e, f** Radiographs taken 30 months after surgery showing the reconstituted lunate

ratio (CHR) were also measured postoperatively. Clinical and radiographic results were judged by the scoring system we devised [22].

Results

The postoperative course was uneventful in all but three patients who underwent radial wedge osteotomy and one patient who underwent radial shortening. Screw loosening in the cast was found 1 month after surgery in two patients who had the radial wedge procedure, and they required cast immobilization for 4 months in order to obtain a solid bony union. One patient complained of persistent neuralgia in the distribution of the radial sensory nerve. One patient, who underwent radial shortening, experienced a delayed union, but healing occurred after 5 months with no further problems.

Radial wedge osteotomy resulted in radial flexion of the radius from 5° to 15°, and from 0 to 2 mm of shortening. The average radial flexion was 10.0° ± 3.0°, and the average radial shortening was 0.8 mm. The radius was shortened from 1 to 8 mm (average 3 mm) by the radial shortening procedure.

Wrist pain improved postoperatively with no or mild pain on strenous activity in all cases (100%) following radial wedge osteotomy, and in 20 cases (87%) after radial shortening. Three patients treated by radial shortening developed ulnar wrist pain postoperatively. All three had a preoperative ulnar variance of more than 0 mm and had undergone radial shortening of more than 4 mm. One patient treated with radial shortening required ulnar shortening to relieve ulnar wrist pain.

Fourteen patients (52%) experienced an improvement of more than 10° in flexion-extension of the wrist after radial wedge osteotomy, and 14 patients (61%) did so after radial shortening. The mean improvement was similar for the two procedures, being 17° with radial wedge osteotomy and 16° with radial shortening. Improved grip strength of more than 5 kg was recorded in 19 patients (79%) after radial wedge osteotomy and in 16 patients (70%) after radial shortening. The percent increase in grip strength, compared to unaffected side, was 19% and 27% with radial wedge osteotomy and radial shortening, respectively. When the results were evaluated by Lichtman's criteria, 25 cases (93%) were rated as being satisfactory following radial wedge osteotomy and 19 (83%) following radial shortening.

Ståhl's index, which indicates the degree of flattening of the lunate, increased in 1 case (4%) by radial wedge osteotomy and in 6 cases (26%) by radial shortening. This indicator decreased in 14 cases (52%) by radial wedge osteotomy and in 16 cases (48%) by radial shortening. The CHR increased in 1 case (4%) by radial wedge osteotomy and in 5 cases (22%) by radial shortening. It decreased in 9 cases (33%) by radial wedge osteotomy and in 8 cases (35%) by radial shortening. Radiographically, sclerosis of the lunate was improved in 12 cases (44%) after radial wedge osteotomy and in 11 cases (48%) after radial shortening; cystic changes improved in 10 cases (37%) and 14 cases (67%), respectively (Figs. 1, 2), while fragmentation improved in 3 cases (11%) and in 10 cases (43%), respectively. Improvements in radiographic findings and measurements of the lunate architecture were more frequent after radial shortening than after radial wedge osteotomy, and deterioration of the lunate architecture was more frequent after radial wedge osteotomy (Table 2).

The results as judged by the scoring system were: excellent, 2 cases; good, 12 cases; fair, 13 cases after radial wedge osteotomy, and excellent, 9 cases; good, 4 cases; fair, 8 cases; and poor, 1 case after radial shortening. There was no difference in the percentage of cases rated as excellent or good, but more patients achieved an excellent result by radial shortening than by radial wedge osteotomy (Table 1). The average score was 17.6 after radial wedge osteotomy and 19.7 after radial shortening.

Discussion

Radial shortening and ulnar lengthening were predicated on Hultén's hypothesis that negative ulnar variance is a major predisposing factor to Kienböck's disease. Radial shortening has also been thought of as an equivalent to ulnar lengthening both in principle and in clinical effect [7]. Biomechanically, radial shortening is believed to redistribute the axial load through the lunate to the radioscaphoid and ulnocarpal joints, as suggested by Perrson [8]. This effect has been confirmed in vitro by Trumble et al. [11], Palmer et al. [23, 24], and Horii et al. [25]. Although both procedures are effective by achieving a decompression effect of the lunate, even in patients with zero or positive variance, radial shortening is believed to be an appropriate surgical procedure for Kienböck's disease with negative ulnar variance. Unlike the cases described in most previous reports, more than one-half of the wrists with Kienböck's disease in our series showed zero or positive variance. In addition, some patients with positive variance of our series who were treated with radial shortening later developed ulnar wrist pain caused by ulnocarpal abutment syndrome. These factors led us to seek an osteotomy other than radial shortening or ulnar lengthening.

In 1982, Tsumura showed that radial wedge osteotomy with reduction of the radial inclination angle unloads the lunate by increasing the load on the radioscaphoid joint without increasing the load on the ulnocarpal joint [12]. We were encouraged by the results of his experimental study and started to treat our cases using radial wedge

Table 2. Postoperative radiographic findings

Procedure	Sclerotic change			Cystic change			Fragmentation			Ståhl's index[a]			Carpal height ratio		
	Improved	Unchanged	Exacerbated	Improved	Unchanged	Exacerbated	Improved	Unchanged	Exacerbated	Increased	Unchanged	Decreased	Increased	Unchanged	Decreased
Lateral closing osteotomy (n)	12 (44%)	9 (33%)	6 (23%)	10 (37%)	8 (30%)	9 (33%)	3 (11%)	16 (59%)	8 (30%)	1 (4%)	12 (44%)	14 (52%)	1 (4%)	17 (63%)	9 (33%)
Radial shortening (n)	11 (48%)	7 (30%)	5 (22%)	14 (61%)	8 (35%)	1 (4%)	10 (43%)	9 (39%)	4 (17%)	6 (26%)	6 (26%)	11 (48%)	5 (22%)	10 (43%)	8 (35%)

[a] The ratio of the lunate height to width as measured on lateral radiograph

osteotomy. Although some workers have questioned the value of radial wedge osteotomy with reduction of radial inclination angle on the bases of experimental studies using pressure-sensitive film [23, 24], and have supported the achievement of the decompression effect by radial wedge osteotomy with increase of radial inclination angle [26], our clinical results were satisfactory in most patients, with relief of wrist pain, improved wrist range of motion, and grip strength.

Unlike radial shortening, radial wedge osteotomy did not increase the axial load applied to the ulnocarpal joint. Therefore, there is no risk of inducing ulnocarpal abutment syndrome, which is sometimes noted after radial shortening. In fact, of the 27 patients who underwent radial wedge osteotomy, none developed ulnar wrist pain.

Because the 2 treatment groups differed in age distribution, stage of illness, and follow-up time, it is not possible to determine which type of radial osteotomy is preferable based on the minor differences observed here. For example, radiographic improvements of the lunate architecture were greater with radial shortening than with radial wedge osteotomy. Therefore, judged by the scoring system, more patients achieved an excellent result by radial shortening than by radial wedge osteotomy. However, this difference in radiographic results may be ascribable to a higher mean age, shorter follow-up time, or a deficiency in the surgical method itself. In any event, the clinical results achieved by radial wedge osteotomy were at least as favorable as the results obtained by radial shortening, and both methods yielded satisfactory results, regardless of the stage of illness.

Of the many treatments recommended for Kienböck's disease, radial osteotomies have the advantage of avoiding the complications associated with arthrotomy and thus do not significantly comprise the wrist function. Although radial osteotomy does not always reconstitute the lunate architecture roentgenographically, progression of the disease process is arrested in most patients and good results have been obtained clinically, irrespective of the stage of illness. Drawbacks associated with radial osteotomy include difficulty in bony union and disturbance of distal radioulnar function. We believe that the step-cut osteotomy is a reliable way to obtain a solid union even though it requires a more meticulous technique than does simple osteotomy. Although some restriction of forearm rotation was noted in our series, no patient complained of pain on the distal radioulnar joint or restriction of forearm rotation.

We now prefer radial wedge osteotomy for the patients with zero or positive variance and radial shortening for the patients with negative variance. In conclusion, both radial wedge osteotomy and radial shortening yield consistently satisfactory results in patients with Kienböck's disease.

References

1. Calandriello B, Palandri C (1966) Die Behandlung Lunatum Malazie durch Speichenverkurzung. Z Orthop 101:531–534
2. Axelsson R (1973) Niveauoperationen bei Mondbeinnekrose. Handchirurgie 5:187–196
3. Rosenmeyer B, Artmann M, Viernstein K (1976) Lunatum-Malacie, Nachuntersuchungs-ergebnisse und therapeutische Erwagungen. Arch Orthop Unfall-Chir 85:119–127
4. Eiken O, Niechajev I (1980) Radius shortening in malacia of the lunate. Scand J Plast Reconstr Surg 14:191–196
5. Ovesen J (1981) Shortening of the radius in the treatment of lunatomalacia. J Bone Joint Surg [Br] 63:231–232
6. Almquist EE, Burns JF (1982) Radial shortening for the treatment of Kienböck's disease: A 5- to 10-year follow up. J Hand Surg 7:348–352
7. Schattenkerk ME, Nollen A, Hussen F (1987) The treatment of lunatomalacia: Radial shortening or ulnar lengthening. Acta Orthop Scand 58:652–654
8. Persson M (1945) Pathogenese und Behandlung der Kienböckschen Lunatummmalazie. Der Fracturtheorie im lichte der erfolge operativer Radiusverkürzung (Hultén) und einer nenen Operationsmethode-Ulnaverlängerung. Acta Chir Scand (Suppl) 92:1–158
9. Armistead RB, Linscheid RL Dobyns JH, Beckenbaugh RD (1982) Ulnar lengthening in the treatment of Kienböck's disease. J Bone Joint Surg [Am] 64:170–178
10. Sundberg SB, Linscheid RL (1984) Kienböck's disease — results of treatment with ulnar lengthening. Clin Orthop 198:43–51
11. Trumble T, Glisson RP, Seaber AV, Urbaniak JR (1986) A biomechanical comparison of the methods for treating Kienböck's disease. J Hand Surg [Am] 10:88–93
12. Tsumura H, Himeno S, Kojima T, Kido M (1982) Biomechanical analysis of Kienböck's disease: It's cause and treatment. Orthop Surg (Jpn) 33: 1400–1402
13. Tsumura H, Himeno S, Kawai T, Kojima T, Kido M (1983) Biomechanical analysis of Kienböck's disease. Orthop Surg Traumatol (Jpn): 26:123–128
14. Tsumura H, Himeno S, An KN, Cooney WP, Chao EYS (1987) Biomechanical analysis of Kienböck's disease. Orthop Trans 11:327
15. Graner O, Lopes EI, Carvalho BC, Atlas SA (1966) Arthrodesis of the carpal bones in the treatment of Kienböck's disease. Painful ununited fractures of the navicular and lunate bones with avascular necrosis, and old fracture-dislocations of carpal bones. J Bone Joint Surg [Br] 48:767–774
16. Ueba Y (1979) Treatment of lunatum malacia by enucleation-tendon insetion method. Orthop Surg (Jpn) 34:1093–1096
17. Nakamura R, Miura T, Araki T, Suzuki M, Kasumi H, Kajta T, Murase T (1981) Operative treatment and its results in Kienböck's disease. Orthop Trauma Surg (Jpn): 24:1847–1855
18. Ståhl F (1947) On lunatomalacia (Kienböck's disease), a clinical and roentogenological study, especially on its pathogenesis and late results of immobilization treatment. Acta Chir Scand (Suppl): 126:1–133
19. Youm Y, McMurtry RY, Flatt AE, Gillespie TE (1968) Kinematics of the wrist. Part I. An experimental study of radial-ulnar deviation and flexion-extension. J Bone Joint Surg [Am] 60:423–431
20. Calandriello B, Palandri C (1966) Die Behandlung der Lunatum Malazie durch Speichenverkürzung. Z Orthop: 101:531–534
21. Lichtman DM, Alexander AH, Mack GR, Gunther SF (1987) Kienböck's disease — update on silicone replacement arthroplasty. J Hand Surg 7:343–347
22. Nakamura R, Imaeda T, Miura T (1990) Radial shortening for Kienböck's disease: Factors affecting the operative results. J Hand Surg [Br] 15:40–45
23. Palmer AK, Werner FW (1988) Biomechanical evaluation of operative procedures performed for the treatment of Kienböck's disease. Presented at the 43rd annual meeting of the American Society for Surgery of the Hand, Baltimore
24. Werner EW, Palmer AK, Utter RG (1988) Distal radial osteotomy for the treatment of Kienböck's disease: a biomechanical study. Orthop Trans 12: 486–487
25. Horii E, Garcia-Elias M, An KN, Bishop AT, Cooney WP, Linscheid RL, Chao Eys (1990) Effect on force transmisson across the carpus in procedures used to treat Kienböck's disease. J Hand Surg [Am] 15:393–400
26. Simmons EH, Dommisse I (1974) The pathogenesis and treatment of Kienböck's disease. Clin Orthop 105:300

An Application of Strut Bone Graft in the Surgical Treatment for Kienböck's Disease

Toshiro Futami, Makoto Yamamoto, and Kazuhito Nakamura[1]

Abstract. A new surgical option (strut bone graft), based on the results of morphological observation and a biomechanical experiment on the lunate, was tried on ten patients in the relatively early stages of Kienböck's disease in which no significant bone collapse had been observed on X-rays. The surgical method consists of thorough curetting of the necrotized portion of the affected lunate followed by tight insertion of a columnar-shaped bone graft into the cavity resulting from the curettage.

Significant improvement of the preoperative clinical symptoms without further bone collapse as seen on X-rays was obtained in nine patients.

Keywords: Kienböck's disease — Surgical treatment — Strut bone graft — Trabecular pattern of the lunate — Biomechanical experiment

Introduction

Many surgical options for Kienböck's disease have been reported in the literature [1–6]. Most of these surgical options for excising the lunate necrosis appear to aim towards biological rather than biomechanical reconstruction. We present an alternative surgical option, strut bone graft, for the treatment of this particular condition. Our method involves a mechanical reconstruction of the lunate by inserting a columnar-shaped bone graft into the lunate. The surgical indications, operative technique, results, and theoretical background of our new method are described from morphological and biomechanical viewpoints.

Surgical Indications and Operative Technique

The strut bone graft was performed for patients who satisfied the following criteria: (1) the patient being highly active at work and sports and desiring swift therapeutic effect, and (2) no evidence on X-rays of apparent bone collapse of the lunate (stage 2) [6].

The following is a description of the surgical technique. Before the operation, an arthroscopical observation of the radiocarpal and mid-carpal joints is always performed in order to confirm that the articular surface is not involved (Fig. 1). The curettage procedure, which starts from the dorsal aspect of the lunate, is critical. Special care is taken during this procedure because of individual variances in the progress of necrosis and in the configuration of the lunate. We usually use an air drill and monitor the surgery with X-ray (Fig. 2).

After sufficient curettage, the bone graft is taken from the proximal portion of the ulna, curved into a column, and fitted snugly into the curetted cavity of the lunate. The grafted bone is implanted parallel to the direction of mechanical stress in the lunate (i.e., along the line connecting the capitate and the lunate) (Fig. 3). In addition, small bone chips are packed tightly around the grafted bone, and two Kirschner wires are introduced percutaneously for temporal fixation. A Scotch cast is then applied for about 6 weeks.

Postoperative management includes allowing active exercise to start after the cast is removed, and patients can resume work and sports approximately 4 months after surgery.

[1] Department of Orthopaedics, Kitasato University East Hospital, 2-1-1 Asamizodai, Sagamihara, Kanagawa 228, Japan

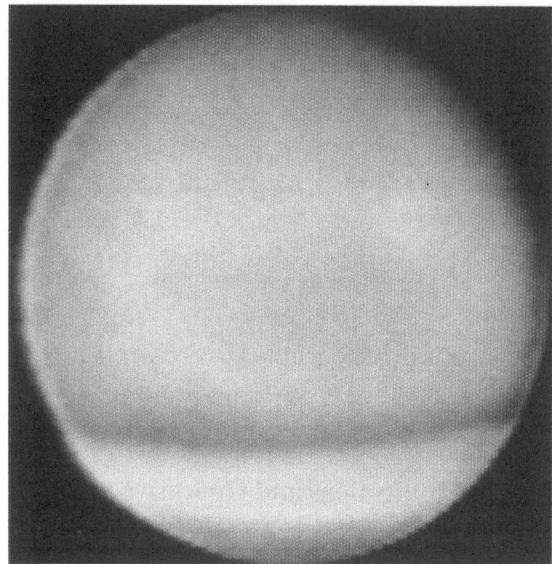

Fig. 1. Before the operation, an arthroscopical observation of the radiocarpal and mid-carpal joint should always be performed in order to confirm that the articular surface is not involved

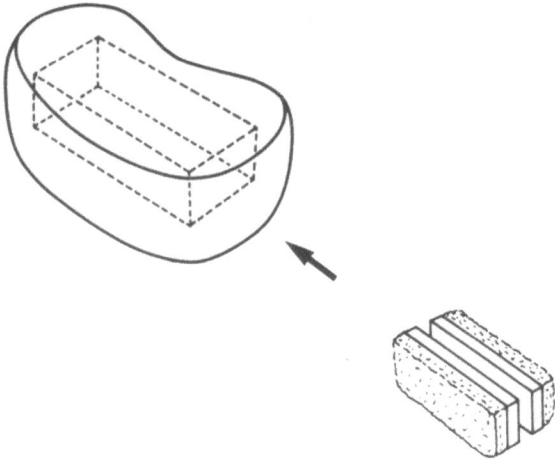

Fig. 3. A schematic illustration of the strut bone graft. The columnar-shaped grafting bone is implanted snugly into the curetted cavity of the lunate

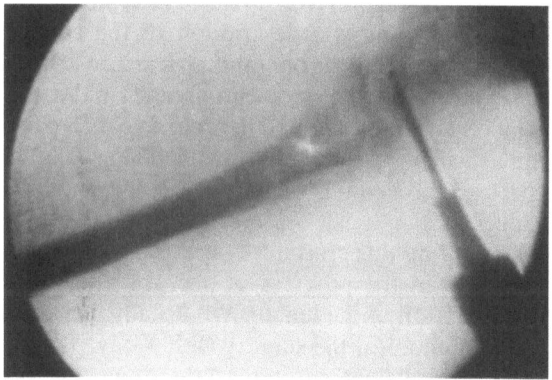

Fig. 2. The curettage procedure is very critical. We usually use an air drill and monitor the surgery with X-ray

Cases and Postoperative Results

Details and results of the operated cases are summarized in Table 1. The age of the patients at operation ranged from 22 to 39 years (mean 31 years). Predisposing causes for the lesions were found to be golf in 4 cases and were occupation-related in 6 cases. The duration of symptoms ranged from 6 to 13 months (mean 9 months) and the follow-up period was from 2.2 to 4.5 years (mean 3.1 years).

The results were evaluated as either satisfactory or unsatisfactory as proposed by Lichtman [6]. Using his criteria, satisfactory results were obtained in 9 cases, and postoperative X-rays of these cases revealed that bone collapse was prevented.

Some representative cases are described below.

Case 1

Preoperative X-ray tomograph showed apparent necrosis (Fig. 4, left). An X-ray tomograph taken 2 years after surgery confirmed that further development of bone collapse was prevented (Fig. 4, right). The results were extremely favorable and the patient now hopes to become a professional golfer.

Case 3

Although some resorptive change around the grafted bone was visible on X-rays taken 2.2 years after surgery, bone collapse was prevented (Fig. 5). Clinical results were also satisfactory.

Case 5

Collapse of the lunate gradually developed 3 months after surgery, and progressed to complete collapse in 6 months (Fig. 6). The clinical results were unsatisfactory.

Table 1. Case details and results

Case no.	Age (years)	Sex	Rt/Lt	Caused by	Duration of symptoms (months)	Follow-up period (months)	Results
1	22	M	Lt	Golf	10	42	S
2	33	M	Rt	Golf	9	36	S
3	22	M	Rt	Occupation	8	54	S
4	35	M	Lt	Occupation	9	24	S
5	38	M	Lt	Golf	6	26	U
6	39	M	Rt	Occupation	8	27	S
7	25	M	Rt	Occupation	13	38	S
8	28	M	Rt	Golf	9	39	S
9	33	M	Lt	Occupation	8	38	S
10	34	M	Rt	Occupation	9	40	S

Rt, Right; *Lt*, left; *S*, satisfactory; *U*, unsatisfactory

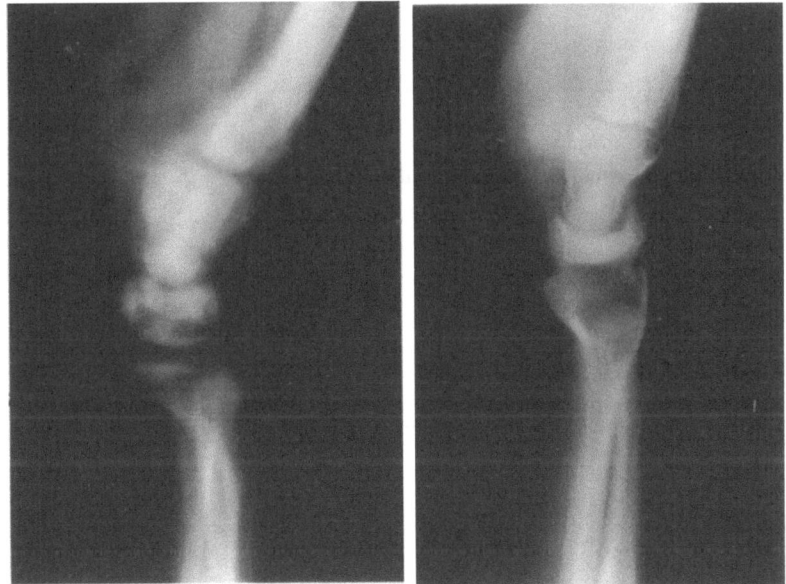

Fig. 4. Case 1. Pre- and postoperative X-rays. Preoperative X-rays tomograph (*right*) showed apparent necrosis. On the X-ray tomograph taken 2 years after surgery (*left*), bone collapse was shown to have been prevented

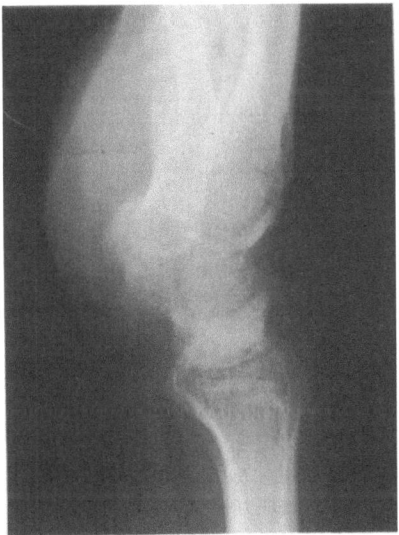
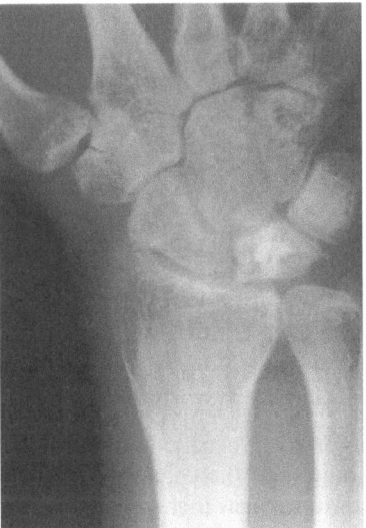

Fig. 5. Case 3. Postoperative X-rays. Although some resorptive change around the grafted bone was noted 2.2 years after surgery, bone collapse had been prevented

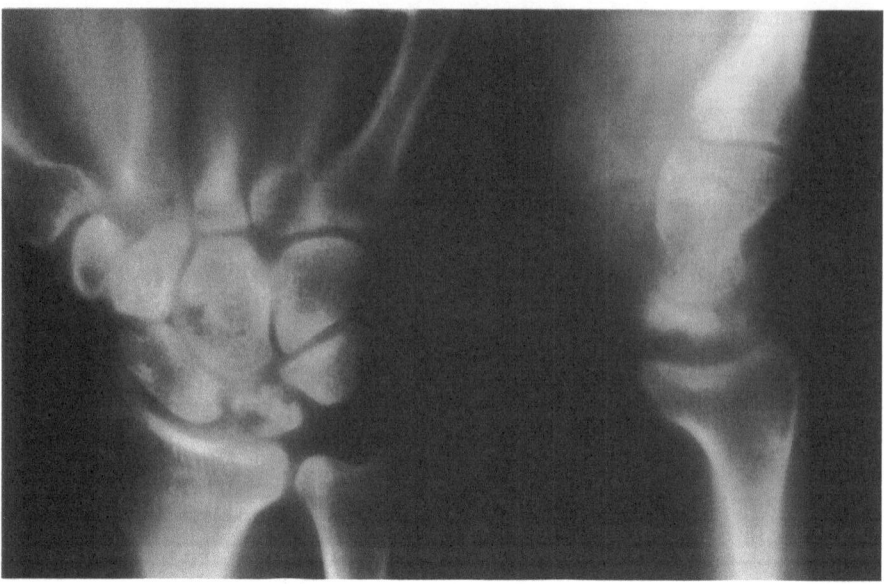

Fig. 6. Case 5. Postoperative X-rays. Collapse of the lunate gradually developed 3 months after surgery, and progressed to bone collapse in 6 months

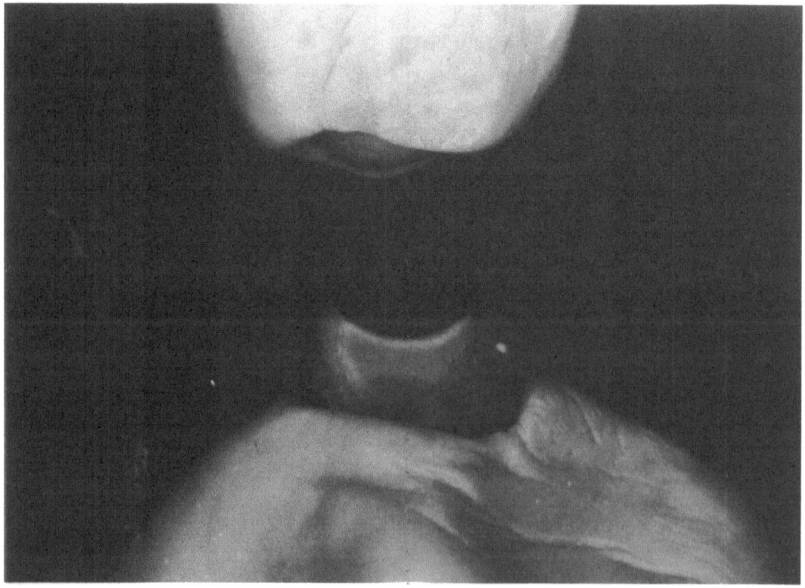

Fig. 7. A static vertical compression load was applied to the lunate

Biomechanical Aspects of the Lunate and Grafting Bone

Mechanical Property

In order to clarify the mechanical property of the lunate and the columnar-shaped grafting bone, a static vertical load was applied to samples taken from cadavers (Fig. 7). The results were micro-fracture of the lunate at 260 kg, collapse of the lunate at 330 kg (Fig. 8), and collapse of the grafting bone at 340 kg.

Trabecular Structure of the Lunate

The trabecular structure pattern in the lunate of normal individuals was examined using Softex X-rays. The prominent trabecular structure in

Fig. 8. The results of applying a static vertical compression load were microfracture of the lunate at 260 kg and collapse of the lunate at 330 kg (*arrows*)

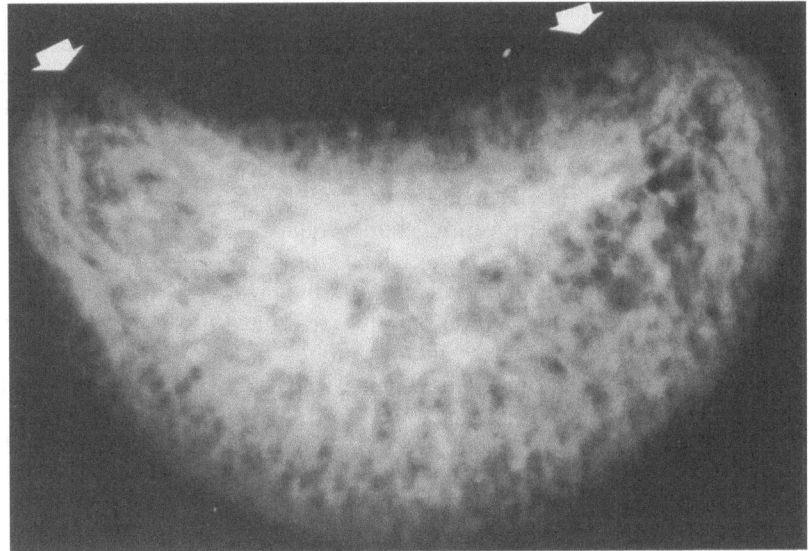

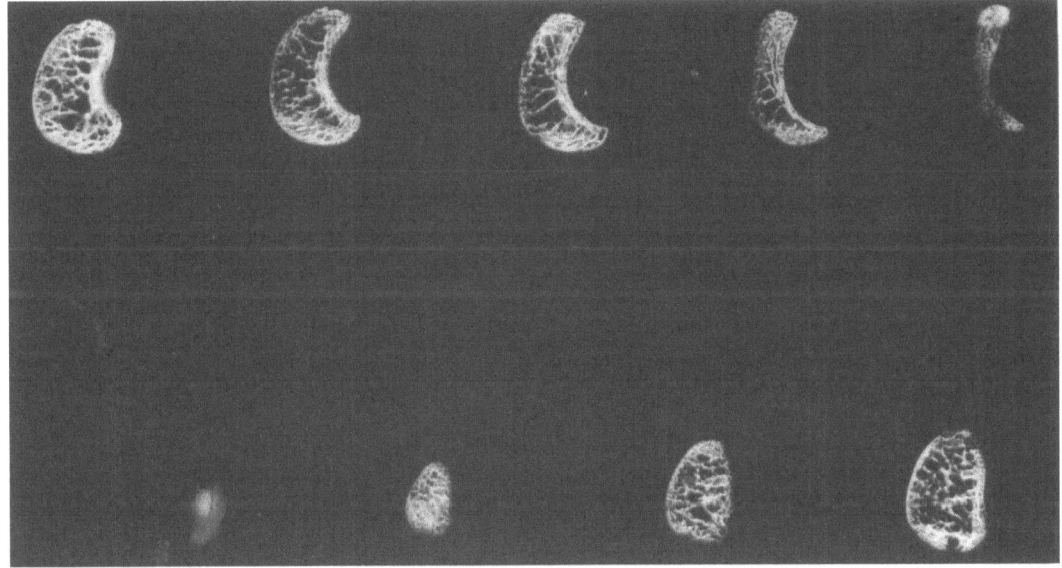

Fig. 9. Trabecular pattern of the lunate in normal individuals. The prominent bone trabecular was found to be oriented along the direction connecting the capitate and radius

the lunate was found to be oriented along the direction connecting the capitate and radius (Fig. 9).

Discussion

Treatment of Kienböck's disease is controversial. Several surgical options have been applied depending upon the patient's background and/or X-ray findings [1–6]. However, some drawbacks to these procedures still remain. We attempted strut bone graft for the following reasons: first, we had been seeking an innovative method that would produce better results than those of conventional surgical procedures, and second, one of the co-authors (M.Y.) had used strut bone graft to treat patients with aseptic necrosis of the femoral head with favorable results in most cases. He stated that conventional surgical procedures for bone necrosis focus on biological rather than on biomechanical reconstruction and that strut bone graft aims to prevent collapse by reconstructing the normal trabecular pattern in the femoral head by inserting a columnar-shaped bone graft oriented in the same direction of the femoral head [7]. We wonder whether this therapeutic strategy of preventing bone collapse by biomechanical reconstruction can be applied to the treatment of Kienböck's disease by inserting the strut bone graft parallel to the direction of mechanical stress in the lunate. In addition, the results of our biomechanical experiment confirmed that the strut bone graft had sufficient mechanical strength to withstand a vertical compression load of 330 kg.

The strut bone graft has been applied in only a small number of cases with limited postoperative observation. More data must be accumulated and further study should focus on clarifing long-term changes in the mechanical strength of the grafted bone before definite conclusions can be reported. However, the evidence that progressive bone collapse was clearly prevented in 9 out of 10 cases indicates that the strut bone graft can be a successful surgical option for treating Kienböck's disease in the relatively early stages.

Conclusions

A preliminary report on a new surgical procedure, strut bone graft, was presented, including its surgical indications, actual operative technique, postoperative results, and theoretical background from a biomechanical viewpoint. This procedure could be a successful surgical option for the patients in the relatively early stages of Kienböck's disease.

References

1. Swanson AB (1970) Silicone rubber implants for the replacement of the carpal scaphoid and lunate bones. Orthop Clin North Am 1:299–309
2. Ishiguro T (1984) Experimental and clinical studies of Kienböck's disease: Excision of the lunate followed by packing of the free tendon. J Jpn Orthop Assoc 58:509–522
3. Hirukawa M, Shirai Y, Iketani M (1985) Long-term results in patients with Kienböck's disease treated by shortening the radius. J Jpn Soc Surg Hand 2:430–434
4. Watson HK, Ryu J, DiBella A (1985) An approach to Kienböck's disease: Triscaphe arthrodesis. J Hand Surg [Am] 10:179–187
5. Yajima H, Tamai S, Inada A (1990) Treatment of Kienböck's disease with vascular bundle implantation and triscaphe arthrodesis. J Jpn Soc Surg Hand 7:747–750
6. Lichtman DM (1977) Kienböck's disease: The role of silicone replacement arthroplasty. J Bone Joint Surg [Am] 59:899–908
7. Yamamoto M (1988) Strut bone graft for aseptic necrosis of the femoral head. The hip: Clinical studies and basic research. Elsevier Science, Amsterdam, pp 185–188

Treatment of the Advanced Stages of Kienböck's Disease by Joint Fusion Between Pro-Lunate Iliac Cortico-Cancellous Graft and Scaphoid, Capitate, and Piramidalis Bones

ALESSANDRO CAROLI and STEFANO ZANASI[1]

Abstract. After a short analysis of the treatment techniques specifically indicated in the different X-ray stages of Kienböck's disease, the authors describe their own variation of Duparc's intercarpal arthrodesis technique for the treatment of the advanced IIIB and IV stages of the disease, according to Lichtman's classification. The modification consists of using small staples instead of a screw for iliac cortico-cancellous bone graft fixation. This method assures perfect graft stability and passive wrist mobilization at the 4th postoperative day, thus obviating the necessity of long immobilization in a plaster cast. The authors present the results at the average follow-up time of 28.5 months in 15 cases treated by substitution of the necrotic lunate bone by autologous implant of iliac bone and intercarpal perineolunate arthrodesis with staples, followed by immediate passive mobilization using the continuous passive motion machine Kinetec (Cogemo S.A., Tournes, France). The constant disappearance of pain coupled with the recovery of good wrist total active movement (TAM average 78°) and excellent stability and grip strength (average 81% of the uninvolved hand) have enabled 13 out of 15 patients to normally resume their former heavy manual jobs. Based on the obtained results, the authors deem this method to be worthy of consideration in carefully selected cases (young patients, heavy manual laborers with advanced Kienböck's disease) as a good alternative to proximal-row carpectomy or wrist arthrodesis.

Keywords: Kienböck's disease — Intercarpal arthrodesis — Autoplastic bone graft — Early mobilization

Introduction

Kienböck's disease treatment should be related to the clinical and X-ray staging of the disease, as suggested by Lichtman [1]. Common to all stages is an intrinsic weakness of lunate bone due to vascular necrosis. According to Taleisnik [2], three factors influence the exact evolutional stage and, consequently, the opportune treatment of the disease: the lunate crushing, the carpal collapse and instability, and the perilunate osteoarthritic changes. When lunate bone has not yet collapsed (stages I and II) it is important to try to unload the bone in order to avoid its collapse. An ideal method, at least from the theoretical point of view, would be the use of an external fixation device in distraction, accompanied with an application of pulsed electromagnetic fields. To unload the lunate bone, if there is a minus variant of ulna, we prefer the radial shortening technique: capitate shortening is advised if the negative variant is not present. In particular, it has been shown on a biomechanical model [3] that radial shortening or, alternatively, ulnar lengthening are methods capable of redistributing loads from the radiolunate joint to the radioscaphoid joint and to the ulnar column, by decreasing the lunate compression by about 40%. Such biomechanical rationale of the validity of the technique is constantly confirmed by clinical data on pain relief and improved X-ray findings of the lunate bone [4, 5]. This also applies to capitate shortening, expecially when it is fused with hamate bone, redistributing loads over the wrist by significantly unloading the radiolunate joint and, conversely, increasing the load at the radioscaphoid joint [3]. This can cause the adjacent triquetrohamate and scaphotrapezial joints to be dramatically overloaded, thus putting the carpus at the theorical risk for further collapse: these effects are not well known to date. These

[1] University of Modena, Orthopaedics Department, Hand Surgery Unit, Largo del Pozzo 71, I-41100 Modena, Italy

methods are, in our opinion, efficacious at stage IIIA. At stage IIIA, B we deem the triscaphoid arthrodesis of Watson [6] to be very useful, especially if it is accompanied by lunate high performance (HP) silicone replacement arthroplasty or better, by a biological spacer in order to avoid silicone intolerance. This method, even if it only minimally unloads the lunate bone, is able to improve carpal stability and to prevent rotatory subluxation of the scaphoid and the consequent carpal collapse. We consider proximal row carpectomy to be a salvage procedure in stages IIIB and IV, despite numerous reports of its good clinical results. In his series, Imbriglia [7] demonstrated that the operation appears to diminish pain, maintain a functional arc of motion, and improve grip strength, even though it leads to a deterioration of the radiocapitate joint. These results were better in Bedeschi and Folloni's series [8] in which the importance of the volar approach is enphasized in order to restore the maximum movement. Naturally, proximal row carpectomy does not fully restore grip strength: for most young patients and heavy manual workers, the operation does not restore sufficient strength to allow them to return to their former jobs even if they can perform the activities of daily living.

In stages IIIB and IV, according to Lichtman, in which the fragmentation and collapse of the lunate bone is associated with a first carpal row diastase and proximal migration of the capitate, limited carpal arthrodesis is correctly indicated. Above all, in the young patient with great wrist functional demands, such techniques are efficacious and able to completely assure the stability that surgery aims to restore as an alternative to proximal row carpectomy or wrist arthrodesis.

Duparc and Christel [9], in stages III and IV, directly replace the lunate bone with a cortico-cancellous bone graft taken from the iliac crest and fixed to the nearby carpal bones with a screw transversely introduced from the pyramidalis, in order to put the proximal carpal row in compression. They then apply a plaster cast for 2 months. This technique assures a stable wrist with a dramatic decrease in pain and a regaining of 80% of grip strength: any significant limitation of active and passive wrist movement conditionates the quality of results. Based on these data, since 1985 Caroli and co-workers have performed an intercarpal arthrodesis by fusing the iliac bone graft to the adjacent carpal bones by mini-staples in young patients who do heavy manual labour, in stages IIIB and IV according to Lichtman (Figs. 1a–c). This method assures an excellent graft stability and, at the same time, permits wrist mobilization on the 4th postoperative day, avoiding the necessity of long immobilization

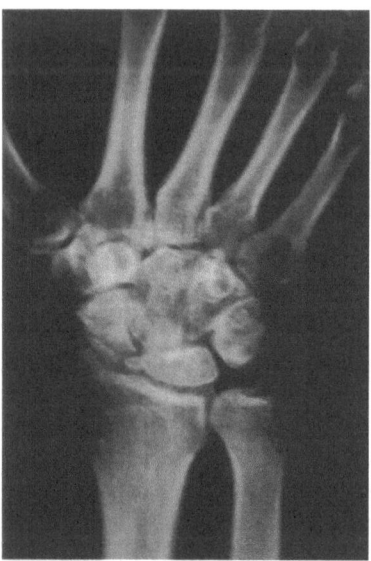 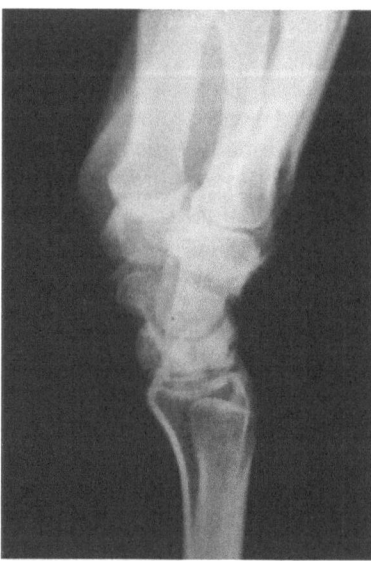 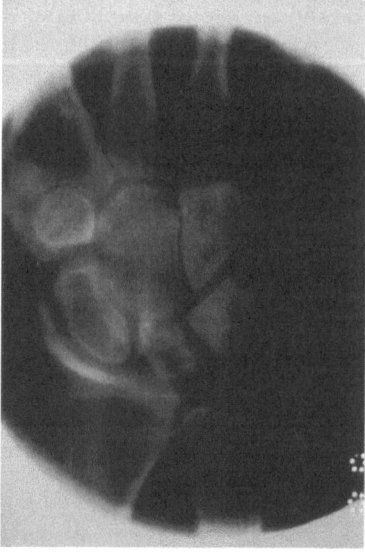

a   b   c

Fig. 1. Preoperative findings in a 21-years-old male laborer. **a, b** Standard orthogonal x-ray films and **c** tomography confirm Kienböck's disease in stage IIIB, according to Lichtman's classification

a
b
c

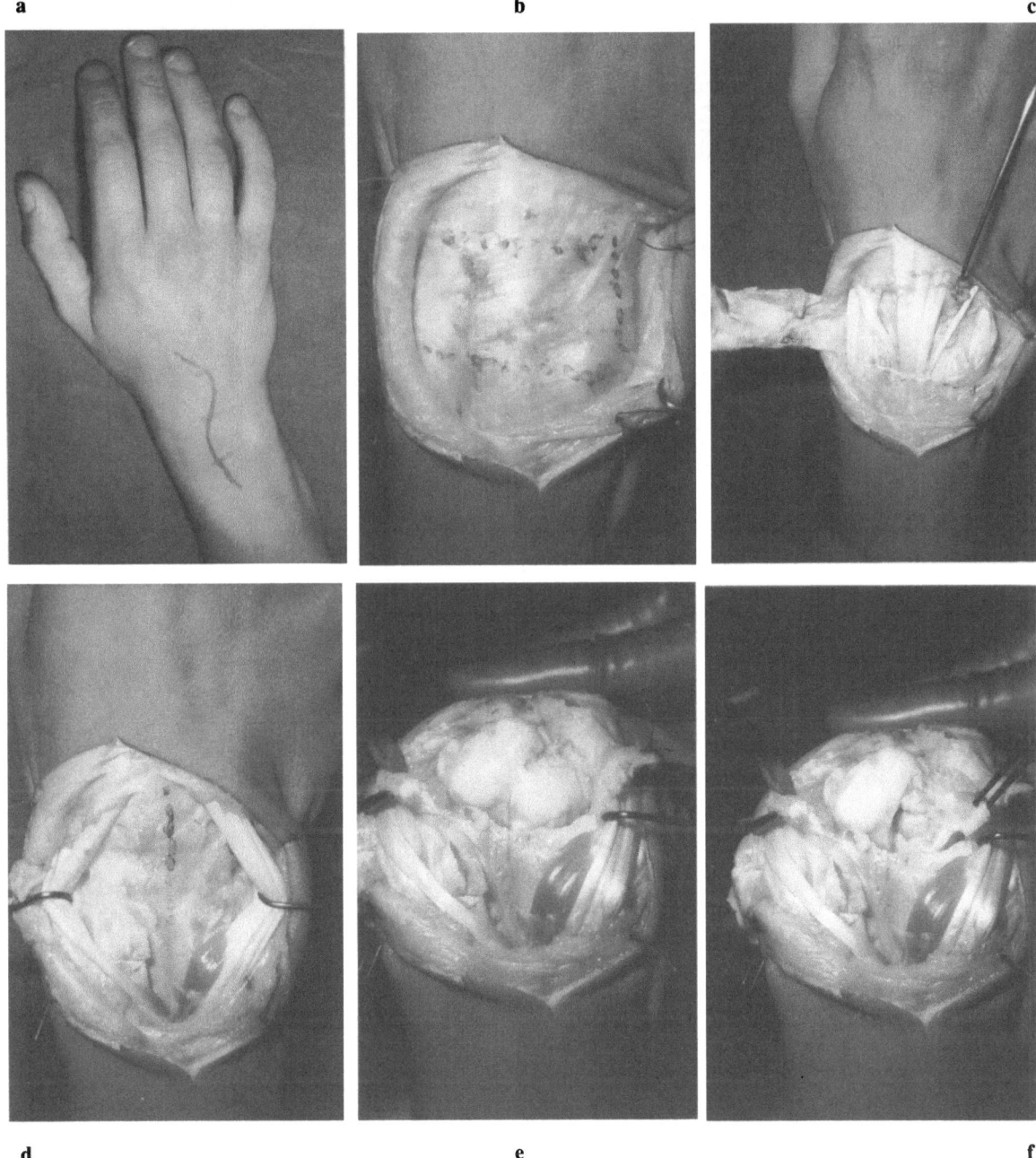

d
e
f

Fig. 2a–o. Surgical technique of joint fusion

in a plaster cast and the consequent wrist stiffness.

Surgical Technique

The wrist is dorsally approached by a lazy "s" surgical incision. (Fig. 2.a). After the elevation of a retinacular flap with a radial base (Figs. 2b, c), a capsular incision is made longitudinally or better (Fig. 2.d), tranversely just proximally to the radiocarpal line in order to maintain a capsular flap that will be easy to resuture. Then, the carpal condyle is exposed by completely flexing the wrist (Fig. 2.e). After excising the lunate in small fragments, taking care to preserve the volar ligaments (Fig. 2.f), the lunate faces of the scaphoid, capitate, hamate, and triquetrum bones are re-g   h   i

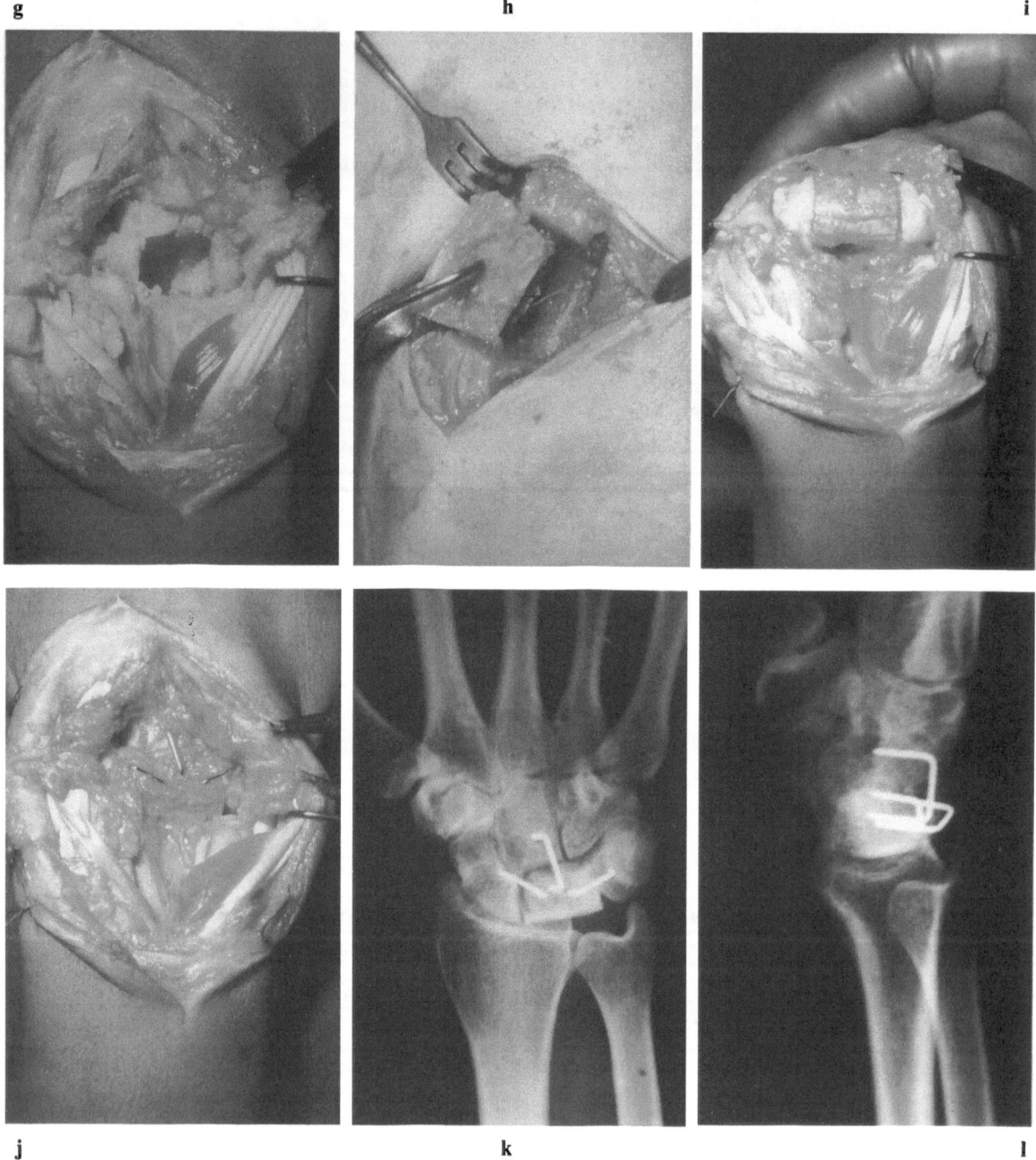

j   k   l

Fig. 2. *Continued*

sected with a power saw (Fig. 2.g). An autoplastic bone graft is taken from the most convex part of the iliac crest (Fig. 2.h). After a very accurate modelling of the bone graft's resection surfaces, it is fitted into the carpal hole by orienting the cortical-free convex surface to the radial glenoid, in order to restore the height and the anatomical convexity of the carpal condyle (Fig. 2.i). The stabilization of the iliac bone graft is assured with three or four ministaples. (Fig. 2.j). This internal device does not require postoperative immobilization, thus differing from Duparc's original compression screw technique, in which the patient must wear a forearm plaster cast for at least 2 months. When the graft is stabilized, it is an opportune time to passively flex and extend the

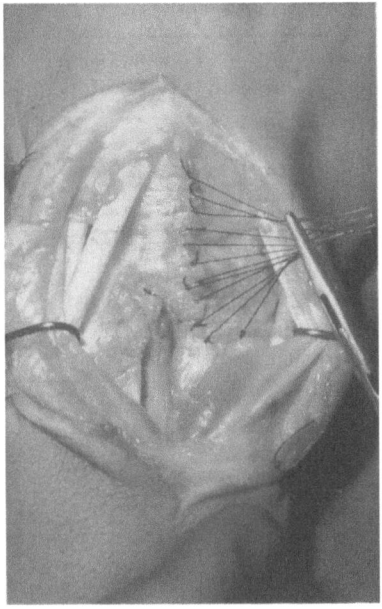 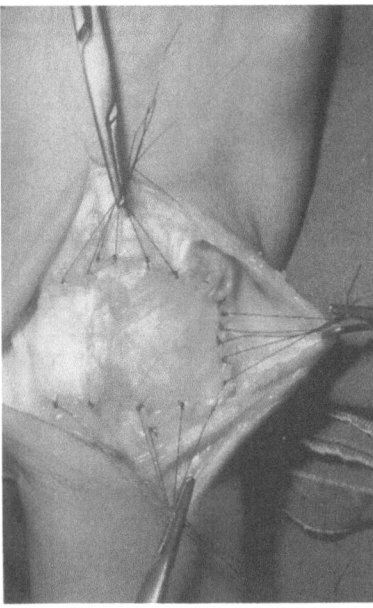 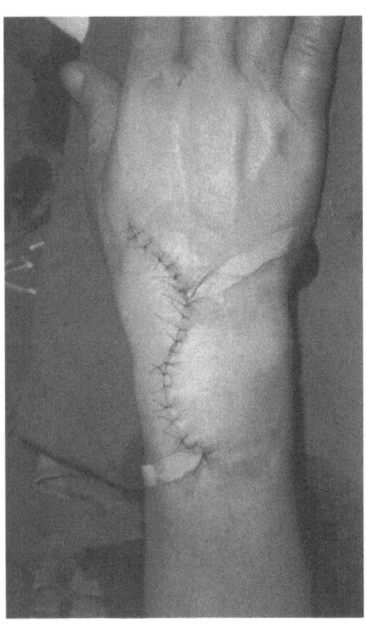

m   n   o

wrist to verify the stability and correct gliding of the carpal condyle over the radial glenoid. X-ray intra-operative anteroposterior and lateral controls permit verification of the correct placement of the graft, the quality of arthrodesis, and the correct placing of the fixative devices (Figs. 2.k, l).

After capsular (Fig. 2.m), retinacular (Fig. 2.n), and skin recontruction (Fig. 2.o), a plaster slab is used for the first 3 postoperative days. On the next day the patient is allowed to passively mobilize the wrist using the hand and wrist continuous passive motion machine Kinetec (Cogemo S.A., Tournes, France) (Figs. 3a, b). This rehabilitation treatment is given 3 times a day to regain the flexion-extension preoperative wrist motility which is progressively restored in 2 weeks. After release from the hospital, patients continue further active and passive mobilization at the rehabilitation department until the first postoperative month.

Case Series

Between January, 1986 and June, 1990 the authors treated 20 patients at the Hand Surgery Unit of the University of Modena with this technique. Of these, 15 (12 males, 3 females)

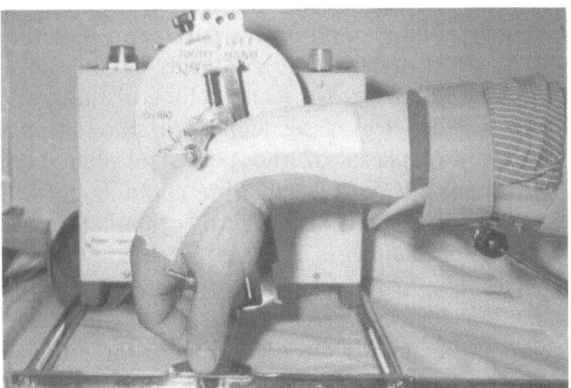 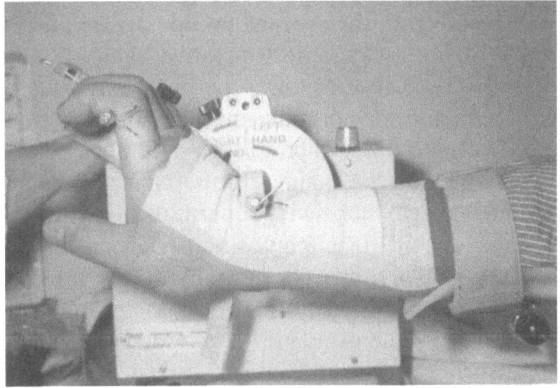

a   b

Fig. 3a,b. Postoperative rehabilitation treatment by Kinetec. Passive wrist mobilization in flexion-extension is started on the 4th postoperative day

Table 1. Total active movement (TAM) (flexion-extension)

Range	Patients (n)	
	Preoperative	Postoperative
0°–40°		
41°–80°	9	9
81°–120°	2	4
121°–160°	4	2
Average TAM	81°	78°

Table 2. Pain

	Patients (n)	
	Preoperative	Postoperative
None		5
Present only under strain		10
Severe	8	
Disabling	7	

Table 3. Grip strength (kg/cm^2)

(expressed as percentage of uninvolved hand)

Preoperative	From	25/65 · 38%	Average value:
	To	75/90 · 83%	58%
Postoperative	From	52/100 · 52%	Average value:
	To	110/110 · 100%	81%

Table 4. Radiographic results

	Patients (n)[a]
Bone graft dislocation	0
Partial graft's reabsorption	7
Osteolysis around staples' stems	10
Non-union with scaphoid	11
Non-union with capitate	6
Non-union with piramidalis	6
Non-union with hamate	7
Remodeling of graft's surface	12

[a] Out of a total of 15 patients

returned for follow-up (average follow-up 28.5 months; range 15–50 months). The mean age at surgery was 38 years (range 26–61 years). All the patients were employed in activities involving heavy manual labor (7 workmen, 4 artisans, 2 farmers, 1 housewife, and 1 gymnastics teacher). The dominant hand was affected in 12 cases out of 15. X-ray findings showed nine patients to be in stage IIIB and six in IV, according to Lichtman's classification.

Results

Criteria for assessment included total active movement (TAM), pain, comparative grip strength, worsening of arthritic changes, and resumption of former employment. TAM in flexion-extension changed from the average preoperative value of 81° degrees to the average postoperative value of 78°, i.e., 96% of the pre-operative average value (Table 1). Preoperative pain was severe and disabling, but was absent (5 cases) or present only under strain (10 cases) postoperatively (Table 2). Grip strength, expressed as percentage of the uninvolved hand, increased from the average preoperative value of 58% to the average postoperative value of 81% (Table 3). These features permitted 13 out of 15 patients to normally resume their former jobs. Radiographically (Table 4), there was a worsening of the main arthritic changes (radiolunate space narrowing, perilunate arthrosis, radial styloid osteophytosis, periarticular calcifications) in only 1 case. There was no case of bone graft dislocation nor was there an occurrence of significant graft reabsorption: slight reabsorbtion occurred in 7 cases out of 15. The rate of non-union with the scaphoid was high (11/15) and less with the capitate (6/15), the piramidalis (6/15), and the hamate (7/15).

Moderate osteolysis around the staples stems occurred (10/15); this is more important at the ulnar side, where the staple stabilizes the graft with the piramidalis bone, and it is probably due to the greater independence of this bone in comparison to the capitate and scaphoid bones. It is interesting to note the constant remodelling of the radial glenoid graft's surface in its ability to perfectly restore the convexity of the carpal condyle (Figs. 4a, b). Remodelling of the graft's free surface was associated with fibrocartilagineous metaplasia of the periosteal iliac bone surface (Figs. 5b, c), which we could assess with arthroscopic and histological examinations of sample specimens.

No cases of infection or of intolerance to the fixation devices were found. Complications were rare and generally did not influence the outcome of the operation. Massive reabsorption occurred in 1 case at the capitate surface of the graft (1/15). A breakdown of one staple between the graft and piramidalis bone occurred when fusion was

Fig. 4. Clinical and X-ray findings at 56 months' follow-up of the patient in Figs. 1–3. **c, d** There is excellent wrist mobility and good fusion of the graft with the scaphoid and triquetrum bones. **a, b** The remodeling of the graft's free surface has perfectly restored the convexity of the carpal condyle

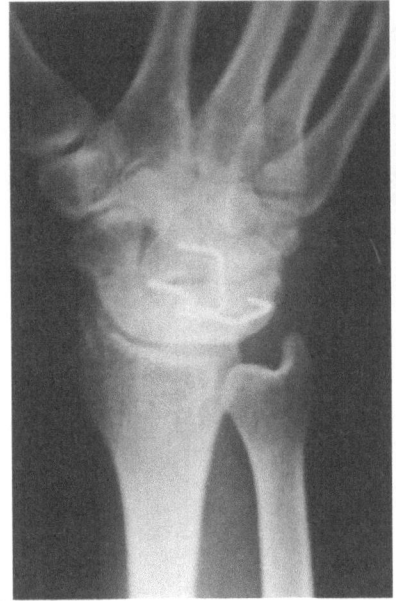

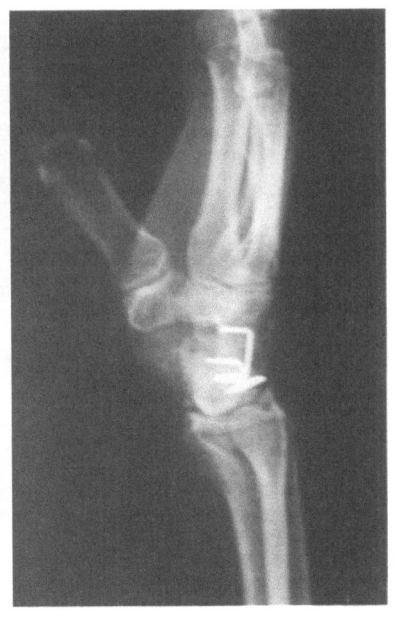

a

b

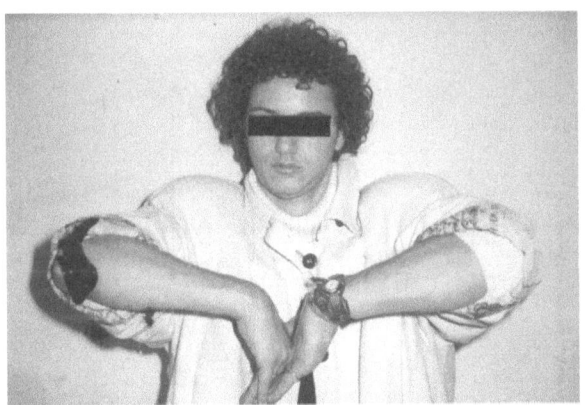

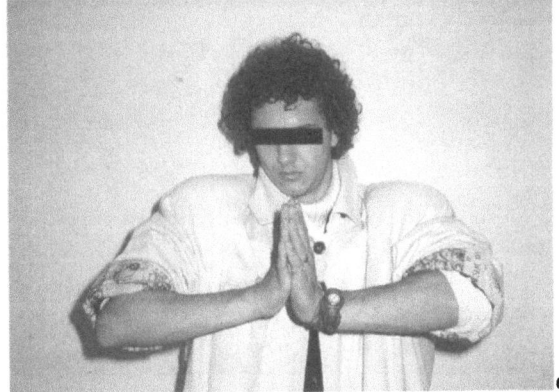

c

d

already completely realized (1/15). Mobilization of one staple which limited wrist extension (Fig. 5a) (1/15) and skin necrosis (1/15) were also found. In these last 3 cases, the problem was solved with staple removal and with a local skin flap, respectively.

Based on the criteria for assessing the standard of functional results shown in Table 5, in which a score between 0–3 or 0–2 or 1 is given according to the different results of the criteria, the authors found 80% of the results to be satisfactory, i.e., 12 out of 15 were excellent (Figs. 4c, d) or good, with only 3 being fair (Table 6).

Discussion

Several methods have been proposed to correct advanced stages of Kienböck's disease. Chuinard and Zeman [10] perform capitate-hamate ar-

throdesis which, in the advanced stages when the capitate has migrated more than 2 mm proximally, is combined with the Swanson silastic prosthesis to prevent further proximal collapse of the capitate: however, this arthrodesis does not include both rows and is unable to allow the shift of the loads ulnarly either alone or in association with Swanson replacement arthroplasty. With time, capitate collapse is associated with the proximal migration of the whole distal carpal row with the hamate and the diastasis of the proximal carpal row [2]. In their biomechanical studies, Trumble et al. [11] confirmed the inability of such a method to decrease the loads over the lunate bone. Hori [3] also confirmed that, due to the hamatotriquetrum joint, this technique is not able to prevent proximal radial translation under compressive load, so that the lunate bone is only minimally unloaded.

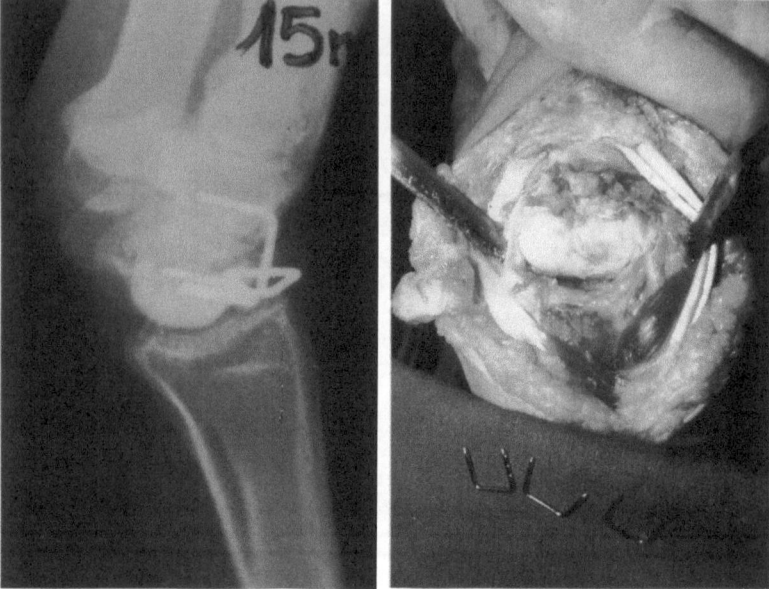

Fig. 5. a X-ray findings at 15-months' follow-up in a 42-year-old male, in which there is a stop of wrist extension due to staples mobilization. **b, c** Intra-operative distal wrist articular surface exposure to remove the staples. The perfect restoration of carpal condyle due to a fibro-cartilagineous metaplastic process of the graft-free surface can be easily appreciated

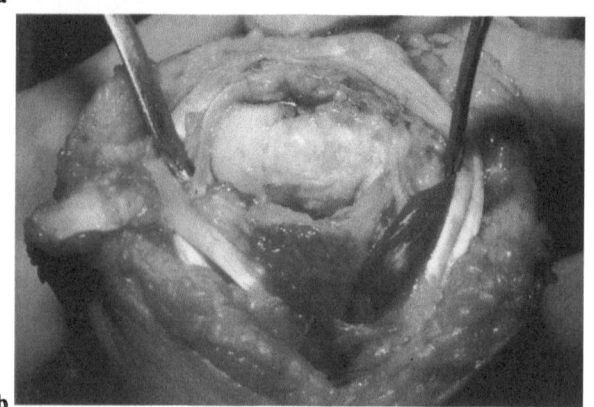

Table 5. Criteria for assessing standard of functional result

Pain	None 3[a]	Under strain 2	Severe 1	Disabling 0
TAM	121°–160° 3	81°–120° 2	41°–80° 1	0°–40° 0
Grip	>90% 3	75%–90% 2	50%–75% 1	<50% 0
Work	Yes 2		No 0	
Arthritis	Yes 0		No 1	

TAM, Total active movement

[a] The numbers represent points in scoring

Capitate shortening combined with both capitohamate fusion and silastic lunate replacement is advised by Almquist [12] in stage IIIA, B in which there has been fragmentation of the lunate including either the radiolunate or the capitolunate surface. The purpose of these combined procedures is to decrease the forces acting on the silastic lunate by shortening the

Table 6. General results of the 15 cases studied

Total score	Evaluation	Cases (n)
From 12 to 10	Excellent	6
From 9 to 7	Good	6
From 6 to 3	Fair	3
Less than 3	Poor	

capitate and fixing it to the ulnar column in order to avoid progressive proximal migration of the capitate. Despite the encouraging clinical results, this technique is not free of complications which are basically linked to the aseptic necrosis of the capitate proximal pole and to silastic material intolerance.

Watson [6] performs scapho-trapezial-trapezoidal (STT) arthrodesis whose rationale is based on the fact that it creates a radial column to the capitolunate axis, which is able to support the loads and unload the lunate bone in such a way as to prevent carpal collapse. Simple triscaphoid arthrodesis can support the wrist loads and may be used in order to maintain the affected lunate bone at the II–IIIA stage. Nevertheless, such a technique can support the carpus and also relieve the pain when the lunate is collapsed (stage IIIB) if it is combined with a Swanson silastic prosthesis [13] or, much better, to a biological spacer in order to avoid complications associated with silicone. Scaphoid rotation overcorrection may cause a significant decreasing of wrist motility and an early radioscaphoid arthrosis. The effectiveness of the method was confirmed by Trumble et al. [11] who verified biomechanically that STT arthrodesis significantly decreases the loads over the lunate bone. However, such a technique becomes inefficacious in wrist ulnar deviation and severely limits wrist motility in radial deviation and extension (less than 30%) because it stabilizes the scaphoid bone, which is mobile in radial deviation, and abolishes its rotation, which normally occurs in extension. Based on more recent studies of biomechanics, Hori [3] verified that such a method unloads the radiolunate joint only by 5%, a value that is obviously not significant, so that the clinical efficacy of this method is not due to its decompressive effect, but, rather, to its improved carpal stability.

Graner [14] suggested performing perilunate arthrodesis in the advanced stages of the disease by using the head of the capitate as lunate osteoplastic and filling the gap in the capitate bone with a bone graft. According to this author, such a technique is indicated only when other classic techniques fail. The great advantage of such a technique is the maintaining a good motility of the radiocarpal joint in the absence of significant pain. Sennwald [15] criticized this method because it is not physiological and may cause necrosis and deformation of the proximal third of the capitate after its devascularization. Furthermore, the radius of the curvature of the capitate head is less than that of the lunate fossa of the radius so that carpal stability may be not good, and progressive arthritic deterioration of the radiocapitate joint with time is unavoidable.

Fusion of the lunate and scaphoid to the radius [12] has the advantage of maintaining an average wrist motion of 40° extension and 20° flexion, with excellent stability and pain relief without silicone replacement. This technique appears to be ideal for patients requiring use of the hands for heavy lifting. However, it is contraindicated when the lunate lacks an adequate surface with which to articulate with the capitate.

Crabbe [16], Inglis [17], Neviaser [18], and Imbriglia [7] reported good results by the proximal row carpectomy technique in stages IIIB and IV. In particular, Bedeschi [8], who uses the anterior approach, reported obtaining a stable wrist which was nearly painfree, with increased grip strength, and having an average TAM of 135°. However, we are in agreement with several other authors who consider this operation as being a salvage procedure in which the results remain somewhat controversial. Criticisms of the results of proximal row carpectomy, as they appear in most of the published series, include inadequate recovery of strength, loss of motion, prolonged rehabilitation, progressive painful arthritis, and for most patients, not enabling the resuming of their former jobs.

The principal contraindication to this procedure is the presence of significant degenerative changes on the proximal pole of the capitate or of the lunate fossa of the radius. As in the Graner technique, the discrepancy between the radii of curvature of the lunate fossa and of the proximal pole of the capitate, even if it is approximately two-thirds of the corresponding value of the lunate [7], causes a greater freedom of movement (the motion of the capitate consists of translation as well as rotation) and a progressive deterioration with time of the radiocapitate joint.

As a salvage procedure, wrist arthrodesis should generally be used after the failure of other methods, and limited to the severe arthritic changes associated with the disease at stage IV. In the Razemon and Fisk series [19], such a technique is performed after an average of 6 years from the appearance of the first signs: the patient recovers a nearly normal grip strength and complete relief of pain both at rest and with exertion at the cost of sacrificing total radiocarpal motility.

In stages IIIB and IV, we deem the substitution of the necrotic lunate bone by autologous implant of iliac bone and intercarpal perineolunate arthrodesis followed by immediate passive mobilization using a Kinetec to be useful as an alternative to proximal row carpectomy and wrist arthrodesis, and, limited to the stage IIIB, as an alternative to STT arthrodesis with a biological spacer. The critical steps of this not very difficult procedure include the remodeling and correct fitting of the iliac bone graft, which should perfectly restore the convexity and the height of the carpus.

Unlike Duparc's original technique, ours allows an early passive mobilization of the wrist. The mini-staples, in fact, assure an excellent graft stability, as we have verified by dynamic X-ray controls (unpublished data). This procedure is capable of correcting carpal collapse and instability, and presents the great advantage of assuring a nearly total relief of pain by restoring excellent wrist stability and grip strength. Intercarpal arthrodesis by its very nature causes a limitation of wrist mobility that remains confined to the radiocarpal joint: nevertheless, early passive mobilization associated with this technique permits complete restoration of motion at this level by assuring an average TAM in flexion-extension of 78°, i.e., in our series, or 96% of the preoperative average wrist TAM. This useful ROM in the absence of pain, associated with a recovery of 81% of the normal grip strength, allowed most patients (13 out of 15) to resume their former heavy manual jobs. Furthermore, it is significant that, at midterm follow-up, there is a slackening in the evolution of arthritic changes in cases associated with preoperative arthrosis: however these data need to be verified using a longer-term follow up period.

References

1. Lichtman DM (1988) The wrist and its disorders. Saunders, Philadelphia
2. Taleisnik J (1985) The wrist. Churchill Livingstone, New York
3. Hori E, Garcia-Elias M, An KN, Bishop AT, Cooney WP, Linscheid RL, Chao EYS (1990) Effect on force transmission across the carpus in procedures used to treat Kienböck's disease. J Hand Surg [Am] 15:393–400
4. Armistead RB, Linscheid RL, Dobyns JH, Beckenbaugh RD (1982) Ulnar lengthening in the treatment of Kienböck's disease. J Bone Joint Surg [Am] 64:170–178
5. Almquist EE, Burns JF (1982) Radial shortening for the treatment of Kienboeck's disease. A 5 to 10 year follow up. J Hand Surg [Am] 7:348–352
6. Watson HK, Ryu J, DiBella A (1985) An approach to Kienboeck's disease: Triscaphe arthrodesis. J Hand Surg [Am] 10:179–187
7. Imbriglia JE, Broudy AS, Hagberg WC, McKernan D (1990) Proximal row carpectomy: Clinical evaluation. J Hand Surg [Am] 15:426–430
8. Duparc J, Christel P (1978) Traitement chirurgical des necroses du semi-lunaire par arthrodese intercarpienne. Ann Chir 32:565–569
9. Bedeschi P, Folloni A (1989) Proximal row carpectomy: Indications, modified technique and results. Paper presented at the BOA-SIOT Combined Meeting, London, 13–15 September
10. Chuinard RG, Zeman SC (1980) Kienboeck's disease: An analysis and rationale for treatment by capitate-hamate fusion. Orthop Trans 4:18
11. Trumble T, Glisson RG, Seaber AV, Urbaniak JR (1986) A biomechanical comparison of the methods for treating Kienboeck's disease. J Hand Surg [Am] 11:88–93
12. Almquist EE (1987) Kienboeck's disease. Hand Clin 3:141–148
13. Alexander AH, Turner MA, Alexander CE, Lichtman DM (1990) Lunate silicone replacement arthroplasty in Kienboeck's disease: A long term follow-up. J Hand Surg [Am] 15:401–407
14. Graner O, Lopes EK, Costa Carvahlo B, Atlas S (1966) Arthrodesis of the carpal bones in the treatment of Kienböck's disease, painful nonunited fractures of the navicular and lunate bones with avascular necrosis, and old fracture-dislocations of carpal bones. J Bone Joint Surg [Am] 48:767–774
15. Sennwald G (1987) The wrist. Springer, Berlin
16. Crabbe WA (1964) Excision of the proximal row of the carpus. J Joint Bone Surg [Br] 46:708–711
17. Inglis AE, Jones EC (1977) Proximal row carpectomy for diseases of the proximal row. J Bone Joint Surg [Am] 59:460–463
18. Neviaser RG (1986) On resection of the proximal carpal row. Clin Orthop 202:12–15
19. Razemon JP, Fisk GR (1983) Le poignet. Expansion Scientifique Francaise, Paris

Replacement of the Lunate by the Pisiform in Kienböck's Disease

MUNEAKI ABE, MUNEKAZU DOI, TSUNEHIKO ISHIZU, TOSHIO HASEGAWA, and TOSHINOBU ONOMURA[1]

Abstract. During the period from 1980 to 1988, 14 patients with stage III Kienböck's disease were treated at our hospital by a modified Saffar's procedure. Thirteen patients were followed-up for an average of 73.2 months (range 13–125 months).

Clinical patterns used in assessment included pain, strength, motion, and X-ray findings. Pain relief after the surgery was achieved in all patients, but four of them complained of mild pain after strenuous activity. Grip strength improved from the preoperative 42.9% of that of the normal side to 73.9% postoperatively. Postoperative dorsiflexion of the wrist joint improved 94.3% of that of the normal side, compared to 57.7% preoperatively. On the X-ray examination, the carpal height ratio showed a significant decrease at follow-up examination, but the carpal-ulnar distance ratio and the radioscaphoid angle did not deteriorate significantly after surgery. Overall clinical results were evaluated according to Lesur, Merle, and Michon's criteria (1989). Four patients were rated as showing excellent results, four were good, and four fair. There were no poor results. All the patients were satisfied with their results.

Periodical X-ray findings of the inserted pisiform showed that reduction in its shape and increased bone density took place in most cases at 6–12 months after surgery, and that nearly normal shape and density returned 1–2 years later. In 3 cases, however, the shape and density of the pisiform decreased and did not return to normal. These findings suggest that vascularity to the pisiform is not sufficient to keep its shape and bone density despite some vascularity expected from the attached flexor carpi ulnaris.

Keywords: Lunate — Kienböck's disease — Treatment — Pisiform transfer — Surgical technique

Introduction

Replacement of the lunate by the pisiform with its vascular pedicle and the flexor carpi ulnaris tendon attached for the treatment of advanced Kienböck's disease was reported by Saffar [1] in 1982. We have used this operation since 1980 as a procedure for treating advanced Kienböck's disease. We present our modified procedure and the long-term results.

Surgical Technique

Under general anesthesia, a tourniquet is inflated without exsanguination and a curved skin incision is made on the ulnar side of the wrist (Fig. 1.a). The pisiform, with its vascular pedicle and the flexor carpi ulnaris (FCU) tendon, is dissected out under magnification (Fig. 1.b). The median nerve and flexor tendons are retracted radially. A distally based rectangular flap of the wrist capsule is outlined and elevated (Fig. 1.c). Excision of the lunate is performed with a small rongeur and the dorsal capsule is carefully preserved. After completion of this dissection, the tourniquet is deflated in order to verify the vascularity of the pisiform, which is then placed into the cavity at a sufficient depth. The reflected capsular flap is put back and sutured into place (Fig. 1.d). When closing the capsular flap over the FCU, care must be taken not to compress the vascular pedicle.

Immediately after surgery, a long arm plaster cast is applied with the wrist in a slightly flexed

[1] Department of Orthopedic Surgery, Osaka Medical College, 2-7 Daigakucho Takatsuki, Osaka 569, Japan

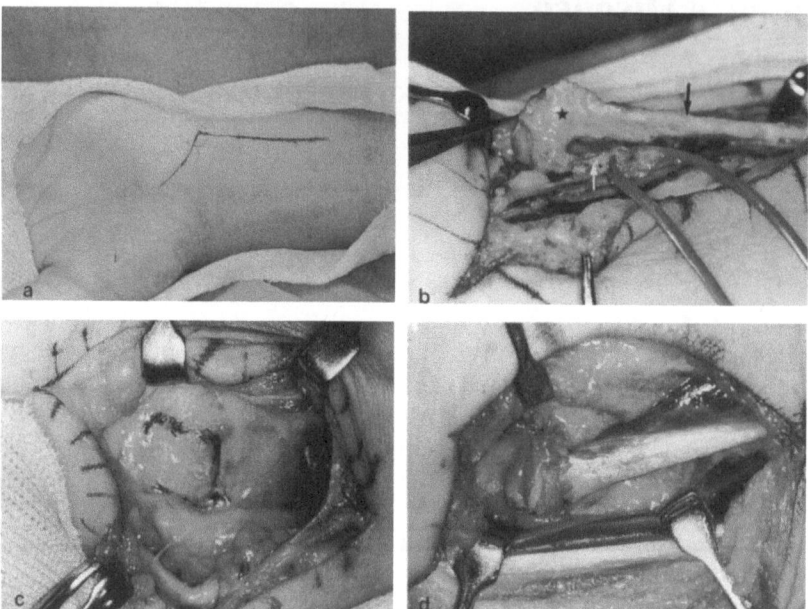

Fig. 1. Surgical technique. **a** Skin incision. **b** The pisi-form (*star*) with its vascular pedicle (*white arrow*) and the flexor carpi ulnaris (FCU) tendon (*black arrow*). **c** Distally based rectangular flap of the wrist capsule. **d** The pisiform is placed into the cavity and the reflected capsular flap is sutured into place

position. The plaster cast is removed after 3 weeks and active range-of-motion exercises are commenced.

Patients and Methods

During the period from 1980 to 1988, 14 patients with Kienböck's disease were treated by Saffar's procedure at Osaka Medical College Hospital, among whom follow-up examination was possible in 13. There were 8 males and 5 females whose average age at surgery was 46.1 years (range 31–65 years) (Table 1). The right wrist was affected in seven patients and the left in six. Nine patients were employed in occupations requiring manual labor, two were office workers, and two were housewives.

Most of the patients complained of loss of wrist motion, pain in the affected wrist, and loss of grip strength. The clinical symptoms developed during an average of 3.9 years before surgery (range 4 months–20 years). The X-ray findings were classi-fied according to Lichtman's criteria as follows: four patients in stage IIIA and nine patients in stage IIIB.

Thirteen patients were followed-up for an average of 73.9 months (range 13–125 months)

(Table 1). Detailed clinical and radiological examinations were performed and compared with presurgical findings and those at review.

Results

Clinical

The clinical patterns used in the assessment in-cluded pain, strength, and motion. A significant improvement was generally achieved in all para-meters. In none of the patients was the wrist worse after surgery.

Pain

At follow-up, all patients stated that pain had either disappeared or was decreased significantly. Seven patients had no pain, two had occasional pain, and four had mild pain or discomfort after strenuous work. In no patients did pain interfere with daily activity.

Ability to Work

Twelve patients returned to their previous oc-cupations, but one patient (case 4), who worked as a truck driver, changed to less strenuous work because of discomfort while steering the vehicle.

Table 1. Patients who underwent pisiform replacement

Case	Age (years)	Sex	Variance (mm)	Stage	Follow-up (months)	Pain at follow-up	Grip strength (%[a]) Preop.	Grip strength (%[a]) Postop.	Extension (%[a]) Preop.	Extension (%[a]) Postop.	Flexion (%[a]) Preop.	Flexion (%[a]) Postop.	Clinical result (score)
1	43	F	0.5	IIIB	125	None	69.4	92.7	52.9	92.9	21.4	64.3	Excellent (10)
2	52	M	0	IIIA	84	None	43.8	81.4	76.5	83.3	57.1	50.0	Good (9)
3	44	M	2.5	IIIB	117	Occasionally	43.3	83.9	71.4	86.7	44.4	72.7	Good (9)
4	31	M	−4.0	IIIB	115	Mild on exertion	30.4	70.7	39.5	80.0	60.3	45.5	Fair (6)
5	48	F	−2.4	IIIB	120	None	25.0	62.5	75.0	120.0	64.3	92.3	Excellent (10)
6	41	M	−2.0	IIIA	111	Occasionally	44.4	78.3	55.6	78.3	50.0	88.9	Good (9)
7	48	F	−1.4	IIIB	78	Mild on exertion	43.5	44.5	83.3	90.0	81.8	50.0	Fair (6)
8	49	M	1.0	IIIB	13	None	46.9	75.0	67.7	100.0	60.0	70.0	Excellent (10)
9	46	M	2.9	IIIB	69	None	79.3	111.5	33.3	116.7	75.0	87.5	Excellent (11)
10	65	F	3.0	IIIA	59	Mild on exertion	11.1	39.5	66.7	91.7	50.0	91.7	Fair (7)
11	40	M	−1.2	IIIB	17	None	25.0		21.4		50.0		
12	39	M	2.0	IIIA	20	Mild on exertion	45.2	77.8	50.0	100.0	18.8	81.3	Good (9)
13	53	F	−1.0	IIIB	33	Occasionally	50.0	68.8	56.3	91.7	66.7	57.1	Fair (7)
Mean	46.1				73.9		42.9	73.9	57.7	94.3	53.8	70.9	

Preop., Preoperatively; *Postop.*, postoperatively
[a] Compared with the normal side

Grip Strength

Grip strength was measured and the results were compared with the preoperative findings in 12 patients (Table 1). Preoperative grip strength was 42.9% of that of the opposite side and improved to 73.9% at follow-up.

Range of Motion

The range of motion was also compared with the preoperative level, and dorsi-flexion was found to be improved in all patients (57.7% preoperatively and 94.3% at follow-up) (Table 1). Improvement was observed for palmar flexion in eight patients but a decrease of palmar motion was noted in four patients. Radial deviation also improved in all patients except for one after surgery. However, a decrease of ulnar deviation was noted in 3 patients. Transfer of the FCU tendon might have influenced the decrease of palmar and ulnar flexion.

Overall Clinical Results

These were evaluated according to Lesur, Merle, and Michon's criteria [2] (Tables 2, 3). Four patients were rated as showing excellent results, four good, and four fair. There were no poor results. All patients were satisfied with their results.

Radiological

Standard dorsopalmar and lateral radiographs of both wrists in the neutral position were made for all the patients. Carpal height, carpal-ulnar

Table 2. Scoring of clinical parameters[a]

Score	Pain	Strength	Movement
4	None	≧90%	≧90%
3	Rare, slight not disabling	≧70%	≧70%
2	Activity slightly limited	≧50%	≧50%
1–0	Activity limited or very limited	<50%	<50%

[a] According to Lesur et al. [2]

Table 3. Scoring and assessment of the clinical results[a]

Assessment	Points	Patients (n)
Excellent	10	4
Good	8–9	4
Fair	6–7	4
Poor	<5	0

[a] According to Lesur et al. [2]

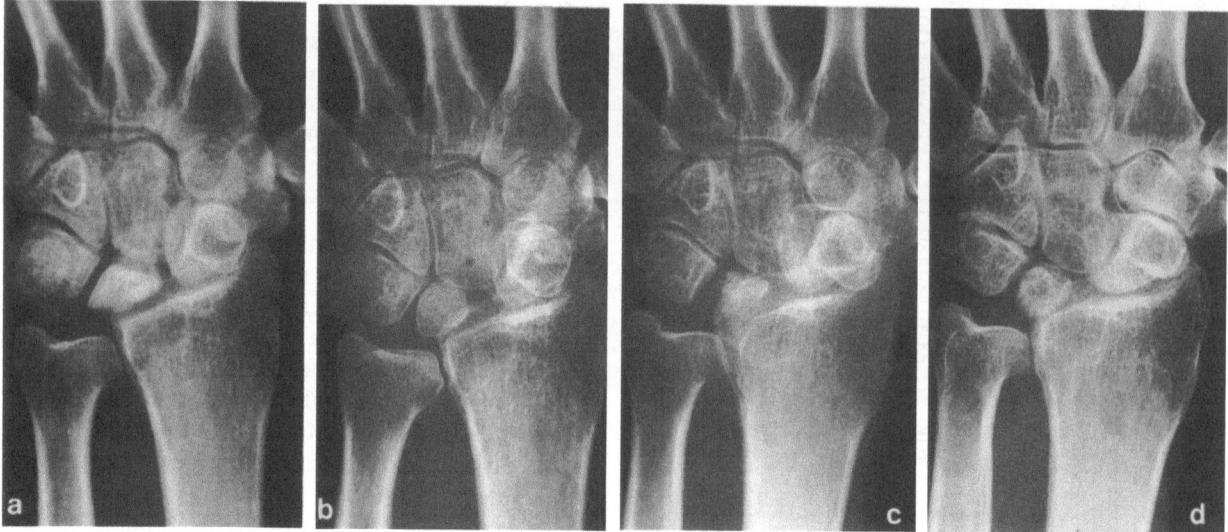

Fig. 2. A 48-year-old housewife (case 5). **a** Before surgery. **b** One month after surgery. **c** Radiograph taken 1 year after surgery shows some reduction of the replaced pisiform and increased bone density. **d** Radio-graph taken 10 years after surgery shows that the nearly normal shape and density of the pisiform have been resumed

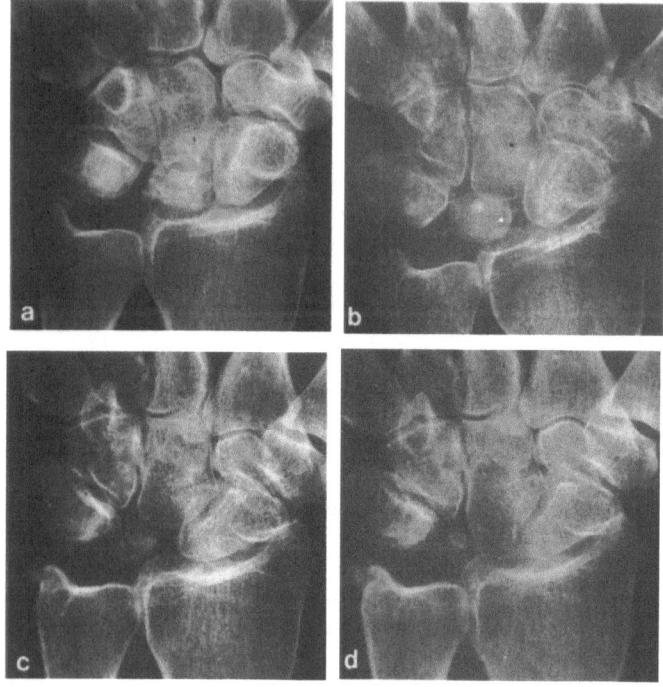

Fig. 3. A 48-year-old female factory worker (case 7). **a** Before surgery. **b** One month after surgery. **c** Radiograph taken 3.4 years after surgery shows that the replaced pisiform has been almost absorbed. **d** Radiograph taken 6.5 years after surgery shows that the normal configuration of the pisiform has not been resumed. In this case, clinical results were evaluated as being fair

distance ratio, and radioscaphoid angles were measured and compared with pre- and postsurgi-cal findings and at the time of follow-up in order to evaluate the carpal alignment [3].

Carpal Height Ratio

The mean value found before surgery was 0.49 (range 0.45–0.55). From 1 to 3 months after surgery, we found a mean index of 0.48 (range

0.42–0.54). The mean value found at follow-up review was 0.47 (range 0.41–0.52). Statistically, the carpal height ratio showed a significant decrease at follow-up examination. However, compared with 1–3 months after surgery, the follow-up review showed no deterioration in the ratio after a longer follow-up period.

Carpal-Ulnar Distance Ratio
The mean value before surgery was 0.31 (range 0.22–0.41) and the mean value at 1–3 months after surgery was 0.29 (range 0.22–0.37). The mean value at follow-up examination was 0.29 (range 0.21–0.38). These data showed that the carpal-ulnar distance ratio did not decrease significantly after surgery.

Radioscaphoid Angle
The mean angle before surgery was 69.2° (range 55°–83°) The mean angle measured 1–3 months after surgery was 74.5° (range 59°–83°). The mean angle at follow-up examination was 71.4° (range 62°–80°). These data showed that the radioscaphoid angle increased significantly immediately after surgery, but that further deterioration of the angle did not occur after a longer follow-up period.

Other Findings
X-ray findings of the inserted pisiform showed reduction in its shape and that increased bone density took place in most cases during 6–12 months after surgery, but the nearly normal shape and density was resumed 1–2 years later (Fig. 2). In case 1, the transposed pisiform fused with the triquetrum and no deterioration of the carpal alignment was observed. In 3 cases (cases 7, 8, and 13) the shape and density of the pisiform decreased and did not return to normal (Fig. 3). Clinical results in these 3 cases were excellent in one and fair in two.

Discussion

Transfer of the pisiform bone as a treatment for Kienböck's disease was reported by Beck [4] in 1971. He reported a case of successful treatment by transfer of the pisiform bone on a vascular pedicle into the excavated lunate bone. In 1982, Saffar [1] reported a new technique for replacement of the lunate by the pisiform together with its vascular supply and while being attached to the flexor carpi ulnaris. We have been using his procedure for the treatment of advanced Kienböck's disease since 1980, because of the superiority of replacing dead bone with living bone instead of using a prosthesis. According to Saffar's description, the main nutrient pedicle of the pisiform seems to be constant and an arterial circle exists around the bone. In our experience, small vascular pedicles to the pisiform were found in 7 out of 13 cases, but a reliable main nutrient pedicle from the ulnar artery was difficult to find in spite of careful dissection under magnification. As previously mentioned, X-ray findings showed that the shape and density of the replaced pisiform decreased during 6–12 months after surgery. This suggests that vascularity to the pisiform is not sufficient to keep its shape and bone density despite some vascularity expected from the attached flexor carpi ulnaris.

In 1985, Saffar [5] recommended other associated procedures, such as shortening of the radius for negative variance and scapho-trapezo-trapezoidal fusion to restore carpal height. We have never carried out any of these associated procedures. The radiological results showed that the carpal height decreased and the radial angle increased immediately after surgery but no further deterioration was observed during the longer follow-up period. Additionally, we have never observed osteoarthritic changes in the radiocarpal joint.

Clinically, some decrease in palmar flexion and ulnar deviation was observed in some patients, but grip strength, dorsiflexion, and radial deviation improved after the procedure. Some patients complained of mild pain or discomfort after strenuous work, but all the patients were satisfied with the results.

We conclude that replacement of the lunate by the pisiform is a useful procedure for treatment of advanced Kienböck's disease. Good long-term results can be achieved even though some deterioration in the carpal height and radioscaphoid angle may occur.

References

1. Saffar P (1982) Replacement du semi-lunaire par le pisiforme. Ann Chir Main 1:276–279
2. Lesur EL, Merle M, Michon J (1989) The limitations of replacement of the lunate by a Swanson prosthesis. French J Orthop Surg 3:328–337

3. McMurtry RY, Youm Y, Flatt AE, Gillespie TE
   (1978) Kinematics of the wrist, II. Clinical applications. J Bone Joint Surg [Am] 60:955–961
4. Beck E (1971) Die Verpflanzung des Os pisiforme

am Gefäßstiel zur Behandlung der Lunatummalazie.
   Handchir 3:64–67
5. Saffar P (1985) Replacement of lunate by pisiform in
   Kienböck's disease. J Orthop Surg Techniques 1:
   61–79

Part III. Scaphoid Fractures

Diagnosis and Management of Acute Scaphoid Fractures

Nicholas Barton[1]

Keywords: Fracture — Scaphoid — Non-union

Introduction

Although a fracture of the scaphoid was described by Janjavay from Paris in his thesis in 1846 [1], it was not until X-rays came into use that the subject began to be studied. However, much that has been written or said about fractures of the scaphoid consists of unproved assertions or what I believe to be incorrect statements. For many years this dogma was, like the teaching of Galen, accepted with hardly any question, but in recent years, we have begun to look at this subject afresh.

The University Hospital in Nottingham treats all the trauma cases for a population of about 750,000, and true fractures of the scaphoid are not as common as I had supposed. We have calculated from our own figures that a hospital serving a population of 250,000 (which is the average in the UK) will only see about three true scaphoid fractures in a month. Many other patients are treated for possible fractures of the scaphoid who never really had one, but it is wise to be on the safe side.

However, in another sense, fractures of the scaphoid are *more* common than we know about, because we only see the tip of the iceberg: often on X-rays of patients who have fallen and hurt their wrist an old un-united fracture of the scaphoid which the patient did not know about is revealed. Thus, we do not know the true incidence of scaphoid fractures, because there are probably a lot of people with old scaphoid fractures who

have *not* fallen and hurt it again and are therefore unaware that they have an un-united fracture.

It may also be that other undiagnosed and untreated fractures of the scaphoid *do* unite, as suggested by McLaughlin and Parkes [2], who believed that undisplaced fractures may have more or less intact articular cartilage which effectively splints the bony fragments which therefore "would heal under almost any circumstances". They distinguished these from cases in which the articular cartilage and supporting soft tissues were also fractured, but only through some part of their circumference, and detected these by aspiration of blood. We have attempted this but found it difficult and unreliable.

Nevertheless, this is a crucial point, because most fractures of the scaphoid are undisplaced and, if McLaughlin and Parkes were right, then neither diagnosis nor treatment is important in many patients. However, I disagree with them for three reasons:

1. I have seen patients with fractures so hard to detect that, when I showed them in an X-ray conference, they were missed by distinguished orthopaedic surgeons. These were certainly undisplaced fractures and may have had intact articular cartilage. They had also been missed by the doctors treating them, had not been treated, and had failed to unite.
2. Langhoff and Anderson [3] studied 285 scaphoid fractures, of which 32 were not detected on the first X-rays and, therefore, were not immobilized immediately. They found that delays of up to 4 weeks did not affect union but "when the delay exceeded four weeks, most fractures had healing complications".
3. I have operated on over 100 cases of nonunion and of these, about two-thirds were never treated by using plaster casts or were only immobilized briefly and inadequately.

[1] Nottingham University Hospital, Queen's Medical Centre, Nottingham NG7 2UH, UK

Diagnosis

The traditional clinical test is tenderness in the anatomical snuff box but this area is always tender because, if enough pressure is applied to the snuff box, it presses on the terminal sensory branches of the radial nerve. It is, therefore, very important to compare tenderness with that of the other wrist. The test of longitudinal compression [4] has the advantage that it can be carried out while the wrist is in a plaster cast, but it is not a reliable test, since it may be positive with other injuries or negative with a fracture of the scaphoid.

Since clinical findings are unreliable, we must depend very heavily on X-rays. The traditional views, ascribed to Russe [5] but actually described earlier by Böhler [6] are the PA, the semi-pronated oblique, the lateral, and the semi-supinated oblique, although the last is the least useful for this purpose. The radius, lunate, capitate, and finger metacarpals all lie in one axis, but the long axis of the scaphoid is flexed in relation to them by 45°–60°. This flexion of the scaphoid is increased during radial deviation, when the base of the first metacarpal must approach closer to the radial styloid; the scaphoid flexes over the fulcrum of the strong radioscaphocapitate ligament (which is seen during the anterior surgical approach to the scaphoid or to ganglia on the front of the wrist). The other mechanism which drives this flexion of the proximal row in radial deviation and extension in ulnar deviation is the helical shape of the joint between the hamate and the triquetrum. To detect a fracture of the scaphoid it is obviously better to study an X-ray which shows the scaphoid from the side rather than end-on, which is why we prefer always to have X-rays with the wrist in ulnar deviation for this purpose.

It is often said that scaphoid fractures may be undetectable on the first X-rays, but become visible after 2 weeks. However, it has been shown [7, 8] that the fracture is nearly always visible, if you look properly, on the original X-ray: the PA and semi-pronated views alone will pick up 97% of fractures. The advantage of waiting 2 weeks and repeating the X-rays is merely that the chances of detecting the fracture are doubled; in addition, the X-rays may, by chance, be taken at a slightly different angle.

Although the fracture may be obvious (Fig. 1), there can be genuine difficulty in diagnosing scaphoid fractures, which may be overlooked even by

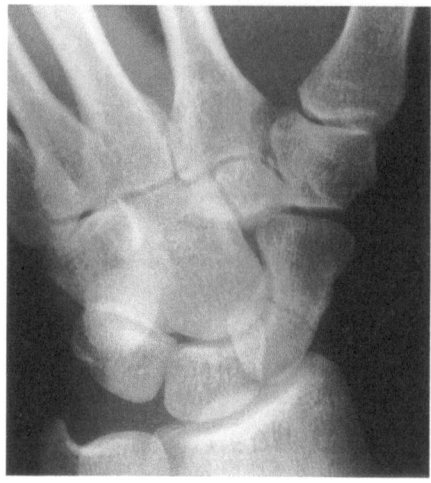

Fig. 1. Not all fractures of the scaphoid are as obvious as this one

an experienced observer. This was proved by Dias et al. [9] who showed 60 sets of scaphoid X-rays to five orthopaedic registrars (residents in training), five senior registrars, five consultant orthopaedic surgeons, and five radiologists: precisely those whose responsibility it is to diagnose scaphoid fractures in practice. The X-rays included original films, additional films taken 2 or 3 weeks later, normal films (of the other, uninjured wrist) and random copies of these films. The number of errors was considerable: those for the original and second X-rays of the fractures are shown in Table 1. The second X-rays did not improve the accuracy of diagnosis, regardless of the seniority of the observer. Of the normal radiographs, 20% were reported as showing a fracture. After an interval, the same observers were shown the same X-rays again: the more experienced doctors were more consistent in their opinions but, unfortunately, not more accurate (Table 2). Thus, there is clear evidence that it can be difficult to diagnose fractures of the scaphoid by just looking at the X-rays: even experienced observers can miss them or see what they imagine to be a fracture where there is none. Herbert, in his excellent book published recently [10], writes "the most important view is the comparative view of the opposite uninjured wrist". It is surprising how seldom this is done, as it seems obvious that when there is any doubt the same view of the opposite wrist at the same angle should be used for comparison. A recent prospec-

Table 1. Percentage errors in the diagnosis of scaphoid fractures. (Modified from Dias et al. [9])

Observers (n)	Radiographs			Mean errors
	Initial films	After 2 or 3 weeks	Both	
Registrars (5)	37	43	37	39
Senior registrars (5)	43	42	39	49
Consultants (5)	42	43	39	41
Radiologists (5)	42	43	43	43
Mean	41	43	40	41

Analysis of variance for groups: DF3× = 0.86, $P = 0.83$; for observers: DF19× = 31.3, $P = 0.04$; for radiographs: DF19× = 297.7, $P = 0.0001$

Table 2. Reproducibility: agreement between first and second viewing by 20 observers. (Modified from Dias et al. [9])

Observers (n)	Right twice	Wrong twice	Changed mind	Kappa value[a]	Standard error
Registrars (5)	27	8	15	0.299	0.143
Senior registrars (5)	29	9	12	0.429	0.139
Consultants (5)	26	13	11	0.528	0.124
Radiologists (5)	34	12	4	0.802	0.094
All	116	42	42	0.513	0.065

[a] Kappa value can vary from −1 (complete disagreement) through 0 (chance agreement) to +1 (complete agreement)

tive study of 200 patients has confirmed the value of this policy [11].

Another useful tip is to alter the angle of the X-ray beam. The usual pictures, whether PA, oblique, or lateral, are all taken with the X-ray beam perpendicular to the long axis of the arm (Fig. 2.a). However, the long axis of the scaphoid is *not* perpendicular to the long axis of the arm; therefore if the beam is tilted appropriately (Fig. 2.b), it is more likely to pass through the fracture and visualize it [12]. We find these tilted views of great value. The Ziter view [13] is another way of doing the same thing, although, again, a similar technique was used much earlier by Böhler and reported by Schnek [14].

What is the value of other methods of investigation? Unfortunately, they are not as helpful in practice as one might expect. Soft-tissue signs on plain radiographs [15, 16], such as the scaphoid fat stripe (Fig. 3), thermography [17], and bone scanning [18] are all non-specific, while ultrasound, as a provocative test, has been found to be unreliable [19].

More elaborate special investigations, such as CT scanning [20] and MRI [21], are specific but many hospitals do not have facilities for them

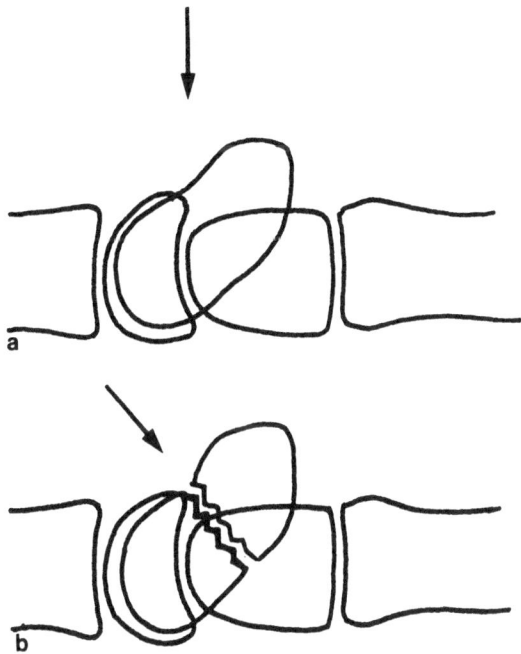

Fig. 2. a All projections of conventional scaphoid radiographs are taken with the X-ray beam perpendicular (*arrow*) to the long axis of the arm. **b** The beam has been tilted (*arrow*) so that it is perpendicular to the long axis of the scaphoid. On the resulting film, the scaphoid looks elongated

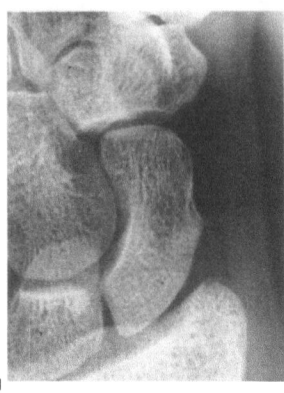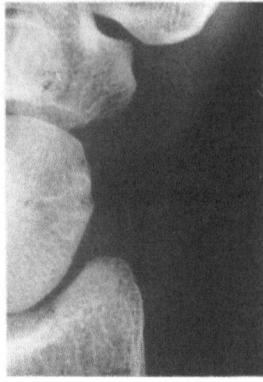

Fig. 3. Scaphoid fat stripe. **a** Normal, with the dark fat stripe forming a straight line. **b** Abnormal, the haemarthrosis from a fracture displacing the fat stripe outwards and giving it a convex margin

and, even in those which do, they are seldom available instantly. We need a test which can be done in the fracture clinic cheaply and, above all, quickly. The clinician needs to know within an hour whether the patient has a fracture that must be treated, and he is obliged to depend on X-rays despite the difficulty of interpreting them correctly and with certainty.

Treatment

Fractures of the scaphoid tuberosity, which need to be only 3 or 4 weeks in a plaster cast, pose no difficulties [22]. The problem is with fractures which go right across the scaphoid: not necessarily at the waist, as some are more proximal and some more distal.

There are surgeons, especially in Japan and the USA, who take the view that fractures of the scaphoid are intra-articular fractures and should therefore be treated by internal fixation. They draw an analogy with subcapital fractures of the femur, which are also intracapsular. I believe this is false: most scaphoid fractures unite with conservative treatment, whereas most subcapital fractures do not. Trans-scaphoid perilunar dislocations certainly require open reduction and internal fixation, not only because the wrist has become so unstable but because we have found that there may be torn capsule interposed between the proximal and distal poles of the scaphoid [23]. I would also accept that operation is

required in significantly displaced fractures which cannot be reduced by manipulation, but such fractures are uncommon. Internal fixation may also be used, *in combination with bone grafting*, in the treatment of non-union and perhaps of delayed union.

However, most scaphoid fractures should, in my view, be treated conservatively in a plaster cast. McLaughlin and Parkes [2] advocated internal fixation in young male breadwinners who might suffer economic catastrophe from prolonged immobilization in plaster. We no longer use such long periods of immobilization and most societies have now evolved systems to provide financial support during a temporary period of unemployment due to physical disability. We must always remember that it is possible, although unlikely, that the patient could suffer even a worse catastrophe from surgical or anaesthetic complications of an unnecessary operation. McLaughlin refers to the "almost universal refusal of the surgeons who advocate prolonged immobilization to submit their own fractured scaphoids to... this plan of treatment", but I would have mine treated conservatively if it did not have one of the indications for operation mentioned above.

However, it is not enough to advocate immobilization in a plaster cast: what kind of a cast should be used and for how long? Many different types of casts have been recommended by different authors. It may be below the elbow or extend above the elbow, in which case the forearm may be supinated or pronated. The wrist may be extended or flexed and in radial or ulnar deviation. The thumb may be included right to the tip of the thumb, or as far as the inter-phalangeal joint, or be left completely free. Some surgeons have even recommended including the fingers.

Immobilization of the Elbow

The first question to be considered is whether the plaster cast should be above or below the elbow. In 1975, Lindstrom [24] reviewed 244 fractures treated in Moberg's unit in Gothenberg, Sweden, and found no difference between the Böhler below-elbow type of cast and the Verdan above-elbow cast as regards frequency of non-union or period of immobilization. In the same year, Alho and Kankaanpää from Finland [25] compared 51 patients treated by below-elbow casts with 41 by above-elbow ones, as a randomized prospective study. After 3 months, there were two non-unions with the below-elbow cast and six non-unions with the above-elbow one. Thus, neither of these papers found any advantage in extending the cast above the elbow.

A more recent paper from the United States by Gelman et al. [26], also a randomized prospective study, was of 51 undisplaced scaphoid fractures: 28 were treated by an above-elbow cast for the first 6 weeks and then by a shorter cast until they were united, while 23 were treated by a below-elbow cast from the beginning. This paper is worthy of serious consideration, because there was adequate follow-up (X-rays of all the wrists were taken after at least 6 months) and the authors define what they mean by union, delayed union, and non-union, which many papers on this subject fail to do. Their conclusion was that the above-elbow cast was superior: there were no nonunions with it, whereas two fractures treated in below-elbow casts failed to unite. However, their numbers were very small and must be set against the Scandinavian papers which reached the opposite conclusion with larger numbers.

Immobilization of the Thumb

In Britain, almost all practitioners use a below-elbow cast, including the thumb to the interphalangeal (I.P.) joint: indeed it is called a "scaphoid plaster" as if there were no alternative (Fig. 4). It is suprisingly difficult to find out why and when this became the standard teaching in Britain. Sir Reginald Watson Jones [27], in the first edition of his famous book on "*Fractures and Joint Injuries*" published in 1940, described a rather curious cast which "covers the first interosseous space and includes the first metacarpal as far as the thenar muscles", but leaves the rest of the thumb free. This advice was unchanged in the second edition. In the third edition of 1943, he wrote "some surgeons also include the metacarpophalangeal joint of the thumb, and even the interphalangeal joint" and in the fourth edition (1955) he recommended this more strongly "including the metacarpal base of the thumb, or perhaps better still, the metacarpophalangeal joint and proximal phalanx". In the fifth edition, published in 1976 after Watson Jones' death, this chapter was not revised but it was re-written by Fisk for the sixth edition (1982) who described what had become the standard British method: the "scaphoid plaster," extending to the neck of the proximal phalanx.

The change seems to have come around 1955 and I think there were two influences which

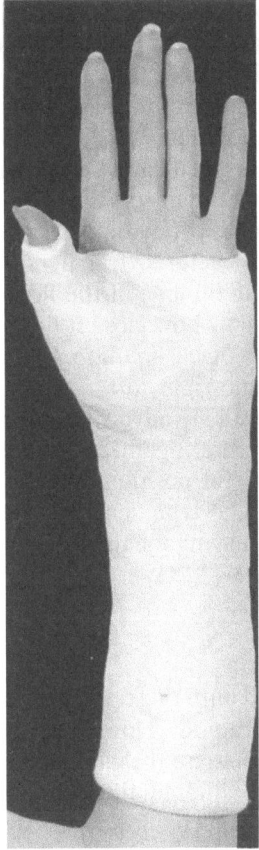 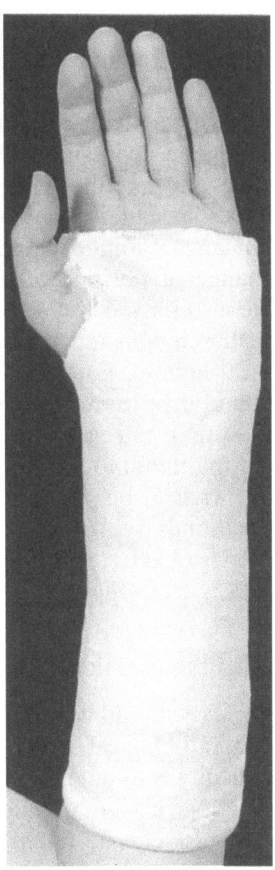

Fig. 4   **Fig. 5**

Fig. 4. Standard "scaphoid" cast

Fig. 5. Plaster cast leaving the thumb free, as used in treating Colles' fractures. The author believes that this is also the best cast to use for a scaphoid fracture

brought it about. The first was the paper by Böhler and others [28] in 1954: this is in German and has only recently come to my attention through the kindness of Professor Lindstrom of Umea in Sweden who translated the relevant part for me. Up to 1942, Böhler left the thumb out of the cast, but he later started including it. In this paper he wrote "it will be interesting to investigate if the times for union are shorter, and if in fact the number of pseudarthroses may be reduced". (That is what we have done, as I will describe below.) The second was another paper published in the same year by Stewart [29] who reported a very large series of fractures from the US army and recommended including the thumb in the cast as far as the inter-phalangeal joint.

However, there are other views about immobilizing the thumb. Soto-Hall [30], also then in the US army, believed that the whole thumb should be included in the cast, including its distal phalanx. His paper contained photographs of X-rays of cadaveric fractures and he specifically stated "in these specimens, any movement of the interphalangeal joint of the thumb produces a definite change of position of the fractured fragments". He also passed a wire along the line of the flexor pollicis longus tendon to show how close it lies to the scaphoid. For him, the logical solution was to immobilize the whole thumb right to the tip. At the other extreme, London [31] advocated leaving the thumb out of the cast altogether: "encase the wrist in plaster in a useful position and with the thumb free", i.e., a similar type of cast to that used for Colles' fractures, leaving the thumb completely free (Fig. 5).

Diagnosis of Union

The cast should be retained until there are clinical and radiological signs of union. However, the difficulty is to determine what are the clinical and radiological signs of union. Union in the tibia, for example, can be tested by mechanical stressing, but the scaphoid is too small for that method. Tenderness is unreliable in an area which may be tender normally and I find that many wrists with non-union are not tender, thus I do not consider this clinical examination to be very helpful.

Special investigations are seldom applicable to routine cases, only for problematical ones. In such cases, conventional tomography or CT scanning [32, 33] may be helpful, but, unfortunately, we often may not know that a particular fracture is a problem at that stage. Real-time ultrasound can determine movement or lack of movement between the fragments [34].

In practice, we must again rely on X-rays in most cases. Watson Jones [27] also felt that the clinician must depend on radiographic evidence, and insisted that the union is not sound until complete obliteration of the line of the fracture can be seen in two views; he repeated the X-rays 3 weeks after the cast was removed. It was perhaps because of this insistence that he was prepared to keep the wrists in casts for many months, in a way which would now be considered unacceptable. Russe [5] stressed that increased density of the bone at the site of the former fracture cleft may be a sign of *union* not, as is commonly thought, a sign of non-union.

Nevertheless, in looking at X-rays taken 8 or 12 weeks after a scaphoid fracture, I have found great difficulty in deciding whether or not union has occured. The more experience I gained, the more difficult I found it, and I began to question my ability. This led to the study by Dias et al. [35] who arranged for eight different observers to review 20 good X-rays taken after 12 weeks of immobilization of a definite scaphoid fracture whose outcome was known. They were asked whether the fracture had united, whether there were trabeculae crossing it, and whether the proximal pole was avascular. These experienced observers, four orthopaedic consultants and four consultant radiologists, did not agree upon the answers to these simple questions. Dias then waited a few months and showed the same X-rays again to the same people, who sometimes did not agree with what they had said the first time. He concluded that "previous published conclusions based on such assessment are open to question". In reality, this means *all* previous publications are open to question, as they include statements like "60% were united in 8 weeks" or "80% were united in 10 weeks", based on radiological judgments which we now know to be unreliable.

Our experience has been that one can, in most cases, be confident of the outcome on X-rays taken 6 months after the fracture occurs, although we have not submitted this to the same rigorous analysis. We therefore use these films to determine the outcome for research purposes. However, even after 6 months, there are some X-rays in which the fracture is still very clearly visible although it appears united: these we call "probable union" (Fig. 6).

We do not want to keep all our patients' wrists in casts for 6 months; so, for practical purposes to decide when the immobilization can be discontinued, we still have to do our best to determine union by clinical and radiological assessment after 2 or 3 months.

What is the rate of non-union after treatment of a scaphoid fracture? According to Leslie and Dickson [7] it is 5% (11 out of 222) after standard British treatment. However, their review was of patients discharged at the end of treatment and it is possible that some of their patients actually had non-union but were not complaining. Herbert and Fisher believe that this is very common and that the incidence of non-union after conservative treatment is around 50% [36]. To determine the correct figure, Dias [37] followed-up 82 patients with definite fractures of the waist of the scaphoid

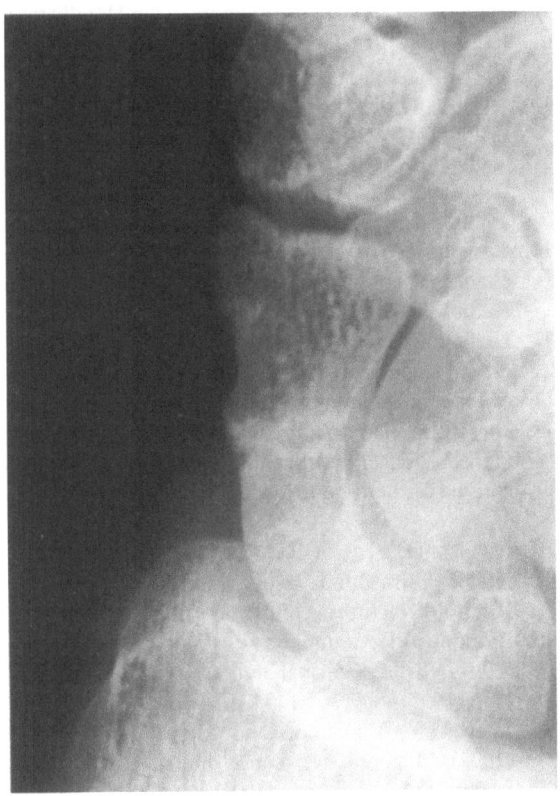

Fig. 6. "Probable" union of the scaphoid. On this X-ray taken 6 months after the injury, the site of the fracture is still clearly visible but appears to be united

treated conservatively and found that the incidence of non-union was 12.3% (making it more than 5% but less than 50%) — and most of these did have symptoms.

Nottingham/Leicester Scaphoid Study

Having defined what I mean by union, I will now describe an investigation done jointly at Nottingham University Hospital and at our sister medical school in Leicester, as we wanted to get a large enough number of patients to be of statistical value. We studied 292 patients, treated over a 2-year period, with definite fractures right across the scaphoid [38]: I would like to stress that these were definite fractures — we did not include any of which it could later be said that there had never been a fracture at all.

The patients were randomly assigned to treatment either in a "scaphoid" cast (including the proximal phalanx of the thumb) or a Colles' type of cast (leaving the thumb free) (Figs. 4, 5). The 2

groups were comparable for age, sex, affected side, time in cast, and also for type and displacement of fracture. For this we wanted a large number, so that these factors would be equalized. However, in our practice, although it seems not to be the same in some other countries, the great majority of our scaphoid fractures are either undisplaced or virtually undisplaced, i.e., we rarely see displaced ones. If a scaphoid fracture was associated with dislocation then it was, of course, operated on and not included in this series.

All the wrists were kept in casts for 8 weeks, after which the casts were removed and the wrists examined. If they were not tender and we thought the X-ray indicated the fracture to be united (bearing in mind the difficulty of being sure), we left the cast off. If there was still tenderness or the X-ray findings were doubtful, we put the wrist back into a cast for another 4 weeks but then left it free and did not repeat the X-ray at that stage. All these patients were reviewed and the wrists X-rayed 6 months after the fracture to achieve a reliable end-point by which to compare these two methods of treatment. We did not succeed in persuading every patient with a fracture of the scaphoid to come back after 6 months: these were young men, sometimes rather irresponsible, and, if they had no symptoms, it was difficult to get them to return for follow-up. However, all the 292 patients described in this series did come back and were followed-up for 6 months.

They were asked questions each time they came about what they could do in the cast (dressing, eating, writing, driving, and so forth) and an activity score was compiled from their answers. As one would expect, those who were in the Colles' cast with the thumb free were able to do more than those whose thumb was included in the cast; but when the cast was removed, the differences evened out very quickly. Similarly, opposi-

Table 3. The Nottingham/Leicester scaphoid study: radiological results 6 months following the injury. (Modified from Clay et al. [38])

	Scaphoid cast Number (%)[a]	Colles' cast Number (%)
Definite union	111 (78)	114 (77)
Probable union	18 (12)	19 (13)
Non-union	14 (10)	15 (10)
	143	148

[a] (Percentages are to the nearest whole number)

tion was better when the wrists were in a Colles' type of cast. There was not much difference between the 2 groups with regard to grip strength and they regained wrist movements equally well after removal of the casts.

Our results are summarized in Table 3. Probable union was almost the same in the 2 groups, and non-union was exactly the same: 10% in each group. We conclude, therefore, that after a scaphoid fracture immobilization of the thumb confers no advantage. The rate of non-union is determined by the nature of the fracture and by the *quality* of the cast, how strong and close-fitting it is, not the area covered by the cast. Since it is more convenient for the patient to have the thumb free, that is what we recommend.

References

1. Janjavay. (1846) Theses de Paris 25, p 25 (quoted by Lindstrom [25])
2. McLaughlin HL, Parkes JC (1969) Fracture of the carpal navicular (scaphoid) bone: Graduations in therapy based upon pathology. J Trauma 9:4:311–319
3. Langhoff O, Andersen JL (1988) Consequences of late immobilization of scaphoid fractures. J Hand Surg [Br] 13:1:77–79
4. Chen SC (1989) The scaphoid compression test. J Hand Surg [Br] 14:3:323–325
5. Russe O (1960) Fracture of the carpal navicular. Diagnosis, non-operative treatment, and operative treatment. J Bone Joint Surg [Am] 42:5:759–768
6. Böhler L (1929) Die Technik der Knochenbruchbehandlung. Wien, Maudrich
7. Leslie IJ, Dickson RA (1981) The fractured carpal scaphoid. Natural history and factors affecting outcome. J Bone Joint Surg [Br] 63:2:225–230
8. Duncan DS, Thurston AJ (1985) Clinical fracture of the carpal scaphoid — an illusionary diagnosis. J Hand Surg [Br] 10:3:375–376
9. Dias JJ, Thompson J, Barton NJ, Gregg PJ (1990) Suspected scaphoid fractures. The value of radiographs. J Bone Joint Surg [Br] 72:1:98–101
10. Herbert TJ (1990) The fractured scaphoid. Quality Medical, St. Louis, p 32
11. Abdel-Salam A, Eyres KS, Cleary J (1992) Detecting fractures of the scaphoid: the value of comparative X-rays of the uninjured wrist. J Hand Surg [Br] 17:1:28–32
12. Lindgren E (1949) Some radiological aspects in the carpal scaphoid and its fractures. Acta Chir Scand 98:538–548
13. Ziter FMH (1973) A modified view of the carpal navicular. Radiology 108:707–708
14. Schnek F (1930) Die Verletzungen der Handwurzel. Ergebnisse der Chirurgie und Orthopädie 23:1–109
15. Dias JJ, Finlay DBL, Brenkel IJ, Gregg PJ (1987) Radiographic assessment of soft tissue signs in clinically suspected scaphoid fractures: The incidence of false negative and false positive results. J Orthop Trauma 1:3:205–208
16. Carver RA, Barrington NA (1985) Soft-tissue changes accompanying recent scaphoid injury. Clin Radiol 36:423–425
17. Hosie KB, Wardrobe J, Crosby AC, Ferguson DG (1987) Liquid crystal thermography in the diagnosis of scaphoid fractures. Arch Emerg Med 4:117–120
18. Jorgensen TM, Andresen J-H, Thommesen P, Hansen HH (1979) Scanning and radiology of the carpal scaphoid bone. Acta Orthop Scand 50:663–665
19. DaCruz DJ, Taylor RH, Savage B, Bodiwala GG (1988) Ultrasound assessment of the suspected scaphoid fracture. Arch Emerg Med 5:97–100
20. Biondetti PR, Vannier MW, Gilula LA, Knapp R (1987) Wrist: Coronal and transaxial C.T. scanning. Radiology 163:149–151
21. Imaeda T, Wakamura R, Miura J, Makino N (1992) Magnetic resonance imaging in scaphoid fractures. J Hand Surg [Br] 17:1:20–27
22. Prosser AJ, Brenkel IJ, Irvine GB (1988) Articular fractures of the distal scaphoid. J Hand Surg [Br] 13:1:87–91
23. Wilton TJ (1987) Soft-tissue interposition as a possible cause of scaphoid non-union. J Hand Surg [Br] 12:1:50–51
24. Lindstrom G (1975) Scaphoid fractures. A survey based on 373 cases over a 7-year period of observation. (in Swedish, with English summary). Thesis. University of Göteborg, Sweden
25. Alho A, Kankaanpää V (1975) Management of fractured scaphoid bone. A prospective study of 100 fractures. Acta Orthop Scand 46:737–743
26. Gellman H, Caputo RJ, Carter V, Aboulafia A, McKay M (1989) Comparison of short and long thumb-spica casts for non-displaced fractures of the carpal scaphoid. J Bone Joint Surg [Am] 71:3:354–357
27. Watson Jones R (1940) Fractures and Joint Injuries (1st edn.). Livingstone, Edinburgh
28. Böhler L, Trojan E, Jahna H (1954) Behandlungsergebnisse von 734 frischen einfachen Brüchen des Kahnbeinkörpers der Hand. Reconstr Surg Traumatol 2:86–111
29. Stewart MJ (1954) Fractures of carpal navicular (scaphoid). A report of 436 Cases. J Bone Joint Surg [Am] 36:5:998–1006
30. Soto-Hall R (1945) Recent fractures of the carpal scaphoid. JAMA 129(5):335–338

31. London PS (1967) A practical guide to the care of the injured. Livingstone, Edinburgh

32. Bush CH, Gillespy J, Dell OC (1987) High-resolution CT of the wrist: Initial experience with scaphoid disorders and surgical fusions. Am J Roentgenol 149:757–760

33. Pennes DR, Johsson K, Buckwalter KA (1989) Direct coronal CT of the scaphoid bone. Radiology 171:3:870–871

34. Dias JJ (to be published) Real-time ultrasound in the assessment of union of scaphoid fractures.

35. Dias JJ, Taylor M, Thompson J, Brenkel IJ, Gregg PJ (1988) Radiographic signs of union of scaphoid fractures. An analysis of inter-observer agreement and reproducibility. J Bone Joint Surg [Br] 70:2:299–301

36. Herbert TJ, Fisher WE (1984) Management of the fractured scaphoid using a new bone screw. J Bone Joint Surg [Br] 66:1:114–123

37. Dias JJ, Brenkel IJ, Finlay DBL (1989) Patterns of union in fractures of the waist of the scaphoid. J Bone Joint Surg [Br] 71:2:307–310

38. Clay N, Dias JJ, Costigan P, Gregg PJ, Barton NJ (1991) Need the thumb be immobilized in scaphoid fractures? A randomized prospective trial of Colles and scaphoid casts. J Bone Joint Surg [Br] 73(5): 828–832

Scaphoid Non-Union: Current Approach to Management

Diego L. Fernandez[1]

Keywords: Scaphoid non-union — Classification — Bone grafting — Screw fixation — Revascularization — Salvage procedures

Introduction

Better understanding of the physiopathology of carpal trauma and its sequelae has, in the past decade, led to a more aggressive treatment of the fractured and non-united carpal scaphoid. This implies the concept of fracture instability [1, 2] with a relative constant displacement pattern of the distal fragment into flexion, ulnar deviation, and perhaps a pronation malalignment as well. If fracture healing ensues, mal-union is the rule; otherwise, the pseudarthrosis progresses to bone resorbtion with additional secondary shortening of the scaphoid. In both instances, the initial associated dorsal carpal instability pattern leads to further carpal collapse, which eventually results in mechanical overload and degenerative changes of the wrist joint.

On the other hand, stable fractures and non-unions without displacement have a more favorable prognosis. The basic aim of the treatment of angulated non-union or severely deformed mal-union is the restoration of normal scaphoid anatomy with interpositional bone grafting techniques and internal fixation. Stable, non-deformed non-unions may, alternatively, profit from conventional inlay bone grafting techniques. However, early rehabilitation of the wrist is only possible with stable internal fixation of the scaphoid, both in the unstable and stable non-union types.

Fractures and non-unions of the proximal pole represent a different therapeutic entity that may be aggravated by the presence of avascular necrosis. Retrograde screw fixation of small proximal fragments through a dorsal approach is our current method of choice. However, if intra-operative findings reveal a complete avascular necrosis of the proximal fragment but no arthritic changes, a revascularization procedure should be attempted in every case and an effort be made to salvage the anatomical integrity of the proximal carpal row.

Diagnosis, Imaging, and Classification of Scaphoid Non-Unions

A non-union of the scaphoid may be *symptomatic* with or without a known history of previous wrist trauma, revealing pain localized at the dorso-radial aspect of the wrist, usually exacerbated at the extremes of flexion or extension of the wrist, and frequently associated with loss of grip strength. Long-standing *asymptomatic* non-unions may well reveal the first symptoms several years after initial trauma, with progressive pain and limitation of motion due to secondary arthritic changes and carpal collapse.

Recent follow-up studies on the natural history of the non-union of the scaphoid [3–5] have clearly proven that initial fracture displacement and carpal instability lead to progressive degenerative changes with a distinct pattern of occurrence. Initially, the degenerative changes are located at the radioscaphoid joint, and later include the scaphocapitate and, finally, the capitolunate joint [5]. Due to progressive shortening and flexion deformity of the scaphoid, a dorsiflexed intercalated segment instability (DISI) pattern is frequently observed, with proximal migration of the capitate and increased dorsiflexion of the

[1] Department of Surgery, Kantonsspital Aarau, CH-5001 Aarau, Switzerland

153

lunate. However, as pointed out by Watson [6], the radiolunate joint "survives" the progressive arthritic pattern of the advanced carpal collapse for many years. Based on the knowledge of the natural history of scaphoid non-unions, asymptomatic patients should be advised of the possibility of late degenerative changes, and an operation to restore scaphoid integrity should be proposed in spite of the absence of symptoms.

Scaphoid non-unions may be localized in the distal third, the waist, or the proximal third. Its recognition is important for the choice of the surgical approach. According to the radiographic appearance and the nature of the interposed tissue, scaphoid non-unions are further classified into *fibrous*, *cystic*, and *sclerotic* types. Loose fibrous tissue with adjacent small cysts are found in *early delayed unions*. With time, bone resorption with larger adjacent cystic cavities, a more organized fibrous tissue, and partial healing of the cartilage envelope are the pathoanatomic findings of the *cystic non-union*. The sclerotic type corresponds to an established *pseudarthrosis*, with disappearance of the cysts, presence of a "false joint" with sclerotic margins and even a cartilage lining, allowing passage of joint synovial fluid between both fragments. Herbert [7, 8] divides the established non-union into 2 types: (1) *fibrous union*, which is a relatively stable non-deformed non-union with variable cystic changes, and (2) *pseudarthrosis* with instability, shortening, deformity, and discrepancy between the size of the bone fragments.

Biomechanically, non-unions of the scaphoid are subdivided into *stable*, undisplaced, or non-deformed, and *unstable*, displaced, or angulated types. An unstable scaphoid non-union shows displacement of the fragments greater than 1 mm and the ulnar deviation views or image intensifier examination shows motion at the non-union site. The lateral wrist X-rays show a dorsal intercalated instability pattern, and lateral trispiral tomograms of the wrist clearly show the flexion or "humpback deformity" of the scaphoid. On the other hand, stable or undisplaced non-union corresponds basically to a delayed union or fibrous non-union with a persistant gap, usually after a trial of conservative treatment for an initially nondisplaced fracture of the waist without the above-mentioned radiographic findings.

From a prognostic standpoint and especially for the choice of the method of treatment, surgical approach, and type of bone grafting procedure, our decision is based on (1) the anatomical local-ization of the non-union, (2) presence or absence of instability or deformity, and (3) the vascular status of the proximal fragment. If these parameters are clearly diagnosed with an AP lateral X-ray of the wrist and comparative films of the opposite wrist to determine and measure any associated carpal instability and the amount of scaphoid shortening in plain navicular views, no further sophisticated imaging of the scaphoid is needed. However, tomograms and CT-scans are valuable diagnostic measures for the evaluation of bone healing and precise determination of post-traumatic scaphoid deformity [9]. Three-dimensional reconstruction provides a high degree of accuracy for the preoperative planning of complex surgical correction of scaphoid deformity in three planes. Finally, magnetic resonance imaging plays an important role in the preoperative evaluation of avascular necrosis of the proximal fragment and for the assessment of restoration of scaphoid vascularity following revascularization procedures [10, 11].

Treatment

Although non-united fractures recognized as early as 3–6 months after injury can be submitted to a trial conservative treatment with prolonged cast fixation combined or not with pulsed electromagnetic fields with a reported union-rate of 80% [12], non-invasive management is not reliable for deformed unstable non-unions and long-standing sclerotic non-unions, because restoration of normal scaphoid length and carpal alignment cannot be achieved in spite of eventual union. Furthermore, with the substantial improvement of union rate with a very short period of wrist immobilization due to modern refinements of stable internal fixation of the scaphoid, a less cumbersome treatment modality with early use of the hand for non-strenous activities can be offered to the patient, resulting in particular benefit to patients not engaged in heavy manual labor and who can profit from free wrist motion long before healing of the non-union [8, 13]. On the other hand, conventional bone grafting techniques without internal fixation still require a minimum of 3 months of wrist immobilization in a cast. Currently, our management protocol for established scaphoid non-unions bases the indication of the particular procedure on the following parameters: (1) established scaphoid non-unions *without secondary degenerative changes* of the wrist, in which union of the scaphoid has to be obtained, (2) scaphoid non-union *with early degenerative changes* of the wrist, in which scaphoid union has to be combined with an additional operation for the initial radioscaphoid arthritic changes in order to guarantee a painless wrist, and (3) scaphoid non-unions *with advanced degenerative wrist disease* for which only a salvage procedure (resection arthroplasty, partial or total fusions) should be elected.

For the first group, surgical indication is based on the concept of stability, the location of the pseudarthrosis, and the presence or absence of avascular necrosis. An unstable, angulated, or displaced non-union of the waist or distal third with a viable proximal fragment are best treated with anterior interpositional bone-grafting techniques and rigid internal fixation. Proximal non-unions with viable proximal fragments, seldom associated with massive deformity and instability patterns, are managed with bone grafting and retrograde screw fixation through a dorsal approach. Non-unions with complete avascular necrosis without degenerative changes, regardless of the location, are given a trial of revascularization combined with bone grafting. Stable non-deformed non-unions or delayed non-unions, that do not require restoration of scaphoid length,

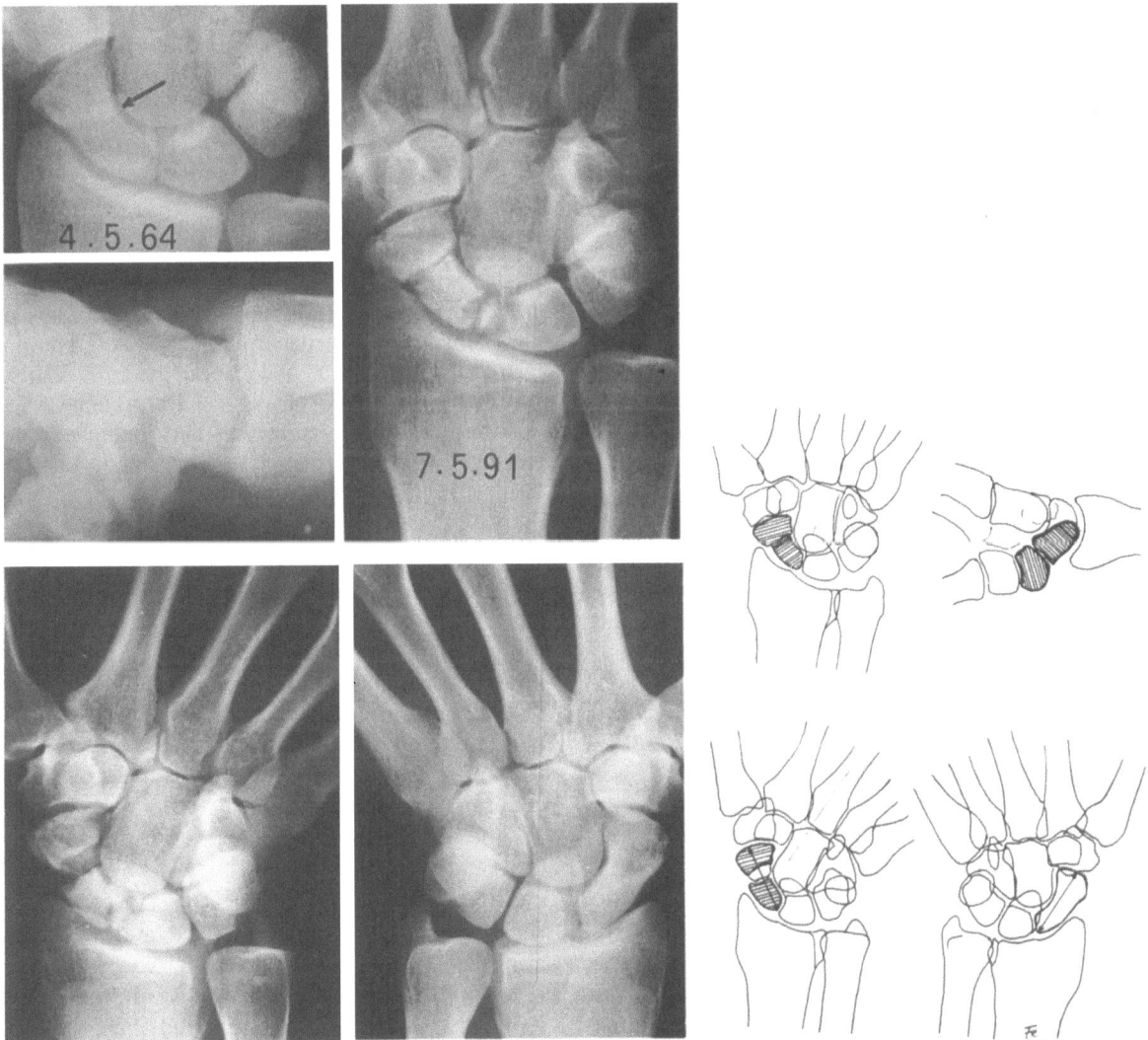

Fig. 1. a Scaphoid pseudarthrosis 27 years after injury. Anteroposterior roentgenogram in maximal ulnar deviation shows widening of the non-union gap. **b** Tracing of the radiographs of the case showed in **a**. This is useful to measure carpal collapse, evaluate DISI deformity, and calculate the length of the scaphoid in the uninjured side

may be treated with conventional inlay bone
grafting techniques [14].

Surgical Procedures

Anterior Interpositional Bone Grafting Technique

This technique originally suggested by Fisk [15]
to correct the "humpback deformity" with radiovolar grafting using a wedge-shaped graft taken
from the radial styloid and followed by cast
fixation, was subsequently modified by various
authors [7, 16–19]. It is the current method
of choice for unstable, deformed, and angulated
non-unions located at the waist or at the distal
third of the carpal scaphoid with a viable proximal
fragment [7, 16, 20]. It is also useful for corrective
osteotomies to treat scaphoid mal-unions associated with carpal instability. Restoration of
normal scaphoid length through distraction of the
non-union restores the "strut" function of the
radial column of the carpus, which, in turn,
controls the initial carpal collapse and the associated dorsal lunate rotation.

To correct angular deformity and restore
normal scaphoid length, the amount of resection
and size of the graft needed are calculated preoperatively by carefully tracing the radiographic
findings in the AP and lateral views of the injured
and of the contralateral wrists [16]. This helps us
to determine the amount of carpal collapse and
the normal and pathological scapholunate and
lunocapitate angles for each case individually.
Particularly in the unstable mobile non-unions,
the pseudarthrotic gap opens in maximal ulnar
deviation. An X-ray of both wrists taken in this
position (Fig. 1) is very helpful for determining
the amount of bone defect that has to be replaced
by the interpositional bone graft in the anteroposterior plane. An X-ray of the uninjured wrist
in the same position is useful to measure scaphoid
length, because the scaphoid rotates to an extended position in maximal ulnar deviation. The
size and form of the graft can be calculated
in millimeters and will vary, depending on the
specific deformity of each particular scaphoid
non-union. If there is no flexion deformity of
the scaphoid, shortening or associated carpal
instability, or collapse, a small rectangular graft
to fit the defect after resection of the non-union
is used. Otherwise, the graft is triangular or
trapezoidal in order to obtain correction of the
flexion deformity in the sagittal plane and the

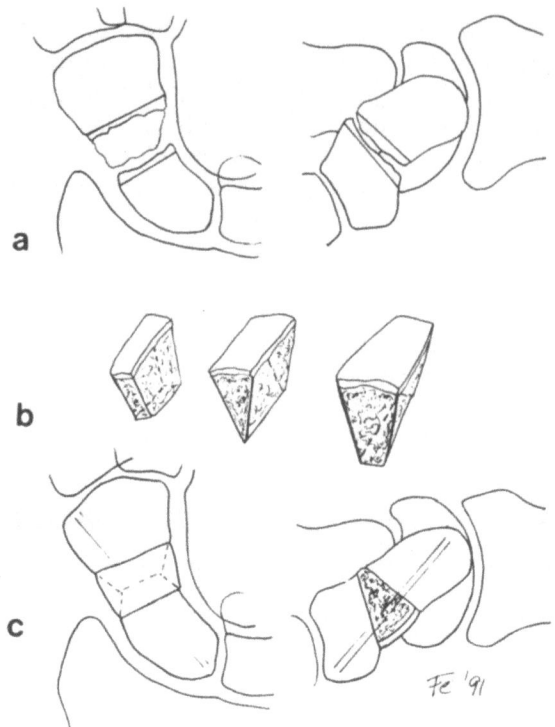

Fig. 2. Preoperative planning for interpositional bone
graft technique. **a** Resection of sclerotic borders of
non-union. **b** Iliac cortico-cancellous bone graft with
rectangular, triangular, and trapezoidal cross-section,
depending on size and shape of defect. **c** Final result
with graft in place, correcting the "humpback deformity" and lunate rotation and showing ideal screw
positioning in the AP and sagittal planes

desired radial angulation in the frontal plane
(Fig. 2).

There is no doubt that three-dimensional computerized imaging offers a more exact calculation
of the graft dimensions. However, it must be
kept in mind that not every hand surgeon has
the possibility to use expensive imaging procedures. Therefore I believe that conventional
preoperative planning using plain X-rays or
tomograms is still a worthwhile and valuable
method.

Non-unions of the distal third and waist are
approached through the classic Russe palmar
incision, which is extended distally into the thenar
eminence with a radially directed 2-cm oblique
limb, making sure that the angle of the incision
lies within the transverse skin crease of the wrist
to avoid hypertrophic scars. The anterior capsule
is incised in line with the skin from the distal
radius to the scaphotrapezoidal joint, taking care

to expose the most palmar-radial corner of the scaphoid without damaging its blood supply. The capsular flaps that contain the strong radio-scaphocapitate ligament are held on both sides with stay sutures to facilitate anatomic closure at the final stage of the procedure. The sclerotic or irregular borders of the non-union site are then resected with a small osciallating saw to offer a perfect surface contact between the graft and the scaphoid fragments. Additional cystic defects are curetted out and filled with small cancellous bone chips. The vascularity of the proximal fragment is checked by counting the bleeding points, as suggested by Green [21]. If the proximal fragment is relatively avascular (one or two bleeding points), multiple 1-mm drill holes are placed within the sclerotic cancellous bone. The flexion deformity and shortening of the scaphoid are corrected by distracting the osteotomy on the palmar radial aspect with a small spreader clamp. As this is done, the surgical assistant simultaneously corrects the dorsal rotation of the lunate by pushing the palmar pole towards the radius with a fine bone spike or by using a Kirschner wire inserted through the palmar pole of the lunate to control rotation, as suggested by Nakamura et al. [22]. Then, the cortical cancellous graft is obtained from the iliac crest and shaped according to the preoperative plan and the dimensions of actual bone defect and is inserted with the cortical part of the graft being oriented palmarly. At this point of the procedure, the image intensifier is useful to control both correct carpal alingment, especially lunate rotation, and implant positioning for internal fixation. If normal lunate rotation cannot be achieved spontaneously by distracting and correcting the scaphoid deformity, a fine Kirschner wire can be inserted through the palmar pole across the lunate fossa of the radius and brought out percutaneously through the dorsal aspect of the forearm, as described by Linscheid et al. [17]. Finally, compression screw fixation of the scaphoid is carried out. We initially performed multiple Kirschner wire fixation [16], but we currently prefer screw fixation by either a conventional lag screw technique with a 2.7 ASIF cortical or a Herbert screw. These implants have been shown to produce adequate inter-fragmentary compression that guarantees undisturbed healing in spite of early functional after-treatment [7, 13]. However, optimal screw placement in line with the long axis of the scaphoid and perfect apposition of well-vascularized bone surfaces are the basic pre-requisites that predict a good result. Careful closure of the palmar capsule completes the operation, and a palmar plaster splint that includes the thumb is applied postoperatively for 2 weeks, at which time the sutures are removed. Wrist immobilization is discontinued at 2 weeks after the operation except in those cases where Kirschner wire fixation of the lunate across the radius is needed. Should postoperative pain persist at 2 weeks, a removable plastic splint or wrist brace may be used for another 2 weeks. The patient is encouraged to use the hand for activities of daily living. However, heavy manual work and strenuous sport activities are forbidden until 8 weeks after surgery. At this time, the first radiographic control using conventional scaphoid views is made. Our criteria to establish healing are (1) the absence of pain, (2) the radiographic evidence of bridging bony trabeculae on both sides of the interposed graft, (3) disappearance of the osteotomy lines in conventional X-rays, and (4) no signs of screw loosening (Fig. 3).

Corrective Osteotomy for Scaphoid Mal-Union

Although seldom routinely recognized, there is increasing evidence [7, 22–24] that healed scaphoid fractures with severe deformity also alter normal carpal kinematics, resulting in an

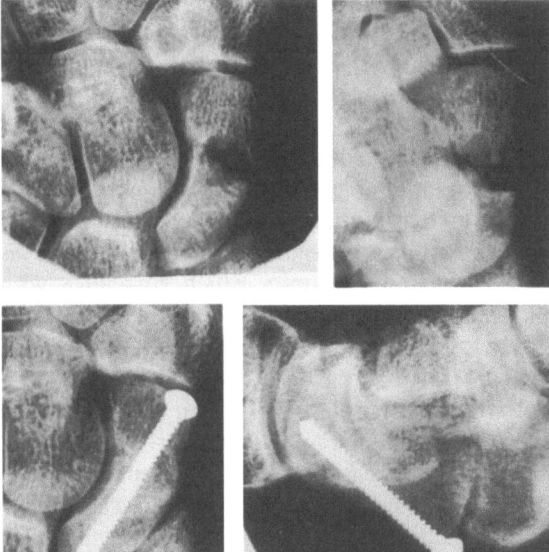

Fig. 3. Unstable cystic non-union treated with interpositional bone graft and lag screw. Result at 3.5 years after operation

unsatisfactory functional outcome associated with a considerable incidence of posttraumatic arthritis of the wrist. The classic deformity of a mal-united scaphoid includes shortening, flexion deformity in the sagittal plane, and radial angulation or ulnar deviation of the distal fragment in the frontal plane. Although not mentioned in the most recent literature, a rotational mal-alignment with displacement of the distal fragment in a pronated position in the horizontal plane may very well be possible. Attempts to measure the degree of mal-union using the radiolunate angle has been suggested by Condamine et al. [24] who classified mal-unions with a radiolunate angle between 10°–20° as moderate and greater than 20° as severe. Amadio and colleagues [23] evaluate the scaphoid mal-union by measuring two intra-scaphoid angles measured in the lateral and AP planes using the trispiral tomogram cut that best shows the whole scaphoid. The lateral scaphoid angle is used to evaluate the "humpback deformity" and is the angle subtended by two perpendicular lines to the proximal and distal articular surface. It has a mean of 24° (range 15°–32°). The anteroposterior scaphoid angle subtended between the perpendiculars to the proximal and distal articular surfaces in the AP view has a mean of 40°. Shortening can be measured, as mentioned previously, using the contralateral wrist in the maximal ulnar-deviated position. It is clear that the most accurate evaluation of a scaphoid mal-union can be readily performed using a three-dimensional computerized reconstruction that may further provide the surgeon with a plastic model in which corrective osteotomy can be planned and actually performed preoperatively. Although some patients remain asymptomatic following a mal-union, others reveal increasing pain due to overload, arthritic changes of the wrist, and scaphoid shortening, as well as flexion deformity which correlates with disabling limitation of wrist extension [7]. For this group of patients, corrective osteotomy should be performed at an early stage to prevent progressive carpal collapse. The surgical technique is summarized in Fig. 4. Angular correction is calculated by measuring the intra-scaphoid angles in the AP and lateral views. The scaphoid is approached through a standard volar approach and fine Kirschner wires inserted from the palmar to the dorsal sides are used to determine the angle of correction in the sagittal plane and are used as "joy sticks" to manipulate the fragments into the corrected position following osteotomy. A

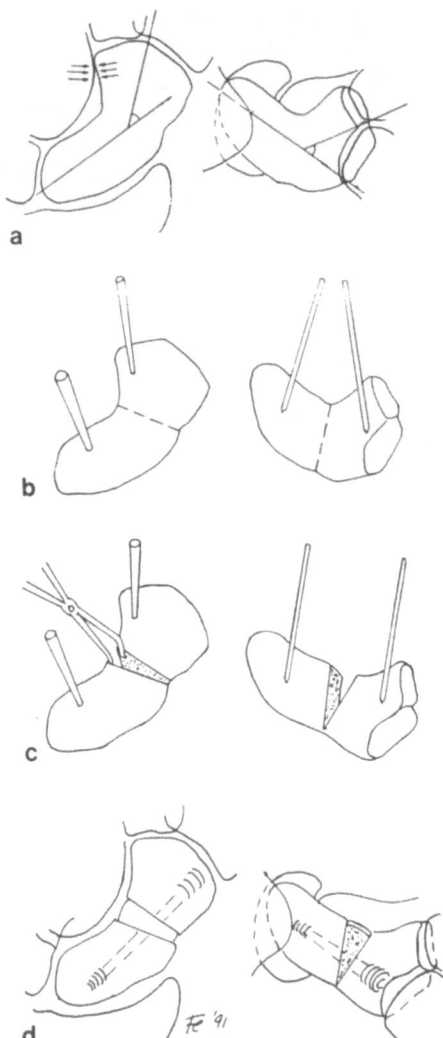

Fig. 4. Technique of corrective osteotomy for scaphoid mal-union. **a** Evaluation of deformity in AP and lateral planes measuring the intra-scaphoid angles. **b** Kirschner wires are useful to mark the angle of correction in the sagittal plane and to manipulate the fragments after osteotomy. **c** Palmar and ulnar opening wedge osteotomy. **d** Final result with wedge graft in place and Herbert-screw fixation

transverse osteotomy at the level of the waist at the maximum point of deformity is performed with a oscillating saw, taking care not to damage the dorsal cartilage envelope that may serve as a hinge, especially for those cases without massive shortening. After having opened the osteotomy volarly, a small spreader clamp is used to correct the deformity in the frontal plane by opening the osteotomy on the ulnar side. Temporary

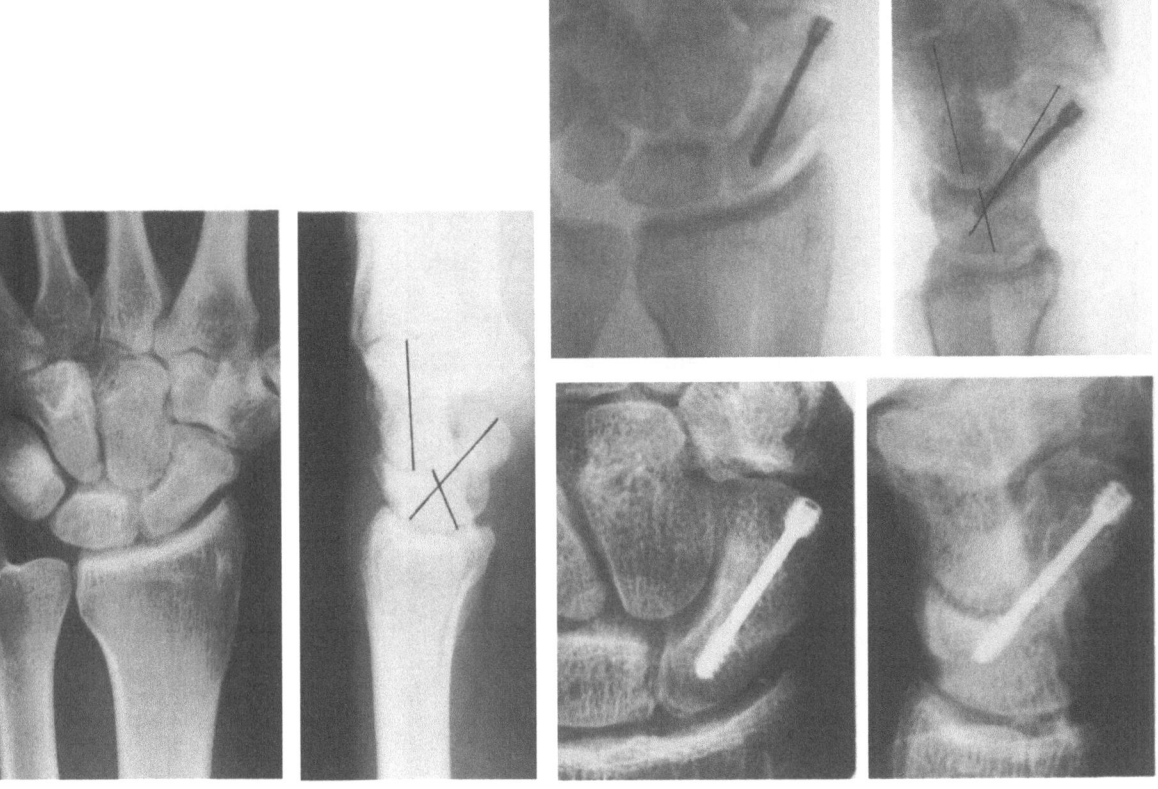

Fig. 5. a Symptomatic scaphoid mal-union 5 years following conservative treatment of a left scaphoid fracture. Notice shortening and slight radial angulation in the AP view and a DISI deformity on the lateral view. **b** Results immediately after and 3 years following corrective osteotomy with the graft taken from the distal radius

Kirschner wire fixation is then performed, and axial correction is assessed in the AP and lateral planes using the image intensifier. A cortico-cancellous wedge graft shaped to fit the defect is taken from the iliac crest and inserted snugly in the osteotomy gap. Internal fixation of the osteotomy with screw fixation completes the procedure (Fig. 5). Postoperative treatment does not differ from the interpositional bone graft technique for non-union.

Dorsopalmar Screw Fixation and Cancellous Bone Grafting for Viable Proximal Pole Non-Unions

Although fractures and non-unions of the proximal third of the scaphoid can be operated on through a palmar approach, complete exposure of the scapholunate junction can only be achieved with an extensive volar capsulotomy. This implies disruption of the most important palmar ligaments of the wrist. Furthermore, internal fixation is far easier and direct for small fragments through a dorsal approach with the wrist flexed than through the classic palmar approach [7, 25]. Another disadvantage is that the point of entry of the implants is situated far away from the non-union site. Also, manipulation and reduction of the small proximal fragment is easily achieved through a small incision with minimal soft tissue disruption. A 3 to 4 cm-long oblique incision beginning at Lister's tubercle parallel to the extensor pollicis longus tendon is used. The joint capsule is exposed between the wrist extensors and the extensor pollicis longus and incised in line with the long axis of the scaphoid. Flexion of the wrist clearly exposes the non-union site and the scapholunate junction. The interposed tissue

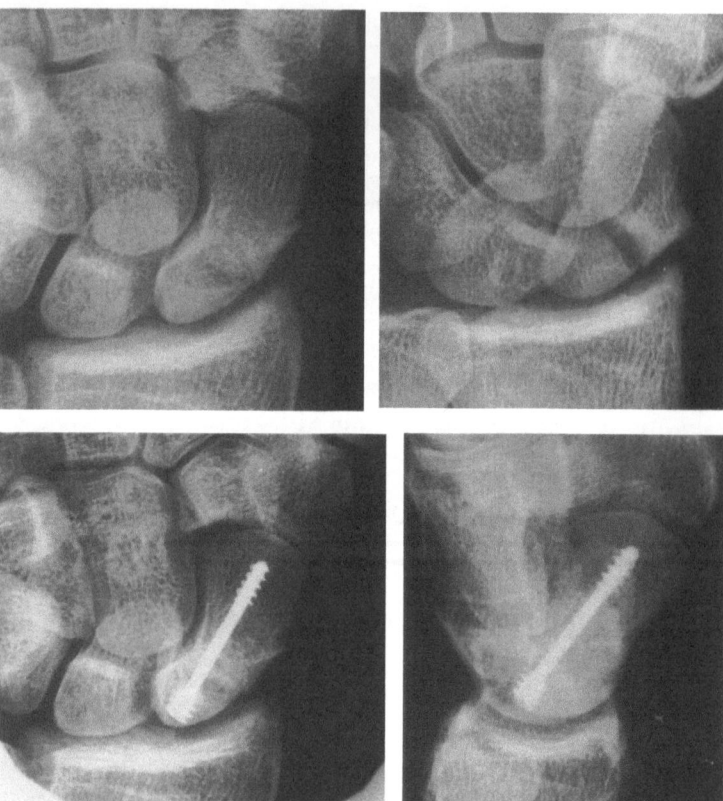

Fig. 6. Radiographs before and 1 year after treatment of a proximal scaphoid non-union with retrograde Herbert-screw fixation and iliac bone grafting

is curetted out, taking care not to damage the cartilage envelope over the dorsoradial aspect of the pseudarthrosis. Due to the limited bone stock of the proximal fragment, bone resection should be minimal; however, if a significant amount of sclerosis is present, multiple drill holes of the proximal fragment should be performed to enhance revascularization. The cavity is then packed with cancellous bone from the iliac crest and the non-union is temporarily stabilized with a fine Kirschner wire. Internal fixation is carried out with a free-handed Herbert screw or with a 2.0-mm ASIF mini-screw, taking care to counter-sink the screw head beneath the cartilage. The advantage of the Herbert screw is that the proximal threads can be completely embedded in the proximal fragment (Fig. 6). The postoperative treatment protocol is basically the same as that for the interpositional bone graft technique. However, if there is any doubt about the stability of fixation or impaired vascularity of the proximal fragment, postoperative cast fixation is used for a period of 6–8 weeks.

Revascularization and Bone Grafting Procedure for Avascular Necrosis of the Proximal Fragment

Due to its vulnerable blood supply, the carpal scaphoid is second to the head of the femur in producing avascular necrosis (AVN) of the proximal fragment following fracture. There is a 30% incidence of AVN in fractures of the waist and 100% incidence in the proximal one-fifth of the scaphoid. As pointed out by Herbert [7], it is important to differentiate between *complete avascular necrosis*, with absence of the normal trabecular structure, cystic changes, and subchondral bone collapse, and *transient ischemia*, with the bone appearing sclerotic on X-rays but without cystic changes and deformity. Ischemic proximal fragments usually revascularize slowly if bony union of the pseudarthrosis occurs [26]. On the other hand, conventional bone grafting techniques have shown a high failure rate in providing bone union and revascularization if the proximal fragment is completely avascular [21].

In the absence of periscaphoid arthritic changes or established carpal collapse, it seems that the logical way to preserve the anatomical integrity of the proximal carpal row is to obtain scaphoid union·and revascularization in one single operation. Recent studies on vascularized bone graft procedures [27, 28] are encouraging, but still not statistically significant due to the small number of patients reported. In view of the acceptable revascularization rate obtained with the vascular bundle implantation procedure described by Hori and others [29–31] for Kienböck's disease, I have adopted this technique in combination with iliac bone grafting to revascularize proximal scaphoid poles. This technique has been successful in 8 out of 10 cases treated between 1981 and 1988, with an average follow-up of 4 years. Although the diagnosis of avascular necrosis is suspected in plain roentgenographs (sclerosis, cystic changes, abnormal trabeculation) and may be further documented as a cold spot in bone scans or by the absence of bone marrow signal with magnetic resonance imaging [11], it is the intra-operative *total absence of bleeding points* in the proximal fragment that confirms the diagnosis [21].

With the patient under general anesthesia and the iliac crest draped free, the scaphoid is exposed through the same dorsoradial incision described for proximal pole non-unions. The capsule is incised, taking care to perserve the dorsal ridge vessels to the distal fragment and the sensory branches of the radial nerve. After having visualized the non-union site, the cancellous surface of the proximal fragment is carefully inspected for punctate bleeding points under magnification. When there is any doubt, the tourniquet may be released and the arm re-exsanguinated. Next, a trough is prepared on the dorsoradial aspect on both scaphoid fragments to receive a cortico-cancellous inlay graft as in the Matti-Russe procedure. A cortico-cancellous bone graft is taken from the iliac crest and inserted in the trough. A single Kirschner wire is used to stabilize the scaphoid, and additional free cancellous bone chips are packed in the non-union gap. The skin incision is then extended distally to the second dorsal web space and the extensor tendons to the index finger are retracted ulnarly (Fig. 7). The second dorsal inter-metacarpal artery and veins are identified and carefully dissected together with the perivascular tissue to the level of the web space, where they are transected and ligated. The vascular bundle is then freed proximally, taking care to ligate small collateral branches found in its course. Following this, a 2.7-mm hole is drilled

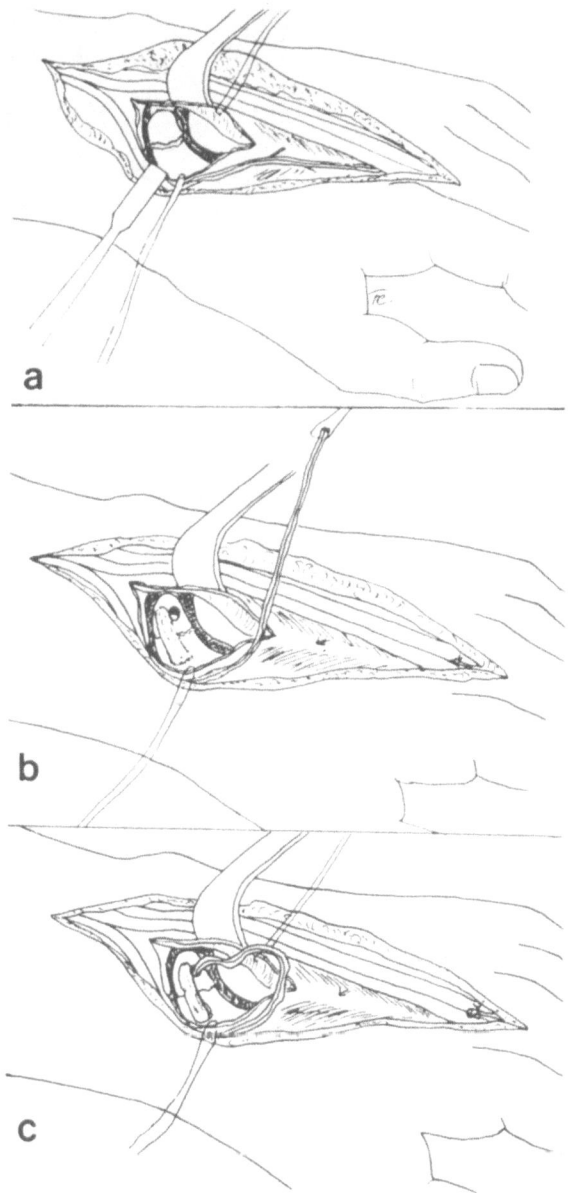

Fig. 7. Revascularization procedure for scaphoid non-union and avascular necrosis. **a** Exposure of non-union and dorsal inter-metacarpal vascular bundle through an "extensile" dorsoradial approach. **b** Pedicle raised from the distal to the proximal borders. Notice the dorsoradial inlay bone graft and position of the drill hole in the proximal fragment. **c** Vascular pedicle entering the drill hole

from the dorsal to the palmar sides across the proximal pole of the scaphoid. The vascular bundle is then passed through the drill hole

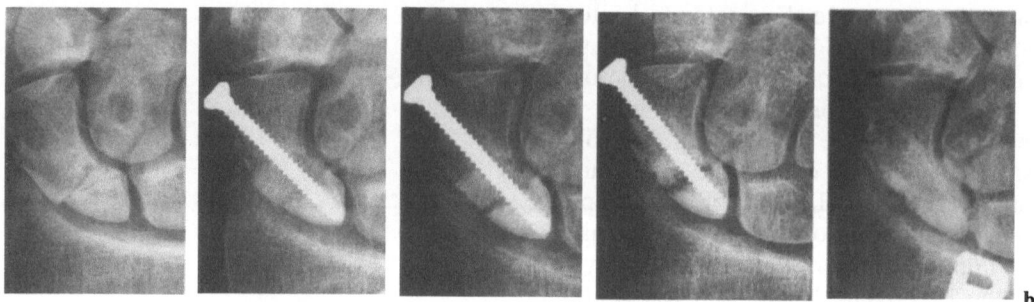

Fig. 8. a Persistant pseudarthrosis following inter-positional bone grafting and screw fixation due to avascular necrosis of the proximal fragment. **b** Non-union healed after screw removal, cortico-cancellous iliac peg grafting of the enlarged screw channel, and revascularization with the Hori procedure

from the dorsal to the palmar direction. This is facilitated by attaching a fine reabsorbable suture to the end of the pedicle and using a straight needle to guide the suture and vascular pedicle through the bone. The suture is retrieved across the palmar aspect of the wrist and tied over the skin. The wrist capsule should be loosely closed around the point of entry of the vascular pedicle. Post operatively, the same guidelines as those for a Russe procedure are used: 4 weeks thumb spica cast that includes the elbow, followed by a short navicular cast for another 6 weeks.

At 10 weeks, the plaster cast is removed and bone healing is evaluated with AP tomograms of the scaphoid following removal of the Kirschner wire under local anesthesia. If vascularity of the proximal pole is re-established, there is a progressive decrease of the sclerosis of the proximal fragment and reappearance of a normal trabecular cancellous structure (Fig. 8). Although not used routinely, magnetic resonance imaging with normalization of the bone marrow signal is a useful diagnostic aid to assess revascularization of the proximal pole.

Salvage Procedures

In presence of a long-standing scaphoid non-union with advanced degenerative changes of the wrist, an operation that will promote union of the pseudarthrosis, will not relieve pain or improve function of the wrist. It is for this group of patients that a salvage procedure is indicated. If the non-union is associated with early degenerative changes which are localized in the radioscaphoid joint with osteophytic changes of the radial styloid, bone grafting of the pseudarthrosis combined with radial styloidectomy is worth con-

sidering before a salvage procedure is indicated. The type of salvage procedure that can be offered to the patient depends basically on the functional requirements of the wrist, the level of pain, age, and occupation. If the functional demands of the wrist are not important (non-heavy manual workers, non-dominant hand), conservative treatment with external wrist supports may be considered. This group of patients also profits from pain-relieving operations, such as denervation [32], osteophyte removal, synovectomy, removal of a small necrotic proximal pole combined with styloidectomy, and inter-positional arthroplasty with a rolled tendon.

For the young heavy-manual worker with dominant-hand involvement and advanced degenerative changes, total wrist fusion is the procedure of choice to guarantee a painless and stable wrist [34]. If the hand is non-dominant and the degenerative changes are basically localized on the radial aspect of the radiocarpal joint with a well-preserved midcarpal joint, a radio-scapholunate fusion with excision of the proximal scaphoid fragment and replacement with an iliac bone graft is worth considering.

If the patient does not accept wrist fusion, a motion-preserving salvage procedure may be indicated. However, in my experience, it is difficult to guarantee complete relief of pain. It should be pointed out to a patient involved in heavy manual work that a external wrist support may become necessary during work and that the wrist may be left free for activities of daily living. If silicon replacement arthroplasty of the scaphoid is elected, an additional intercarpal fusion to unload the prothesis should be performed at the same time, to prevent carpal collapse and, theoretically, to reduce the incidence of silicon synovitis [6, 7, 18]. If the articular surface of the capitate does not show advanced degenerative arthritic changes and the lunate fossa of the distal radius is well preserved, proximal row carpectomy [33] may be considered as an alternative motion-preserving procedure. A failed arthroplastic procedure can always be salvaged with total wrist fusion at a later date.

Conclusions

Successful treatment of scaphoid non-union depends basically on the correct choice of the specific treatment modality for each non-union type. Other factors that will equally influence the final outcome are the proper selection of the patient, precise knowledge of the technique including its limitations and pitfalls, correct surgical performance, as well as the appropriate postoperative protocol, rehabilitation, and careful interpretation of the radiographic follow-up results.

Although delayed union may be treated with prolonged immobilization and stable non-unions with conventional inlay bone graft techniques, given the predictable results that can be obtained today with stable internal fixation of the scaphoid, there is a general tendency to treat these conditions with compression screw fixation in order to allow early motion of the affected wrist.

Interpositional bone graft techniques for unstable non-unions and mal-unions are technically demanding procedures. Therefore, in my view, a meticulous preoperative plan with precise measurements of the resection, form, and size of the graft, the desired final angular correction, and implant positioning is mandatory. If the scaphoid non-union is associated with vascular impairment of the proximal fragment, the surgeon should be aware that, at least in young patients without associated degenerative changes, a revascularization procedure should be attempted in an effort to save the scaphoid and preserve the anatomical architecture of the carpus. Careful preoperative and intra-operative assessment of the vascularity of the proximal pole depends on the surgeon's own personal judgement and experience as well as on the correlation of the radiographic findings in plain X-rays, tomography, scintigrams, and magnetic resonance imaging. Finally, for the treatment of degenerative wrist disease associated with scaphoid non-union, it must be stressed that there is still a place for conservative treatment and that the long-term results of resection arthroplasty with or without implant interposition with regard to complete pain relief, stability, and grip strength are still questionable. Conversely, wrist fusion offers a painless and strong wrist at the expense of loss of function. Therefore, the advantages and disadvantages of each salvage procedure should be carefully considered by the surgeon before recommending them to the patient.

References

1. Smith DK, Cooney WP, An KN, Linscheid RL, Chao EYS (1989) The effects of simulated unstable scaphoid fractures on carpal motion. J Hand Surg [Am] 14:283–291
2. Weber ER (1980) Biomechanical implications of scaphoid waist fractures. Clin Orthop 149:83–89
3. Leslie IJ, Dickson RA (1981) The fractured carpal scaphoid. Natural history and factors influencing outcome. J Bone Joint Surg [Br] 63(2):225–230
4. Mack GR, Bosse MJ, Gelberman RH, Yu E (1984) The natural history of scaphoid non-union. J Bone Joint Surg [Am] 66:504–509
5. Ruby LK, Stinson J, Belsky MR (1985) The natural history of scaphoid non-union. A review of fifty-five cases. J Bone Joint Surg [Am] 67:428–432
6. Watson HK, Ballet FL (1984) The SLAC wrist: Scapholunate advanced collapse pattern of degenerative arthritis. J Hand Surg [Am] 9:358–365
7. Herbert TJ (1990) The fractured scaphoid. Quality Medical, St. Louis, pp 121–138
8. Herbert TJ, Fisher WE (1984) Management of the fractured scaphoid using a new bone screw. J Bone Joint Surg [Br] 66:114–123
9. Sanders WE (1988) Evaluation of the humpback scaphoid by computed tomography in the longitudinal axis plane of the scaphoid. J Hand Surg [Am] 13:182–187
10. Gillespy T III, Genant HK, Helms CA (1986) Magnetic resonance of osteonecrosis. Radiol Clin North [Am] 24:193–208
11. Trumble TE (1990) Avascular necrosis after scaphoid fracture: A correlation of magnetic resonance imaging and histology. J Hand Surg [Am] 15:557–564
12. Frykman GK, Taleisnik J, Peters G, Kaufman R, Helal B, Wood VE, Unsell RS (1986) Treatment of nonunited scaphoid fractures by pulsed electromagnetic field an cast. J Hand Surg [Am] 11:344–349
13. Fernandez DL (1990) Anterior bone grafting and conventional lag screw fixation to treat scaphoid nonunions. J Hand Surg [Am] 15:140–147

14. Russe O (1980) Die Kahnbeinpseudarthrose, Behandlung und Ergebnisse. Unfallheilkunde 148: 129–134

15. Fisk GR (1979) Operative surgery. Part II. In: Bentley G (ed) Orthopaedics. Butterworth, Kent, p 540

16. Fernandez DL (1984) A technique for anterior wedge-shaped grafts for scaphoid non-unions with carpal instability. J Hand Surg [Am] 9:733–737

17. Linscheid RL, Dobyns JB, Cooney WP (1982) Volar wedge grafting of the carpal scaphoid in non-union associated with dorsal instability patterns. Proceedings of the Seventh Combined Meeting of the Orthopaedic Associations of the English Speaking World, Cape Town, South Africa, March 1982. J Bone Joint Surg [Br] 64:632–633

18. Mack GR, Lichtman DM (1988) Scaphoid non-union. In: Lichtman DM (ed) The wrist and its disorders. Saunders, Philadelphia, pp 314–318

19. Taleisnik J (1988) Fractures of the carpal bones. In: Green DP (ed) Operative hand surgery, 2nd edn. Churchill Livingstone, New York, pp 826–830

20. Cooney WP, Linscheid RL, Dobyns JH, Wood MB (1988) Scaphoid non-union: Role of anterior interpositional bone grafts. J Hand Surg [Am] 13:635–650

21. Green DP (1985) The effect of avascular necrosis on Russe bone grafting for scaphoid non-unions. J Hand Surg [Am] 10:597–605

22. Nakamura R, Hori M, Horii E, Miura T (1987) Reduction of the scaphoid fracture with DISI alignment. J Hand Surg [Am] 12:1000–1005

23. Amadio PC, Berquist TH, Smith DK, Ilstrup DM, Cooney WP, Linscheid RL (1989) Scaphoid malunion. J Hand Surg [Am] 14:679–687

24. Condamine JL, LeBourg M, Raimbeau G (1986) Pseudarthroses du scaphoïde carpien et intervention de Matti-Russe. Annales Orthop De L'Ouest 18:23–31

25. Alnot JY, Bellan N, Oberlin C, De Cheveigné C (1988) Les fractures et pseudarthroses polaires proximales du scaphoïde carpien. Ostéosynthese par vissage de proximal à distal. Ann Chir Main 7:101–108

26. Verdan C, Narakas A (1968) Fractures and pseudarthrosis of the scaphoid. Surg Clin North [Am] 48:1083–1095

27. Guimberteau JC, Panconi B (1990) Recalcitrant non-union of the scaphoid treated with a vascularized bone graft based on the ulnar artery. J Bone Joint Surg [Am] 72:88–97.

28. Kuhlmann JN, Mimoun M, Boabighi A, Baux S (1987) Vascularized bone graft pedicled on the volar carpal artery for nonunion of the scaphoid. J Hand Surg [Br] 12:203–210

29. Foucher G, Saffar PH (1982) Revascularization of the necrosed lunate. Stages I and II with a dorsal intermetacarpal arteriovenous pedicle. J Chir Main 1:259

30. Hori Y, Tamai S, Okuda H (1979) Blood vessel transplantation to bone. J Hand Surg [Am] 4: 23–33

31. Tamai S, Yajima H, Mizumoto S, Hori Y (1990) Treatment of Kienböck's disease with vascular bundle implantation. In: Book of Abstracts of the 45th Annual Meeting American Society for Surgery of the Hand, September 26, 1990, Toronto

32. Wilhelm K (1966) Die Gelenkdenervation und ihre anatomischen Grundlagen. Ein neues Behandlungsprinzip in der Handchirurgie. Hefte Unfallheilk 86:1–109

33. Neviaser RJ (1983) Proximal row carpectomy for post-traumatic disorders of the carpus. J Hand Surg [Am] 8:301–305

34. Fernandez DL, Bamert P (1980) Técnica y resultados de la artrodesis de muñeca con placa de compresión. Rev Esp Cirugia de la Mano 7: 29–39

Psychological Aspects of Scaphoid Fractures

J. Paul Ryley[1]

Abstract. Sociodemographic, clinical, and psychological variables were examined prospectively in 92 patients with scaphoid fracture. The patients appeared to be fairly representative of the general population. Knowledge of the injury predicted attendance at 6-month follow-up, but possibly more important was the attention given to them by the surgeon. Suggestions for improving patient compliance are proposed.

Keywords: Scaphoid — Fracture — Psychological — Compliance — Personality

Introduction

The clinical impression of patients with scaphoid fractures has been that they are irresponsible young men who rarely attend follow-up to the desirable 6-month point, perhaps 70% dropping out by then, and who do not take adequate care of their cast. There has been thought to be a high rate of non-union with presumably subsequent morbidity from arthritis, but this has been difficult to estimate due to the low rate of successful follow-up. It could, therefore, be most useful if non-attendance and/or non-union could be predicted, or even prevented, and we considered that such treatment failures might be identified by using psychological variables.

Previous work has examined scaphoid fracture outcome retrospectively. Barr et al. [1] examined 39 veterans with fractures sustained in military service. An unstandardized interview and questionnaire were used and, although six were thought to have "personality factors which played a definite role" in their injury, there was

no clear pattern. Kim et al. [2] studied 30 patients with scaphoid non-union treated by bone grafting and found psychiatric disorder in 9 out of 13 patients with a poor clinical result and in 1 out of 17 patients with a good result. Unfortunately, evidence of psychiatric involvement was based solely on orthopedic case notes in 22 patients, including 16 out of 17 in the "good result" group, and there were numerous other methodological flaws [3]. We therefore conducted a prospective study using standardized instruments.

Patients and Methods

There was a suspicion that this type of patient may comply poorly with a psychiatric assessment, so it was decided that assessment should be by personal interview, be slanted to the psychological rather than the psychiatric (i.e., avoiding questioning about mental illness), be brief, and be conducted on only one occasion.

The hypotheses to be tested included:

1. Are patients who fracture their scaphoid really irresponsible (and ignorant) young men?
2. Do they differ from the general population, or from a control sample of patients with other fractures, on measurable personality traits or psychiatric morbidity?
3. Can any of the above measures predict non-attendance, non-union, or maltreatment of their cast?

Method

A total of 92 patients were seen on their routine clinic visit as part of the Nottingham-Leicester study of the effectiveness of different types of casts used in the treatment of scaphoid fractures [4].

[1] University Department of Psychiatry, Nottingham University Hospital, UK

According to the protocol of the orthopedic study, they were placed in a backslab in the Accident and Emergency department and seen the following day in fracture clinic when randomization of the cast type was made. Two weeks later, they were reviewed in fracture clinic, at which point (wherever possible) they were assessed by the author. The lesions comprised a consecutive series of fractures of the body of the scaphoid.

Questions on socio-demographic variables and knowledge of and attitudes towards the injury and its treatment were asked. The Eysenck Personality Questionnaire (EPQ) [5] and the General Health Questionnaire (GHQ) in its 30 — item form [6] were administered. The EPQ measures four personality dimensions: P, "toughmindedness"; E, "extraversion"; N, "emotionality"; and L, "tendency to see oneself in a good light". The GHQ-30 measures the likelihood of a subject having a psychiatric disorder; sensitivity and specificity are over 70% when the usual cutoff score is employed. It was hoped that patient compliance would be improved by using the shorter 30-item version rather than the full 60 items. Furthermore, as many of the excluded items concern somatic symptoms, this should reduce the false — positive rate.

Patients were then randomized with one-half receiving a 5-minute explanation of their injury. This covered its name and nature (using an articulated skeleton of the hand, a separate scaphoid bone, and the patient's X-rays); the rationale of treatment, including the reasons for the 6-month appointment scheduling; and the consequences of non-union. It should be noted that all patients had been seen by a surgeon on at least two previous occasions and would have already been given this information.

Table 1. Social class distribution of the patients according to the standard Registrar-General's classification (UK)

Class	Definition	Percentage of patients
I	Professional	3.3
II	Managerial	16.3
III NM	Clerical	7.6
III M	Skilled manual	19.6
IV	Semiskilled manual	16.3
V	Unskilled manual	8.7
—	Unclassified	28.3

NM, nonmanual; M, manual

Three outcome measures were assessed from case notes at 6 months: attendance at follow-up, union of fracture, and damage to casts as recorded by the surgeon at 2, 4, and 8 weeks.

An age-sex matched control group ($n = 92$) was recruited from patients with other fractures and sprains of the upper limb or lower leg sustained within the preceding 2 months, plus some who underwent knee arthroscopy. They all completed the EPQ and GHQ-30.

Results

There were no refusals to being tested and complete data were obtained on 91 out of the 92 patients seen, with 65% having been seen within 3 weeks of the injury and 85% within 1 month.

Sociodemographic Features

Males comprised 75% of the scaphoid fracture group and the median age was 26 years: however, 28% were over age 37 years, as the age distribution was highly skewed to the left. The whole of this skew was due to the male patients. Social class distribution of the patients was as shown in Table 1. Figures for the catchment area population were only available for head of household, against which this sample contained an excess of class II and unclassified and a deficit of class III NM. The unclassified group consisted largely of students and a few housewives. In general, this sample seemed to be in above-average levels of occupation; 26% had education to "A" levels or higher and only 16% admitted to significant misbehavior at school (e.g., frequent punishments, truancy, suspension, etc).

Clinical Features

Most (74%) had sustained the injury in a fall on the hand in an outstretched position. In 14% it was caused by a twisting/kickback mechanism and in only 3.3% did it occur in a fight. While 19% had consumed alcohol within the 3 hours preceding the injury, only two (2.2%) were drunk and only another two had had over 2 pints of beer.

It emerged that 63% knew they had broken the scaphoid bone and could localize it fairly accurately. While 80% knew that the cast had been applied to help the bone knit, only 11% realized it was also for pain control. In spite of this reasonable level of knowledge, 26% had a significantly damaged cast when seen for this study as did 54% when that assessment was combined with those of the surgeons in the first 8 weeks. There was no association between sex or age and damage to the cast. In the latter part of the study, once this high rate of damage had been noted, fiberglass resin was used instead of plaster of Paris.

Only 55% gave the correct answer (8–12 weeks) when asked how long the bone would take to heal. There seemed to be a tendency for Accident and Emergency doctors to give the patients an estimated recovery period of 6–8 weeks, in spite of the orthopedic trial protocol. Long-term problems were expected by 17%, such as weakness in the wrist, and a further 44% thought that they might have such problems.

The median time spent in the Accident and Emergency department was 170 minutes, but 34% spent more than 4 hours there. Forty per cent were definitely dissatisfied with their waiting time, and this dissatisfaction correlated highly with the actual waiting time ($P < 0.001$), but neither measure correlated with attendance at 6 months.

Psychological Features

Compared with EPQ data from the general population with a similar age-sex distribution, patients with scaphoid fracture were significantly more extravert ($P < 0.01$) and had higher L-scores ($P < 0.001$). However, the magnitude of the differences were small, being 13.0 vs 14.5 for E and 7.0 vs 9.3 for L, both scores with a range of 0–21. The higher L scores were particularly prominent among females. There were no significant differences compared to the control group.

The mean GHQ score was 6.8, 48% scoring above the 4/5 cutoff. The control group had a mean score of 5.4, which was not significantly different, and 47% scored above the cutoff. These rates of "caseness" are quite high, being typically around 25%–40% in other outpatient samples [7].

The clinical impression of this group of patients was that there was little to suggest unusual personality patterns among the vast majority of them. However, a few did seem clinically unusual. One appeared depressed and sullen, and, while otherwise co-operating fully with the interview,

refused to fill in the questionnaires. Nevertheless, he attended 8 out of 10 follow-up appointments (his fracture united). A second patient who sustained the injury playing street football while he was drunk had completely destroyed the cast after 2 weeks due to his lifting frozen food in his job at a freezer center. However, he attended all 6 appointments (his fracture was united). A third went swimming in his cast at 3 weeks. The fracture achieved union at 3 months at which point he was discharged (in error), having attended six out of seven follow-up evaluations.

Outcome

A total of 62 (76% of those with available data) attended the 6-month follow-up appointment and a further 8 were erroneously discharged early. This attendance rate was achieved with no extra encouragement to attend beyond the sending of up to three routine further appointments. Only 20 (22%) failed to attend. Three fractures were known to have non-union.

The only factor associated with attendance was how much the patient knew about the injury ($P = 0.0005$), but there were trends ($P = 0.06$) towards greater attendance if patients knew that the plaster was applied to hold the bone still so it could heal and if P scores were lower. The extra explanation of the injury, received by one-half of the patients, had no effect.

There were too few non-unions (three) to make comparisons truly meaningful, although, interestingly, their L scores (mean, 13.7) were nearly double the normal population mean (7.0) ($P = 0.04$) and well above the sample mean (9.3).

As regards care of the cast, patients damaged Colles-type casts more than scaphoid-type casts ($P = 0.03$) and also damaged them more if they perceived them as having a *low* nuisance rating on a visual analogue scale ($P = 0.016$). There was a trend for scaphoid-type casts to be perceived as more of a nuisance ($P = 0.13$).

The attendance rate at follow-up on a comparison sample of 100 consecutive patients from the trial before psychological assessments were begun was 51%, even after up to three personal letters, plus telephone calls, in addition to the routine "further appointment" letters. The rate in the Leicester-based arm of the trial, where all patients were seen by the same surgeon on each occasion in a special clinic for patients in this trial, was 100% ($n = 192$).

Discussion

Although this group of patients with scaphoid fractures does contain a relatively high proportion of young men and produces scores on a personality questionnaire which are significantly different statistically from the normal population, the magnitude of the differences is small and the clinical impression is that of a normal group. In particular, they did not differ from patients with other fractures, they were highly co-operative with the researcher, and tended to have higher educational achievements. The adverse clinical impression of the group (mentioned in the Introduction) is likely to have been obtained from the few patients who did behave irresponsibly. (It is interesting that the three most memorable "irresponsible" patients all attended follow-up until they were discharged and all had union of their fractures). The psychological and knowledge tests did not provide for prediction of outcome.

Further study of patients with non-union would be useful in order to replicate the work of Kim et al. [2] but using stricter methodology. The suggestion of a high rate of psychological morbidity has also been made in patients with recurrent voluntary dislocation of the shoulder [8] and industrial injury [9]. Methodological problems are present in both papers, but psychological morbidity appeared to be associated with operative failure (particularly multiple failed procedures) and prolonged disability, respectively.

Although individual clinical features were disappointing as predictors of outcome (except for knowledge about injury with regard to attendance and perhaps the L-score for non-union), attendance rates varied greatly between the clinical estimate (30%), rate in the orthopedic-only phase in Nottingham (51%), rate in this study (76%) and rate in the Leicester-based arm (100%).

The differences between the latter 3 groups are highly significant statistically ($P < 0.01$) and are also very large clinically. It seems that just as the fact of being in a research study increases compliance (the Hawthorne effect), so the extra attention of the psychological assessment (a 20-minute interview) or the personal attention of the surgeon (in Leicester) may improve this still further. It is interesting that increasing factual knowledge imparted to one-half of this sample had no effect on patient compliance.

Attendance dropped off during the latter part of this study, a mid-point split giving rates of 87% against 70%. This may be related to the discontinuation of inclusion of patients in the orthopedic trial numbers, although randomization and data collection continued. It is likely that there would be a reduction in orthopedic interest during this time.

Since scaphoid-type casts are damaged less by patients (in spite of being perceived as being more of a nuisance) and since cast type does not affect attendance at follow-up, this type of cast may be advantageous. However a similar result may be achieved by using a more robust material, such as fiberglass resin.

Overall, there seem to be two ways in which compliance could be increased in these patients. The first might be to improve the communication of accurate information when the patient is first seen, especially information about the nature of the injury, and why the long-time confinement in plaster and long follow-up is therefore necessary. This information is no doubt imparted, but not necessarily assimilated at present.

Secondly, although this could cause great logistical problems, it would seem that patients would be more likely to attend if they could always see the same surgeon. This might also improve job satisfaction with surgeons getting to know patients better, and would reduce the time they spend in updating themselves from notes and X-rays.

Further work is indicated, including evaluation of the group of patients with scaphoid non-union to see if psychological differences (as were suggested by the high L-scores in the three patients reviewed herein) can be ascertained.

References

1. Barr JS, Elliston WA, Musnick H, Delorme TL, Hanelin J, Thibodeau AA (1953) Fracture of the carpal navicular (scaphoid) bone. An end-result study in military personnel. J Bone Joint Surg [Am] 35:609–625
2. Kim WC, Shaffer JW, Idzikowski C (1983) Failure of treatment of ununited fractures of the carpal scaphoid. The role of noncompliance. J Bone Joint Surg [Am] 65:985–991
3. Cooney WP (1984) Letter. J Bone Joint Surg [Am] 66:1145–1146
4. Clay NR, Dias JJ, Costigan PS, Gregg PJ, Barton NJ (to be published) Need the thumb be immobilised in scaphoid fractures? A randomised prospective trial of Colles and "Scaphoid" casts. J Bone Joint Surg [Br]

5. Eysenck HJ, Eysenck SBG (1975) The manual of the Eysench personality questionnaire. Hodder and Stoughton, Sevenoaks, Kent, UK

6. Goldberg DP (1972) The detection of psychiatric illness by questionnaire. Oxford University Press, London

7. Berrios GE, Ryley JP, Garvey TPN, Moffat DA (1988) Psychiatric morbidity in subjects with inner ear disease. Clin Otolarygol 13:259–266

8. Rowe CR, Pierce DS, Clark JG (1973) Voluntary dislocation of the shoulder. A preliminary report on a clinical, electromyographic and psychiatric study of twenty-six patients. J Bone Joint Surg [Am] 55:445–460

9. Beals RK, Hickman NW (1972) Industrial injuries of the back and extremities. Comprehensive evaluation — An aid in prognosis and management. A study of one hundred and eighty patients. J Bone Joint Surg [Am] 54:1593–1611

Natural History of Chronic Scaphoid Fractures

Yoshifumi Nagatani,[1] Kotaro Imamura,[1] and Eiji Hirano[2]

Abstract: The dorsiflexed intercalated segment instability (DISI) pattern can usually be detected in chronic scaphoid fractures. We reviewed the roentgenographic findings of 75 chronic scaphoid fractures (21 delayed unions and 54 non-unions) in order to assess the incidence and severity of the DISI pattern and degenerative changes of the wrist. In the cases of delayed union, 3 out of 4 (75%) distal third fractures and 1 out of 16 (6%) middle third fractures had a DISI pattern; it was absent in the 1 proximal third fractures. In the cases of non-union, 9 out of 10 (90%) distal third fractures and 10 out of 35 (29%) middle third fractures had a DISI pattern. Thus, the DISI pattern was found most frequently in distal-third fractures and more frequently in chronic cases. In the patients whose duration of non-union was less than 10 years, the incidence of degenerative changes of the wrist was 15%. However, when the duration of non-union was more than 20 years, all the patients had arthrosis.

It is well known that chronic scaphoid fracture sometimes results in dorsiflexed intercalated segment instability (DISI) and degenerative arthritis. However, details related to the occurrence of these complications are not clear. The purpose of this study was to clarify the factors which cause DISI deformity and degenerative arthritis in chronic scaphoid fracture.

Keywords: Scaphoid fractures — DISI (dorsiflexed intercalated segment instability)

[1] Department of Orthopaedic Surgery, Nagasaki University, School of Medicine, 7-1 Sakamoto-machi, Nagasaki 852, Japan
[2] Department of Orthopaedic Surgery, Aino Memorial Hospital, Nagasaki, 854-03 Japan

Subjects

Seventy-five patients with chronic scaphoid fractures, excluding lunate and perilunate dislocations, who were referred to Nagasaki University between 1983 and 1990, were divided into 2 groups (Table 1). One group consisted of 21 cases of delayed union and the other 54 cases of non-union.

The subjects in the delayed union group had been injured between 2 and 6 months (average 3 months) before the first examination in our clinic. Their ages ranged from 17 to 59 years (average 28 years). Those in the non-union group had been injured between 6 months and 40 years before examination (average 7 years 5 months). Their ages ranged from 12 to 62 years (average 34 years). The times of fracture occurrence were not clear in 5 cases.

All the patients in both groups had not received any treatment for fractured scaphoid between the time of injury and the first examination.

Methods

At the first examination, the range of motion (ROM) of the wrist was measured, and standard posteroanterior and lateral views and dynamic series of roentgenograms were taken.

The radiolunate angle was measured in a lateral X-ray view [1]. In this study, 10° or more of radiolunate angle dorsiflexion was considered as being DISI [2]. Scaphoid length was measured in a ulnar-deviated PA view and compared with the non-affected scaphoid [3].

According to the extent of the degenerative changes evidenced in roentgenographic findings, osteoarthritis (OA) was classified into 2 groups [2, 4]. The OA(+) group showed a pointing of the radial styloid (Fig. 1.a). The OA(++) group

171

Table 1. Subjects in this study

	Wrists (n)	Average duration of fracture	Average age (years)
Delayed unions	21	3 Months (2–5)	28 (17–59)
Non-unions	54	7 Years 5 months (6 months–40 years)	34 (12–62)

Table 2. Correlation between the incidence of DISI and the site of scaphoid fractures

	Distal third	Waist	Proximal third	Total
Delayed unions	3/4	1/16	0/1	4/21
	(75%)	(6.3%)	(0%)	(19%)
Non-unions	9/10	10/35	1/9	20/54
	(90%)	(28.6%)	(11.1%)	(37%)

showed a narrowing of the radioscaphoid joint space and sclerosis of the carpal bones (Fig. 1.b).

Based on the above-mentioned clinical and radiographical findings, the following correlations were made and investigated: (1) between the incidence of DISI and the site of scaphoid fractures, (2) between the radiolunate angle and the scaphoid length, (3) between the ROM of the wrist and the grade of carpal instability, and (4) between the extent of OA changes and the duration of the non-union. The second and third correlations were investigated only for the non-union group because, in the delayed union group, bone absorption was not sufficiently advanced and the

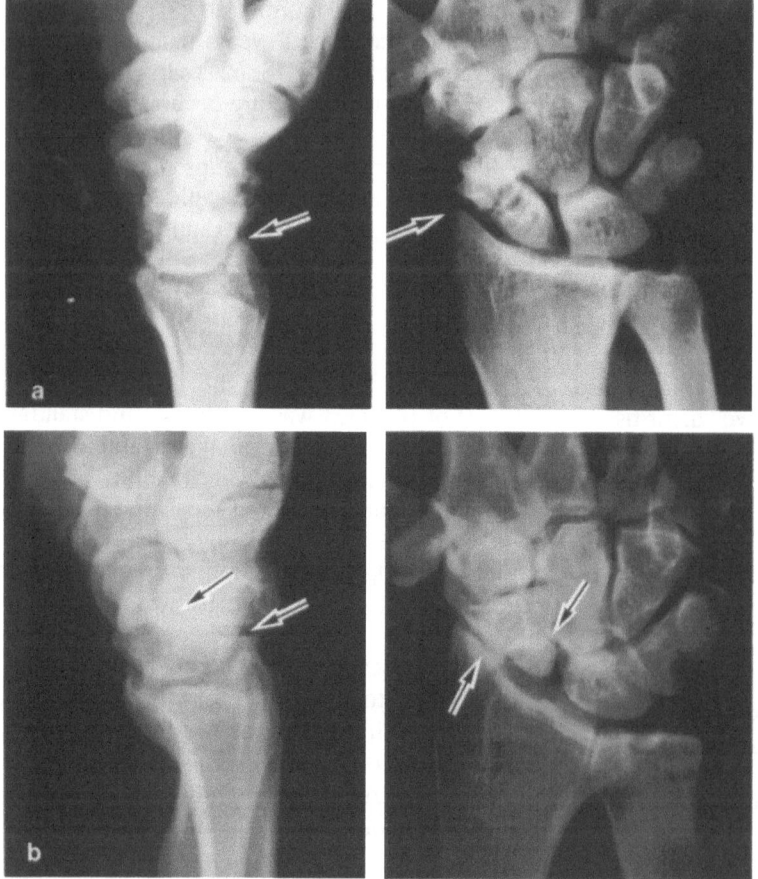

Fig. 1. Radiological findings of **a** the OA(+) group showing a pointing of the radial styloid (*arrow*) and **b** the OA(++) group showing narrowing of the radioscaphoid and midcarpal joint (*arrow*)

ROM of the wrist could not be measured precisely due to pain.

Results

Correlation Between the Incidence of DISI and the Sites of Scaphoid Fractures (Table 2)

In the 21 cases in the delayed union group, 4 had a fracture in the distal third, 16 in the middle third, and 1 in the proximal third. DISI deformity was observed in 3, 1, and 0 of them, respectively.

In the 54 cases in the non-union group, 10 had a fracture in the distal third, 35 in the middle third, and 9 in the proximal third. DISI deformity was observed in 9, 10, and 1, respectively. The incidence of DISI was highest for distal third fractures.

Correlation Between the Radiolunate Angle and Scaphoid Length

There was a significant association between the radiolunate angle and the scaphoid length, with a correlation coefficient (r) of -0.66 ($P < 0.001$) (Fig. 2).

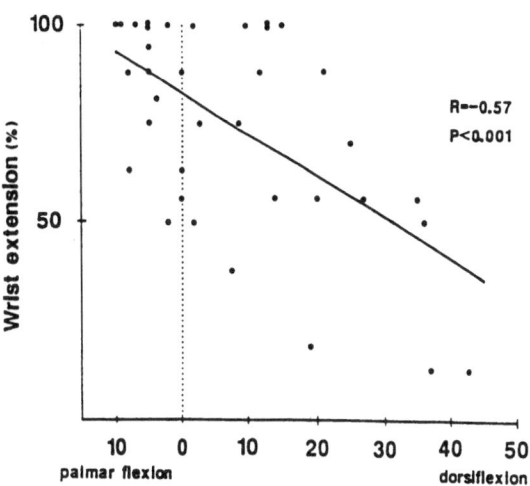

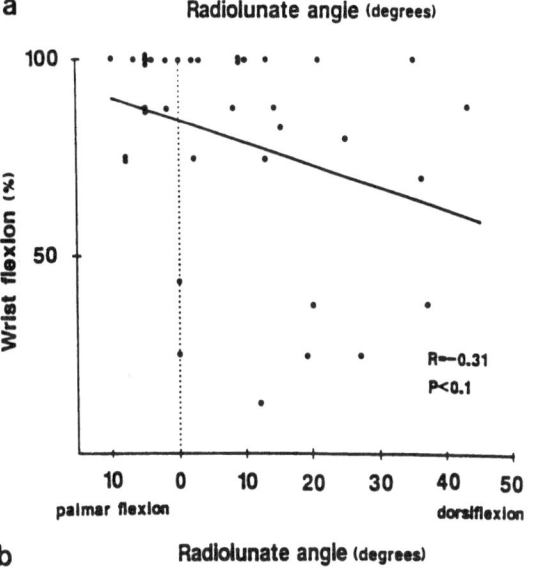

b

Fig. 3. Correlation between the **a** radiolunate angle and wrist extension, and **b** the radiolunate angle and wrist flexion

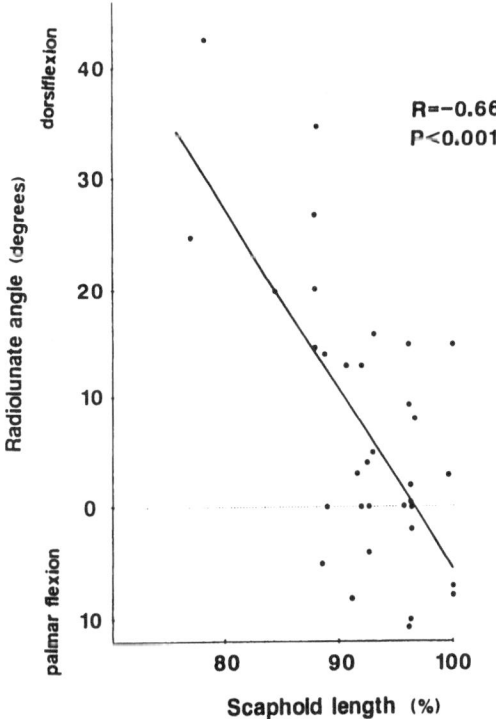

Fig. 2. Correlation between the radiolunate angle and the scaphoid length

Correlation Between the ROM of the Wrist and the Grade of Carpal Instability

The correlation between the wrist extension and the radiolunate angle is shown in Fig. 3.a. The wrist extension became smaller as the radiolunate angle increased. There was a significant association between wrist extension and the radiolunate angle ($r = -0.57$, $P < 0.001$).

The correlation between the radiolunate angle and wrist flexion is shown in Fig. 3.b. The correlation was less than that seen in wrist extension.

Table 3. Radiographically confirmed degenerative changes in chronic scaphoid fractures

	2–6 Months	6–12 Months	1–4 Years	5–9 Years	10–19Years	>20 Years	Total wrists (n)
OA (−)	21	10	15	3	2		51
OA (+)		2	1	1	3	3	10
OA (++)				1	1	7	9

OA, Osteoarthritis

Correlation Between the Extent of OA Changes and the Duration of Non-Union (Table 3).

No OA changes were found in the delayed union group. In the cases in which duration of the non-union was less than 5 years, OA was deteced in 3 out of 28 cases (10.7%), while OA was present in 14 out of 16 (87.5%) of the cases in which duration of the non-union exceeded 10 years.

Discussion

In this study, DISI was present in 19% of cases of delayed unions and in 37% of those of non-union, which is twice that of delayed unions. According to Fisk [5], Cooney [6], and Nakamura [7], the more time that elapses, the higher is the incidence of DISI due to bony absorption on the anterior aspect of the fracture site. We measured the

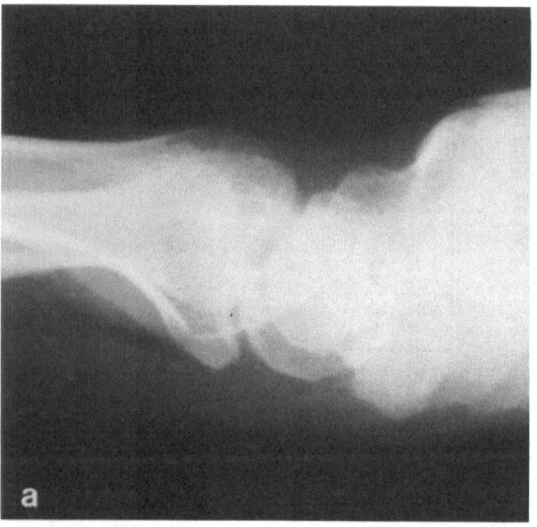

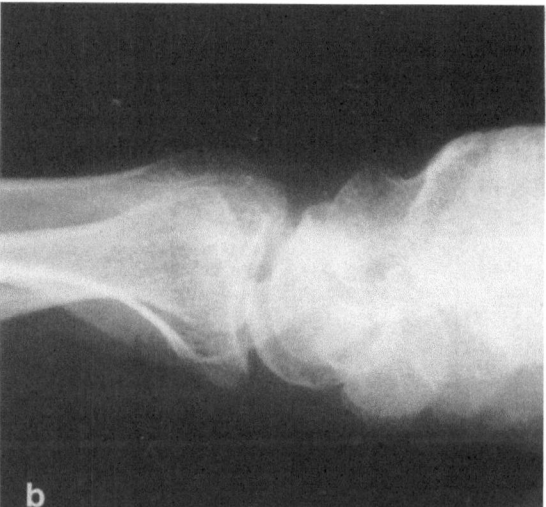

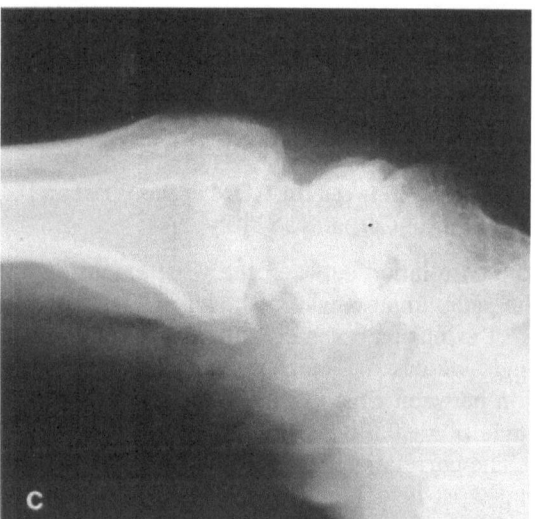

Fig. 4. Lateral dynamic series of roentgenograms in an 18-year-old male patient with severe DISI. **a** Lunate dorsiflexion of 37° in maximum extension. **b** Lunate dorsiflexion of 35° in neutral position. **c** Lunate palmar flexion of 6° in maximum flexion

scaphoid length in order to confirm this theory. The results showed that there is a significant relationship between the radiolunate angle and the scaphoid length. Therefore, we agree that the shortening of the scaphoid due to the bony absorption is one of the most important factors related to the occurrence of DISI.

Another factor related to DISI may be the fracture site. In fractures in the distal third of the scaphoid, the incidence of DISI was 90%, in middle third it was 28.6%, and in the proximal third, 1.1%. The radiocapitate ligament runs obliquely over the waist of the scaphoid. The scaphoid rotates on this ligament during wrist flexion and extension. In the distal third fractures, however, the distal part becomes free from the control of the ligament and flexes easily. We consider this to be the reason for the incidence of DISI to be much higher in the distal third fractures of the scaphoid.

What effect does DISI produce on the ROM of the wrist? In severe DISI cases with limitation of wrist extension, the lunate is locked in a dorsiflexed position, even when the wrist is in a neutral position, and the lunate cannot be dorsiflexed further (Fig. 4). Therefore, the midcarpal joint plays the main part of active motion in wrist extension. That may be the reason for the limitation of wrist extension in cases of DISI.

Degenerative change in scaphoid non-union has been addressed by Mack [2] and Vender [4]. Mack found the statistical incidence of displacement and degenerative change to increase greatly after a duration of 10 years [2].

In this study, the incidence and degree of degenerative arthritis were most significantly related to the duration of the non union. This finding supports those of Mack [2] and Vender [4]. The duration of non-union may be the most important factor for the degenerative arthritis.

Conclusions

The incidence of DISI in the non-union group was much higher than that of delayed union group. In the distal third fracture of the scaphoid, the incidence of DISI was also much higher. The site of fracture was shown to play an important role in the occurrence of DISI.

The shortening of the scaphoid due to bony absorption is the major risk factor is DISI, and wrist extension becomes limited in severe DISI cases.

The incidence of degenerative arthritis was shown to increase greatly after a duration of 10 years.

References

1. Sarrafian SK, Melamed JL, Goshgarian GM (1977) Study of wrist motion in flexion and extension. Clin Orthop 126:153–9
2. Mack GR, Bosse MJ, Gelberman RH (1984) The natural history of scaphoid non-union. J Bone Joint Surg [Am] 66:504–9
3. Fernandez DL (1984) A technique for anterior wedge-shaped grafts for scaphoid nonunions with carpal instability. J Hand Surg [Am] 9:733–7
4. Vender MI, Watson HK, Wiener BD, Black DM (1987) Degenerative change in symptomatic scaphoid nonunion. J Hand Surg [Am] 12:514–9
5. Fisk GR (1984) The wrist. J Bone Joint Surg [Br] 66:398 407
6. Cooney WP, Dobyns JH, Linscheid RL (1980) Nonunion of the scaphoid: Analysis of the results from bone grafting. J Hand Surg [Am] 5:343–54
7. Nakamura R, Imaeda T, Tsuge S, Watanabe K (1991) Scaphoid non-union with DISI deformity. A survery of clinical cases with special reference to ligamentous injury. J Hand Surg [Br] 16:156–61

The Treatment of Scaphoid Fractures Using Free-Hand Insertion of a Herbert Screw

SATOSHI TOH, SEIKO HARATA, RYUJIROU NAKAMURA, SADAHIRO INOUE, KEIRYO NAKAHARA, and KENJI TSUBO[1]

Abstract. Surgical techniques and clinical indications for free-hand Herbert-screw insertion for scaphoid fractures are described. Eleven patients were treated by this method. The fractures included 3 of the acute stable type, 4 of the acute unstable type, and 4 of delayed union. Three cases were complicated by fractures of the distal radius and one by the fracture of the proximal radial head. In 1 case, bony fusion was not achieved due to malalignment: an additional bone graft was performed, and a good bony union was achieved. In the other 10 cases, a solid union and good clinical results were achieved. This method is recommended for acute stable scaphoid fracture complicated by concomitant fractures requiring early mobilization, patients with acute stable fractures who wish to avoid long-term external fixation, acute unstable fractures in which trial reduction is perfect, cases of delayed union not requiring bone graft, and when the fracture is in the small proximal pole.

Keywords: Scaphoid fracture — Herbert screw — Free hand insertion

Introduction

From 1984 to date, we have treated 54 cases of scaphoid fracture using Herbert screws [1]. In the Herbert-screw system, the use of an alignment guide is important for inserting the screw properly [2]. However, in certain cases, we have performed free-hand insertion of the screw without an alignment guide. The following is a discussion of the surgical techniques and operative indications for this method.

Patients

Eleven patients were treated by free-hand Herbert-screw insertion. They included ten males and one female, ranging in age from 15 to 73 years. According to Herbert's classification, 3 fractures were of the acute stable type (type A), 4 of the acute unstable type (B), and 4 were cases of delayed union (C). All delayed union fractures were so-called late fractures, with the patients presenting 1 month or more after injury. Three cases were complicated by fractures of the distal radius and one by the fracture of the proximal radial head (Table 1).

Operative Methods

We performed free-hand insertion using a palmar approach in 10 cases, and in the remaining case, that of a proximal pole fracture, the screw was inserted in a retrograde manner, as described by Herbert [2].

Detailed Description of the Operative Procedure in Our Palmer Approach

A 1-cm transverse skin incision is made over the scaphotrapezium joint. The joint is identified, and its capsule is incised transversely (Fig. 1.a). Trial reduction of the fracture is carried out using an image intensifier. First, the fracture is stabilized temporarily by a Kirschner wire inserted in exactly the same direction as the intended line of the screw. Next, a second wire is inserted ulnarward and parallel to the first wire. The barrel of the guiding jig is placed onto the distal scaphoid

[1] Department of Orthopaedic Surgery, Hirosaki University, School of Medicine, 5-Zaifu-cho, Hirosaki, Aomori 036, Japan

Table 1. Characteristics of the patients and results of surgery

Patient no.	Age (years)	Sex	Cause of injury	Time from injury to surgery	Type of fracture[a]	Follow-up time (months)	Patient's satisfaction	Result[b] Clinical result	Radiographical result	Comment
1	16	M	Fall	5 days	B2	37	0	0	0	Complicated by fracture of head of radius
2	21	M	Snow board accident	1 days	A2	15	0	0	0	Complicated by fracture of radius end
3	18	M	Car accident	5 weeks	A2	31	0	0	0	Complicated by fracture of radius end
4	19	M	Fall	2 months	C	36	3	3	3	Revision Russe's operation, union
5	15	M	Fall	4 weeks	B2	16	0	0	0	
6	15	M	Football	4 weeks	C	37	0	0	0	
7	67	M	Fall	4 weeks	C	30	0	0	0	
8	73	F	Fall	2 days	B1	20	1	1	1	
9	19	M	Fall	1 day	B2	10	0	0	0	
10	28	M	Fall	2 weeks	A2	8	0	0	0	
11	34	M	Car accident	2 months	C	31	0	0	0	Complicated by fracture of radius end

[a] Type of fracture: Accoding to Herbert's classification [2]
[b] Result: According to Herbert's grading [2]

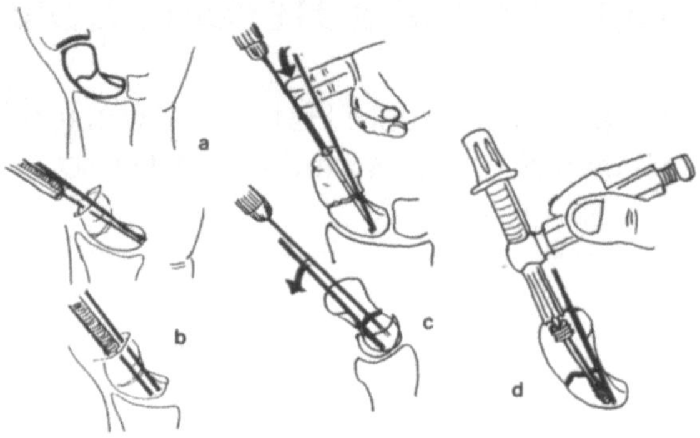

Fig. 1. Operative procedures. **a** Small transverse skin incision at the scaphotrapezium joint. **b** A Kirschner wire is inserted in the same direction as the intended line of the screw and a second wire is then inserted ulnarward and parallel to the first wire. The barrel is placed around the first Kirschner wire. **c** When it is difficult to insert the first wire in the same direction as the intended line of the screw, a first wire is inserted ulnarward and pulled volarward, and a second wire is then inserted along the intended line of the screw. **d** The first wire is removed and the screw is inserted in a free-hand manner

around the first Kirschner wire (Fig. 1.b). When it is difficult to insert the first wire in the same direction as the intended line of the screw, a first wire is inserted ulnarward and pulled volarward and a second wire is then inserted along the intended line of the screw (Fig. 1.c). After removing the wire and using the pilot drill, the main drill, and the tap, the screw is inserted in a free-hand manner (Fig. 1.d). If there is no problem with stability of the fracture site, the second Kirschner wire is removed. It is important that the screw be inserted perpendicular to the fracture line. It is possible to insert the screw in the proper position even though only a small incision is created.

For most patients, we permit gentle active movement of the wrist at 2 weeks after the operation. In cases which were complicated by other concomitant fractures, exercise can be started 3 weeks postoperatively.

Results

The length of follow-up ranged from 8 to 37 months (mean 25 months). In one case, bony fusion was not achieved due to malalignment: an additional bone graft was performed, and a good

Fig. 2. A 16-year-old male with a type-B2 scaphoid fracture and a right-sided fracture of the. head of the radius. **a** Preoperative roentgenograms. *Arrow*, fracture site. **b** Roentgenograms taken 6 months after the operation

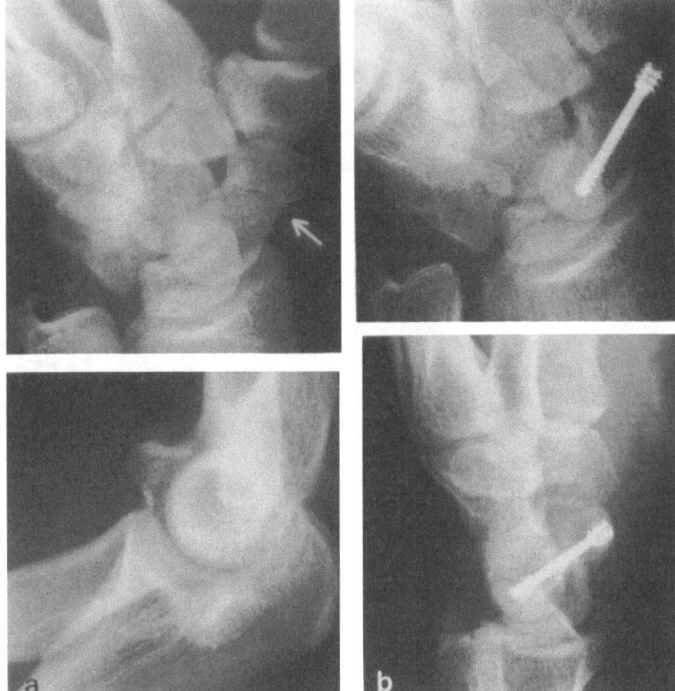

bony union was achieved. In each of the other 10 cases, there was a solid union and good clinical results (Table 1).

Case Reports

Case 1

A 16-year-old male with an acute unstable scaphoid fracture was referred with a right-sided fracture of the head of the radius and scaphoid. Five days after injury, we fixed both fractures simulataneously using Herbert screws and free-hand insertion for the scaphoid. Active range-of-motion exercise of all parts of the arm was begun after 3 weeks. Presently, 37 months after the operation, he has no complaints, and wrist range-of-motion and grip power are almost normal (Fig. 2).

Case 2

A 19-year-old male suffered an acute stable scaphoid fracture of the left hand. Wrist roentgenograms revealed an intra-articular fracture of the end of the radius. We initially applied external fixation, and Kirschner wires were used to fix the fragments of the intraarticular fracture. Then, a Herbert screw was inserted to stabilize the scaphoid fragments. Four months later, the patient was able to return to work (Fig. 3).

Case 3

An 18-year-old male suffered a fracture-dislocation of the wrist joint with a concomitant acute stable scaphoid fracture. Osteosynthesis using Kirschner wires was performed immediately at another hospital. He was referred to us 5 weeks after the trauma. We used free-hand insertion of a Herbert screw to stabilize the scaphoid fracture. Ten days later, the patient began active exercise of the wrist, and he was able to return to his assembly line job in a factory after 4 months (Fig. 4).

Case 4

This is the only case in which poor results required a second operation. A 19-year-old male suffered a type C (delayed union) scaphoid fracture, and the initial operation was performed 2 months after the injury. Unfortunately, the fracture was not perfectly repositioned before fixation was performed, resulting in non-union. Four months later, a second operation was performed using the Russe method [3]. Postoperatively, the patient's wrist was immobilized by external fixation for 2 months. Six months after the second

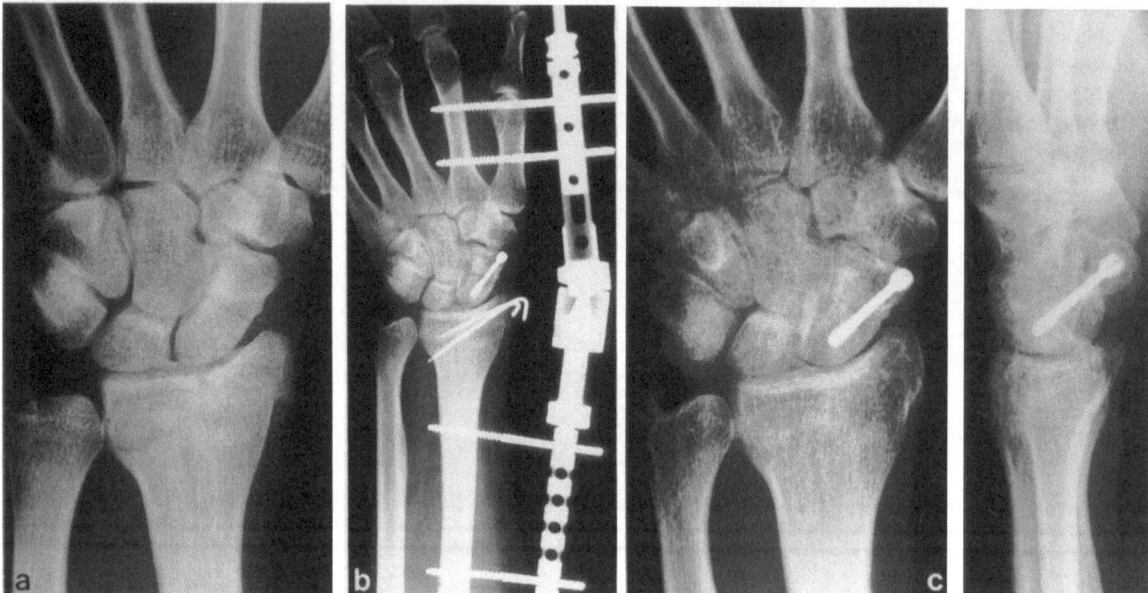

Fig. 3. A 19-year-old male with a type-A2 scaphoid fracture. **a** Wrist roentgenograms revealed an intra-articular fracture of the end of the radius. **b** External fixation and Kirschner wires were used for the inter-articular fracture. A Herbert screw was inserted to stabilize the scaphoid fragments. **c** The patient was able to return to work 4 months later

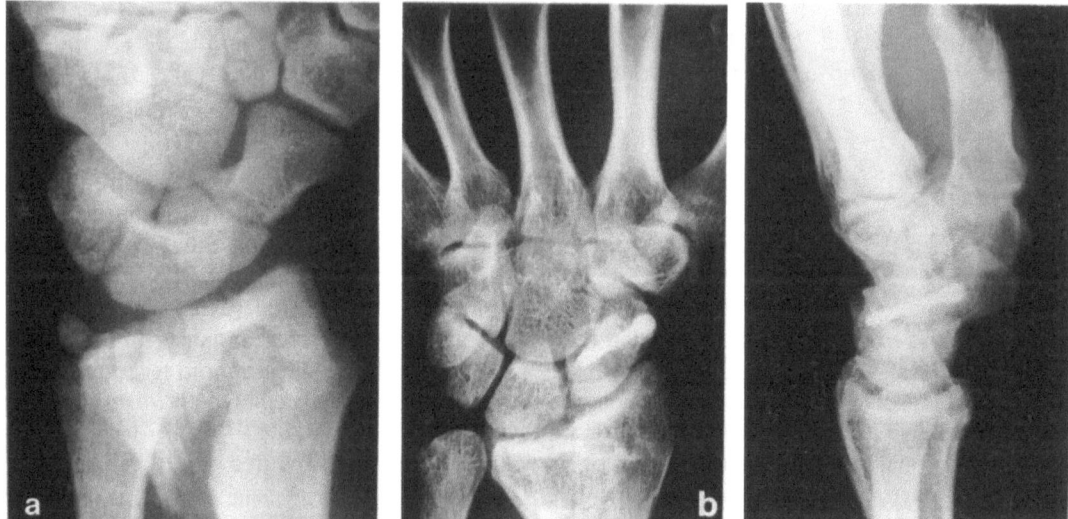

Fig. 4. An 18-year-old male. **a** Fracture-dislocation of the wrist joint with a concomitant type A2 scaphoid fracture. **b** Roentgenograms 1.5 years after the opera-tion. He was able to return to his assembly line job in a factory 4 months after the initial operation

operation, the range of motion of the wrist and grip power were almost normal (Fig. 5).

Discussion

Some controversy exists as to whether acute stable fractures should be treated surgically [4, 5]. Based on our experience, we recommend surgical inter-vention for 3 types of patients: those who cannot accept long-term immobilization, those who de-sire to return to athletic activities as soon as possible, and those who also have a fracture of the radial head or distal end of the radius. We especially recommend this procedure for the last group because of the danger of joint contracture associated with long-term immobilization. Even

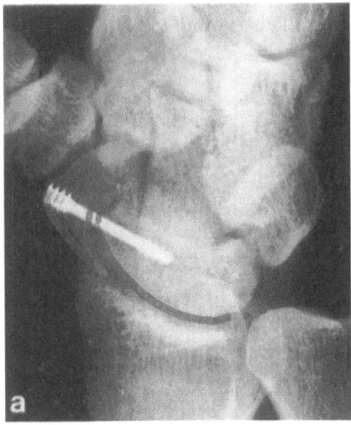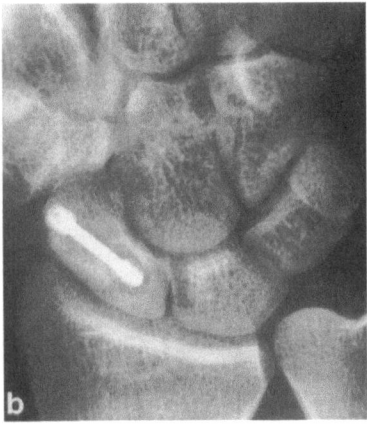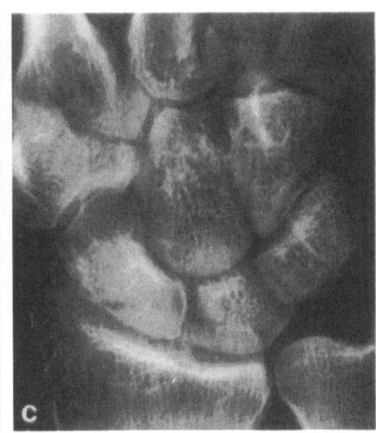

Fig. 5. A 19-year-old male who suffered a type-C scaphoid fracture. **a** Unfortunately, the fracture was not repositioned perfectly. **b** Roentgenograms 4 months after the operation revealed a ring sign surrounding the screw. **c** The second operation was performed using Russe's method and bone union was achieved 5 months afterwards

in acute unstable fractures, we feel this method can be used when a trial reduction is perfect. It can also be used in cases of delayed union when the alignment is good and a bone graft is unnecessary. In addition, as mentioned by Herbert, it is, of course, a good method in cases in which the fracture is in the small proximal pole.

An important advantage of this method is that osteosynthesis can be performed through a small skin incision. In theory, excessive dissection could compromise the blood supply to the scaphoid [6], whereas the blood supply is not disrupted in this method. Another advantage of this method is that no ligaments are cut, thereby enabling mobilization much earlier than with the usual Herbert-screw procedure. One disadvantage of this method is that it necessitates the use of an image intensifier. Another is that it is sometimes impossible to achieve adequate compression of the fracture site without an alignment guide. However, if good alignment can be preserved during the operation, the screw alone provides adequate compression.

References

1. Toh S, Harata S, Tsubo K, Inoue S, Nakahara K (1989) Clinical results of Herbert's method for scaphoid fracture. J Jpn Soc Surg Hand 6:727–730
2. Herbert TJ, Fisher WE (1984) Management of the fractured scaphoid using a new bone screw. J Bone Joint Surg [Br] 66:114–123
3. Russe O (1960) Fracture of the carpal navicular. Diagnosis, nonoperative treatment, and operative treatment. J Bone Joint Surg [Am] 42:759–768
4. Dickson RA, Leslie IJ (1988) Conservative treatment of the fractured scaphoid. In: Razemon JP, Fisk GR (eds) The wrist. Churchill Livingstone, Edinburgh, pp 80–87
5. Cooney WP, Dobyns JH, Linscheid RL (1980) Fractures of the scaphoid: A rational approach to management. Clin Orthop 149:90–97
6. Botte MJ, Mortensen WW, Gelberman RH, Rhoades CE, Gellman H (1988) Internal vascularity of the scaphoid in cadavers after insertion of the Herbert screw. J Hand Surg [Am] 13:216–221

Treatment of Acute Stable Scaphoid Fracture Using the Herbert Screw with a Small Skin Incision

Kotaro Imamura, Yoshifumi Nagatani, and Eiji Hirano[1]

Abstract. Acute stable scaphoid fracture (Herbert type A2) is generally managed conservatively with a plaster cast. However, long-term immobilization causes inconveniences of daily living and, more importantly, prohibits an early return to work even for the person who is not a heavy laborer and could resume working had the wrist not been fixed in a cast. Since the Herbert bone screw gives rigid internal fixation of bone fragments and allows early mobilization of the wrist, acute stable scaphoid fracture is treated using this screw, without requiring a cast, in order to solve the problems mentioned above. The screw is inserted into the scaphoid through a small skin incision just over the scaphotrapezial joint using a free-hand procedure monitored under an image intensifier. Thirteen wrists of 13 patients were operated upon from May, 1988 until November 1990. The average age of the patients was 29.4 years. The average time for returning to work after surgery was 3.2 weeks (range 1 day to 6 weeks). The average hand-grasping power was 94.6% and the average range of motion of the wrist was 98.1% compared with the non-affected side. According to Herbert's assessment system, the results of all the cases were graded as excellent.

Keywords: Scaphoid fracture — Acute stable fracture — Herbert screw — Small skin incision

Introduction

Acute scaphoid fracture, especially the stable type (Herbert type A2) [1], is managed conservatively as a rule. However, long-term immo-bilization in a plaster cast causes not only joint contracture but also significant limitations in daily living. Since the Herbert screw gives rigid internal fixation and allows early motion of the wrist, we have treated acute stable fractures by using a Herbert screw without a cast as of 1988, in order to reduce inconveniences in daily living and to achieve an early return to work.

This is an introduction of the surgical technique and a discussion of its usefulness.

Surgical Technique

The skin just over the scaphotrapezial (ST) joint is incised about 1.0 cm longitudinally under the axillar block (Fig. 1.a). The thenar muscle is divided parallel to its fiber and the joint is exposed by incising the capsule transversely (Fig. 1.b). Under the image intensifier, a Kirschner wire (1.2 mm) is inserted into the scaphoid from the ST joint to the proximal pole in order to confirm the direction and length of the screw (Fig. 1.c). To avoid a misdirected insertion of the Kirschner wire, it is vital to be familiar with the shape of the scaphoid which twists like a pretzel. A drill guide is pushed onto the distal articular surface of the scaphoid (Fig. 1.d) after which the Kirschner wire is removed. Taking care not to change the position and direction of the drill guide, the Herbert screw is inserted into the scaphoid through the articular surface using the free-hand procedure (Fig. 1.e). The drilling, tapping, and screw insertion should be carried out under monitoring by an image intensifier because repeated misdirected drilling causes failure of rigid fixation. A shorter Herbert screw than that previously measured should be chosen because the head of the screw is deeply buried from the articular surface into the bone. No postoperative plaster cast is applied. Active

[1] Department of Orthopaedic Surgery, Nagasaki University School of Medicine, 7-1 Sakamoto-machi, Nagasaki 852, Japan

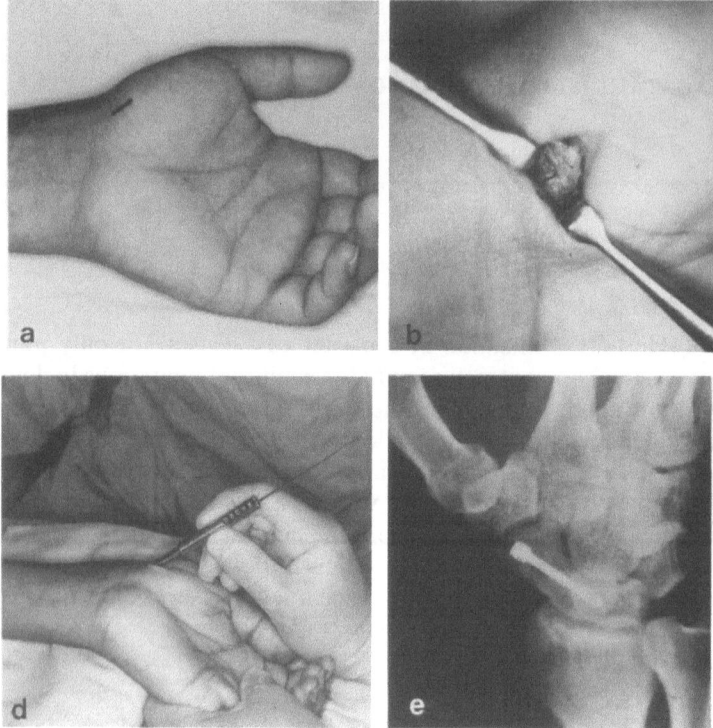

Fig. 1. a A small incision just over the scaphotrapezial (ST) joint. **b** Exposure of the ST joint. **c** Insertion of a Kirschner wire under monitoring by an image intensifier. **d** A drill guide is pushed onto the distal articular surface of the scaphoid to keep the same direction as the Kirschner wire. **e** Insertion of a Herbert screw

Table 1. Patient data

Case	Age (years)	Side involved	Time between inj.-op. (days)	Occupation	Return to work (days)	Union of fracture (months)	Pain	Limitations in ADL	HGP (%)	ROM (%)	Follow-up period (months)
1	29	L	9	Banker	14	2	(−)	(−)	80	100	12
2	31	L	19	Driver	30	2	(−)	(−)	100	100	8
3	15	L	2	Student	2	1	(−)	(−)	100	100	12
4	26	R	11	Driver	30	2	(−)	(−)	87	100	7
5	34	L	4	Office worker	30	2	(−)	(−)	86	100	4
6	36	L	17	Sailor	30	1.5	(−)	(−)	77	75	5
7	17	L	11	Student	5	2	(−)	(−)	92	100	13
8	63	L	5	Farmer	42	1.5	(−)	(−)	100	100	5
9	30	L	3	Policeman	8	1	(−)	(−)	100	100	6
10	17	R	6	Student	13	1	(−)	(−)	105	100	17
11	25	L	7	Cook	42	2	(−)	(−)	90	100	12
12	35	R	10	Driver	17	2	(−)	(−)	120	100	10
13	24	L	20	Student	1	2	(−)	(−)	93	100	7

Inj.-op., Injury and operation; *ADL*, activities of daily living; *HGP*, hand-grasping power (compared to non-affected side); *ROM*, range of motion (compared to non-affected side)

movement of the wrist may be permitted 1 week after the operation.

Patients and Methods

Thirteen wrists of 13 male patients were operated from May, 1988 to November 1990. The average age of the patients was 29.4 years (range 15–63 years). There were 3 right and 10 left wrists. All the cases were stable fractures of the middle third of the scaphoid (Herbert type A2). The subjects' occupations were students (4), taxi drivers (3), banker (1), sailor (1), policeman (1), farmer (1), office worker (1), and cook (1).

The average interval between the time of injury and the operation was 8.7 days (range 2–19 days).

At follow-up examination, we interviewed the patients concerning wrist pain and disturbances in the activities of daily living, measured the range of wrist motion and hand-grasping power, and evaluated the radiographic findings.

The mean postoperative follow-up period was 9 months (range 4 months–1 year 5 months).

Results

After removal of the stitches, each patient could wash his face without any difficulty. The average time for returning to work was 3.2 weeks (range 1 day–6 weeks). The students went back to school after a few days. However, the farmer and the cook, who were heavy manual workers, were not allowed to resume working before 6 weeks in order to avoid displacement of the wrist fragments as a result of excessive load. Bone union was achieved in all cases within 1–2 months (average 1.7 months). At follow-up, none of these patients had wrist pain or limitations in

daily living. The average hand-grasping power was 94.6% (range, 77%–120%) compared with the non-affected side. The average range of motion of the wrist was 98.1% (range, 75%–100%). According to Herbert's assessment system, the results in all cases were graded as excellent (Table 1).

Case Presentation

A 26-year-old taxi driver (case 4) injured his right wrist in a traffic accident. A general practitioner diagnosed his injury as a scaphoid fracture (Fig. 2.a) and a plaster cast was applied. Expressing his desire for an early return to work, he was referred to our hospital. The operation was carried out on an out-patient basis 11 days after the accident (Fig. 2.b). No plaster cast was applied and active motion of the wrist was encouraged 1 week after surgery. He returned to his usual work 1 month after surgery. The fracture was healed without

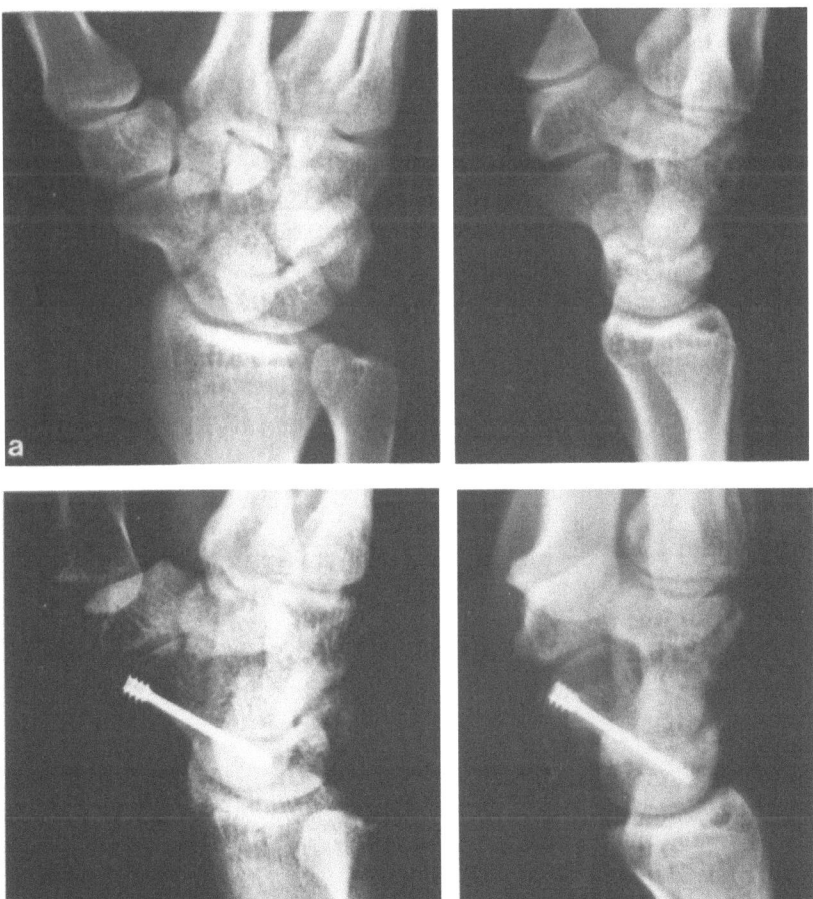

Fig. 2. a The wrist of a 26-year-old taxi driver (case 4). A middle-third scaphoid stable fracture was diagnosed. Herbert screw fixation through a small incision was carried out 11 days after the accident. **b** When reexamined 7 months after the operation, the fracture was seen to be healed without any complications

any complications 2 months after the operation. When re-examined 7 months after surgery, he had no wrist pain and no limitations in daily living. He had a full range of wrist motion and hand-grasping power was 53 kg.

Discussion

Cast immobilization has been the usual treatment for acute stable fractures. The period of immobilization is advised as being 6 weeks by Russe [2], 8 weeks by Watson-Jones [3], and 12 weeks by Stewart [4]. We also have immobilized the wrist with a plaster cast for an average of 8 weeks (range 5–11 weeks). Cast immobilization restricts many simple but necessary daily activities and also delays the return to work. On the other hand, it has been advocated that the Herbert screw provides the necessary rigid internal fixation for fracture of the scaphoid and that a plaster cast was rarely required, thus permitting early active wrist motion.

In Herbert's original procedure, the skin incision is larger than that of our procedure so that the fragments of the scaphoid can be held with a jig, and the radiocapitate and radiolunate ligaments can be incised. Consequently, the original procedure necessitates the immobilization of the wrist with a plaster cast until the incised ligaments heal. In our technique, however, it is unnecessary to incise the above-mentioned ligaments except for a small part of the scaphotrapezial ligament. Therefore, no plaster cast is necessary whatsoever and active wrist motion can be achieved earlier. Furthermore, another advantage of this technique is that the blood supply to the scaphoid from the surrounding soft tissue is not disturbed because of the small size of the skin incision. This may well be favorable to achieving bone union.

Conclusion

Herbert screw fixation through a small skin incision is useful for acute stable scaphoid fractures because it frees the patient from the inconvenience of wearing a plaster cast and enables an early return to work.

References

1. Herbert TJ, Fischer WE (1984) Management of the fractured scaphoid using a new bone screw. J Bone Joint Surg [Br] 66:114–123
2. Russe O (1960) Fracture of the carpal navicular. J Bone Joint Surg [Am] 42:759–768
3. Watson-Jones R (1934) Inadequate immobilization and non-union of fracture. Br Med J May 26, p 937
4. Stewart MJ (1954) Fractures of the carpal navicular (scaphoid). J Bone Joint Surg [Am] 36:998–1006

Vascularized Bone Graft Pedicled on the Dorsal Innominate Artery for Scaphoid Non-Union

Yuichi Hirasé and Tadao Kojima[1]

Abstract. Zaidemberg reported on a new vascularized bone graft for scaphoid non-union in 1989. This is a pedicled vascularized bone graft from the dorsum of the distal radius combined with the innominate artery and is approached dorsally. We used this technique in 4 cases of non-union of the scaphoid. All 4 cases exhibited radiographic union, 3 within 6 weeks, and 1 at 9 weeks postoperatively. Wrist pain was diminished remarkably in all patients. Although the dorsal approach to the scaphoid has some disadvantages for hand surgeons, this treatment offered a higher union rate in comparison with conventional bone grafts. We believe that this procedure should be recommended as a new vascularized bone graft for scaphoid non-union. Additionally, it may also have the potential for use as a procedure for avascular necrosis of lunate.

Keywords: Vascularized bone graft — Scaphoid non-union — Scaphoid fracture — Bone graft — Scaphoid

Introduction

Inlay bone graft in the volar approach and Herbert-screw fixation currently seem to be well established as the successful choices for scaphoid non-union. However, even with these procedures more than 10% of cases cannot achieve adequate union. Recently, some new methods of pedicled vascularized bone grafts have been introduced. The pronator quadratus pedicled bone graft from the distal radius was first described by Braun [1] and Chacha [2], and Kawai and Yamamoto [3]

subsequently modified this method. Kuhlman et al. [4] reported on their experience with vascularized bone graft pedicled on the volar carpal artery for non-union of the scaphoid. In 1991, Zaidemberg and associates [5] reported on a new pedicled vascularized bone graft from the dorsum of the distal radius and its use in 9 cases of non-union of the scaphoid. We now report its advantages and disadvantages based on our experiences with this method in 4 cases of scaphoid non-union.

Anatomical Study and Surgical Procedure

The vascularization of the distal radius is based on a consistent retrograde branch from the radial artery which provides blood supply to its dorsoradial aspect. This artery is anatomically described as the innominate artery branching from the radial artery around the wrist. It ascends deep into the radiocarpal ligament at the level of the radiocarpal joint and turns to lie on the dorsoradial aspect of the distal radius at the level of the radial styloid (Fig. 1). A bone fragment with the overlying vascular pedicle can be harvested for graft. Zaidemberg and associates [5] studied 20 cadaverous specimens and reported that this anatomical arrangement was found in all of them.

In the surgical procedure, a dorsal approach is chosen for achieving exposure, and an oblique incision on the radiodorsal aspect of the wrist is made (Fig. 2). The extensor retinaculum is exposed and divided taking care not to injure the dorsal sensory branch of the radial nerve. The first dorsal compartment, comprised of the extensor pollicis brevis and abductor pollicis longus, is retracted volarly, and the extensor carpi radialis longus and extensor communis tendons are reflected ulnarly. By retracting these

[1]Department of Plastic and Reconstructive Surgery, Jikei University School of Medicine, 3-25-8 Nishi-Shinbashi Minato-ku, Tokyo 105, Japan

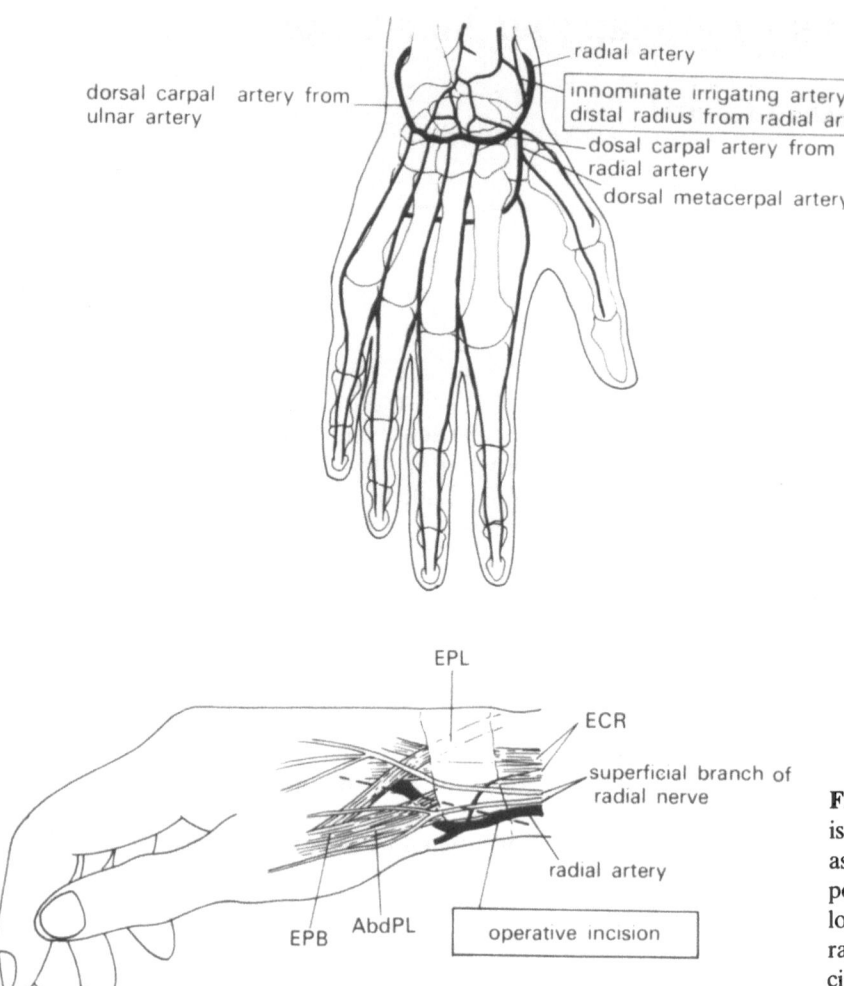

. The innominate branch the radial artery lies on orsoradial aspect of the radius at the level of the styloid

Fig. 2. An oblique incision is made on the radiodorsal aspect of the wrist for easy exposure. *EPL*, Extensor policis longus; *ECR*, extensor carpiradialis; *EPB*, extensor pollicis brevis; *AbdPL*, abductor pollicis longus

tendons, the irrigating artery is easily identified as overlying the distal radius. The vascularized bone graft can be transposed and enough length of the vascular pedicle to the scaphoid can be harvested without isolating the irrigating vessel from the radial artery. The non-union of the scaphoid is exposed to the fresh sclerotic bone ends by a drill. A cavity 20 mm in length is made in the scaphoid in the same manner as in the conventional bone graft technique. A bone graft with the same size as the scaphoid cavity is harvested from the distal radius together with the vascular pedicle. The bone graft is fitted into place with Kirschner wires. The skin is closed and a long arm cast with a thumb spica is applied for 1 month, followed by a short arm cast with a thumb spica for 2 weeks.

At about 6 weeks, when stable bony union is confirmed by X-ray, excercise is begun.

Clinical Cases

We treated four patients with scaphoid non-union associated with chronic wrist pain. The fracture had been initially missed in three patients and the length of immobilization time had not been sufficient to achieve union in the fourth.

Case 1

This 20-year-old male suffered a scaphoid fracture in a traffic accident and his wrist was immobilized for 10 weeks. On X-ray, union was seen to be unsuccessful and a cystic shadow was detected (Fig. 3). An operation was performed and an aseptic cyst was resected in the scaphoid fracture for purposes of reduction. A pedicled vascularized bone was harvested and transposed for Kirschner-wire fixation (Fig. 4).

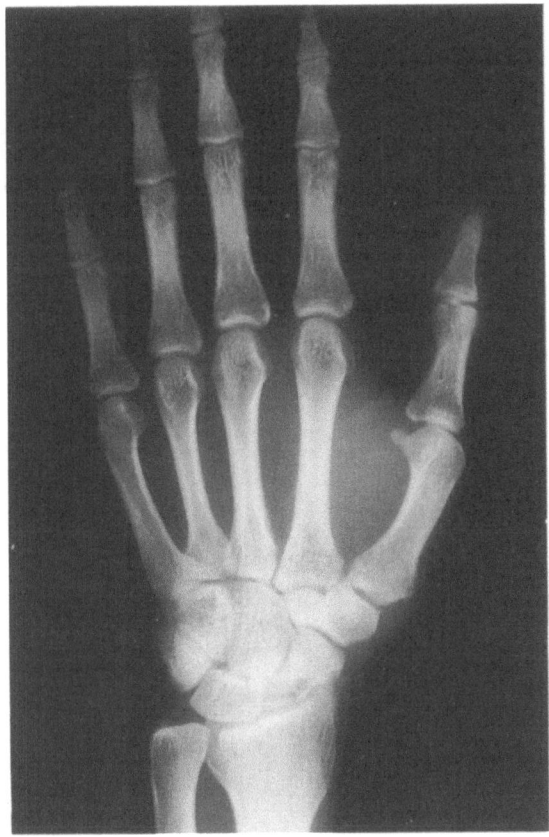

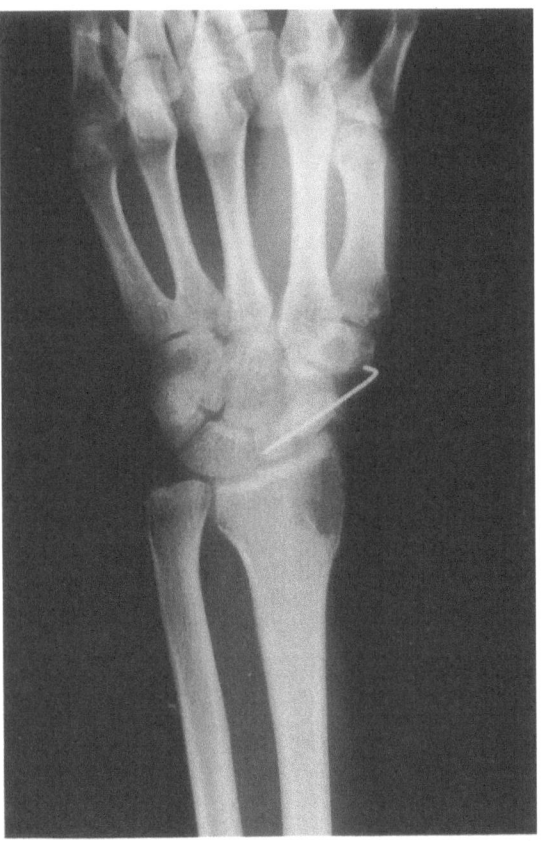

Fig. 3. Case 1. A cystic shadow was detected on X-ray but bony union was absent

Fig. 5. Bony union was confirmed on X-ray at the 5th week postoperatively (case 1)

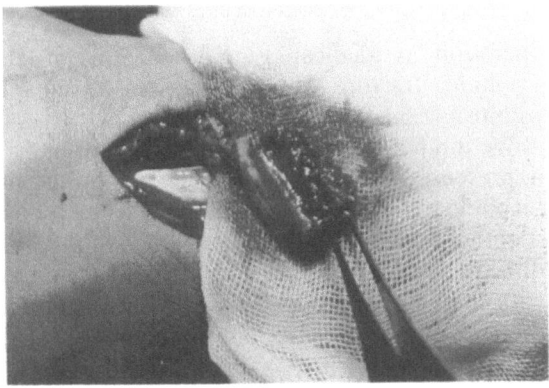

Fig. 4. A pedicled vascularized bone graft was elevated from the distal radius (case 1)

Five weeks later, union was confirmed on X-ray (Fig. 5). Excercise was begun and range of motion was improved remarkably. Wrist extension increased by 60° and flexion increased by 50° (Fig. 6).

Case 2

This 23-year-old male injured his wrist playing soccer and it was immobilized for several weeks for relief of wrist pain. Two years later, however, he still had chronic pain in his wrist and was referred to our hospital because of pseudo-arthrosis (Fig. 7). A vascularized bone graft was performed and bony union was confirmed on X-ray only 6 weeks later (Fig. 8). At 3 months postoperatively, the Kirschner wire was removed and the range of motion increased by 50° in extension and by 40° in flexion, both without pain (Fig. 9).

Bony union was confirmed radiographically in all four patients. The length of immobilization was 5–9 weeks (average 6.75 weeks). Chronic wrist pain at rest was completely relieved in all patients. Motion pain was eliminated in three patients and remarkably diminished in the fourth. The increased range of motion was 40°–60° in extension and 30°–50° in flexion.

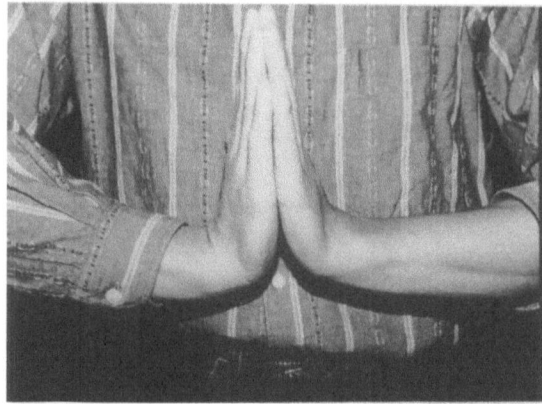

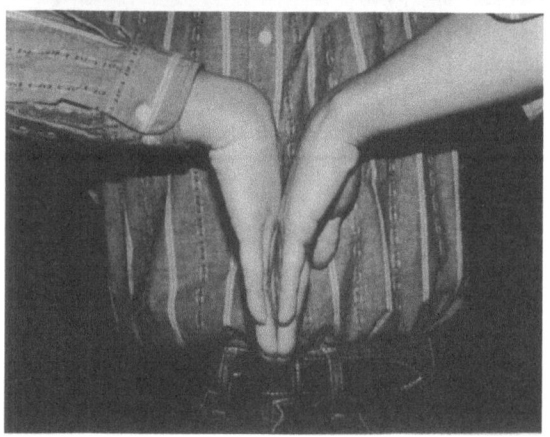

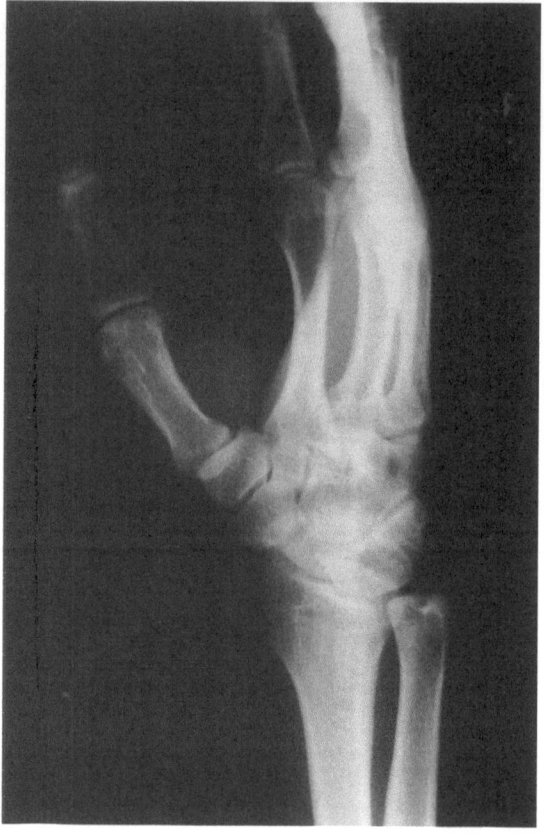

Fig. 6. Improved range of motion (case 1)

Fig. 7. This case was referred introduced to our hospital 2 years after injury because of pseudoarthrosis of the scaphoid (case 2)

Discussion

While treating these cases, we discovered the advantages and disadvantages of this method. The biggest advantage is the shorter period of immobilization and an apparently higher union rate. Zaidemberg used this method on 9 cases which failed to achieve union by the conventional (free) bone graft [6]: union was clearly successful within 6 weeks in all 9 cases and the patients were free of wrist pain. He described that the combination of vascularized bone graft and Herbert-screw fixation was particularly appealing in that it allowed mobilization as early as 4 weeks following surgery.

Another advantage is the ease of the technique for elevating the osseous flap, taking only 20 minutes at most. The direct arterial supply to the distal radius can invariably be seen under the extensor retinaculum. Almost all the time of

operation is dedicated to reduction of the scaphoid fracture, and surgery is complete within 2–2.5 hours at most.

We prefer the volar approach in general as it preserves the original vascular supply of the scaphoid. The dorsal approach of this method is slightly disadvantagous for us; reduction is a little difficult because the lack of space as compared with the volar approach. However, this problem can be solved if a little bigger incision is made and the intraoperative X-ray image is used. We believe that the advantages are much more important than the disadvantages in this method.

In addition to its application for scaphoid non-union, this pedicled vascularized bone graft may have a potential use in avascular necrosis of lunate. If the radiocarpal ligament is divided to elevate the flap, the proximal portion of the irrigating vessel can be dissected from the ligament to achieve a longer pedicle.

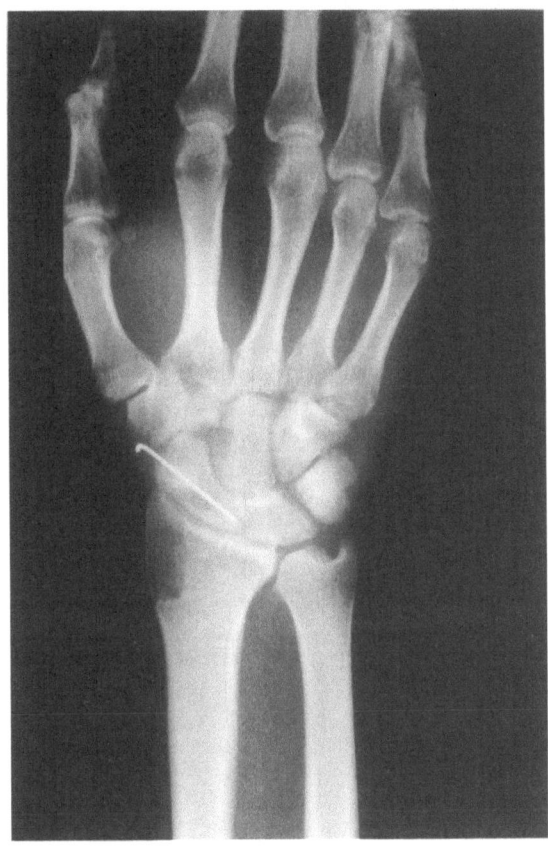

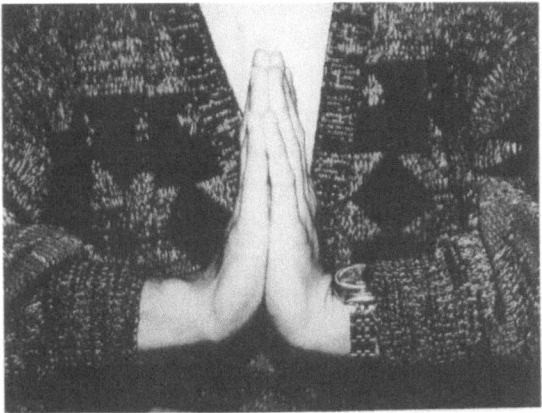

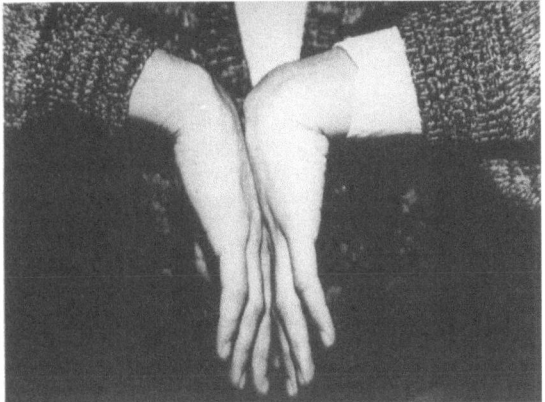

Fig. 8. Bony union was confirmed on X-ray 6 weeks later (case 2)

Fig. 9. Improved range of motion (case 2)

This procedure should be considered as a new technique for vascularized bone grafting around the wrist.

References

1. Braun RM (1983) Pronator pedicle bone grafting in the forearm and proximal carpal row. Orthop Trans 7:35
2. Chacha PB (1984) Vascularized pedicular bone grafts. Int Orthop 8:117–138
3. Kawai H, Yamamoto K (1988) Pronator quadratus pedicled bone graft for old scaphoid fractures. J Bone Joint Surg [Br] 70:829–831
4. Kuhlmann JK, Mimoun M, Boabighi A, Baux S (1987) Vascularized bone graft pedicled on the volar artery for non-union of the scaphoid. J Hand Surg [Br] 12(2):203–210
5. Zaidemberg C, Siebert JW, Angrigiani C (1991) A new vascularized bone graft for scaphoid non-union. J Hand Surg [Am] 16:474–478
6. Russe O (1960) Fractures of carpal navicular. Diagnosis, nonoperative and operative treatment. J Bone Joint Surg [Am] 42:759–768

Part IV. Distal Radius Fracture

Current Management of Intra-Articular Fractures of the Distal Radius

Diego L. Fernandez[1]

Keywords: Distal radius — Articular fractures — Limited open reduction — Results

Introduction

Among the wide spectrum of complications associated with fractures of the distal end of the radius [1–16], reflex sympathetic dystrophy and post-traumatic osteoarthritis due to residual articular incongruity are the two conditions that lead to permanent disability, resulting in an unsatisfactory functional outcome. Although reflex sympathetic dystrophy is relatively infrequent [6, 17, 18], the incidence of post-traumatic osteoarthritis is significantly high [17, 19, 20]. For this reason, the primary aim in the management of displaced intra-articular fractures, at least in the young manually active individual, is anatomic reduction of the joint surface both at the radiocarpal and radioulnar levels.

Although restoration of the joint surface can be obtained by a variety of treatment modalities, such as closed reduction, traction, percutaneous manipulation, or formal open reduction, prevention of secondary displacement of the articular fragments in the first 4 weeks constitutes the key to a successful result. This is achieved with minimal internal fixation with Kirschner wires or plates in simple fractures types with relatively well-sized fragments and absence of metaphyseal comminution. Otherwise, an external fixator that will neutralize axial loading of the carpus on the comminuted surface of the radius in combination with primary bone grafting of the bone defect with autologous iliac bone for a period of 5 weeks becomes mandatory.

Modern classification systems of fractures of the distal radius based on the analysis of the mechanism of injury [6, 17], number of fragments [21], stability [22], displacement pattern [23], and degree of joint and metaphyseal involvement [24] have become a valuable aid in deciding on the best possible type of treatment for each fracture type. Furthermore, these classifications have included a prognostic parameter, by separating simple and complex articular fractures that readily orient the surgeon toward the election of the appropriate method for each fracture. The AO classification of fractures of the distal forearm, outlined by the author and Müller, is a very detailed classification organized in order of increasing severity of the bone and articular lesion [25]. It divides the fractures into extra-articular (type A), simple articular (type B), and complex articular (type C) (Fig. 1). Further subdivisions into main and subgroups and the introduction of additional lesions of the distal ulna produced 144 different combinations of fractures occurring at the wrist level. It is, therefore, very useful for standardized computerized documentation of fractures, and may, in the future, provide a solid basis for comparing results of large series treated in different institutions.

On the other hand, assessment of the mechanism of injury is of great interest not only because manual reduction and realignment of the fracture is usually achieved by applying the opposite force which produced the injury, but also associated ligamentous lesions, subluxations, and fractures of the neighboring carpal bones and concomitant soft tissue damage are in direct relationship to the quality and degree of trauma sustained. Since the basic mechanical features of each fracture is strictly dependent on the mechanism of injury, I prefer to classify the fractures of the distal radius as follows:

[1] Department of Surgery, Kantonsspital Aarau, CH-5001 Aarau, Switzerland

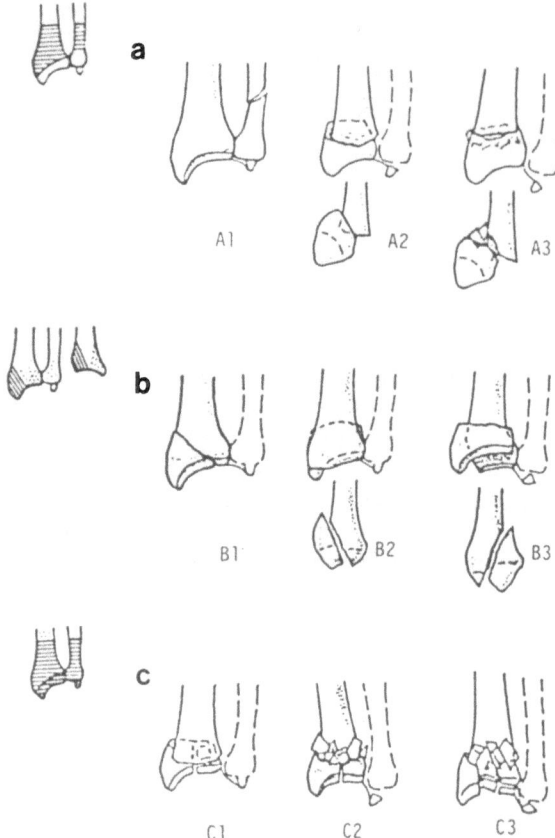

Fig. 1. AO-Classification of fractures of the distal forearm (main groups). **a** *Extra-articular:* isolated extra-articular fracture of the ulna (*A1*); extra-articular fracture of the radius (*A2*); extra-articular fracture of the radius with varying degrees of metaphyseal comminution or impaction (*A3*). **b** *Simple articular:* cuneiform articular fracture (*B1*); dorsal marginal fracture (Barton's) (*B2*); volar marginal fracture (reversed Barton's) (*B3*). **c** *Complex articular:* articular fracture with a simple intra-articular component (two fragments and no metaphyseal comminution) (*C1*); articular fracture with a simple intra-articular component and metaphyseal comminution (*C2*); comminuted articular fracture of the radius (*C3*)

1. Type I: *bending fractures* of the metaphysis in which one cortex fails under tensile stresses and the opposite one undergoes a certain degree of comminution (extra-articular Colles' or Smith's fractures)
2. Type II: *shearing fractures* of the joint surface (Barton's, reversed Barton's, radial styloid, simple articular fractures)
3. Type III: *compression fractures* of the joint surface with impaction of the subchondral and metaphyseal cancellous bone (intra-articular

comminuted fractures of the distal radius, complex articular fractures, "pilon radial")
4. Type IV: *avulsion fractures* of ligament attachments (ulnar-radial-styoid, radiocarpal fracture dislocations)
5. Type V: *combinations* of bending, compression, shearing, or avulsion mechanisms (*high velocity injuries*)

Using this simple classification, the ideal method of fixation is easily recognized. *Bending fractures* are best treated by a counterforce to that which produced the injury, i.e., one that will excert tension forces on the side of the concavity of the angulation. This is achieved in cases with adequate bone quality and absence of metaphyseal comminution with a well-molded three-point contact cast. *Shearing fractures* usually occur in hard cancellous bone (young individuals), are extremely unstable due to the obliquity of the fracture line and, therefore, suitable for internal fixation (lag screws, buttress plating). Realignment and reduction of *compression fractures* of the joint surface can be achieved in most cases by applying tension to the joint capsule with finger traps, external fixators, or pins and plaster cast techniques. In certain cases, however, disimpaction of cartilage-bearing fragments may require limited or extensile open reduction and replacement of the cancellous defect with a bone graft. *Avulsion fractures* are, in fact, ligamentous lesions resulting after an important wrist sprain in which rotational forces are part of the mechanism of injury. Therefore, additional ligament carpal disruption should be ruled out. Tension wiring or screw fixation may be useful if such fractures are severely displaced. Finally, if a fracture presents with one or more of the above-mentioned features (*bending, compression, shearing, avulsion*) a combined method of repair will be selected for treatment.

Further recognition of fragment stability, displacement pattern, and associated soft tissue lesions in these 5 fracture types will also influence the treatment modality.

Current Management of Fractures Affecting the Articular Surface of the Distal Radius

Shearing or Simple Articular Fractures

The basic common feature of these fractures is that a portion of the metaphyseal and epiphyseal areas of the distal radius is intact and in continuity with the non-affected portion of the joint surface. It is for this reason that the ultimate prognosis and functional outcome in this fracture group is predictable, because the displaced articular fragment can be exactly reduced and solidly fixed to the intact distal column of the radius. They usually occur in young individuals with hard cancellous bone that offers ideal holding power for internal fixation material. Since there is no transverse metaphyseal fracture nor massive comminution, shortening with respect to the ulna is not a problem. However, due to the obliquity of the fracture plane, these fractures are very difficult to "hold out to length" with conservative measures, or with joint distraction using external fixators. Ligamentotaxis may restore the joint level but usually fails to close the articular gap, resulting in volar or dorsal radiocarpal subluxation.

Fractures of the radial styloid are ideally treated by closed manipulation and percutaneous pinning. However, if anatomic reduction can not be accomplished, open reduction is performed through a dorsoradial approach. Isolated dorsal marginal fractures are rare, in contrast to the frequent combination between a dorsal marginal fracture and a radial styloid fragment (Fig. 2). If closed manipulation and percutaneous pinning fails to provide anatomical congruity of the joint surface, open reduction is carried out using a dorsal incision between the third and fourth extensor compartments. Usually, the radial styloid fragment is easily reduced and can be pinned to the metaphyseal area. Depending on the size of the associated dorsal rim fracture, either a small T- or L plate can be used with a buttressing effect.

Fractures of the volar margin are intrinsically unstable and the volar fragment may show a variable amount of comminution. The widely accepted method of treatment is open reduction and internal fixation by means of a volar buttress plate [26–30].

Compression or Complex Articular Fractures

This group is characterized by the affectation of both the metaphyseal area and the joint surface by the fracture. Traction X-ray views of the wrist following reduction, tomograms, and CAT scans are useful for determining the exact number of fragments and extent of displacement and comminution.

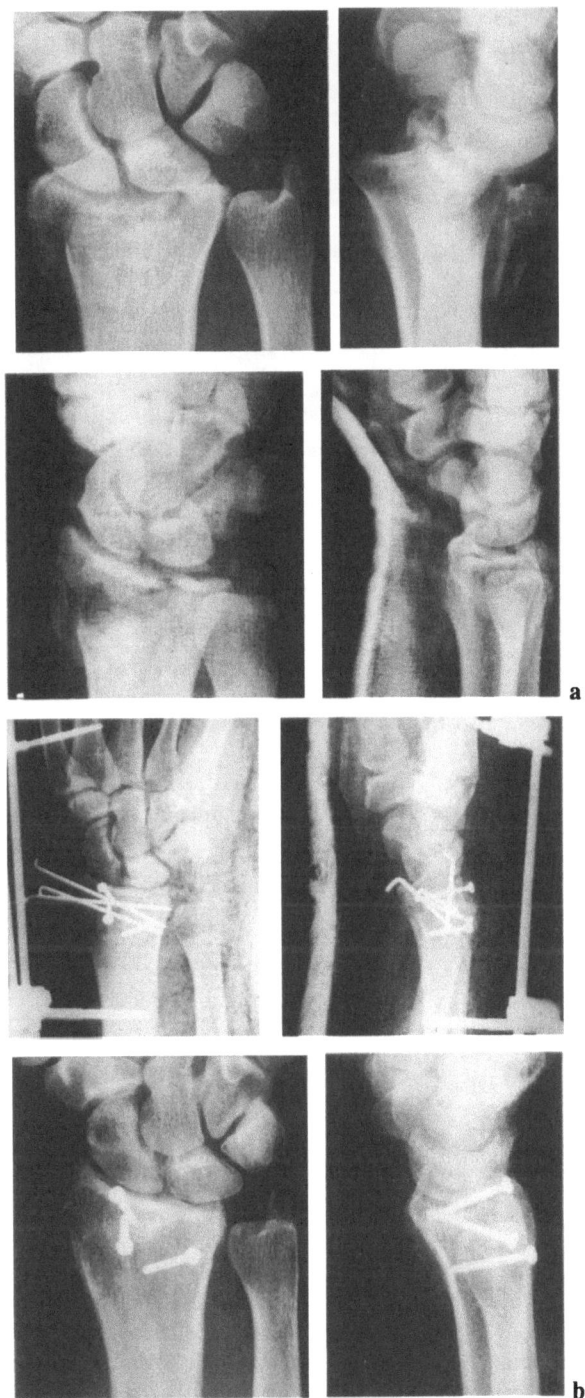

Fig. 2. **a** Combined radial styloid and dorsal margin fracture showing unacceptable joint surface congruity after closed reduction. **b** Radiographs immediately after open reduction and internal fixation with Kirschner wires for the styloid fragment and with lag screws for the dorsal fragment. A wrist fixator was used as a neutralization frame to permit open wound care for 4 weeks. Follow-up at 5 years shows a well-preserved joint space

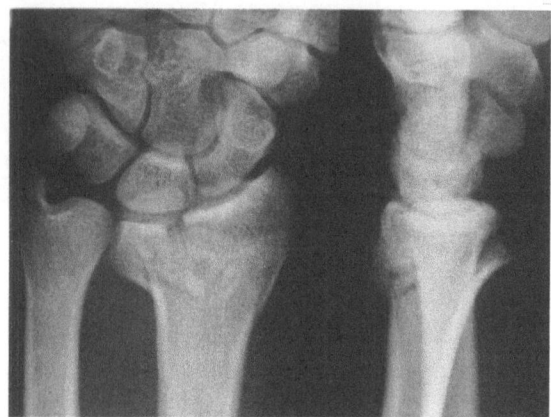

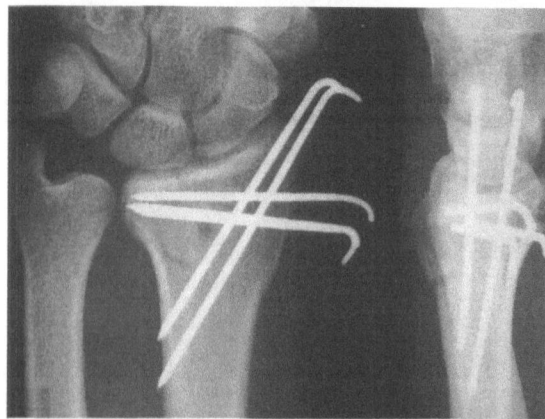

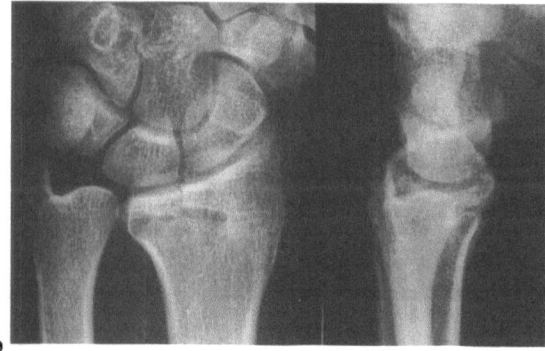

Fig. 3. a Intra-articular displaced two-part fracture in a young adult. **b** Anatomic reduction obtained with closed manipulation and percutaneous reduction and pinning of the ulnar fragment. Follow-up films at 3 years show absence of degenerative changes in the radiocarpal joint

In contrast to the shearing fractures described previously, treatment not only includes the effort to restore articular congruity, but also the correction of the metaphyseal angulation and maintenance of the radial length with respect to the distal ulna. If the fracture has a simple intra-articular component (*two-part fracture*) and

no metaphyseal comminution, it usually responds to both closed and percutaneous reduction and seldom needs formal open reduction (Fig. 3). A *percutaneous reduction* implies the manipulation of cartilage-bearing fragments with an awl or a periosteal elevator inserted through a small skin incision with minimal soft-tissue dissection and done under fluoroscopic or arthroscopic guidance [31, 32].

If the fracture presents with a simple articular component but extensive metaphyseal comminution, external fixation is the method of choice to control radial shortening and metaphyseal angulation. If articular congruity is not adequately restored after the application of the external fixator, a percutaneous or limited open reduction in combination with bone grafting is advocated for this group.

For *three- and four-part* articular fractures with increasing degrees of metaphyseal comminution, open reduction together with bone grafting becomes progressively necessary, because joint distraction with the external fixator does not always disimpact small cartilage-bearing fragments or accomplish reduction of severely rotated volar ulnar lip fragments in the so-called four-part fractures [32–35]. Finally, these injuries are the result of high-velocity trauma with a higher incidence of associated fractures of the distal ulna, resulting in increased instability of the distal forearm that may require additional specific treatment. Furthermore, these fractures are frequently associated with carpal ligament injuries (partial or total tears of the scapholunate ligament).

A displaced complex articular fracture should be treated in the operating room under adequate anesthesia with the iliac crest draped in a sterile manner. A tourniquet is applied in the event that a limited or extensile open reduction should become necessary. A classic closed manipulation with traction, palmar flexion, and ulnar deviation is attempted, and the quality of reduction is assessed under fluoroscopy. An alternative method is to apply longitudinal traction using sterile finger traps after having performed routine surgical preparation of the skin. The use of the finger-trap traction frees both hands of the surgeon for manipulation and pinning. Restoration of radial length, volar tilt, and articular congruity is then assessed. If there is no metaphyseal comminution and reduction of the joint fragments is acceptable, a conventional percutaneous pinning is carried out by inserting two 1.6-mm

Kirschner wires across the radial styloid into the dorsomedial cortex of the radial shaft. If reduction of the medial fragment is anatomic with no articular step-off, percutaneous pinning from the radial styloid towards the sigmoid notch is performed with a 1.2-mm Kirschner wire, taking care not to enter the distal radioulnar joint.

If a satisfactory reduction of the dorsomedial fragment (die-punch) cannot be achieved by radial deviation of palmar flexion, as suggested by Mortier et al. [36, 37], a 2 cm-long incision is placed between the fourth and fifth dorsal compartment through which an awl is introduced to manipulate the dorsoulnar fragment against the lunate under fluoroscopic control. Should a sagittal gap persist between the two fragments, a bone forceps introduced through the skin incision and placed over the skin overlying the radial styloid is applied (Fig. 4). With the forceps in place, transverse percutaneous pins are introduced across both fragments. When the medial fragment is split into volar and dorsal components and the volar fragment cannot be reduced anatomically due to its tendency to rotate dorsally when tension is applied to the volar capsule, open reduction is mandatory. An extended incision for carpal tunnel release is used in this particular situation. The volar ulnar corner of the radius is exposed between the ulnar artery and nerve and the flexor tendons. A partial incision of the pronator quadratus is needed for complete exposure of the fragment. Reduction is achieved without additional soft tissue dissection in order not to disturb the important attachments to the triangular fibrocartilage complex. Usually, a single Kirchner wire introduced obliquely from the volar to the dorsal sides and retrieved through the dorsal skin of the forearm offers sufficient stability. However, for bigger fragments, screw or plate fixation is an alternative method of fixation. After having fixed the volar ulnar fragment, reduction of the dorsoulnar fragment is achieved by applying tension to the dorsal radiotriquetral ligament with gentle palmar flexion and radial deviation of the wirst. If this accomplishes reduction anatomically, an oblique Kirschner wire is inserted from the dorsal cortex to the volar radial shaft to stabilize this fragment. If the fragment is too small to accept internal fixation material, it should be buttressed against the lunate with subchondral cancellous bone grafts. This implies a limited open reduction for this fragment through a small incision between the fourth and fifth dorsal compartments. If the fracture presents with a considerable degree of metaphyseal and even diaphyseal comminution, external fixation is the most reliable method of stabilization to prevent radial shortening in these situations. However, if radiocarpal and radioulnar joint congruity cannot be achieved with external fixation alone, percutaneous or formal open reduction of the joint surface should be used in combination with external fixation (Fig. 5).

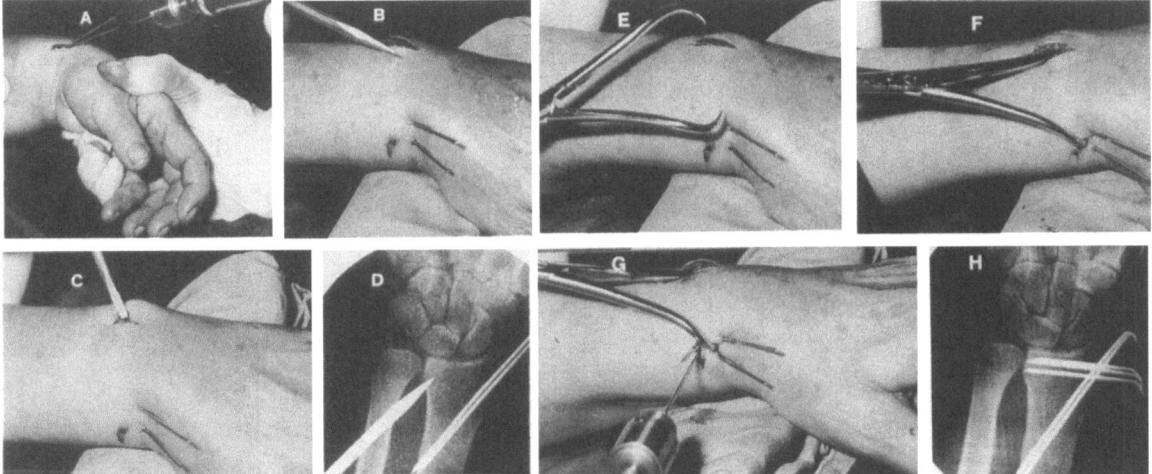

Fig. 4. Technique of percutaneous reduction of articular fractures of the radius. **A** Percutaneous Kirschner-wire fixation of radial styloid fragment. **B–D** The dorsoulnar fragment is reduced with an awl introduced through a skin incision and controlled under image intensifier. **E, F** A pointed reduction clamp may be used to close the fracture gap. **G, H** The ulnar fragment pinned transversely

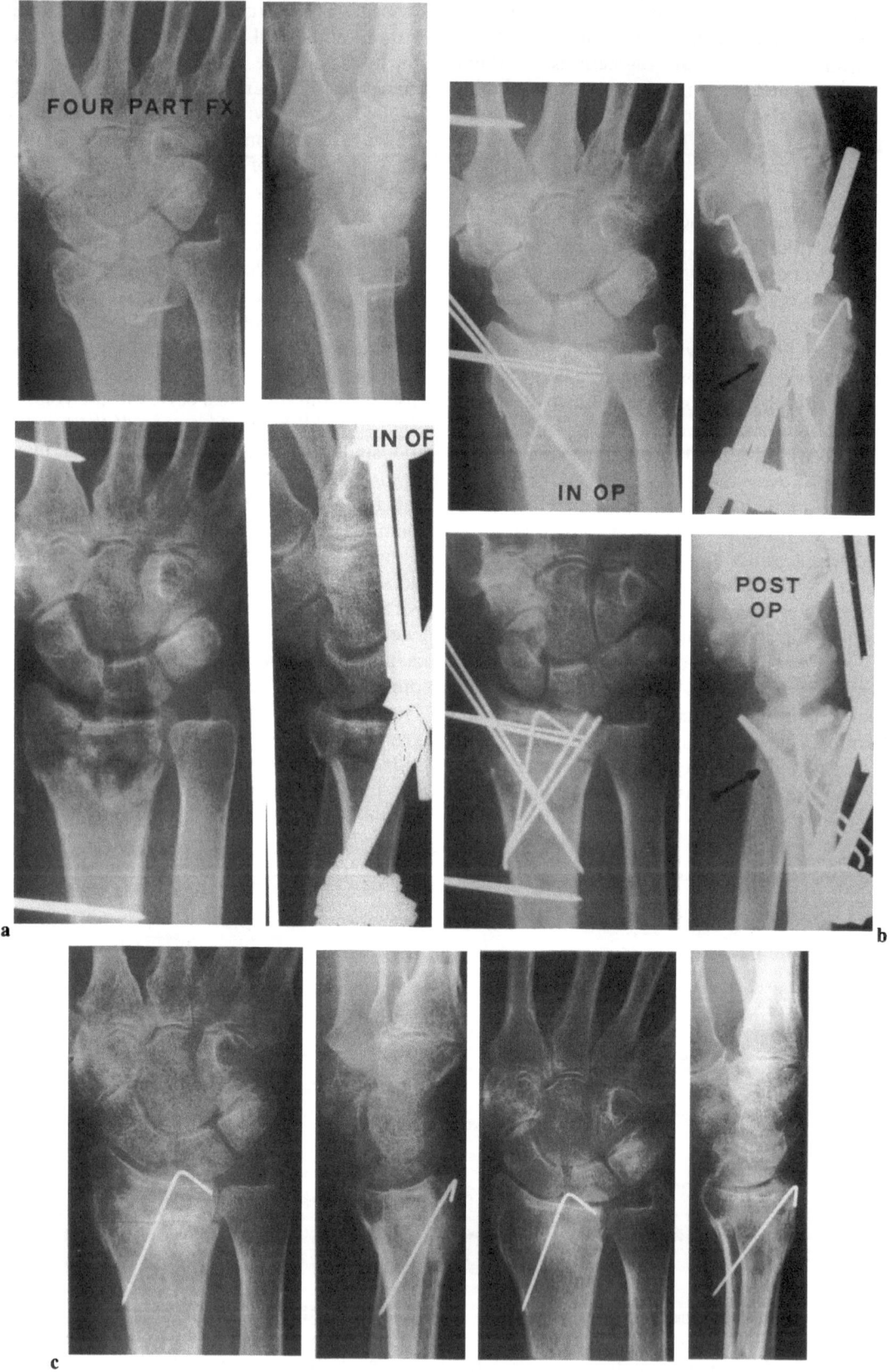

Following application of the wrist fixator, the fixator clamps are tightened and the quality of joint reduction is assessed under fluoroscopy. If articular congruity is unacceptable, a percutaneous or a formal open reduction, as described previously, is carried out with the fixator in place. The choice of the surgical approach depends on the localization of the fragments needing additional reduction. The most commonly used approach is between the third and fourth extensor compartments. Through a transverse capsulotomy of the wrist, the displaced fragments are elevated and reduced against the scaphoid and the lunate. The use of Kirschner-wire fixation introduced transversely from the radial styloid towards the distal radioulnar joint depends on the size of the fragments. The remaining bone defect after reduction is systematically grafted with autologous cancellous iliac bone to provide additional mechanical support of the articular fragments and accelerate bone healing. This permits early removal of the fixator after 5 weeks without danger of secondary displacement, thus allowing for early rehabilitation of the wrist. For high velocity injuries with associated fractures of the distal ulnar shaft, rigid internal fixation with a plate is advocated in every case provided that the soft tissue coverage is adequate. Skeletal fixation of the ulna is performed first, and radial length is then adapted to the ulna with an external fixator applied radially. If the head of the ulna is severely comminuted, no attempt to achieve anatomic reduction is made initially. However, we do not advocate distal ulnar excision but, instead, allow for remodelling of the head with early forearm rotation exercises. A resection arthroplasty of the distal ulna may be performed at a later date if the patient become symptomatic [38]. Primary fixation of the fracture of the base of the ulnar styloid or reattachment of the trian-gular fibrocartilage complex is only indicated in the acute situation when massive anteroposterior instability of the distal ulna persists following reduction and fixation of the distal radius, or in radiocarpal dislocations in order to guarantee primary ulnar stability of the carpus [39]. A figure-of-eight tension wire with or without additional Kirschner wires is our method of choice.

Postoperatively, the wrist is supported by either a sugar-tong splint or an external fixator. A sugar-tong splint is applied for 2 weeks for all cases treated with percutaneous pinning or in fractures that underwent internal fixation with Kirschner wires and small plates. To avoid pin-tract infections, generous skin incisions are made, and the patient receives instructions for personal pin care. At 2 weeks, a short arm cast with a window to enable pin care is maintained for another 3 weeks. Cast and pins are removed at 5 weeks following reduction.

For cases treated with external fixators, a sugar-tong splint to control pronation and supination in the first 3 weeks may occasionally be used in cases with severe distal radioulnar disruption. However, most of the cases do not need additional plaster cast support. Wrist fixators can be removed at 5 weeks provided that the fracture has been grafted; otherwise, the fixators should be left in place for as long as 6–7 weeks. After removal of the fixator, supervised physiotherapy is recommended for another 2 weeks and exceptionally dynamic splints my be used if joint contractures are present.

Clinical Material

Between 1979 and 1986, 40 patients with articular fractures of the distal radius in which restoration of the joint surface could not be achieved by closed reduction or joint distraction, were treated with a combination of percutaneous and/or open reduction. The average age was 37 years (range 18–23 years) and the follow-up period averaged 4 years (range 2–8 years). Twenty-six patients were males and fourteen were females. The fracture distribution is shown in Table 1. According to this classification, there were 9 simple articular fractures and 31 complex articular fractures [24]. Out of 40 fractures, 4 were open and 36 were closed. Restoration of articular congruity was achieved in 21 patients with percutaneous reduction, out of which 17 were stabilized by

◁—————————————————————

Fig. 5. a Residual joint incongruity, dorsal tilt, and metaphyseal bone defect are seen following closed reduction and external fixation of a four-part articular fracture. **b** Intra-operative (*IN-OP*) roentgenograms following open reduction, pin fixation, and bone grafting of radial styloid and dorsoulnar fragments (*top*) still show displaced volar-ulnar fragment (*arrow*). Post-operative roentgenograms (*bottom*) after anatomic reduction and pinning of the volar-ulnar fragment through a "limited" volar approach. **c** Follow-up X-rays at 5 weeks and 24 months demonstrate no residual step-offs, shortening, or metaphyseal angulation

Table 1. Fracture distribution[a] of the 40 patients studied

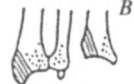 *B* *Simple Articular*[b] Fracture affects a portion of the articular surface, but the continuity of the metaphysis and epiphysis is intact

 Complex articular Fracture affects the joint surfaces (radioulnar and/or radiocarpal) and the metaphyseal area

9 *B1* Cuneiform articular fracture of the distal radius

31 Articular fracture of the radius with simple intra-articular component (2 fragments and no metaphyseal comminution)

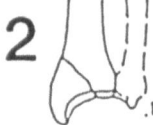 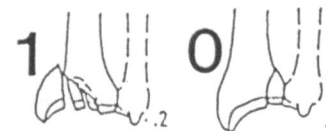 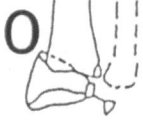

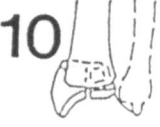 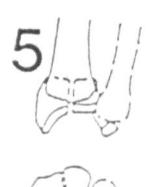

1. Radial styloid
2. Comminuted radial styloid
3. Ulnar "wedge" fracture

1. Colles' fracture affecting the radioulnar joint
2. Colles' fracture with dorsoulnar articular fragment
3. T-Fracture in the sagittal plane

B2 Dorsal margin fracture (Barton's fracture)

C2 Articular fracture of the radius with simple intra-articular component and metaphyseal comminution

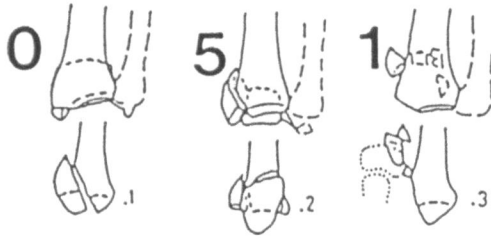

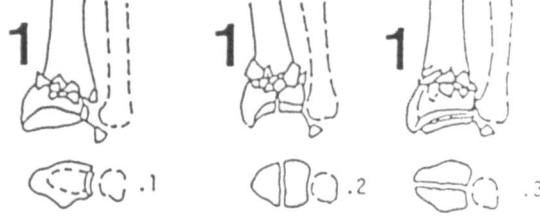

1. Simple
2. Associated with radial styloid fragment
3. Associated with radio-carpal dorsal dislocation

1. Colles' fracture affecting the radioulnar joint
2. T-Sagittal fracture
3. T-Frontal fracture

B3 Volar margin fracture (reversed Barton's, Letenneur)

C3 Comminuted articular fracture of the radius

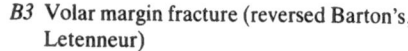 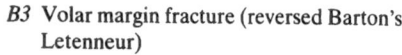

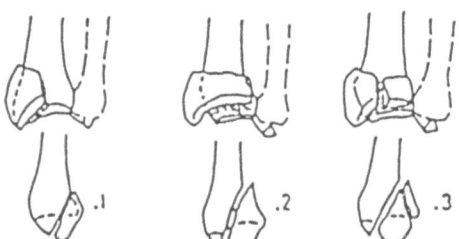

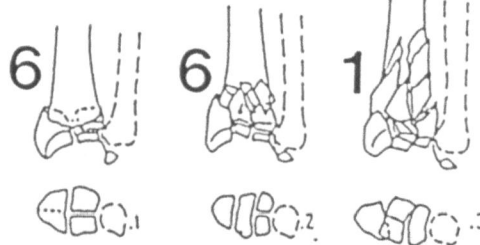

1. Volar-radial fragment (sigmoid notch intact)
2. Volar fragment (affecting sigmoid notch)
3. Comminuted volar fragment

1. Without metaphyseal comminution ("4-part-fracture")
2. With metaphyseal comminution
3. With metaphysodiaphyseal comminution

[a] Represented by the numbers in bold print
[b] Italicized items refer to the classifications in Fig. 1

percutaneous pinning and 4 by percutaneous pinning combined with an external fixator. The remaining 19 patients were treated with open reduction, 9 had internal fixation with Kirschner wires, 5 had a combination of Kirschner-wires and external fixation, and 5 patients had external fixation alone. Eleven of the nineteen patients with open reduction had additional bone grafting of the metaphyseal defect. Three patients underwent internal fixation of their associated ulnar fractures, and a small volar plate to buttress anteromedial fragments was used in two patients.

Radiographs of all 40 patients were evaluated in a retrospective analysis before reduction immediately after and at later follow-up. This included measurements of the inclination of the articular surface in the sagittal and frontal planes, the radial shortening, and articular congruity which was assessed by measuring the residual articular step-off. Detailed information of the pre- and postoperative results are presented in Table 2. Assessment of the functional results was performed at later follow-up in 31 patients who could be retrieved for a later control study (average 3.1 years). The functional evaluation parameters included wrist motion, power grip, key pinch, digital motion, residual pain, and working ability.

Radiographic Results

The radiographic follow-up showed that the fractures in 28 patients had healed, with an average volar tilt of 5.6°, four 0°, and 8 with a residual mean dorsal tilt of 8.8°. The ulnar tilt for all 40 patients averaged 18.5°. Loss of correction between the postoperative and follow-up radiographs was observed in 11 patients, and was invariably found in fractures with metaphyseal comminution that were treated with percutaneous pinning and cast fixation alone. However, in the external fixator group, no loss of initial reduction was observed as of the time of removal of the fixator. Of these 11 patients with loss of correction, 8 had minimal loss of the initial volar tilt ranging from 2°–5°. Secondary displacement of a postoperative dorsal tilt of 2° to a follow-up value of 6° was observed in one patient. Two elderly patients with a neutral tilt postoperatively developed a dorsal tilt of 8° and 9°. A minimal loss of correction ranging from 2°–5° was observed in the frontal plane in ten patients.

Assessment of the anatomic reduction of the articular surface showed that, at last follow-up, 15 patients showed a joint depression ranging

between 1–3 mm, and 25 revealed no articular step-off. Of these 15 patients, 12 had a joint depression of 1 mm, 2 patients 2 mm, and 1 patient 3 mm. Therefore, 37 patients (92.5%) had an articular depression of 1 mm or less at later follow-up.

Assessment of radial shortening (radioulnar index) showed that eight patients (28%) had some amount of radial shortening ranging from 1 to 4 mm immediately after surgery. At later follow-up, 12 patients (30%) exhibited radial shortening ranging from 1 to 7 mm. However, radial shortening did not exceed 3 mm in 10 out of these 12 patients.

Functional Results

Out of the 31 patients who could be retrieved for clinical control, 15 had percutaneous joint reduction and 16 had open reduction of the distal radius fracture. The overall mean range of motion of the wrist for the patients reviewed was 62.5° of extension (range 55°–80°), 59.5° of flexion (range 50°–75°), 77° of pronation (range 55°–85°), 72.5° of supination (range 40°–90°), 25° of ulnar deviation (range 15°–30°), and 9.5° of radial deviation (5°–15°). The average loss of grip strength was 50% (range 5%–50%), the average loss of power pinch was 13%, and the average digital motion for all patients measured by the total arm movement (TAM) index was 240%. Out of 31 patients, occasional mild pain was present in 3, moderate in 4, and severe in 2, while the remaining 22 were relieved of pain. Subjective complaints and functional results showed a direct correlation with the radiographic findings, so that a residual dorsal tilt was responsible for loss of palmar flexion and a radial shortening of more than 4 mm was associated with decreased forearm rotation. Radiocarpal pain with articular incongruity was detected in three out of four patients with residual moderate pain and in one of two patients with severe pain. Of these two patients, one developed a rapid post-traumatic arthritis with narrowing of the joint space in spite of an anatomic reduction of the joint surface: due to progressive pain, a total wrist arthroplasty was performed 2 years after injury. The rapid onset and progression of the arthrosis in this patient with an anatomic reduction of the joint surface could be explained either by important primary cartilage abrasion of the joint surface or by a sub-clinical low-grade infection following open reduction (case 36). The other patient showed proximal migration of the lunate

Table 2. Pre- and postoperative results

Case	Year of treatment	Age (years)/sex	Fracture classification (Fig. 1)	Open (O)/closed (C)	Additional injuries	Type of treatment[d]	After treatment[c]	Time of immobilization	Preop. Volar tilt (°)	Preop. Dorsal tilt (°)	Preop. Articular gap (mm)	Preop. Articular step-off (mm)	Preop. Radioulnar index (mm)	Post red. Volar tilt (°)	Post red. Dorsal tilt (°)	Post red. Ulnar tilt (°)	Post red. Articular gap (mm)	Post red. Articular step-off (mm)	Post red. Radioulnar index (mm)	Follow-up Volar tilt (°)	Follow-up Dorsal tilt (°)	Follow-up Ulnar tilt (°)	Follow-up Articular gap (mm)	Follow-up Articular step-off (mm)	Follow-up Radioulnar index (mm)	Time until union (weeks)	Extension	Flexion	Ulnar	Radial	Pronation	Supination	Power grip % loss	Key pinch % loss	Digital motion TAM (index)	Pain[b]	Working ability (%)	Complications	Occupation
1	1979	40M	B$_{1-2}$	O		ORIF	STS	3		10	0	4	−1	5		15	0	0	−1	5		15	0	0	−1	6													
2	1979	20M	B$_{1-1}$	C		ORIF	UPS	3	8		1	0	0	8		14	0	0	0	8		14	0	0	0	3													
3	1979	24M	C$_{1-1}$	C		PRPP	VPB	4		32	0	0	6	2		22	0	0	3	3		20	0	0	3	4													
4	1979	35F	C$_{1-2}$	C		PRPP	VPS	4		20	0	2	0		4	20	0	0	0		4	18	0	0	0	4													
5	1980	23M	C$_{1-2}$	C		ORIF	VPS	4		7	2	2	0		2	22	1	0	0		6	19	1	0	0	4													
6	1980	28M	C$_{1-1}$	C		PRPP	VPS	4		8	2	0	3	8	7	19	0	0	0	8	7	23	0	0	5	5													
7	1981	29M	C$_{1-1}$	C		PRPP	VPS	4		22	2	2	2	5		25	2	0	0	5		20	1	0	11	4													
8	1981	24M	C$_{1-1}$	C		PRPP	VPS	4		35	2	0	6	10		20	0	0	0	10		15	1	0	3	4													
9	1981	33F	C$_{1-1}$	C	*	PRPP	VPS	4		24	0	3	2	4		16	0	0	2	4		20	0	0	0	4													
10	1982	20M	B$_{2-3}$	O		ORIF	STS	4		0	1	0	0	5		24	0	0	−2	5		22	0	0	−2	4	−70	60	30	13	80	85	10	5	245	None	100		Mechanic
11	1982	18M	C$_{1-1}$	C		PRPP	VPS	4		14	2	2	0	8		26	0	0	−2	8		20	0	0	−2	4	70	55	30	12	80	85	15	5	245	None	100		Student
12	1982	38M	C$_{1-2}$	C		PRPP	VPS	4		20	0	3	0	0	0	20	0	0	−1	0	0	20	0	0	0	4	60	65	25	8	80	80	5	10	235	None	100		Mason
13	1982	28M	C$_{1-2}$	C		PRPP	VPS	4		25	1	3	8	8	0	22	0	0	−2	3	0	10	0	0	+1	4	70	50	30	11	85	80	10	5	250	None	100		Painter
14	1982	22M	C$_{3-1}$	C		PRPP (EF)	EF	6		14	0	0	−1	0	0	18	0	0	−2	0	0	20	0	0	−1	6	60	60	25	11	85	65	15	20	210	None	100		Police officer
15	1983	35F	B$_{1-2}$	C		PRPP	VPS	4		30	0	0	0	8		26	0	0	0	8		26	0	0	0	4	65	60	25	11	85	80	10	5	245	None	100		Housewife
16	1983	18M	C$_{1-1}$	C		PRPP	VPS	6		22	3	3	4	7		17	1	0	−1	5		17	1	0	1	5	65	55	30	7	75	85	15	10	250	None	100	Pintrack	Farmer
17	1984	22M	C$_{3-2}$	C		OREF (BG)	EF	6		14	6	5	0		7	20	2	1	0		17	20	2	1	0	6	70	50	30	11	85	80	10	5	250	Moderate	100		Truck driver
18	1984	20M	B$_{2-2}$	C		ORIF (EF)	EF	6		5	0	4	2	7		20	1	0	4	7		20	1	0	4	6	60	65	25	6	65	65	10	15	265	None	100		Pianist

No.	Year	Age/Sex	Type	Red.	Treatment	Fix.	Imm.	Radiographic measurements [a]	Range of motion	Grip	Pain [b]	%	Complications	Occupation
19	1984	19 M	B_{1-1}	C	ORIF	VPS	3	20 10 1 0 10 20 0 0 0 8 0 20 0 0 0	70 60 30 13 85 75 10 15	240	None	100		Mason
20	1984	27 M	B_{2-2}	C	ORIF	VPS	3	20 1 2 10 25 0 0 0 10 0 25 0 0 0	70 60 30 13 85 75 10 15	245	None	100		Machine operator
21	1984	33 F	C_{2-1}	C	PRPP (EF)	EF	6	0 3 4 0 15 0 0 -2 0 0 15 0 0 -2	60 55 20 6 75 75 10 5	250	None	100	Pintracks (2)	Nurse
22	1984	61 F	C_{1-1}	C	PRPP	VPS	4	15 2 5 3 18 0 0 0 5 0 20 0 0 0	55 65 25 9 75 75 10 10	220	None	100		Housewife
23	1985	48 F	C_{3-2}	O*	OREF (BG)	EF	7	15 5 6 0 18 1 -3 3 5 0 18 1 -3 3	60 60 25 11 75 75 20 10	240	Moderate	100		Housewife
24	1985	31 M	C_{3-2}	C	OREF (BG)	EF	7	15 4 5 5 18 0 0 -2 0 10 18 0 0 -2	60 55 25 7 70 70 5 15	240	Moderate	100		Carpenter
25	1985	46 M	B_{2-2}	C	ORIF BG, EF**	EF	6	20 0 2 0 5 25 0 0 -2 5 0 25 0 0 -2	65 60 30 7 80 65 15 10	260	None	100		Gym teacher
26	1985	25 M	C_{1-1}	C	PRPP	VPS	4	10 4 2 4 10 22 0 0 0 6 0 20 0 0 0	55 70 30 13 75 65 10 10	260	None	100		Mason
27	1985	32 M	C_{1-2}	C	PRPP (EF)	EF	6	15 0 5 4 10 12 1 0 0 10 0 10 1 0 0	55 65 25 10 80 70 20 10	250	Mild	100		Clerk
28	1985	70 M	C_{1-1}	C	PRPP (EF)	VPS	4	32 0 3 5 5 25 1 -1 -1 5 0 25 1 0 -1	60 60 20 11 80 70 20 10	250	Mild	100		Retiree
29	1986	25 M	C_{3-2}	C	ORIF (BG)	VPS	4	35 1 2 -1 5 22 0 0 0 0 0 10 0 0 0	65 55 25 8 85 85 9 25	250	None	100	CTS	Electrician
30	1986	63 F	C_{3-1}	C	PRPP	VPS	4	36 2 2 9 0 16 0 0 2 0 9 16 0 0 2	60 65 25 10 80 70 15 15	235	None	100		Housewife
31	1986	56 F	C_{3-1}	C	PRPP	VPS	4	25 2 4 4 0 15 0 0 0 0 8 15 0 0 0	60 44 20 10 70 65 25 20	240	None	100		Housewife
32	1986	70 F	C_{3-2}	C	PRPP	VPS	4	30 3 2 18 0 15 1 2 4 0 10 15 1 2 4	55 55 25 12 65 70 20 10	240	None	100		Housewife
33	1986	30 M	B_{2-2}	C	ORIF BG, EF	EF	6	45 0 6 2 10 20 1 0 3 10 0 20 1 0 3	80 75 30 15 90 90 5 10	260	None	100		Farmer
34	1986	63 F	C_{2-3}	C	OREF (BG)	EF	8 5	2 0 8 5 15 0 1 2 5 0 15 0 1 2	60 65 25 6 80 75 15 5	235	Mild	100	Neuroma	Housewife
35	1986	62 F	C_{3-3}	O	OREF** (BG)	EF	6 15	0 3 0 0 0 0 0 0 0 0 10 0 0 0	60 50 25 7 70 70 25 10	255	None	100		Secretary
36	1986	73 F	C_{3-1}	C	ORIF BG, EF	EF	6	35 2 1 3 5 18 0 -1 5 20 0 0 -1	55 50 15 51 45 35 35 35	190	Severe	50	OA	Housewife
37	1986	54 F	C_{3-1}	C	ORIF (BG)	VPS	4	32 1 1 7 5 18 1 0 0 3 0 18 1 0 0	55 55 25 9 75 65 10 10	260	None	100		Housewife
38	1986	39 M	C_{3-2}	C	ORIF (BG)	VPS	5	0 2 3 2 5 18 1 0 2 0 0 18 1 0 2	55 65 20 9 75 70 10 20	235	None	100		Manager
39	1986	44 M	C_{3-1}	C	ORIF (EF)	EF	4	0 1 2 5 5 12 0 0 0 5 0 12 0 0 0	60 60 25 8 75 75 15 5	230	None	100		Housewife
40	1986	37 M	C_{2-1}	C	PRPP (EF)	EF	7	5 4 7 6 6 17 3 2 2 6 2 7 17 3 2 2	60 50 15 9 60 40 50 30	200	Severe	50	OA, Pintracks (2)	Computer operator

* Ulnar head

** Ulnar shaft

*** Damage

OA, Osteoarthritis. CTS, carpal tunnel syndrome

[a] The radiographic measurements were made according to Castaing's modification of the method of Gartland and Werley. Radial deviation of the articular surface of the radius is defined as the difference between the average ulnar tilt (25°) and the radial inclination of the tilted articular surface with respect to the perpendicular to the radial shaft in the frontal plane. A negative value for ulnar tilt means that there is no ulnar inclination of the articular surface of the radius, but instead there is radial inclination so that the radial articular surface forms a negative angle with respect to the perpendicular of the radial shaft

[b] Pain in the wrist was graded as mild, moderate, or severe. Mild pain was present only at the extremes of the active range of motion of the wrist, and the patient was neither physically nor psychologically disturbed by the pain; moderate pain occurred during heavy manual labor and caused the patient to be disturbed physically, psychologically, or both; severe pain occurred during activities of daily living and even at rest

[c] STS, Sugar-tong splint; VPS, volar plaster splint; EF, external fixation

[d] PRPP, Percutaneous reduction, percutaneous pinning; ORIF, open reduction and internal fixation; OREF, open reduction and external fixation; (BG), bone grafting; (EF), external fixation

caused by the settling of the medial fragment with an articular step-off of 3 mm, resulting in narrowing of the radiocarpal joint space (case 40).

Except for the two patients with severe pain, all patients returned to their prior occupation with 100% working ability and had no limitation in activities of daily living (Table 2). Complications included 1 carpal tunnel syndrome, 5 pintract infections, and 1 iatrogenic lesion of the superficial radial nerve.

Radiographic evidence of degenerative changes, such as narrowing of the joint space, subchondral sclerosis, and osteophyte formation, were not present at the last follow-up in any but the two patients mentioned above.

Conclusions

The main goals of the treatment of intra-articular fractures of the distal radius are *anatomic reduction of the joint surface* and *prevention of secondary intra-articular displacement*. However, the final outcome depends not only on the articular congruity of the radiocarpal joint but also on the residual extra-articular angulation of the joint surface, the radial shortening, and on the absence of associated soft-tissue complications.

The management of displaced comminuted articular fractures of the distal radius has been significantly improved with percutaneous pinning [20, 37, 40–44], with external fixators [22, 45–54], and with percutaneous or open reduction techniques [31–34]. These last two measures should be applied when, in spite of joint distraction, articular congruity cannot be sufficiently restored due to impaction of the articular fragments in the metaphyseal cancellous bone. Although the correlation between the residual incongruity of the distal radius and the high incidence of late post-traumatic arthritis has been clearly shown by Knirk and Jupiter [19], only a few reports have documented the effectiveness of open reduction techniques [33–35, 55].

Analysis of our results of 40 articular fractures, in which anatomic reduction of the joint surface could not be obtained by closed manipulation or "ligamentotaxis" with external fixators, showed a satisfactory extra-articular alignement in 85% of the cases treated, and there was a residual articular incongruity of 1 mm or less at later follow-up in 92.5%. In one-half of the patients, articular realignement was achieved with percutaneous manipulation and with open reduction in the other half. Percutaneous reduction proved to be successful for simple intra-articular fractures (radial styloid, T-fractures and Colles' fractures with associated die-punch fragments) with well sized fragments. Open reduction became necessary for smaller impacted joint fragments and for displaced volar medial fragments. Conversely, the radial styloid fragment responded very well to closed reduction and percutaneous pinning. Although the average follow-up in this study was 4 years, radiographic evidence of radiocarpal arthritis was present in only 5% of the cases at later follow-up. The clinical results correlated with the radiographic findings in the vast majority of the patients. Furthermore, there was a strict parallelism between the clinical results and the severity of the articular comminution, and the incidence of post-traumatic arthritis seemed to depend on the ability to restore the best possible articular congruity. However, other factors equally important for a satisfactory functional outcome in terms of wrist motion included the minimal soft-tissue disruption (made possible by percutaneous and limited open reduction through small incisions), the use of small implants that do not interfere with extensor tendon gliding, and the short period of wrist immobilization. Bone grafting of comminuted fractures played an important role in accelerating bone healing and in allowing for early removal of wrist fixators and early hand rehabilitation [52].

Although anatomical restoration of the joint surface of the lower end of the radius still remains a difficult problem, the past decade has seen important contributions to the understanding of the anatomy of the fracture, and efforts to classify the different fracture types with prognostic and therapeutic implications have succeeded. Since a wide choice of treatment methods to achieve reduction is available, the surgeon should remain flexible in the election of the appropriate technique for each individual case. With a correct indication, precise diagnosis, better technical skills, and selective treatment of associated carpal ligament tears and other soft tissue lesions, the predictability of obtaining satisfactory results in the treatment of articular fractures of the distal radius can be further improved.

References

1. Bacorn RW, Kurtzke JF (1953) Colles' fracture: A study of two thousand cases from the New York State Workmen's Compensation Board. J Bone Joint Surg [Am] 35:643–658

2. Cole JM, Obletz BE (1966) Comminuted fractures of the distal end of the radius treated by skeletal transfixion in plaster cast: An end-result study of thirty-three cases. J Bone Joint Surg [Am] 48:931–945

3. Cooney MP, Dobyns JH, Linscheid RL (1980) Complications of Colles' fractures. J Bone Joint Surg [Am] 62:613–619

4. Fernandez DL (1982) Correction of post-traumatic wrist deformity in adults by osteotomy, bone grafting and internal fixation. J Bone Joint Surg [Am] 64:1164–1178

5. Fernandez DL (1988) Radial osteotomy and Bowers arthroplasty for malunited fractures of the distal end of the radius. J Bone Joint Surg [Am] 70:1538–1551

6. Frykman G (1967) Fractures of the distal end of the radius, including sequelae-shoulder, hand, finger syndrome, disturbance in the distal radio-ulnar joint and impairment of nerve function. Acta Orthop Scand (Suppl) 108:1–155

7. Gartland JJ, Werley CW (1951) Evaluation of healed Colles' fractures. J Bone Joint Surg [Am] 33:895–907

8. Knirk JL, Jupiter JB (1985) Late results of intra-articular distal radius fractures in young adults. Orthop Trans 9:456

9. Martini AK (1986) Die sekundäre Arthrose des Handgelenkes bei der in Fehlstellung verheilten und nicht korrigierten distalen Radiusfraktur. Akt Traumatol 16:143

10. McQueen M, Caspers J (1988) Colles fracture: Does the anatomic result affect the final function? J Bone Joint Surg [Br] 70:649–651

11. Scheck M (1962) Long-term follow-up treatment of comminuted fractures of the distal end of the radius by transfixation with Kirschner wires and cast. J Bone Joint Surg [Am] 44:337

12. Smaill GB (1965) Long-term follow-up of Colles' fracture. J Bone Joint Surg [Br] 47:80–85

13. Stewart HD, Innes AR, Burke FD (1985) Hand complication in Colles' fracture. J Hand Surg [Br] 10(1):103–106

14. Villar RN, Marsh D, Rushton N, Greatorex RA (1987) Three years after Colles' fracture. J Bone Joint Surg [Br] 69:635–638

15. Weber SC, Szabo RM (1986) Severely comminuted distal radial fracture as an unsolved problem: Complications associated with external fixation and pins and plaster techniques. J Hand Surg [Am] 11:157–165

16. Younger CP, DeFiore JC (1977) Rupture of flexor tendons to the fingers after a Colles' fracture. A case report. J Bone Joint Surg [Am] 59:828

17. Castaing J (1964) Les fractures recentes de l'extrémité inférieure du radius chez l'adulte. Rev Chir Orthop 50:581–696

18. Moberg E (1963) Shoulder-hand-finger syndrome, reflex dystrophy, causalgia (abstract). Acta Chir Scand 125:523

19. Knirk JL, Jupiter JB (1986) Intra-articular fractures of the distal end of the radius in young adults. J Bone Joint Surg [Am] 68:647–659

20. Ruiz GR (1981) Percutaneous pinning of comminuted Colles' fractures. Clin Orthop 195:290

21. McMurtry RY, Jupiter JB (1991) Fractures of the distal radius. In: Browner B, Jupiter J, Levine A, Trafton P (eds) Skeletal trauma. Saunders, Philadelphia

22. Cooney WP, Linscheid RL, Dobyns JH (1979) External pin fixation for unstable Colles' fractures. J Bone Joint Surg [Am] 61:840–845

23. Melone CP (1984) Articular fractures of the distal radius. Orthop Clin North Am 15:217–236

24. Fernandez DL (1987) Avant-bras segment distal. In: Mueller ME, Nazarian S, Koch P (eds) Classification AO des fractures. Les os longs. Springer, Berlin, pp 106–115

25. Müller ME, Nazarian S, Koch P (eds) (1987) Classification AO des fractures. Springer, Berlin, pp 106–115

26. DeOliveira JC (1973) Barton's fractures. J Bone Joint Surg [Am] 55:586–594

27. Ellis J (1968) Smith's and Barton's fractures — a method of treatment. J Bone Joint Surg [Br] 47:724–727

28. Fernandez DL (1980) Smith Frakturen. Hefte zur Unfallheilk 148:91–95

29. Fernandez DL, Maeder G (1977) Die Behandlung der Smith-Frakturen. Arch orthop Unfallchir 88:153–161

30. Fuller DJ (1973) The Ellis plate operation for Smith's fracture. J Bone Joint Surg [Br] 55:173

31. Axelrod T, Paley D, Green J, McMurty RY (1988) Limited open reduction of the lunate facet in comminuted intra-articular fractures of the distal radius. J Hand Surg [Am] 13:372–377

32. Fernandez DL, Geissler WB (1991) Treatment of displaced articular fractures of the radius. J Hand Surg [Am] 16:375–384

33. Axelrod TJ, McMurtry RY (1990) Open reduction and internal fixation of comminuted intra-articular fractures of the distal radius. J Hand Surg [Am] 15:1–11

34. Bradway JK, Amadio PC, Cooney WP (1989) Open reduction and internal fixation of displaced comminuted intra-articular fractures of the distal end of the radius. J Bone Joint Surg [Am] 71:839–847

35. Melone CP (1986) Open treatment for displaced articular fractures of the distal radius. Clin Orthop 202:103–111

36. Mortier JP, Kuhlmann JN, Richet C, Baux S (1986) Brochage horizontal cubito-radial dans les fractures de l'extrémité inférieure du radius comportent un fragment postéro-interne. Rev Chir Orthop 72:567–571

37. Mortier JP, Baux S, Uhl JF, Mimoun M, Mole B (1983) Importance du fragment postéro-interne et son brochage spécifique dans les fractures de l'extrémité inférieure du radius. Ann Chir Main 2:219–229

38. Bowers WH (1985) Distal radioulnar joint arthroplasty: The hemiresection-interposition technique. J Hand Surg [Am] 10:169–178

39. Fernandez DL (1981) Irreducible radiocarpal fracture-dislocation and radioulnar dissociation with entrapment of the ulnar nerve, artery and flexor profundus. II — V. Case report. J Hand Surg [Am] 6:456–461

40. Clancey GJ (1984) Percutaneous Kirschner wire fixation of Colles' fractures. A prospective study of thirty-five cases. J Bone Joint Surg [Am] 66:1008–1014

41. Epinette JA, Lehut JM, Cavenaile M, Bouretz JC, Decoulx J (1982) Fracture de Pouteau-Colles: Double embrochage intrafocal en berceau selon Kapandji. Ann Chir Main 1:71–83

42. De Palma AF (1952) Comminuted fractures of the distal end of the radius treated by ulnar pinning. J Bone Joint Surg [Am] 34:651–662

43. Roth B, Müller J, Lusser G, Barone C, Bachmann B (1977) Erfahrungen mit der perkutanen Spickdrahtosteosynthese bei distalen Radiusfrakturen. Helv Chir Acta 44:815–820

44. Stein AH, Katz SF (1975) Stabilization of comminuted fractures of the distal inch of the radius: Percutaneous pinning. Clin Orthop 108:174–181

45. Anderson R, O'Neil G (1944) Comminuted fractures of the distal end of the radius. Surg Gynecol Obstet 78:434–440

46. Cooney WP (1988) Distal radial fractures: External fixation. In: Barton NJ (ed), Fractures of the hand and wrist, vol 4. Churchill Livingstone, Edinburgh, pp 290–301

47. Fernandez DL, Jakob RP, Büchler U (1983) External fixation of the wrist. Current indications and technique. Ann Chir Gynaecol 72:298–302

48. Grana WA, Kopta JA (1979) The Roger Anderson device in the treatment of fractures of the distal end of the radius. J Bone Joint Surg [Am] 61:1234

49. Green DP (1975) Pins and plaster treatment of comminuted fractures of the distal end of the radius. J Bone Joint Surg [Am] 57:304–310

50. Howard PW, Stewart HD, Hind RE, Burke FD (1989) External fixation or plaster for severely displaced comminuted Colles' fractures? J Bone Joint Surg [Br] 71:68–73

51. Jakob RP, Fernandez DL (1982) The treatment of wrist fractures with the small AO external fixation device. In: Uhthoff HK (ed) Current concepts of external fixation of fractures. Springer, Berlin, pp 307–314

52. Leung KS, Tsang HK, Chiu KH,   (1990) An effective treatment of comminuted fractures of the distal radius. J Hand Surg [Am] 15:11–17

53. Vaughn PA, Lui SM, Harrington IJ, Maistrelli GL (1985) Treatment of unstable fractures of the distal radius by external fixation. J Bone Joint Surg [Br] 67:385–389

54. Vidal J, Buscayret C, Connes H (1979) Treatment of articular fractures by 'ligamentotaxis' with external fixation. In: Brooker A, Edwards CC (eds) External fixation. The current state of the art. Williams and Wilkins, Baltimore

55. Wagner HE, Jakob RP (1985) Operative Behandlung der distalen Radiusfraktur mit Fixateur externe. Unfallchirurg 88:473–480

Reconstruction of Distal Radius Fractures and Associated Carpal Problems

H. Kirk Watson and Danny Fong[1]

Keywords: Degenerative arthritis — SLAC — Colles malunion — Ulnar impingement syndrome — Implant silicone — Darrach failed — Instability midcarpal

Midcarpal Instability

One of hand surgery's most common problems is the post-Colles' fracture [1]. This fracture is made up of two components: one is the fracture through the radius, which often results in the shortening of and dorsal articular tilt to the radius. That has one set of problems. The other component is subluxation or dislocation of the distal radioulnar joint and the change in the angulation of the radius sulcus. It is, after all, a groove into which the column of the ulna fits and, if you tip that groove backwards after a Colles' fracture, the ulna no longer fits into that sulcus. The ulna is also often too long because of the shortening effect. We'll discuss the radius problem first, although the easier problem is the handling of the distal ulna. In the distal radius problem, it changes the carpal mechanics. Julio Taleisnik and I published a paper in which we called this a form of midcarpal instability [2]. In ulnar deviation power grip, that is when we grasp a golf club, a tennis racket, or an ax in our hand, the proximal row displaces and rotates. If your ulnar deviates, your scaphoid tends to move in line with the long axis of the forearm and the

lunate tips dorsally. The lunate also slides downslope as it rotates dorsally. Those two motions in the power grip result in the capitate remaining aligned and positioned over the radius. If we fracture the radius and tip that surface dorsally, the lunate will still dorsiflex. It will still tip in a power grip dorsally, but now the downslope has become upslope, and what used to be a slide downhill for the lunate is now a run uphill and it can't do it. You get only part of the normal carpal motion. The capitate and the entire hand are now dorsal to the load-bearing axis of the radius, and that produces an overload phenomenon that occurs at the midcarpal joint. We call it a midcarpal instability, but don't confuse it with a ligamentous type of midcarpal instability which flexes in the opposite direction, i.e., VISI. This problem, then, is an overload phenomenon that occurs only after a younger, active person begins to use the wrist, so it takes several months before you begin to see the intercarpal component of a dorsally tipped radius.

Trapezoidal Osteotomy

To treat this problem, we suggest a local bone graft osteotomy technique [3] (Fig. 1). Through a transverse dorsal incision, one performs an osteotomy of the distal radius. Cut the distal radius across parallel and 1 cm proximal to the radial articular surface. Mark out a trapezoidal-shaped graft proximal to the osteotomy. If you make it wider distally, then you can also lengthen the radial side as you turn the graft. If you don't need to lengthen it, that is, if in the PA view the radius has its normal radial-ulna tilt, then you can make a rectangular graft. Take the graft out, turn it 90°, pry open the distal articular surface, and put the graft in. It is important to maintain the

[1] Connecticut Combined Hand Surgery Service, Hartford Hospital, University of Connecticut, Newington Children's Hospital, Hartford, Connecticut, Yale University, New Haven, Connecticut, and University of Massachusetts, Worcester, Massachusetts, USA

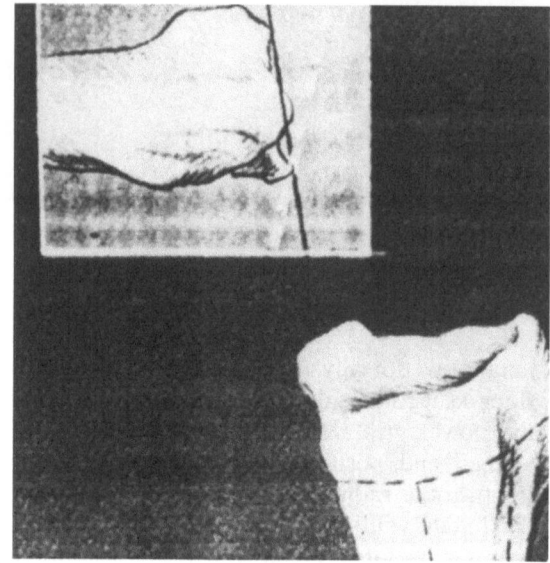
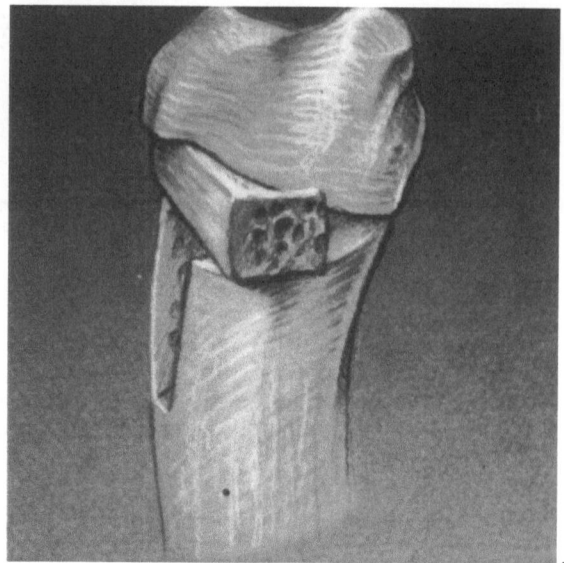

a   b

Fig. 1. a The trapezoidal-shaped graft is outlined proximal to the osteotomy site. It is shaped to restore dorsal and radial tilt. **b** The graft is turned 90° and wedged into the osteotomy site. The corners of the graft donor site are maintained to lock it in tightly. A fixation pin may be added

two distal corners from which the graft came. Protect those two corners when you cut the graft. The graft locks in very tightly. You may want to add a fixation pin running through Lister's tubercle, through a corner of the graft, and out through the radius. We call it a caging pin. It prevents rotation of the graft, but it is often usually not necessary. Some cancellous bone may be pushed under the graft. This is a simple procedure. Adjustment is easy. One needs only move the graft volarly to increase the angulation of the radius articular surface.

There are some people who have ligaments that are tight enough and strong enough that they can support a scaphoid on this backwards slope of the radial articular surface, but the re-establishment of the length and the volar angle of the radius is usually necessary for those carpals to support themselves.

Matched Ulnar Arthroplasty

Let's look at the easier part of this problem, that of the distal ulna. Frequently, the patient you are treating is older and does not require the osteotomy repair of the radius. They may not be athletic, but they have a wrist that is painful, will not supinate and pronate fully, and is limited in flexion and extension, all on the basis of the long

ulna following the Colles' — type fracture. This is a very simple repair. We already talked about the fact that usually one can't just shorten the ulna because the sulcus of the radius has been tipped. If you figure you normally have 14° or so of volar radius tilt and it becomes tipped dorsally 10° or 20°, you are up to 35° of angular deformity in the sulcus of the radius for the ulna. Usually the ligaments have also been attenuated, with or without tear of the triangular fibrocartilage support mechanism for the ulna. Resection is the suggested approach, but the Darrach procedure, which simply cuts off the distal ulna, produces terrible results [4], often with symptomatic winging and painful impingement of the ulna against the radius which is painful. The patient never knows exactly when it is going to hit, but when it hits, they drop what they are holding. It is a significantly limiting phenomenon. The problems are twofold: one is the impingement phenomenon of the ulna against the radius. The other is the winging or the lack of support for the ulna which produces symptomatic volar and dorsal migration. The best approach is the matched ulna arthroplasty [5] (Fig. 2). Bill Bowers and I have both been doing a form of this procedure for 15–20 years. Both of our published papers were almost all on rheumatoid arthritic patients (around 70%). I have just submitted a paper to the *Journal of Hand Surgery* looking at

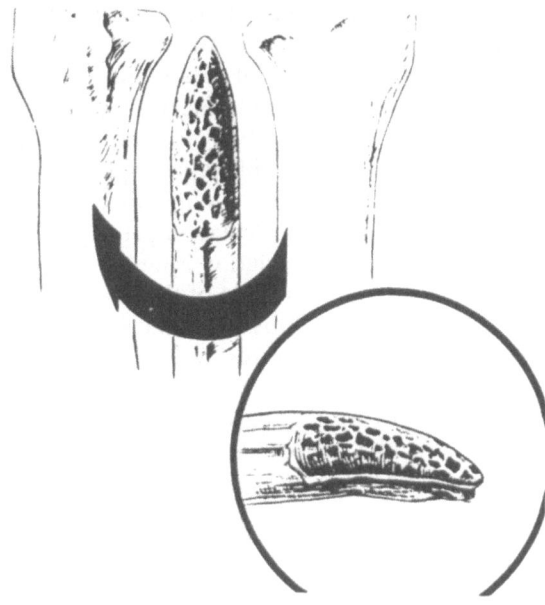

Fig. 2. The distal 5–6 cm of the ulna are reshaped to match the slope of the radius from full pronation to full supination. The distal-most ulna lies just proximal to the articular surface of the radius

all of our *non*rheumatoid, young healthy people with matched ulna. We're pleased with it. The principle is to reshape the distal ulna so that it matches the slope of the radius and to leave it long enough to be held by the ulna sling mechanism. If you just cut off the head of the ulna, the ulna will gradually move radially. What was enough room between the styloid and carpals becomes not enough room. The styloid will now strike the carpals as it moves radially. So, you can't just cut the head off and try to put soft tissue in there. You have to reshape the ulna and the principles are that you reshape it over 5–6 cm and you match it in pronation, in neutral, and in supination to the radius. The length of the distal ulna is left at the level of the radius articular surface. The reshaping is a little like an eccentrically sharpened pencil or perhaps your finger. You shape it a little like your finger, but sharper. The nail of your finger is the retained cortex, all the way to the tip that would be on the most ulnar aspect with the wrist in a neutral position. The ulna is cut away, all around the pulp of the finger shape, so from full pronation to full supination there is no impingement. If these surfaces are relatively parallel, there is no need for soft tissue interposition. They cannot strike each other by virtue of their parallelism. The ulna is left long

enough so that it reattaches itself to the ulnar sling mechanism. It reattaches to the collagen. We don't sew it back. Most of the time the deep layer of the sheath of the extensor carpi ulnaris is still attached to the cortex and that contributes to the initial stability.

Failed Darrach

What do we do with a failed Darrach procedure? Basically, the failed Darrach can be converted into a matched ulna. This is done with a step-cut osteotomy, advancing the most ulnar cortex which is going to represent the fingernail of our finger-shaped or resected ulna. It is necessary to get it up long enough so that it can attach to the ulnar sling mechanism and then reshape it so that it matches the shape of the radius. This is a very successful way of solving the Darrach problem.

The three principles of match ulna arthroplasty are: (1) cut the ulna to match the shape of the radius, a 5–6 cm length of resection; (2) leave the distal ulna at the level of the distal radius, and (3) that means almost always removing the ulna styloid. Again, it is not necessary to sew or fix the ulna back into the ulnar sling mechanism. The cancellous or raw bone gets trapped or grabbed by the healing mechanism and fixes itself so the ulna no longer wings.

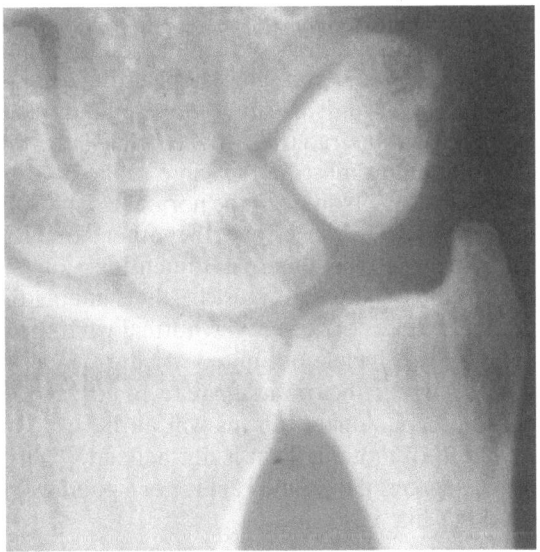

Fig. 3. If the sulcus joint of the radius is reversed, the proximal part of the joint must be resected to provide a parallel surface

Occasionally, the sulcus joint of the radius is more prominent proximally than distally when seen on a PA X-ray (Fig. 3). That is, when moving distally, the joint slopes away from the ulna rather that toward it. When this is present, the proximal part of the joint must be resected to provide a matching or parallel surface on the radius.

Let's look briefly at reconstructive problems of the distal radius. When there is a healed fractured step in the distal radius, the analysis for the reconstruction depends on whether the angulation of the cortex needs to be considered in the repair. When the displaced articular surface is parallel to its normal position, the osteotomy can be parallel to the long axis of the radius, that is, perpendicular to the articular surface because you are just going to slide that piece distally. It is just displaced. If, on the other hand, the articular surface is not congruous, then you design an osteotomy that will result in it being congruous. You would cut a curved osteotomy. As the step is elevated, the fragment rotates so that the surface becomes aligned as the step is corrected. The third way of approaching these radial steps is to resect them.

Let's look at some problems that are not so easily solved. If the die punch fracture has destroyed the radiolunate joint, in other words, you have destruction of the key support joint of the wrist, then a radiolunate arthrodesis is indicated. Note: this follows the basic principle of limited wrist arthrodesis [6]. That basic principle is that the external dimensions of the unit you fuse must be of the same size and same shape as the original unit. In other words, if I fuse the scaphoid to the trapezium and trapezoid, when finished this three-bone unit must be the same shape and the same size as it would be in the normal wrist [7–9]. Otherwise, it will overload the other joints in the wrist. So the external dimensions of the fused radius and lunate must be the same as the external dimensions are in the normal wrist. That is the basic principle of limited wrist arthrodesis.

Wrists with either radiolunate or radioscaphoid or radioscapholunate fusions will all have about 60° or 70° of motion. That is not percent. That is 60–70 *degrees* of motion. That is not a good wrist. We don't like it.

A radioscaphoid arthrodesis several years later is a painless wrist with good function but, again, with only 60° or 70° of motion and that is not as good a wrist as we can have. When the radioscaphoid joint is destroyed, we've a much better

way out of that problem. There are a lot of things that will destroy the joint between the radius and the scaphoid. Fracture of the radius, scaphoid non-union [10], an avascular necrosis or Preiser's disease — all will destroy the radioscaphoid articulation. A rotary subluxation is another and probably the commonest etiology of destruction of the radioscaphoid articulation [11, 12]. When the radioscaphoid articulation is destroyed, there is collapse on the radial side of the wrist with the loss of cartilage resulting in a collapse phenomenon that leads us into what we call SLAC wrist [13–15].

SLAC wrist is the destruction between the radius and the scaphoid and follows a very specific, repeatable pattern. Then it jumps to the capitolunate joint and finally to the hamate-lunate joint, but notice: *never, never*, involves the radiolunate joint — no matter how long it has been there or how severe it is, the radiolunate joint is never destroyed (Fig. 4).

We looked at arthritis of the wrist in around 4,000 X-rays and analyzed how arthritis occurs in

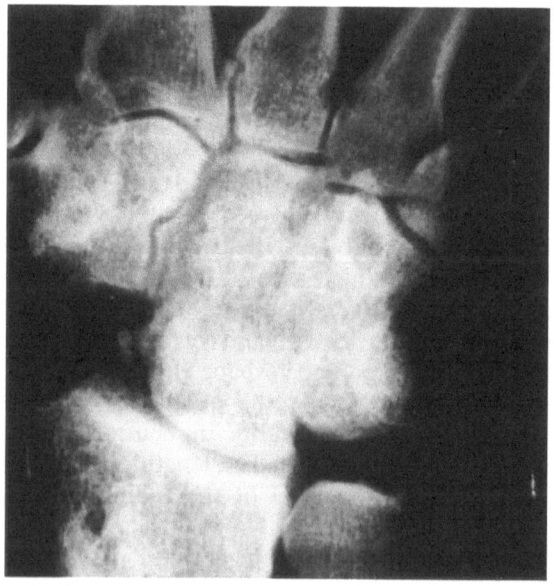

Fig. 4. SLAC wrist secondary to non-union of the scaphoid. There is destruction between the radius and the distal scaphoid joint. The capitate then drives off the radial edge of the lunate, resulting in capitolunate joint destruction followed by hamate-lunate joint destruction. The radiolunate joint is always preserved. The proximal scaphoid fragment acts as a lunate and the proximoscaphoid joint of the radius is also preserved

humans [14]. What we found was that a little over one-half of arthritis of the wrist occurs as SLAC wrist, that is, the destruction pattern between the radius and the scaphoid. About one-quarter of arthritis of the wrist occurs only at the triscaphe joint. Kusunoki has written a paper analyzing triscaphe degenerative arthritis [16]. I think arthritis here is the result of a form of rotary subluxation of the scaphoid that we haven't described. I think there are three types of rotary subluxation of the scaphoid. The first type is the common scapholunate dissociation. Then, I think there are two other types: there is a lateral displacement of the distal scaphoid which produces shear damage only at the triscaphe joint. This has nothing to do with carpometacarpal (CMC) degenerative arthritis. The other is an axial rotation along the scaphoid long axis. Neither of those two destroy the radioscaphoid joint. Neither of those two are rotary subluxation of the scaphoid as we have always talked about it.

We found that one-quarter of arthritis occurs as pure triscaphe, having nothing to do with thumb column collapse, nothing to do with any other abnormalities in any other joints, but just pure triscaphe, and around another 10% occurred as a combination of radioscaphoid and triscaphe degenerative joint disease, meaning that around 90% of arthritis as it occurs in our wrist is a scaphoid problem. The scaphoid is truly the wrist's Achilles heel.

SLAC

One of the criticisms of the 4,000 X-ray review study was that we saw only one X-ray on each patient in time. How do we know there is actually a progression? We now have several cases that are well documented demonstrating wrists with dynamic rotary subuxation of the scaphoid progressing to full SLAC wrist 10–12 years later. Typical SLAC wrist is a loss of radial columnar height, with arthritis between the radioscaphoid, then the destruction occurs between the capitate and lunate because of shear force. Cartilage will tolerate nearly anything in perpendicular loading, even very small areas taking very large loads, but cartilage will not tolerate shear. There is total preservation of the spherical, perpendicularly loaded radiolunate joint. We call the pattern *s*capho-*l*unate-*a*dvanced *c*ollapse. In English, slack also implies a laxity, e.g., "The rope is tight or the rope has some slack in it". We chose a

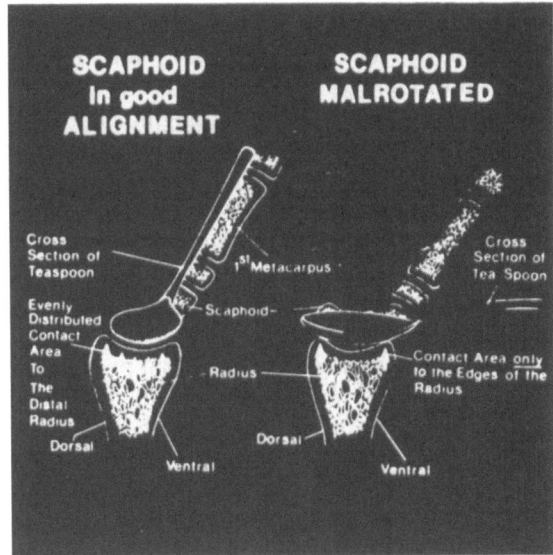

Fig. 5. The radioscaphoid joint is analagous to two spoons nesting in one another. When the handles of the two spoons are together, the contact surface is maximal and congruent. As the spoon handles are moved apart, as in rotary subluxation, the contact is on the center of the upper spoon and on the edges of the lower spoon. In rotary subluxation, this position results in radioscaphoid joint destruction. (From [15] with permission)

phrase which represents the bones and also implies the etiology.

Dynamic Rotary Subluxation of the Scaphoid

The distal end of the radius has a spherical fossa for the lunate and an elliptical egg-shaped fossa for the scaphoid. The scaphoid normally has total contact, but, in the scapholunate dissociation type of rotary subluxation of the scaphoid, the elliptical rotation destroys the continuity and then destroys the joint. The lunate, because it is spherical, can be in DISI or VISI or ulnar position and it will not destroy the radiolunate joint. An analogy is two spoons (Fig. 5): if the handles of two nested spoons are together, we can move the upper spoon any way we want and the contact surface remains total. If, however, I move the spoon handles apart, the upper spoon will rise out of the lower one because it is elliptical. It is egg-shaped and it rises, and now all of the rub, the contact, is on the center of the upper spoon and on the edges of the lower spoon, and that rotation, that particular position, is not tolerated by the radioscaphoid joint. All the other positions of the scaphoid are perfectly acceptable, so there are only alignments of the scaphoid that are intolerable and that destroy the joint. Spoons are a simple analogy. If we cut the spoon in half transversely, we are going to end up with the tip of the spoon being like a little lunate. It is detached from its handle. We now have an analogy of a scaphoid non-union. Late end-stage scaphoid non-union types of destruction all look the same. The proximal pole, big or little, is always treated like a lunate. Being treated like a lunate, it *never* undergoes destruction of its radius-proximal pole articulation. The distal pole rotates and destroys the joint between the radius and the distal scaphoid fragment. The capitate will destroy its joint between the capitate and the lunate. We'll discuss that in a moment, but the proximal scaphoid pole-capitate joint undergoes destruction just as that which occurs between the lunate and the capitate.

An experimental model is a patient with a silicone scaphoid. The capitate sits nicely on the lunate at rest, but without load. As soon as the person makes a fist, for example then the capitate drives into the hole, between the scaphoid and lunate. It skids and drives off the radial side of the lunate producing high shear loads. This destroys the cartilage between the capitate and the lunate. This, then, is the second component of SLAC wrist.

To treat SLAC wrist, the basic principle in the beginning was to fuse the capitate to the lunate, to place the load on the radiolunate, joint take the scaphoid out, and replace it with a silicone implant [13, 17]. We then added the hamate. We added the triquetrum and we added the hamate and triquetrum. We find that once you have the capitate fused to the lunate, it does not matter whether you add these or not, your range of motion is the same. Once you have a capitolunate arthrodesis, the range of motion in the wrist is going to be the same. There are two distinct advantages to including the hamate and triquetrum. Number one is obvious. You are going to have a large cancellous surface area for fusion and your non-union rates are going to go down. The second is that once you add these two bones, you may disobey the rule of limited wrist arthrodesis. You no longer have to obey the rule that says the external dimensions must be the same after the fusion as before. That is because no other joints are now affected. When you include the hamate and triquetrum, no other joints are affected by that fusion and you can then allow collapse to occur. If I were to just fuse the capitolunate, joint then I have to maintain the total height and space between them because it would affect the ulnocarpal joints.

Silicone Implants

There is no place in the human wrist for a silicone scaphoid or a silicone lunate. You have heard that by this time; but from my position, they can stop making them.

We used to use the silicone scaphoid. We are calling back our people with SLAC wrist and doing 15 and 16-year follow-ups. We are looking for particulate synovitis and we are finding it. We are finding little cysts. No big problem with the patient, but we are finding little changes even though we had a fusion and thought the fusion would protect them and we could use plastic even after we began to recognize particulate synovitis. That is not true and they are coming out. For SLAC reconstruction in the past 4 years, we have simply removed the scaphoid and put nothing in its place (Fig. 6).

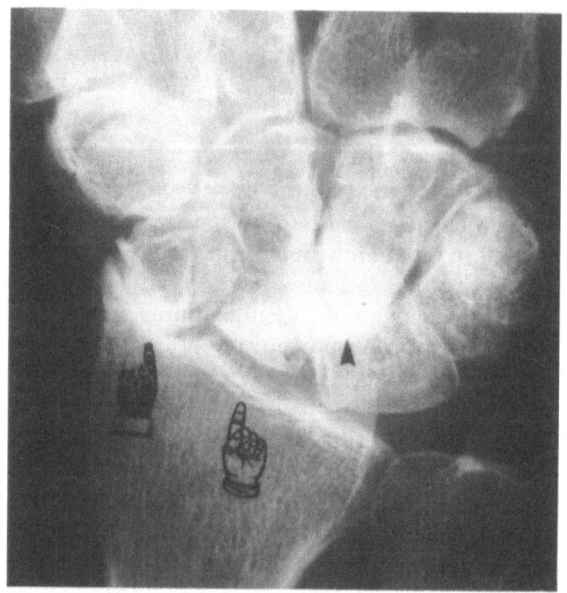

Fig. 6. In treating SLAC wrist, the capitate, lunate, hamate, and triquetrum are fused. The scaphoid is removed with no tendon or other material replacement. The wrist articulates on the normal radiolunate joint

Tendon Implants

Let me make a point. When you are talking about putting tendon interposition anywhere, there are two concepts. One is putting a rolled-up piece of tendon between raw bone ends to prevent contact. If I do an anchovy or tendon interposition between my thumb metacarpal and my trapezium, it is useful; it is good because it is an interposition that prevents the bones from touching. There is, however, no point ever in rolling up a tendon or iliotibial fascia and sticking it in place of a missing carpal bone. Rolled up tendon will not take support. One must make the distinction. Implanting a tendon to take support is useless. Implanting a tendon as a fascial or collagen interposition between bones is effective. If, for example, one implants a rolled-up tendon in place of a lunate and then loads the hand, the capitate compresses both the scaphoid proximal pole and the tendon ball. As soon as loads reach anything over minimum, all of the load shifts to the bone which has stopped compressing before the tendon stops compressing. There is then no function for the tendon ball. From my point of view, there is never a reason to roll up a tendon and fill a space. The body will do that better than you can. In SLAC reconstruction just take the scaphoid out, do your surgery, and leave. The wrist does not tip into radial deviation. The hand is maintained in position by motor tone. For tendon use, the basic decision process is "Am I doing an interposition to keep raw bone ends from touching?", then use it. If I'm putting it in to share load-bearing with bones, then forget it.

We have reviewed our initial SLAC series. We now have just under 200 SLAC that we are following, the oldest dating back 18 years. At 1–2 years, grip strength was 78% of normal. In the 2–4 year follow-ups, the grip strength was 83% of normal. By the time we get over 4 years post-SLAC reconstruction, the grip strength is approaching normal, in the 92nd percentile. Any time you have a procedure on the wrist which shows you that progressive pattern as the years go by, you have a procedure to rely on. Remember, these patients frequently have not been able to use their wrists for many years prior to repair. That is an important pattern. We are on our way to 25-year follow-ups of wrists that are painless with a reasonable range of motion and proven durability. Your average range of flexion-extension with SLAC wrist will be 55% to 60% of the normal side.

In 23 years of practice, I have performed about a dozen wrist fusions, only about a dozen. I think there is almost always a way to avoid a wrist fusion. The key to successful SLAC surgery is correction of the DISI. You must correct the displacement of the lunate. If not, the capitate strikes the radius when the patient tries to dorsiflex. So, the key of the surgery is to displace the capitate volarly on the lunate. As you push the capitate volarly, the lunate will kick into slight VISI or volar flexion position.

Proximal Row Carpectomy

The reason proximal row carpectomy works is because the ligaments drop the capitate into the lunate fossa and we know the lunate fossa has normal cartilage. The problems are these: firstly, the proximal capitate is often destroyed in SLAC wrist (Fig. 4). Secondly, the radial curvature of the proximal capitate is much smaller than the lunate fossa. It is like putting an egg into a rice bowl. The capitate is much sharper and usually destroys the joint. The third and most compelling reason to avoid proximal row carpectomy is that you have just thrown away the proximal articular surface of the lunate. You have thrown away one-half of the normal joint on which, with SLAC reconstruction, the wrist will function well for the rest of the patient's life.

References

1. Watson HK, Gross SC (1991) Wrist instability secondary to distal radius fractures. Complications in Orthop 6(1):9–16
2. Taleisnik J, Watson HK (1984) Midcarpal instability caused by malunited fractures of the distal radius. J Hand Surg [Am] 9(3):350–357
3. Watson HK, Castle TH (1988) Trapezoidal osteotomy of the distal radius for unacceptable articular angulation after Colles' fracture. J Hand Surg [Am] 13(6):837–843
4. Watson HK, Brown RE (1989) Ulnar impingement syndrome after Darrach procedure. J Hand Surg [Am] 14(2) Part 1:302–306
5. Watson HK, Ryu J, Burgess RC (1986) Matched distal ulnar resection. J Hand Surg [Am] 11(6): 812–817
6. Watson HK, Goodman, ML, Johnson TR (1981) Limited wrist arthrodesis. Part II. The triscaphoid joint. J Hand Surg [Am] 6(3):223–233

7. Watson HK, Hanley EN, Boland DM (1983) Intercarpal arthrodesis for rotary subluxation of the scaphoid. Orthop Consult 4(7):1–9

8. Watson HK, Hempton RF (1980) Limited wrist arthrodesis. Part I. The triscaphoid joint. J Hand Surg [Am] 5(4):320–327

9. Watson HK, Ryu J, Akelman E (1986) Limited triscaphoid intercarpal arthrodesis for rotary subluxation of the scaphoid. J Bone Joint Surg [Am] 68(3):345–349

10. Vender MI, Watson HK, Wiener BD, Black DM (1987) Degenerative change in symptomatic scaphoid nonunion. J Hand Surg [Am] 12(4):514–519

11. Brenner LH, Watson HK (1987) Degenerative disorders of the carpus. In: Lichtman DM (ed) The wrist and its disorders. Saunders, Philadelphia, pp 286–292

12. Howard FM (Moderator), Lichtman DM, Taleisnik J, Watson HK (1982) Symposium: Carpal instability. Contemp Orthop 4(1):107–144

13. Watson HK, Ballet FL (1984) The SLAC wrist: Scapholunate advanced collapse pattern of degenerative athritis. J Hand Surg [Am] 9(3):358–365

14. Watson HK, Brenner LH (1985) Degenerative disorders of the wrist. J Hand Surg [Am] 10(6) Part 2:1002–1006

15. Watson HK, Ryu J (1986) Evolution of arthritis of the wrist. Clin Orthop 202:57–67

16. Kusunoki M, Kamano M, Nakamoto T, Kazuki K, Satoh T (1991) Incidence of scaphotrapezal trapezoidal osteoarthritis in elderly Japanese. International Symposium on the Wrist, March 6–8, Nagoya, Japan

17. Watson HK, Vender MI (1988) Wrist and intercarpal arthrodesis. In: Chapman MW (ed) Operative orthopaedics. Lippincott, Philadelphia, pp 1291–1305

Treatment of Distal Radius Fractures by Intra-Focal Pinning with Arum Pins

Abstract. Distal radius fractures are the most frequent among all the types occurring in the wrist. The treatment by reduction and immobilization using a cast is often unsatisfactory, so that many surgeons use osteosynthesis with Kirschner-wire pinning which cannot prevent secondary displacement. Therefore, we proposed a new kind of osteosynthesis, the intra-focal pinning technique, and, as an improvement, the use of special pins (arum).

The principle of intra-focal pinning is very simple: through short skin incisions and after a manual reduction, simple K-wire pins, are inserted directly *into the fracture line*, pushed perpendicularly and then upwardly (oblique), and fixed into the opposite wall. A secondary displacement is thus made impossible by the bumping of the distal fragment directly on the pins which are *working as an abutment*. No cast is fitted, thereby allowing immediate rehabilitation and better functional results. Three pins are needed to be inserted into very precise points laterally, posterolaterally, and posteromedially. With smooth pins, however, a secondary pin displacement is possible since the pin's blunt severed edge may damage the tendons. Consequently, we changed these pins for threaded ones so as to ensure their tightening into the opposite wall of the radius. We invented a new pins, 20/10 mm in length, threaded, and fitted with a special nut which we named "arum" (because it is shaped like an arum flower) to avoid the pin from pricking under the skin. Thanks to its special conical shape, it penetrates the fracture line like a wedge and has a "hyper-reduction effect" which compensates the posterior compression in advance. The tendons cannot be

further damaged because of both the rounded shape of the nut and the housing of the pin's sharp edge within the base of the nut. The third pin is indispensable for controlling the postero-medial fragment which jeopardizes the distal radioulnar joint function. Finally, thanks to the third pin and contrary to what might have been expected, *multi-fragment fractures* are better controlled.

The three pins are set through short incisions, carefully made in order to not damage neural branches and tendons which are separated with the tips of a small forceps. After manual reduction, the fracture line is easily detected by using the forceps. The pin is firmly held with a specially designed pin-holding chuck and is first introduced perpendicularly into the fracture line, then obliquely (45°) upwards until it makes contact with the opposite wall, then pointed, and finally screwed into it with alternative rotatory motion. The arum nut is screwed while its cone is penetrating safely between the tendons and then between the two edges of the fracture, creating the "reduction effect". Screwed in volarly slightly over 2 mm, the arum nuts can be later unscrewed after cutting the pin with special shears: this allows the freshly cut pin-end to house itself into the base of the nut so that it will be harmless to tendons, and the skin is closed with an intra-dermal suture. Then, frontal and lateral radiographs can be taken to check the final result. The pins are removed after 5 weeks, at which time the arum nut is unscrewed from the pin. General or regional anesthesia is used and a *tourniquet* is indispensable because of the risk of neural damage with local anesthesia.

The objective criteria of a good evaluation of the X-ray results are given. Normally, the bi-styloid line is +10°–15° on the horizontal line, the front glenoid line (radial inclination angle) is +24° on the horizontal line, the ulnar variance is

---

[1] Clinique de l'Yvette, 43, Route de Corbeil, 91160 Longjumeau, France

−2 mm, and the side glenoid line is +15°. These values may be noted on an individual form.

The results were first evaluated in a work issued at Lille (France) in 1980, based on 72 cases treated with intra-focal pinning without using arum pins. The mobility was good or excellent in 88% and the occurence of neuro-dystrophy was reduced threefold. After 3–6 months, the pain had totally disappeared in 95%, the strength of the grip was normal in 67%, and the finger mobility was normal in 80%. Previous activities were again undertaken in 80% of the cases after 4–8 weeks. Secondary displacements were less frequent than seen in the usual procedures (25%), *but even when they occurred, the functional results were better because of the possibility of immediate rehabilitation.*

With the arum pins there are no longer pin expulsions nor damage to the tendons, but neuromas are always possible. Radiological results are excellent and good in 70% of the cases. Mal-unions may occur in 29%, but the functional results are better than in usual procedures, except when the distal radioulnar joint is involved. The patients are satisfied by having excellent results in 75% of the cases and by good results in 13%, a total of 88%. There are only 1.5% of poor results and 10.5% of bad results. The superiority of the intra-focal procedure has been confirmed by recent publications.

The indications with the most potential benefit are Colles' fractures with only one distal fragment. The three-fragments fractures, T-shaped in the frontal or sagittal planes, are also good candidates. Even multi-fragment fractures may be treated with unexpectedly good results. Some anteriorly displaced fractures may be fixed with an anterior pin inserted just laterally from the flexor carpi radialis tendon. It is also possible to fix fractures of the distal extremity of the radius *and* ulna, and also reduce mal-unions in children after Salter II fractures.

Only comminutive fractures must be excepted from this procedure. In some cases, it is possible to combine plate fixation with one or two pins in order to avoid lateral displacement.

Keywords: Colles fracture — Intrafocal pinning — Secondary displacement — Reduction of distal radius fracture — Osteosynthesis — Distal radius fracture

Introduction

Distal radius fractures are the most frequent of all types that occur in the wrist. The treatment by reduction and application of a cast is not always satisfactory, so that many surgeons use osteosynthesis with Kirschner wire pinning which cannot prevent secondary displacement [1–10]. For this reason, we proposed a new kind of osteosynthesis, the intra-focal pinning technique [7–8], and, as an improvement of this method, the use of special pins ("arum").

The Principle of Intra-Focal Pinning

Traditionally, fractures of the distal end of the radius were fixed with pins, after manual reduction drilled through the distal fragment and stuck into the proximal one (Fig. 1). Because of the

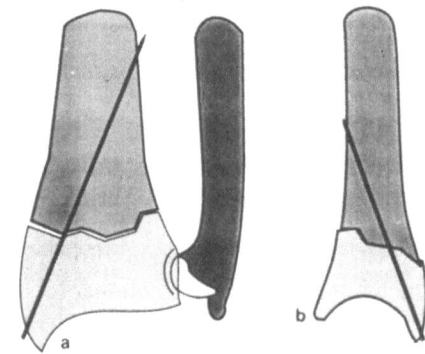

Fig. 1. Classical pinning of distal radius fractures. Note that the pin, inserted in the distal part, is located far away from the edge of the proximal part. **a** Frontal view. **b** Lateral view

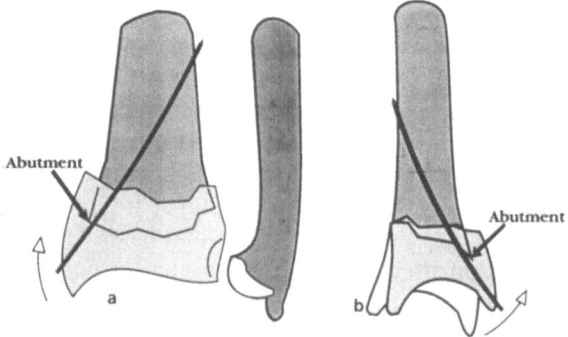

Fig. 2. The secondary displacement after classical pinning. The pin bends slightly until it stops on the wall of the proximal part which constitues an impassable abutment (*black arrow*). **a** Frontal view. **b** Lateral view

pins's flexibility, the distal fragment very quickly moves back until the pins bump into the inferior edge of the proximal fragment (Fig. 2).

In performing intra-focal pinning, first a K-wire is inserted through a short skin incision and, after a manual reduction, smooth K-wires are directly inserted into the fracture line, first, perpendicularly and then upwardly/obliquely, and finally fixed into the opposite wall (Fig. 3).

In this way, any subsequent tilt of the distal fragment is prevented, because a secondary displacement is made impossible by the immediate bumping of the distal fragment on the pins

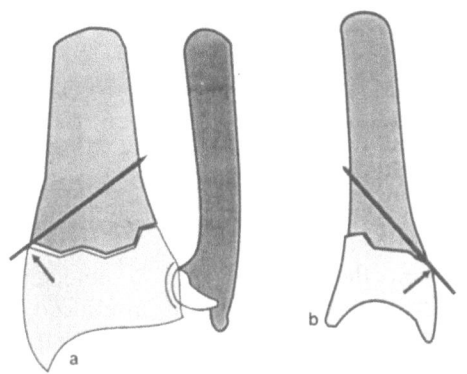

Fig. 3. Principle of intra-focal pinning. The pin, directly set in the fracture line, makes an immediate abutment to the secondary displacement of the distal part. **a** Frontal view. **b** Lateral view

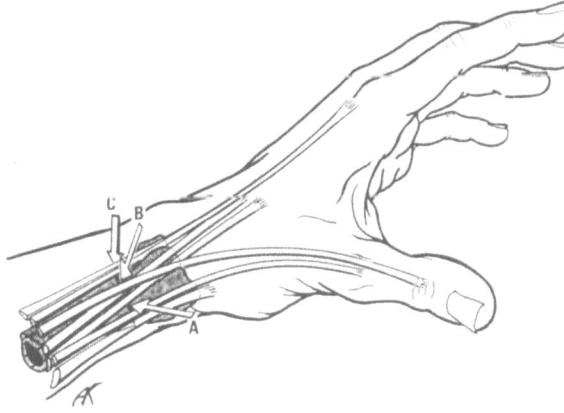

Fig. 4. The three penetrating points of the pins. On this schematic representation, the three points are defined in relation to the tendons. **A** The lateral pin is set between the extensor carpi radialis brevis and the extensor pollicis brevis. **B** The posterolateral pin is set between the extensor pollicis longus and the extensor indicis. **C** The posteromedial pin is set medially in relation to the extensors digitorum, and sometimes between the extensors of the fourth and the fifth fingers.

which are working as an abutment, not as a resistance component. This makes an additional cast superfluous, thus allowing immediate rehabilitation and, therefore, better functional results.

A good fixation needs three pins which are inserted in very precise points (Fig. 4). The first pin is inserted laterally between the tendons of the extensors carpi radialis and the tendon of the extensor pollicis brevis; the second pin is inserted posterolaterally close to the Lister tubercle, taking great care to avoid the extensor pollicis longus; the third is inserted posteromedially, passing between the extensors digitorum and the extensor carpi ulnaris.

Unfortunately, with the traditional method, it is possible that one of the pins will move either into the mass of the bone or towards the surface where it threatens the skin's integrity. Therefore, we exchanged smooth pins for threaded ones, using first full-length then only end-threaded ones, and this in such a way as to ensure their tightening into the opposite wall of the radius.

With this improvement, any secondary displacement of the pins no longer occurs. However, a last and important problem remained to be solved: that of the damage to the tendons caused by the blunt severed edge of the pin. A tentative solution was tried by using little metal or plastic caps "hooding" the undesirable spike of the pin-pointing under the skin, but the positioning of these caps was difficult, they were often dislodged, and ultimately migrated under the skin.

Using Arum Pins

The simultaneous solution to all these problems has now been found thanks to a new conception of intra-focal pins, the arum pins (Fig. 5). These are 20/10 mm in length and are threaded to fit with a special nut named for its resemblance to the shape of an arum flower. Being threaded, the

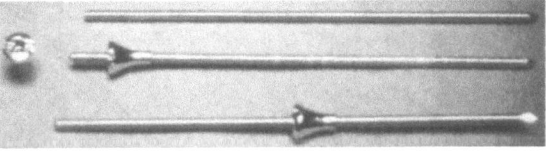

Fig. 5. The arum pins. The pins are 20/10 mm in length, threaded, and fixed with a special arum nut (named after its resemblance to the shape of an arum flower)

pin cannot be expelled. The advantages of the nut are twofold: (1) as it penetrates like a wedge into the fracture line, it has a "hyper-reduction effect" on the fracture, which compensates for the posterior compression in advance (Fig. 6), and (2) whereas the sharp end of an ordinary pin was potentially very damaging to the tendons, both the rounded shape of the arum nut and the housing of the pin's sharp edge within the base of the nut protect the tendons from any damage (Fig. 7).

We now insist on the necessity of using three pins, and not two as we proposed at the onset of our experiment. In fact, there is often a third posteromedial fragment which jeopardizes the distal radioulnar joint (DRUJ) function and needs its own fixation with a third pin in a posteromedial location (Fig. 8). Moreover, the posterior blocking of the distal fragment is better obtained with two posterior pins rather than with only one. Finally, and contrary to what might have been expected, multi-fragment fractures are better controlled with three pins.

Setting the Arum Pins

These pins are set in the following manner:

1. For the displaced fracture, the manual reduction is the same as before (Fig. 9).
2. The setting of each pin is made through three short incisions (7–8 mm), so as to render the tendons visible as is done in the other techniques.
3. Only the skin is cut, and the sub-cutaneous tissues are separated in order to prevent sectioning of the sub-cutaneous nerves.
4. Tendons are separated with the tips of a small forceps (Halstedt type) introduced into an inter-tendinous space.
5. As the tips of these forceps are widened, a second one is inserted between the tendons.
6. The second (closed) forceps scratches the bone up and down in order to find the fracture line, as the reduction motion is improved (Fig. 10.a).
7. When the fracture line is detected, this second forceps is gently introduced in the space and its tips are widened so that the pin may be introduced between them into the fracture (Fig. 10.b).
8. Prior to being firmly positioned in the pin holder, each threaded pin is prepared with

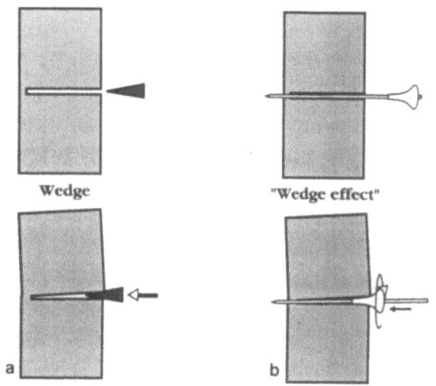

Fig. 6. The "wedge effect" of the arum pin. **a** A regular wedge inserted between two fracture sections widens the space between them. **b** When the conical nut of the arum pin is screwed into the fracture line, it widens this space and makes a hyper-correction

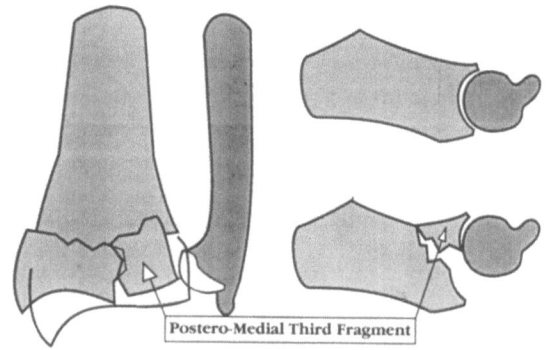

Fig. 8. A third postero-medial fragment, splitting the sigmoid notch, is seen very frequently and must be fixed with a third pin

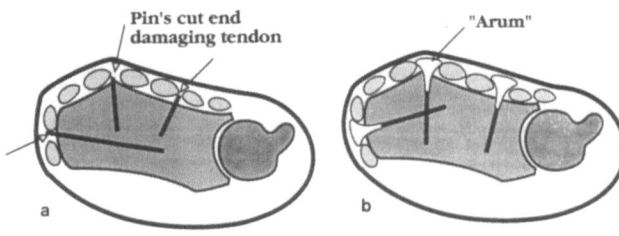

Fig. 7. Damaging of the tendons. **a** In the original intra-focal pinning procedure, the rough, cut end of the pins are damaging to the tendons. **b** The smooth shape of the arum nut cannot wound tendons

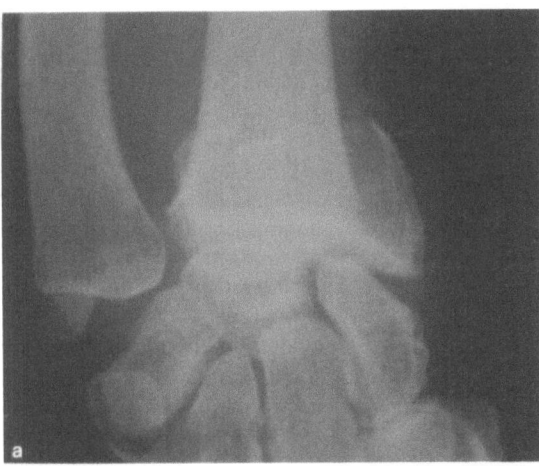

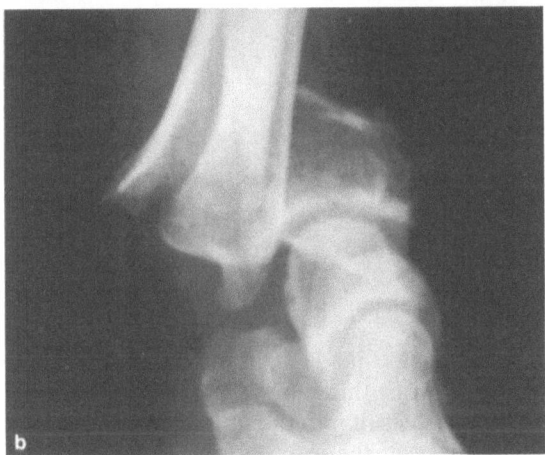

Fig. 9. Radiographs of a Colles' fracture before "arum" intra-focal pinning. **a** Frontal view. **b** Lateral view

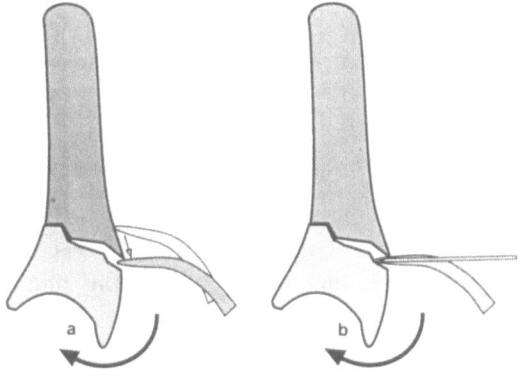

Fig. 10. Introducing the pin into the fracture line. **a** Scratching the dorsal aspect of the radius with a small forceps permits the location of the fracture line. **b** The pin is slipped between the two branches of the forceps which had been introduced into the fracture

the arum nut so as to ensure that the latter is situated at least 1 cm away from the thickness of the bone and in line with the proposed direction of the pin which can be visualized on X-ray.

9. It must be understood that the pin segment caught in the pin holder becomes unusable, because the threading is squeezed by the chuck. Consequently, the part between the arum nut and the chuck will be rendered unusable after being seized by the chuck.

10. The pin thus prepared is used in the same manner as the previously used pins.

11. Schematically, *there are 6 different stages* (Fig. 11): from the initial position (Fig. 11.a) the fracture is reduced manually and the pin inserted, first perpendicularly (Fig. 11.b) into the bone (stage 1), and then obliquely (45°) upwards (Fig. 11.c) until contact is made with the opposite wall (stage 2), pointed, and screwed into the opposite wall (Fig. 11.d) with alternating rotatory motions (stage 3). Then, no back displacement is possible (Fig. 11.e) and the edges of the two bones' fragments are blocked by the pin. The arum nut is screwed (stage 4) while fracture reduction is improved (Fig. 11.f): the cone of the arum is now penetrating safely between the tendons and further between the two edges of the fracture, creating the "reduction effect". The arum nut is introduced into the bone so that the narrow part of the cone will be completely inside; if a greater widening of the fracture edges is desired, it is possible to insert the beginning of the larger part of the cone. Determining the specific optimal width is a matter of experience. Note that the nut must be screwed in intentionally, slightly over 2 mm, by an additional three or four turns. We have made a special pin-holdering chuck with a fitting on the screwdriver (Fig. 12): when the pin is correctly mounted, it is possible to do the pinning without changing the position. The advantage is that the pin is firmly held as the arum nut is either screwed or unscrewed. With our special shears, it is possible to adjust the depth of the pin cut: incompletely cut, the pin may be held during the unscrewing of the nut; then, the pin may be bent and completely broken off. The pin is cut (Fig. 10.g) with special shears (Fig. 14) fitted with asymmetrical jaws (stage 5), cutting it very close to the nut (2 mm). With the special screwdriver repositioned, the

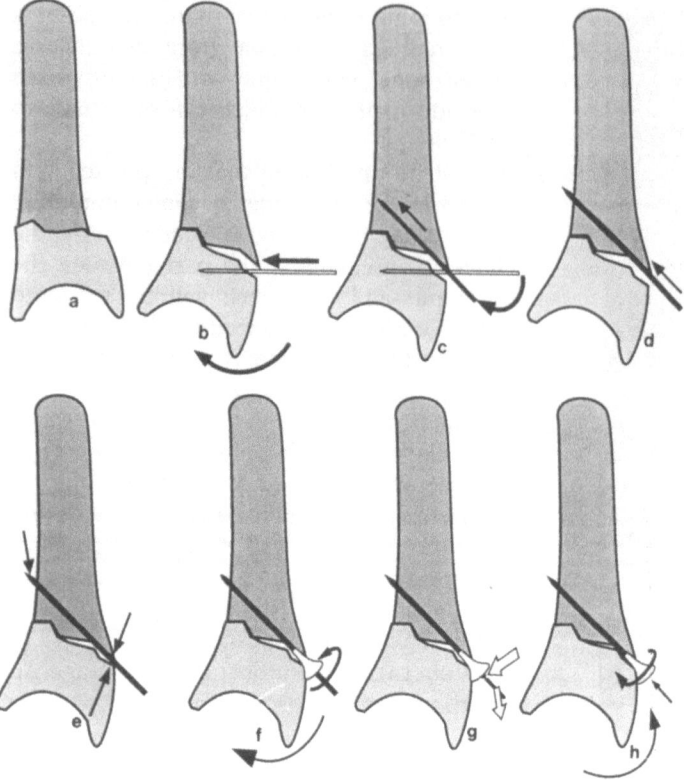

Fig. 11. The stages of the intra-focal pinning technique (side views). **a** The displaced fracture is first reduced. **b** The pin is introduced, first perpendicularly, and then **c** Obliquely upwards until it touches the opposite wall. **d** It is screwed into the bone with some alternating rotation motions. **e** This prevents and further posterior displacement. **f** The arum nut is screwed into the fracture line; the reduction is improved. **g** The pin is cut as close as possible to the nut. **h** The arum nut is unscrewed until the cut end of the pin is housed within the bottom of the nut

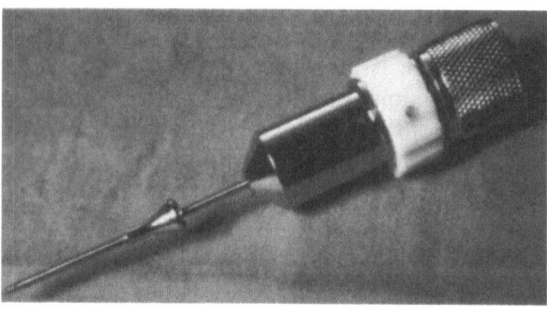

Fig. 12. Our specially designed pin-holder that may be firmly held in the palm of the hand and also be combined with a screwdriver

arum nut (Fig. 11.h) is slowly unscrewed in three turns: this allows the freshly cut pin-end to house itself into the little space prepared in the base of the arum nut (Fig. 15) so that it will be harmless to tendons (stage 6). If the adjustment has been properly effected, the base of the arum is now located at the precise level of the sub-cutaneous tissues. Then, the skin is closed with an intradermal suture, which is not only an esthetic mode of closure, but also the most innocuous because contrary to the stitches, it does not require a large amount of skin on each side; thus the cutaneous perimeter is not diminished and the risk of edema is reduced.

The sketches in Fig. 13 show the correct positioning of the three pins. At this point, frontal and lateral radiographs can be taken in order to check the final result of the pinning (Fig. 16). A very important point is that when the pins are removed after 5 weeks, the unscrewing of the arum lifts out the pin at the same time, because the squeezed threading is blocked within the nut. General or regional anesthesia and *tourniquet* are necessary for this procedure, because of the risk of neural damage if made with local anesthesia.

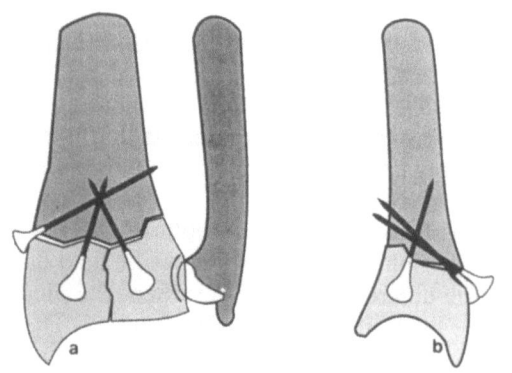

Fig. 13. The ideal location of the three arum pins. **a** Frontal view. **b** Lateral view

Fig. 14. Our specially designed shears with asymmetrical jaws can cut the pin as close as possible to the nut

Fig. 15. The base of the arum nut where there is a small amount of room where the cut end of the pin may be completely hidden

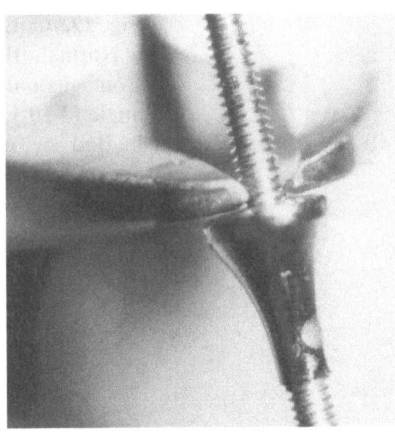

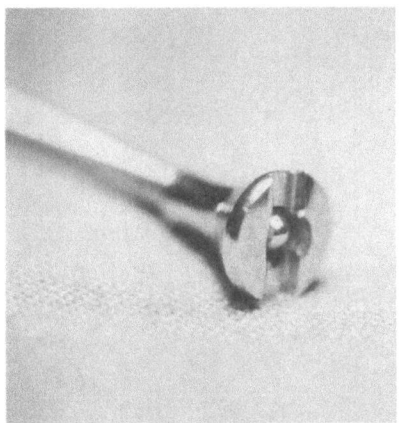

Fig. 14

Fig. 15

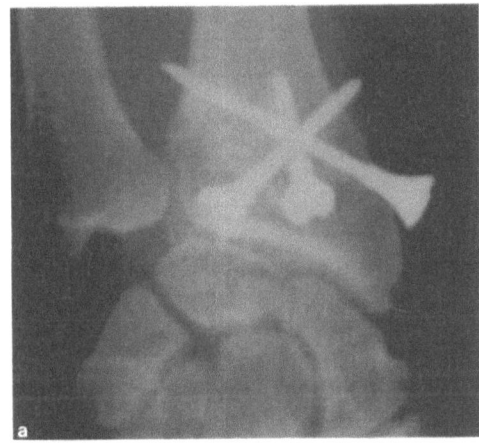

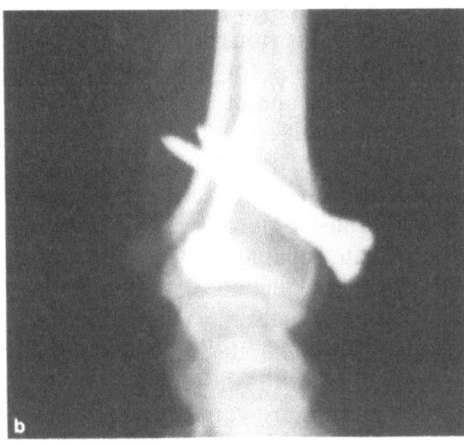

Fig. 16. Radiographs of a Colles' fracture after "arum" intra-focal pinning. **a** Front view. **b** Side view

Evaluation of the Surgical Results

In order to achieve a good evaluation of the X-ray results, it indispensable to use objective criteria with regard to angles and millimeters.

On *frontal radiographs* (Fig. 17.a), the normal (or anatomically reduced) radius is seen with:

1. The bi-styloid line (in French, LBS) tilted at $+10°-15°$ on the horizontal line.
2. The front glenoid line (in French, LGF), also called *radial inclination angle* [2], tilted at $+21°-24°$ on the horizontal line.
3. The ulnar variance (in French, IRCI) is normally equal to $-2\,mm$ (the negative value is taken when the level of the ulnar head is located above the one on the inferior edge of the sigmoid notch).

The imperfect reduction is characterized by the following features:

1. The bi-styloid line becomes horizontal or inverted in negative values (Fig. 17.b).
2. The front glenoid line, or radial inclination angle, also tends to be horizontal or even inverted (Fig. 17.b).
3. The ulnar variance (UV) becomes positive, indicating a compression of the distal part of the radius.
4. A radioulnar diastasis (d) may be eventually noted, indicating a rupture or a tearing of the triangular fibrocartilage complex (TFCC).

On the *lateral radiographs* (Fig. 18) the normality criterion (a) is that the side glenoid line (in French, LGP) is $+15°$, thus the glenoid surface of the radius is oriented downward and slightly forward.

The imperfect reduction (Fig. 18.b) is characterized by:

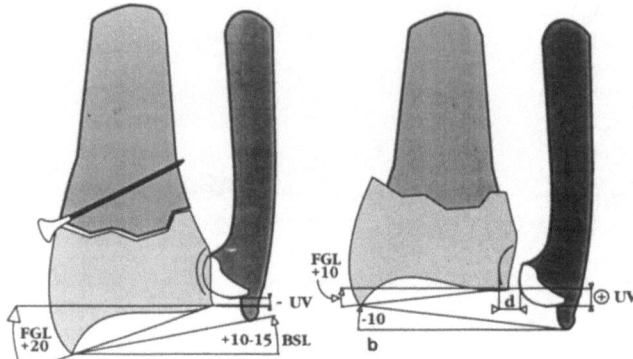

Fig. 17. Criteria of reduction (frontal view). **a** Normal. Bi-styloid line (*BSL*) (+10°–15°), front glenoid line (*FGL*) or radial inclination angle (+20°), Ulnar Variance (*UV*) (−2 m/m). **b** Bad or non-reduction. *BSL* is inverted, and may become negative, the value of *FGL* diminishes or becomes negative, the *UV* becomes positive

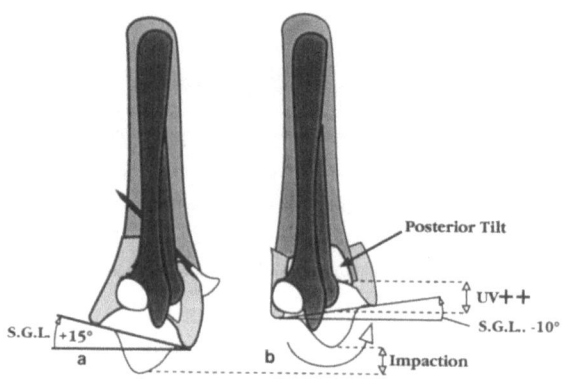

Criterias	BiStyloid Line	Radial Inclinaison Angle	Ulnar Variance	Side Glenoid Line
Before Pinning				
After Pinning				
After Removing				

Fig. 19. Individual patient data form for detecting secondary displacement

Fig. 18. Criteria of reduction (side view). **a** Normal. The side glenoid line (*SGL*) is 15° so the glena faces downwards and slightly forwards. **b** Bad or no reduction. The *SGL* becomes negative and the *UV* becomes positive, as an impaction, associated with a posterior tilt, is visible

1. The tilting of the side glenoid line (SGL), which becomes horizontal or oblique in a backward direction. At that point, its value −10°, which indicates a posterior tilt. (Note that even a zero value of the SLG indicates a posterior tilt.)
2. At the same time, when the UV becomes positive, this allows the measurement of the compression degree of the distal fragment.

These values may be noted on a form (Fig. 19) for each patient which facilitates the evaluation of the various angles and secondary displacements.

Results

The results were first evaluated in a work issued at Lille (France) in 1980 [5] based on 72 cases treated with the original procedure. The most important results were that mobility was good or excellent in 88% of the cases and that the incidence of neuro-dystrophy was reduced by two-thirds.

After 3–6 months, the pain had totally disappeared in 95% of the cases, the strength of the grip was normal in 67%, and finger mobility was normal in 80%. Previous activities were resumed in 80%, at 4 weeks for 21% of these cases at 6 weeks for 53%, and at 8 weeks for 93%.

Secondary displacements were less frequent than in the usual procedures (25%), but even when they occurred, the functional results were better [9] because of having afforded the patients with immediate rehabilitation.

With the introduction of arum pins, there are no longer expulsions of pins nor damage to tendons, although it is always necessary to be very careful with the subcutaneous nerves because neuromas are very serious complications which may be avoided.

Mal-unions may occur in 29% of the patients undergoing the new procedure, but the functional results are better than in the usual procedure, except when the distal radioulnar joint is involved. Radiological results are thereby excellent and good in 70% of the cases.

The patients are satisfied by excellent (75%) and good results (13%), with only 1.5% being poor and 10.5% rated as bad. The superiority of the intra-focal procedure has been confirmed by recent publications [2–4].

Indications

The indications with the most potential benefit are Colles' fracture with only one distal fragment; this is the only case where the use of two pins is possible. The three-fragment fractures, T-shaped in the frontal or sagittal planes, are also good candidates. Even treatment of multi-fragment fractures may be tried with this procedure which can give unexpectedly good results. Some anteriorly displaced fractures may be fixed with an anterior pin inserted just laterally from the flexor carpi radialis tendon. It is also possible to repair fractures of the distal extremity of radius *and* ulna with this procedure.

Only comminutive fractures must be excepted from this procedure. In some cases, it is possible to combine plate fixation with one or two pins in order to avoid lateral displacement. In children, Salter II fractures must be treated by orthopedic reduction and confinement in a cast, but if a secondary displacement does occur, the use of two arum pins kept in place for only 2 weeks can be beneficial.

Conclusion

The results of the treatment of the distal radius fractures have been greatly improved by the arum pinning procedure because of the possibility of immediately embarking on rehabilitation thanks to a much better, precise, and firm fixation not requiring a wide approach and easy to execute.

References

1. Castaing J (1964) Les fractures récentes de l'extrémité inférieure du radius chez l'adulte. Rapport de la 39 ème Réunion Annuelle de la SOFCOT. Rev Chir Orthop 50, 581–666
2. Bleton R, Boulate M, Alnot J-Y (to be published) Etude comparative de trois traitements de fractures de l'extrémité inférieure du radius. Ann Chir Main
3. DiBenedetto MR, Lubbers LM, Ruff ME, Nappi JF, Coleman CR (1991) Quantification of error in measurement of radial inclination angle and radial-carpal distance. J Hand Surg [Am] 16 (3) 399–400
4. Dunaud JL (1983–4) L'embrochage intra-focal "en berceau" des fractures de l'extrémité inférieure du radius. Incidence de ce traitement en matière de réparation des dommages corporels. Memoire pour le CES de réparation juridique du dommage corporel (N° 02100 Saint Quentin), Université R. Descartes Paris V
5. Epinette JA, Lehut JM, Cavenaille M, Bouretz JC, Decoulx J (1982) Fractures de Pouteau-Colles: Double embrochage intra-focal "en berceau" selon Kapandji. A propos d'une série homogène de 72 cas. Ann Chir Main 1:71–83
6. Grumillier P (1976) Fractures de l'extrémité inférieure du radius. Thèse de Médecine (Nancy)
7. Kapandji A (1976) Ostéosynthèse par double embrochage intra-focal. Traitement fonctionnel des fractures non articulaires de l'extrémité inférieure du radius. Ann Chir 30:903–908
8. Kapandji A (1987) L'embrochage intra-focal des fractures de l'extrémité inférieure du radius dix ans après. Ann Chir Main 6:57–63
9. McQueen M, Caspers J (1980) Colles' fractures: Does the anatomic result affect the final function? J Bone Joint Surg [Br] 70:649–51
10. Petit J, GECO (1976) Fractures de l'extrémité inférieure du radius. Rapport de la première réunion du Groupe d'Etude de Chirurgie Osseuse

Rotation of the Forearm in Fracture of the Distal Radius: Clinical and Experimental Studies

Shin Munesada, Yoshinori Oka, Hiroshi Terada, and Nobuyuki Rokuuma[1]

Abstract. The relation between residual deformity in the fracture of the distal radius and the rotation of the forearm is reviewed clinically and experimentally.

The clinical study included 45 cases of closed fracture in patients aged 15 years and over. Assuming that the rotational range on the opposite side was 100%, the average range of pronation-supination was 92.3%. The rotational ranges in the operated cases and in the fracture involving the distal radioulnar (DRU) joint were unsatisfactory. The incidence of symptomatic complaints was high in the cases with a rotational range of under 92%. There was no difference between the rotational range and the radiologically confirmed residual deformity.

Experimentally, we used 4 human upper-extremity cadaver specimens leaving the joint capsule and the interosseous membrane. After making extra-articular fractures, we measured the rotational range and the radiological angle of tilt for each fracture. Experimental results showed that the rotatory range decreased with each change of the angle of tilt.

We consider that the soft tissue problems caused the rotational disturbance in the operated cases because the fractures upon which we operated had severe displacement or comminution. It may be that the loss of rotation in the experiment was related to maladaptation in the DRU joint and change of tension of the soft tissue around the joint. However, this cannot explain the rotational disturbance in relation to the angle of tilt. We must be careful to provide a good alignment of the DRU joint at reduction procedure in order to prevent rotatory disturbance.

Keywords: Distal radius fracture — Distal radioulnar joint — Pronation — Supination — Forearm rotation — Residual deformity

Introduction

Fracture of the distal radius is a common trauma which has been discussed in many reports and clinical reviews. In describing the range of motion of the affected wrist joint, authors have concentrated mainly on dorsiflexion and palmar flexion. However, there is insufficient data on the rotation of the forearm after healing of this fracture. We report a clinical review and the results of a small-scale experiment on the rotation of the forearm in fractures of the distal radius.

Patients and Methods in the Clinical Study

The clinical series consisted of 45 patients with closed fracture in the distal radius. These patients included 23 males and 22 females. We excluded from this series those patients who were under 15 years of age at the time of injury. The ages of the patients varied from 16.6 to 86.9 years (average 43.0 years), and follow-up periods ranged from 0.4 to 6.7 years (average 2.6 years). We analyzed the following features: (1) fracture type at the time of the injury, (2) the method of treatment, (3) present symptoms, (4) present range of rotation, and (5) X-ray measurements on follow-up X-ray films.

Fractures were grouped into 8 types according to Frykman's classification [1]. The basic consideration of this classification depends upon whether or not there is a fracture involving any of the following 3 parts; the radiocarpal joint, distal radioulnar joint, and the ulnar styloid.

In principle, we treated these patients conservatively. The patient's wrist was immobilized

[1] The Department of Orthopaedics, Tokai University, Bohseidai, Isehara, Kanagawa 259–11, Japan

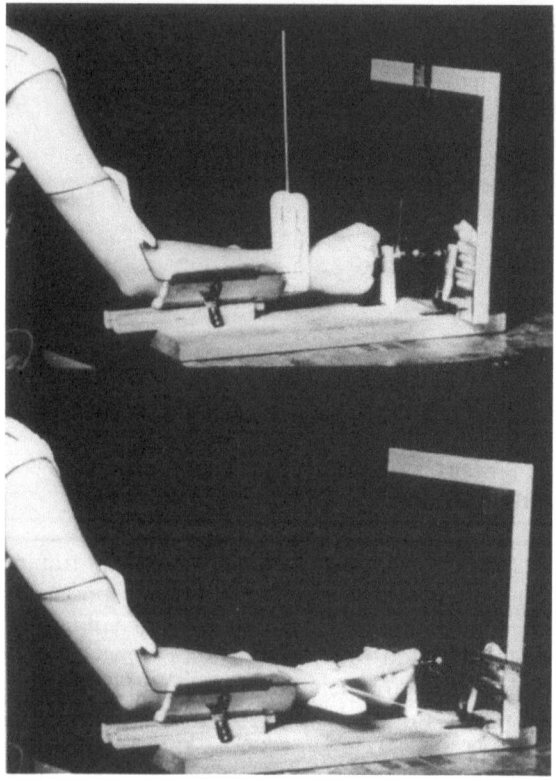

Fig. 1. Measurement of the rotational range using an original instrument

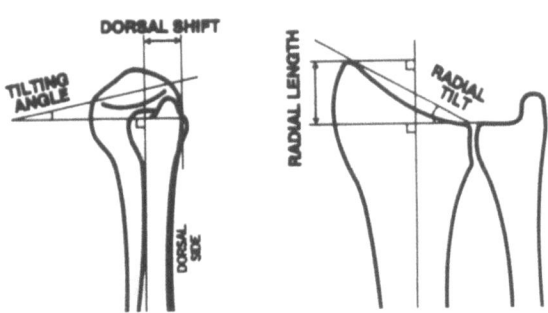

Fig. 2. X-ray measurements of four common parameters

with long-arm or sugar-tong splints immediately after undergoing closed reduction. Range of motion (ROM) exercise was started after immobilization and continued for 5 or 6 weeks. In this series, five patients were operated upon. Internal fixation with Kirschner wires or plates was used in all the operations. We have also used external fixation for the past few years but these cases were excluded from this study because of insufficient follow-up time.

Using our original instrument (Fig. 1), the range of rotation at follow-up was measured actively under 90° flexion of the elbow joint. The range of rotation on the affected side was expressed by comparison of the range of rotation on the opposite side, which was considered to be normal (100%).

In order to evaluate the residual deformity of the affected wrist, we measured four common features using follow-up X-ray films (Fig. 2). The angle of tilt indicated dorsal or volar tilt, the dorsal shift indicated the degree of lateral displacement to the dorsal side, the radial tilt showed the degree of radial or ulnar inclination, and the radial length indicated the grade of shortening. We measured these parameters by comparing the differences to the opposite side.

Clinical Results

Table 1 shows the fracture type at the time of injury. The incidence of type I was 44%, the most frequent type in our study.

At the time of examination, 15 patients (33%) complained of various symptoms in the affected wrist. The most frequent complaint was pain during motion (11 cases), and other complaints were loss of grip power (2), limitation of motion (1), and numbness (1). However, all complaints were slight, which did not cause any trouble in daily life.

The average range of rotation was 92.3% (Fig. 3). Twelve patients scored 100%, the same as that of the opposite side. The average range of supina-

Table 1. Fracture type according to Frykman's classification

Type	Radiocarpal joint	Distal radioulnar joint	Distal ulna	Case (n) (%)
I[a]	−	−	−	20 (44.4)
II	−	−	+	3 (6.6)
III	+	−	−	8 (17.8)
IV	+	−	+	0 (0.0)
V	−	+	−	5 (11.1)
VI	−	+	+	1 (2.2)
VII	+	+	−	4 (8.9)
VIII	+	+	+	0 (0.0)
Others				4 (8.9)

[a] Type I is an extra-articular fracture without a distal ulnar fracture

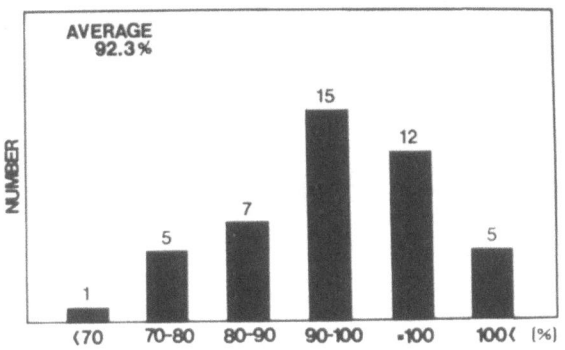

Fig. 3. Average range of rotation (pronation-supination)

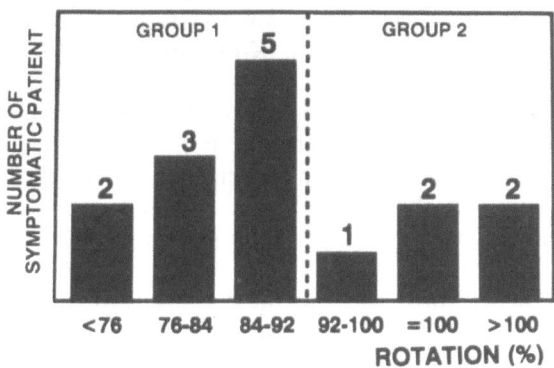

Fig. 5. The symptomatic patients in each group. The patients with a range of under 92% were assigned to group 1, and those over 92% to group 2

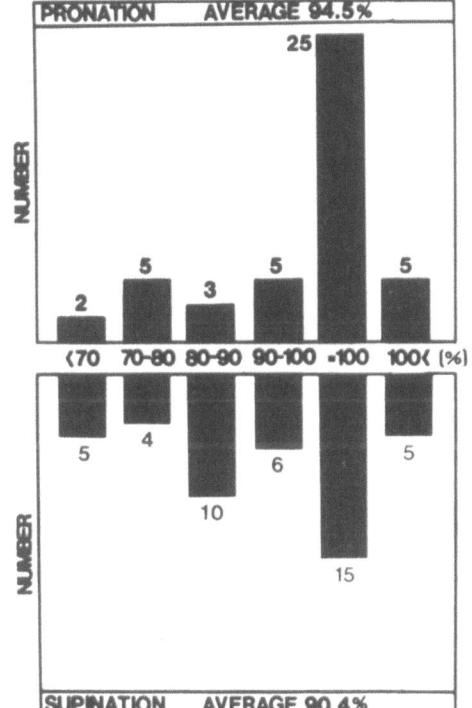

Fig. 4. Average range of pronation and supination

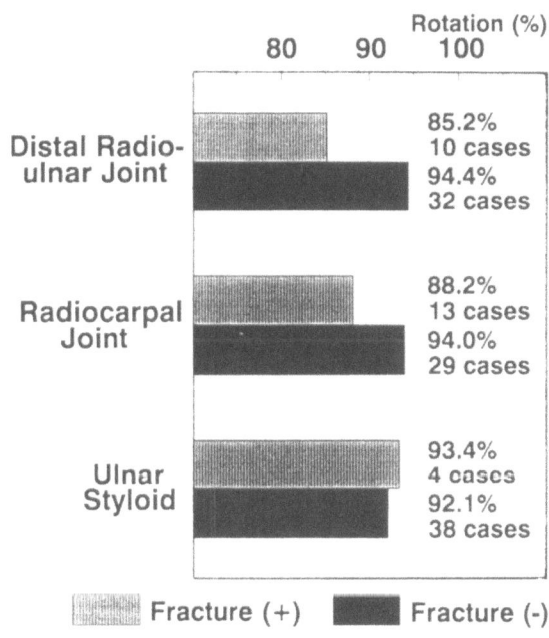

Fig. 6. Range of rotation of the 3 anatomical categories in Frykman's classification

tion was 90.4%, while that of pronation was 94.5%. The loss of supination was, therefore, more marked than that of pronation (Fig. 4).

The average range of rotation in cases of conservative therapy was 94.3 percent. Surgery was conducted in 1 case each of types I, III, and V, and 2 cases of type VII. The postoperative average range was 76.4%.

The average values of our measurements were as follows: the angle of tilt increased by 10.2° to the dorsal side, the dorsal shift increased by 2 mm,

the radial tilt decreased by 6°, and the radial length decreased by 3.3 mm. There was no significant relationship between the range of rotation and the values of each measurement.

We divided all the patients into 2 groups according to the range of rotation being greater or less than 92% because the proportions of symptomatic patients differed most significantly when patients were grouped according to this figure. The patients with a range of under 92% were assigned to group 1, and those over 92% to group 2 (Fig. 5).

We could not detect any significant difference for each value of the X-ray measurements in either group. Additionally, we found no significant difference of the range of rotation among the 8 types of Frykman's classification. Of the 3 anatomical categories in Frykman's classification, however, the average range of rotaiton in fractures involving the distal radioulnar joint was more decreased than in the other 2 sites (Fig. 6). The fractures involving the distal radioulnar joint comprised 38.5% of group 1, while, it was 17.2% of group 2 (Fig. 7). The proportional difference in both groups was most remarkable in these cases.

Materials and Methods in the Experimental Study

On the basis of these clinical results, small-scale experiments were designed to study the relationship between the rotation of the forearm and the residual deformity.

We used four preserved human upper-extremity cadaver specimens. These specimens were grossly

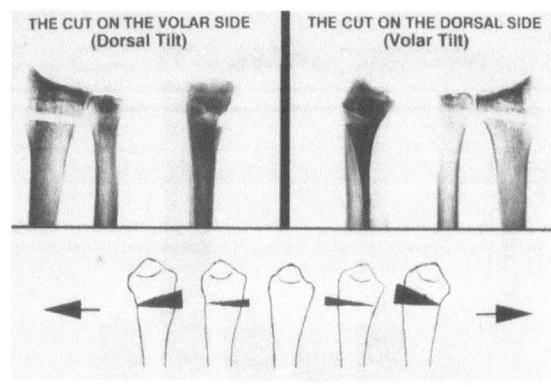

Fig. 8. Experimental method

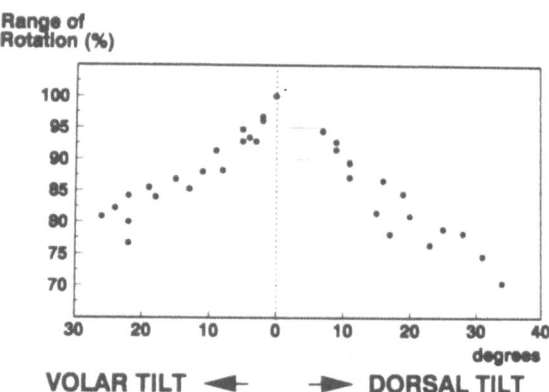

Fig. 9. Experimentally caused deformities

Distal Radioulnar Joint

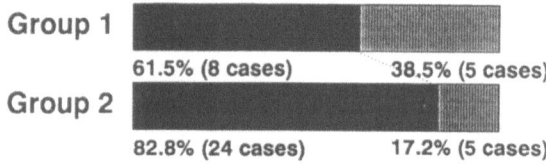

Group 1
61.5% (8 cases)   38.5% (5 cases)

Group 2
82.8% (24 cases)   17.2% (5 cases)

Radiocarpal Joint

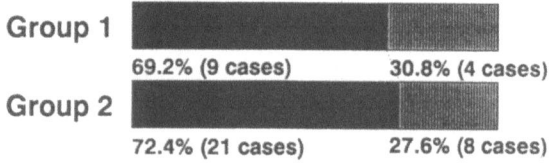

Group 1
69.2% (9 cases)   30.8% (4 cases)

Group 2
72.4% (21 cases)   27.6% (8 cases)

Ulnar Styloid

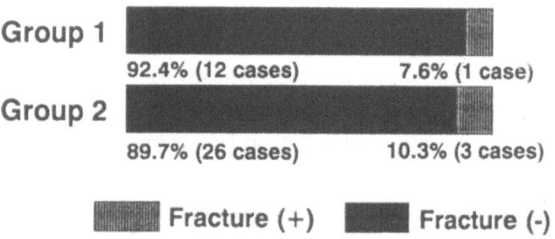

Group 1
92.4% (12 cases)   7.6% (1 case)

Group 2
89.7% (26 cases)   10.3% (3 cases)

░░░ Fracture (+)   ■■■ Fracture (−)

Fig. 7. The fracture involving the distal radioulnar joint comprised 38.5% of group 1 and 17.2% of group 2

Fig. 10. Experimental results

normal and X-ray film confirmed the absence of any apparent bony deformity. We amputated the hand at the wrist and excised the soft tissues of the specimen, leaving the interosseous membrane, the capsule and ligamentous tissue of the elbow joint, and the proximal radioulnar and distal radioulnar joints intact. The specimen was fixed as shown in Fig. 8, providing a stage that was parallel to the line from the radial head to the ulnar styloid process. We made a cross cut to the longitudinal axis of the radius at the proximal capsular attachment of the distal radioulnar joint on either the volar or dorsal side, leaving the opposite cortex intact. Experimental deformities were created with the inclining distal end of the radius by one of several angled wedged blocks that was inserted into the cut (Fig. 9). The range of rotation and the angle of tilt as demonstrated on X-ray were measured in each angle.

Experimental Results

The experimental results are shown in Fig. 10. We defined the initial range of 0° angle of tilt as 100%. Experimental results indicated that the range of rotation decreased together with an increase of both dorsal and volar tilts.

Discussion

In the clinical study, conspicuous loss of rotation appeared in cases of internal fixation. This was because we operated upon patients who had unstable fractures with severe displacement or comminution. We consider that the factors involved in causing limitation of rotation in the operative cases are the damage of soft tissue and the scar formation or adhesion around the fracture site.

Patrick [2] pointed out problems involving soft tissue and reported that the limitation of supination and pronation and the associated pain in patients with Colles' fracture were produced by adhesion or fibrosis of the displaced triangular fibrocartilage, and that there appeared to be no relationship between the degree of the original displacement and the extent of loss of rotation. In Gartland and Werley's analysis of a series of healed Colles' fractures [3], limitations of supination were seen in the cases showing loss of integrity of the distal radioulnar joint.

In our cases of the fracture involving the distal radioulnar joint, the clinical results were unsatisfactory. Therefore, it seems that the rotational disturbance was mainly related to the articulation on the distal radioulnar joint more than to the other two lesions in Frykman's classification.

The experimental fractures included only 1 type of fracture of the distal radius (Frykman's type I). However, experimental results have suggested that change of the angle of tilt induces loss of rotation. We suspect that a loss of rotation in the experiment could be mainly related to the maladaptation of the distal radioulnar joint and change of tension of the soft tissue around the joint. However, this relation was not made clear in the clinical study, and the rotational disturbance cannot solely be explained in relation to the angle of tilt. We suppose that all damaged soft tissues participate in rotational disturbance of the forearm in clinical cases.

Conclusions

We could not clinically determine any specific factors of rotational disturbance. However, based on experimental results, it seems that the fracture involving the distal radioulnar joint is a factor in causing the loss of rotation. Therefore, in order to prevent rotational disturbance, we urge clinicians to use caution while making the alignment of the distal radioulnar joint at the time of reduction procedure.

References

1. Frykman G (1967) Fracture of the distal radius including sequelae — shoulder-hand-finger syndrome, disturbance in the distal radio-ulnar joint and impairment of nerve function. A clinical and experimental study. Acta Orthop Scand Suppl 108
2. Patrick J (1946) A study of supination and pronation, with especial reference to the treatment of forearm fractures. J Bone Joint Surg [Am] 28:737–748
3. Gartland JJ, Werley CW (1951) Evaluation of healed Colles' fractures. J Bone Joint Surg [Am] 33:895–907

Bone Cementing in the Treatment of Distal Radius Fracture in Elderly Patients

Yoshiro Kiyoshige[1]

Abstract. The fracture of the distal end of the radius in elderly patients (more than 75 years of age) were treated with internal fixation by filling the cavity with bone cement.

A longitudinal dorsal incision exposed the fracture between the ECR and FPL tendons. Reduction was secured with a K-wire and the dorsal cortical bone was fenestrated and filled with bone cement. After cementing, the fenestrated dorsal cortical bone was replaced on top of the cement.

After surgery, the wrist remained free from external fixation. The results were evaluated in terms of wrist motion (ROM: range of motion), finger motion (PPD: palp palm distance), grip strength, and bone atrophy. Bone atrophy was measured with the MD method (2nd metacarpal bone density).

Compared with the conventional cast-wearing method (including percutaneous pinning) PPD remained normal, ROM recovered early, and bone atrophy was minimal after using our technique. Grip strength was regained in proportion to the decrease in pain. As an example of fine motor ability, some patients could comfortably use chopsticks to eat their breakfast on the morning after the operation.

The cementing procedure appears to be a superior therapy in view of the patient's quality of life.

Keywords: Bone cement — Treatment — Fracture — Distal radius — Elderly patient

Introduction

Fracture of the distal end of the radius is being encountered with growing frequency in daily practice because of recent increases in the percentage of the elderly within the total population. The fracture is usually treated by manual reduction followed by cast fixation. If the fracture is comminuted, open reduction followed by internal fixation or else extra-skeletal fixation is performed. In elderly patients, however, the alignment after reduction is difficult to preserve. Furthermore, firm internal fixation is difficult due to the tendency towards osteoporosis of the bones in these patients. Finally, if the external fixation is prolonged, the onset of severe bone atrophy or reflex sympathetic dystrophy (RSD) sometimes makes it difficult to use to the affected hand even when bony fusion has been successfully achieved.

For these reasons, we treated this fracture in the elderly by surgery (intramedullary cement fixation) without using external fixation, and instructed the patient to actively use the hand immediately after the operation. This technique has produced excellent results.

Patients and Methods

The ages of the five patients ranged from 75 to 87 years (mean 81.2 years) and all were females. The right side was affected in three cases and the left side in the other two. All patients were right-handed (Table 1).

Intramedullary fixation with bone cement was performed within 2 days of the injury. In all cases, manual reduction was performed under an axillary block, and the reduced position was transcutaneously maintained with a K-wire. A dorsal longitudinal incision was made to separate the extensor carpi radialus (ECR) and extensor pollicis longus (EPL) tendons. When necessary, the proximal portion of the extensor retinaculum was partially dissected in order to expose the fractured area. The dorsal cortex of the fracture area was fenestrated (about 15×10 mm), while the

[1] Department of Orthopaedic Surgery, Saiseikai Yamagata Hospital, 2-3-1 Koshirakawa, Yamagata 990, Japan

Table 1. Cases

No.	Age (years)	Sex	Affected side	Comment
1	77	F	Lt	Volar sprint in place for 4 weeks
2	87	F	Rt	
3	75	F	Rt	
4	83	F	Lt	
5	84	F	Rt	Also distal ulnar fracture

Lt, Left, *Rt*, right

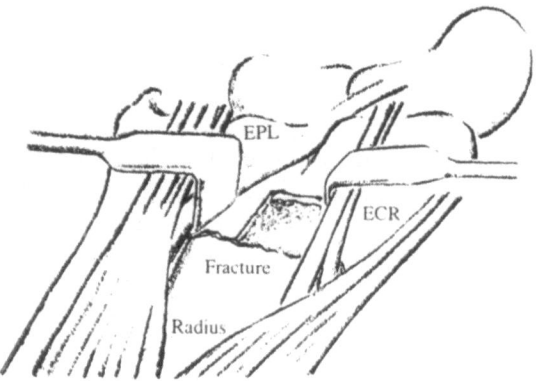

Fig. 1. Surgical procedure. Under axillary block, the fracture was reduced and temporarily fixed with a K-wire. The fracture was exposed between the extensor carpiradialus (*ECR*) and extensor pollicis longus (*EPL*) tendons. The dorsal cortex of the fracture area was fenestrated and the medullary bone deficiency was filled with bone cement. The dorsal cortex was returned on top of the cement

periosteum was preserved as much as possible. The fracture now had the appearance of a bony window. Because the bone in these elderly patients was porotic, the cancellous bone in the fractured area had already collapsed. The medullary cavity was enlarged with a sharp spoon so that a sufficient amount of cement could be introduced. After careful washing and removal of blood through suction, the cavity was filled with bone cement. The dorsal cortical bone which had been removed to create the fenestra was put back on top of the cement (Fig. 1). In earlier cases, we cut the K-wire (used for maintaining the reduced position) at a point very close to the cortex, and the remaining piece of wire was left within the bone to serve as a "core". In recent cases, however, we have removed the K-wire completely before the cement had hardened. Next, as much of the periosteum as possible was sutured in order to create a covering for the fenestra. Finally, the wound was closed. After the operation, a splint was used for 4 weeks in the first case according to the procedure of Nilsson [1] and Schmalholz [2]. For the remaining 4 cases, only elastic bandage was used after the oparation. All patients were instructed to go through the full range of motions as long as these could be performed without pain; they were told, however, not to raise themselves by pushing down on the operated wrist. Active ROM exercise was started within the framework of physical therapy, and the patients could return to normal activities without the need for passive ROM exercise.

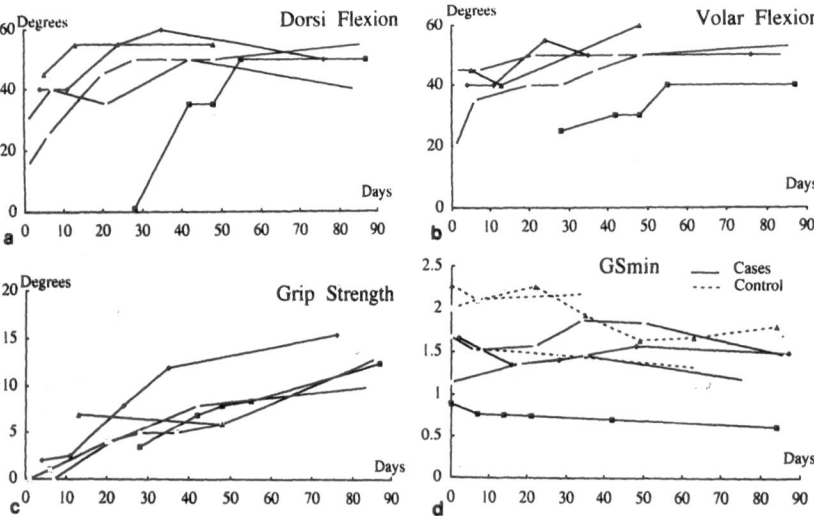

Fig. 2a–d. Range of motion recovered rapidly except for case 1 in which a splint was worn for 4 weeks. Grip strength was regained in proportion to the decrease in pain. Bone atrophy was measured with the micro-densitometry (MD) method. The decrease in the value of GS min for patients treated with cementing was minimal compared with that for control patients who were middle-aged and had worn a cast for 4 weeks

Results

In all cases, X-ray films were used to examine the time course of wrist joint ROM (dorsi-flexion, volar-flexion, radial deviation, ulnar deviation, pronation, and supination), grip strength, palp palm distance, and bone atrophy.

In all but one patient (who wore a splint for 4 weeks), maximum ROM for dorsi- and volar flexion and radial and ulnar deviation was achieved in about 2 weeks (Fig. 2a, b) and maximum ROM for pronation and supination in about 3 weeks. The grip strength tended to improve following the disappearance of pain, this occurring slightly later then ROM improvement. In these 4 cases, palp palm distance reached 0 mm for all fingers within 1 week after the operation. Bone fusion, as observed on X-ray films, was completed in 6–7 weeks, while callus formation occurred simultaneously around the cortex of the fenestra (Fig. 3.c). The postoperative alignment on the surface of the distal radius was preserved throughout the follow-up period. When the extent of bone atrophy was assessed with the microdensitometry (MD) method (GS min, which reflects cancellous bone density), the results for our cases were comparable

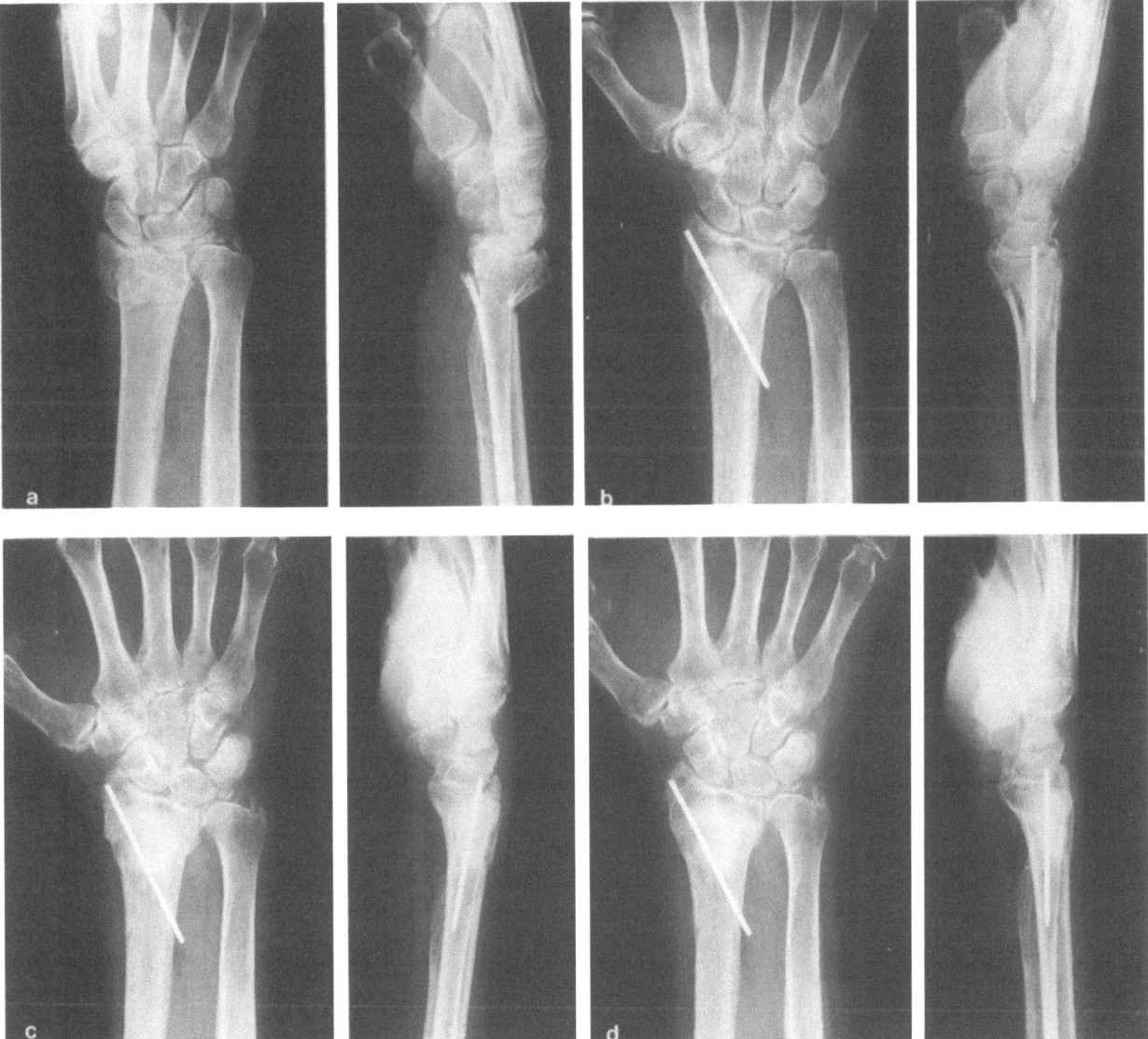

Fig. 3a–d. Case 2 (an 87-year-old female). **a** Preoperative X-rays of the distal radius fracture. **b** Immediately after the operation. **c** Seven weeks postoperatively. The cement is surrounded by cortical bone. **d** There is no sign of bone atrophy

to those for cast-wearing middle-aged patients (Fig. 2.d). X-ray film of the carpal bone also showed no sign of bone atrophy (Fig. 3.d).

Discussion

The use of bone cement in the treatment of fracture of the distal end of radius was first reported by Charnley in 1970 [3]. At present, its clinical use is restricted to some of the northern European countries [1, 2, 4].

The recent sharp increase in the percentege of the elderly in the general population has led to a proportional increase in the number of patients with osteoporosis. In the year 2000, the number of patients in Japan with this disease is estimated to reach 5.3 million, with the annual incidence of fracture of the distal end of radius estimated at 115,000 cases. Conventional treatment of this fracture in the elderly, however, may lead to several problems. Wearing a cast on the wrist for a long time causes RSD and shoulder contracture. Even when bone fusion is achieved, these complications can make it impossible for the individual to use the hand. Furthermore, external fixation sometimes causes elderly patients to be excessively concerned about their condition, leading to exaggerated protection of the affected hand which, in turn, increases the incidence of RSD.

Taking into account the attitudes and the quality of life of the elderly, we suggest that our technique, one which does not require postoperative external fixation, should be considered for these patients.

Conclusions

Fractures of the distal end of the radius in elderly individuals were treated with surgery in which bone cement was used. Wrist joint ROM, grip strength, and PPD were judged as excellent early in the postoparative period, and no bone atrophy was observed postoperatively. Therefore this technique seems to be especially suitable for elderly patients in terms of enhancing their quality of life.

References

1. Nilsson MH (1979) Bone cementing in the treatment of Colles' fracture. Opuscula Medica 24:123–125
2. Schmalholz A (1989) Bone cement for redislocated Colles' fracture. A prospective comparison with closed treatment. Acta Orthop Scand 60:212–217
3. Charnley J (1970) Acrylic cement in orthopedic surgery. Churchill Livingstone, Edinburgh, pp 67–71
4. Kofoed H (1983) Communited displaced Colles' fracture: Treatment with intramedullary methyl metacrylate stabilization. Acta Orthop Scand 54:307–311

Part V. Carpal Instability and Wrist Pain

Carpal Instability — A Review

JAMES H. DOBYNS[1]

Keywords: Wrist — Carpus — Injury — Dislocation — Subluxation — Instability

Introduction

The concept of carpal instability has been discussed for many years [1–12] but it has assumed greater importance as it became obvious that many management problems were directly related to instability [1, 3–5, 7, 8, 10–16]. The unique anatomy, kinetics, and kinematics of the wrist joint [9, 14, 17–38] have intrigued many generations of investigators. In an attempt to simplify the pathomechanical mechanisms of injury, the wrist has been likened to a series of interdependent, roughly parallel joint systems, lying transversely in the coronal plane [19–24, 26, 27, 31, 36–38]; they include a series of columns which assist thumb function radially, flexion-extension centrally, and forearm rotation ulnarly [11, 12, 29]; a ring of bones, the proximal and distal carpal rows, with potential instability between each bone and between the rows [12, 39], and combinations of all these mechanisms [1, 12, 14]. Historically, little attention was paid to problems of carpal instability because they were not recognized except sporadically [2, 9, 29, 40, 41], particularly as they affected the healing of the very common fracture of the scaphoid [4, 5, 42]. Dislocations with and without fractures were recognized as being unstable, but their residual instabilities and the similar instabilities that developed without obvious dislocation were identified by few investigators [2, 5, 9, 29, 41]. Beginning in the 1970s, a few articles [3, 4, 6, 7, 21, 28, 34, 43, 44] attracted attention; a torrent of anatomic, laboratory, and clinical investigation has resulted worldwide. It even became apparent that the oldest problem of all, that of scaphoid delayed, non- and mal-union was commonly associated with instability [1, 4, 10, 11, 13, 45]. The first instability, not due to fracture or dislocation, was the ligamentous analogue of the scaphoid fracture, scapholunate dissociation [2, 3, 6, 7, 28, 34, 43, 46]. Other specific instabilities were swiftly identified [1, 8, 10–12, 15, 39, 47–50]. Since the wrist appears to function and to dysfunction in all the ways suggested, some investigators [1, 14] have tried to classify them by naming the emerging clinical entities by their unique characteristics and anatomic sites, and by fitting them into the old classic categories of fracture, sprain, dislocation, and fracture-dislocation. This will be presented later in table form, but first, with a new terminology having been gradually developed, the author's definitions of the terms used in this review will be given.

General Terminology and Definitions

Carpal Instability

This refers to the loss of natural relationships, anatomic or kinematic, of carpal bones to each other or to the skeletal elements just proximal or distal to the carpus. The following are injuries that may cause carpal instability.

Fracture: a discontinuity of trabeculae, either cortical or cancellous. Most instability seen with a fracture is due to associated or to pre-injury ligamentous laxity or damage. However, a fracture with sufficient loss of bone or of configuration may lead to immediate instability of the carpus. Even if originally stable, secondary loss of bone substance or bone configuration may lead to secondary instability; furthermore, chronic

[1] The Hand Center of San Antonio, 7940 Floyd Curl Drive #900, San Antonio, TX 78229, USA

inflammation at the fracture site may lead to capsuloligamentous attentuation, which will also lead to secondary instability.

Sprain: a discontinuity of ligamentous fibers. Like fracture, the damage may be insufficient to cause immediate instability or it may be sufficient to immediately change the relationships of the carpal elements to any degree less than dislocation. Like fracture, pre-existing damage or laxity or secondary attenuation will affect the presence and degree of instability. Instability developing from a sprain is called a *subluxation* or *partial dislocation*.

Dislocation (luxation): also a discontinuity of ligamentous fibers, but with sufficient instability that two or more normally related and congruent joint surfaces have lost contact and alignment.

Fracture-dislocation: similar to a dislocation except that one or more major fracture fragments (>5 mm in greatest dimension) are present. The anatomical locations of carpal instability are: *radiocarpal* (RC), *perilunate* (pL), *mid-carpal* (M-C), *axial* (AX), *axial-radial* (AX-R) and *axial-ulnar* (AX-U). The collapse positions or positions of deformity are:

1. *Dorsal intercalated segment instability (DISI)*: an extension position of the lunate or of the entire proximal carpal row (PCR). If all elements of the PCR are linked normally and are in extension as a group, the deformity is classified as CIND-DISI; if the PCR elements are dissociated, the deformity is CID-DISI.
2. *Volar intercalated segment instability (VISI)*: a flexion position of the lunate or of the entire proximal carpal row. As with DISI, this deformity may be a CIND-VISI or CID-VISI.
3. *Ulnar translation (UT)*: an ulnar shift of the lunate position vis-à-vis the radius (the normal percentage of the lunate articulating with the radius is about 80% according to Razemon [30] although the spectrum of normal may range as far as 50% — this should be judged by the opposite wrist). The lunate and triquetrum of the PCR may shift in isolation, leaving the scaphoid in its standard position, UT with SLD, or the entire PCR may shift in unison.
4. *Dorsal translation (DT)*: a dorsal shift of the entire proximal carpal row, usually of the entire carpus.
5. *Palmar (or "volar" or "ventral") translation*: a palmar shift of the proximal carpal row, usually of the entire carpus.

Other Descriptive Terms That Are Often Used

Static: an abnormal relationship of the carpal elements, as visualized on standard PA and lateral X-rays, present at rest as well as with motion or other stress.

Dynamic: an abnormal relationship of the carpal elements as visualized by any imaging method, provoked by any stress, i.e., from motion, gripping, compression, etc.

Carpal Instability Dissociative (CID): loss of the natural relationships of individual carpal bones to each other. Although not exclusively, this is usually seen in the PCR as either scapholunate dissociation (SLD) or triquetrolunate dissociation (TLD), or both.

Carpal Instability Non-Dissociative (CIND): loss of the natural relationships of proximal or distal carpal rows to each other or to the skeletal elements, just proximal or distal to the carpus. The usual deformities seen are excessive extension or flexion, but others are possible, i.e., translational or rotational. The most common problems are seen at the radiocarpal or midcarpal level or both. Except for a few references [1, 14, 47], the literature discusses these problems as some form of midcarpal instability [11, 39, 40, 49, 50], but exactly the same deformity; CIND-VISI, CIND-DISI or alternating between the two, can be produced by radiocarpal instability or a combination of RC and M-C instability. Severe radiocarpal lesions, however, nearly always have some degree of ulnar translation as well.

Carpal Instability Combined or Complex (CIC): many carpal injuries, either initially from the severity of the stress or secondarily from increasing ligament attenuation, show elements of more than one category of wrist injury, such as CID and CIND or CID and UT. Indeed, current research suggests that the late or extreme stages of most carpal instabilities show such combined damage [15]. Nevertheless, an understanding of the characteristic damage responsible for the early deformity of each lesion is well worth knowing for both diagnostic and treatment purposes.

Carpal Instability Potential (CIP). There are certain higher risk factors to be found in many wrists. These include the "lax" wrist, whether accompanied by generalized systemic laxity or only involving certain joints, many osseous developmental differences, such as ulna positive or negative configuration, alterations of radial slope, lunate positioning on the radius, carpal coalitions, and others. Disease, infection, tumor, and other pathologies also place the carpus at increased risk, but, above all, the effect of prior trauma or continuing trauma adds to the risk potential for carpal instability. *Carpal instability potential traumatic (CIPT)* is, therefore, a frequent factor in determining the extent of a developing carpal instability.

Other Terms and Abbreviations

These are mostly straightforward anatomic terms: radiocarpal joint (RC or RCJ), mid-carpal joint (M-C), carpometacarpal joint (CMC), distal radioulnar joint (D/RU), ulnocarpal joint (UC), proximal carpal row (PCR), distal carpal row (DCR), radioscaphoid joint (RS), radiolunate joint (RL), scapholunate joint (SL), triquetrolunate joint (TL), capitolunate joint (CL), triquetrohamate joint (TH), scaphotrapezio-trapezoidal joint (STT), capitohamate joint (CH), scaphocapitate joint (SC), radius (R), ulna (U), triangular fibrocartilage (TFC), scaphoid (S), lunate (L), triquetrum (T), capitate (C), hamate (H), pisiform (P), trapezoid (Tzd), trapezium (Tzm), radial styloid (RSty).

The term "trans" is used to indicate discontinuity through bone, as in trans-scaphoid. The term "peri" is used here to indicate "around bone" as in perilunate. Anatomical terms are used to indicate the site of injury; diagnostic terms are used to indicate the type of injury. Some terms in common use such as "rotary subluxation of the scaphoid" are thought to be redundant and are not used here.

Additional Terminology and Definitions

Specific Dislocations [10–12, 28, 48]

It is difficult to understand the language of carpal instability without an understanding of the most frequently occurring forms of carpal instability, the dislocations and fracture-dislocations. The patterns formed by these high-energy injuries indicate the areas of strength and of weakness of the delicately balanced carpal support systems. By far, the most common stress injury is that of loading in extension, resulting in traction stresses applied along the palmar aspect of the wrist and impaction and shear stresses along the dorsal aspect. The most common injury involving the

carpus is tension rupture of the palmar cortices of the radius. This may involve bone alone, such as in, Colles and Smith's fractures, but often involves the ligamentous origins of the palmar radiocarpal ligaments, sufficiently so that the most common type of radiocarpal dislocation is a fracture-dislocation. There are many types of these but the most common are the radialstyloid fracture-dislocation (fx-dn), the volar (or palmar) Barton's fx-dn, and the dorsal Barton's fx-dn. Of the three, the radial styloid fx-dn is more apt to be associated with a perilunate fx-dn than a radiocarpal fx-dn, because the strong ligamentous investment between the radius and lunate often remains partially intact. This stronger support of the lunate, compared to the scaphoid, is the reason that the most common type of carpal dislocation is the perilunate pattern, which is a combination of radiocarpal and midcarpal dislocations. Since the scaphoid, unique within the proximal carpal row, extends to and participates in formation of the mid-carpal joint, it too is subjected to inordinate tension stresses and fractures, more commonly than any regional bone other than the radius. The most common of all carpal dislocation patterns, then, is the trans-scaphoid, perilunate fracture-dislocation. Again, at the carpometacarpal level, ligament support is so sturdy that the most common dislocation pattern is that of fracture-dislocation. The same is true of the axial or longitudinal dislocation patterns for the same reason. At any of these levels, RC, pL, M-C, CMC, and AX, pure ligamentous dislocations are possible, although rare, with the following sequence representing the clinical incidence: pL > RC > CMC > AX > M-C.

Carpal Instability Tables

A table could be constructed for the possible variations of instabilities associated with the fractures of the wrist bones, but such was not part of this presentation and will not be given here. Suffice it to say that there are many interesting ways in which fractures may affect carpal instabilities in addition to the most common reason, that of associated ligamentous damage at the time of bone injury. Radial fractures, as they collapse, alter the surface available for normal carpal conjunct rotations and translations to occur; the altered movement patterns strain, stretch, and attenuate ligaments, which may already be

Table 1. Categories of carpal instability*

Site	Ligament/injury			Ligament/bone injury
	Subluxation	Dislocation		FX-SBLX/DN
RC	CIND-DISI CIND-VISI Both, alternating UT DT PT	Dorsal Palmar Ulnar Radial		Volar Barton's Dorsal Barton's Radiostyloid (may be CID, CIND, UT) Lunate fossa (may be CID, CIND, UT, DT, PT)
pL	CID-DISI (SLD) CID-VISI (TLD)	pL to Lunate (Stages I-V)		Trans-osseous pL t-RSty-pL, t-S-pL, and many others
M-C	CIND-VISI, CIND-DISI (or alternating but due to an MCI cause at TH, CL, STT, or all)	Dorsal Palmar		Trans-osseous M-CI Doral Palmar
CMC +MC +DCR	Axial (not yet observed)	Axial		Axial Axial-radial Axial-ulnar Combinations

* All instabilities within or between categories may be combined. Definitions of the abbreviations are in the text

damaged, and subsequent additional collapse patterns may occur. Fractures of the bones of the proximal carpal row, if they are sagittal plane fractures, introduce a dissociative type of instability until they stabilize by either fibrous or bony healing, after which a continuing instability pattern becomes more like a non-dissociative or a combined pattern. If the PCR fracture is in the coronal (frontal) plane, it is more likely to destabilize in a non-dissociative pattern. Sprains, like fractures, may not be severe enough to cause destabilization, at least right away, but like stable fractures, they are still symptomatic and deserve treatment to facilitate healing and to prevent them from progressing to the point of instability. When sprains do permit instability, they are called subluxations; when there are associated fractures, an appropriate term is that of fracture-subluxation. These fracture-subluxations are identical to ligamentous subluxations, except that major fracture fragments are present and are the same as fracture-dislocations, but dislocation has not yet occurred. Axial disruptions, which are much more common as fracture-dislocations, are the result of high-energy forces applied to the palmar, dorsal, or both surfaces in such a way as to flatten out the carpal arch. As expected, this usually results in collapse of the carpal canal and, in longitudinal or axial disruption of the carpus, splitting it into columns. Metacarpals are usually involved along with the distal carpal row and the proximal carpal row is sometimes involved as well. The number of units involved is variable, but the injuries can be sub-categorized as axial-radial, axial-ulnar, or combinations. Table 1 summarizes the clinical carpal instabilities that have been identified.

Diagnosis of Carpal Instabilities

The usual judicious mix of history, clinical findings, and imaging will usually confirm or strongly suggest the diagnosis. However, the condition occasionally is so insidious that it is not authenticated until arthroscopy, surgery, secondary surgery, or with the passage of time with the development of more characteristic findings. Since the degree of damage varies from moderate sprains to near amputations, it is obvious that the specifics of case history and the definitive nature of both clinical and imaging studies are highly variable. The more dramatic problems of dislocation and fracture-dislocation are usually identified, although the complexities of each are still missed on many occasions. In most centers where wrist problems are common, the static subluxation instabilities are also fairly well recognized even by radiologists who were late in becoming interested in this field. The principal diagnostic problems currently concern the dynamic group of carpal instabilities, where diagnosis often depends on a provocative maneuver, either by the patient or by an examiner, or on a special imaging study or clinical visualization at arthroscopy or surgery. While MRI shows promise for the future, particularly with enhancement of ligaments, the best diagnostic yield is currently obtained from video imaging of both wrists by carrying out a complete range of motion, followed by gripping and any other provocative maneuvers known to the patient or designed by the investigator, followed by a three-compartment arthrogram with motion and grip stress utilized after each dye introduction. Arthroscopy is also often worthwhile to confirm the video findings, but particularly to assess the state of the articular cartilage, which is very important in the planning of treatment. Regardless of the diagnosis, pre-operative assessment should include functional evaluation of wrist capability after rest and appropriate strengthening, after alteration of the provocative activities, and with or without any support that may be available or can be specifically devised for the particular problem. This point is made because there are many individuals with carpal instability who are able to maintain near-normal activity by lifestyle alteration or selective protection. Until surgical/rehabilitation management catches up with diagnostic capability, this type of symptom control is well worth considering. The specifics of diagnosis for each clinical entity are beyond the scope of this review but are available [1, 10, 11, 48].

Treatment of Carpal Instabilities

As referred to previously in the "diagnosis" discussion, many patients with CI are quite satisfied with controlled or protected wrist activity; many do not even seek medical attention until they are past the possibilities of repair/reconstruction and can only be considered for salvage surgery. It does not help this situation that there is still considerable controversy in the most informed circles about both the methods and the effectiveness of the treatments. It is fair to say that surgical

management is still in the developmental stage. Again, it is beyond the scope of a review article to cover the many conditions and the many treatments in detail, but the following is an outline of the conditions and the usual treatments will also be provided [1, 10, 11, 39, 46, 48, 51, 52].

Carpal Instability — Current Name (N), Category (C), and Treatment (T)

N Ulnar translation (UT)

C Radiocarpal instability, UT type

T Early: ligaments identifiable, joint satisfactory. Reduce, repair/tighten all ligaments, palmar and dorsal; control with IF, EF, or both types of fixation for 8–12 weeks.

Late: difficult or unstable reduction or ligaments are a mass of scar. Radiolunate or radioscapholunate fusion.

Late: severely limited range of motion (ROM) and radiocarpal damage but fair to good lunate sulcus and capitate head; proximal row carpectomy (PRC).

N Dorsal translation (DT)

C Radiocarpal instability, DT type

T If associated with mal-union of a radial fracture (extension slope of the distal radial articular surface), this is not a true RCI but merely positional (in Europe "adaptive carpus"); treat with corrective radial osteotomy. If true RCI, treat as in UT, i.e., reduce and repair, if feasible; consider RC fusion or PRC, if not.

N Palmar Translation (PT)

C Radiocarpal instability, PT type

T If associated with mal-union of distal R fx. (flexion slope of the radial articular surface), treat with a corrective osteotomy of the radius (as with the other type of radial mal-union, bone graft is usually needed).

N Scapholunate Dissociation (SLD)

C Perilunate instability: radial component

T Early: easily reduced and maintained; joint surfaces in good condition. Treat with soft-tissue reconstruction. Several different ones are available [1, 11, 12]; the author's favorite is: (1) repair of the SL interosseous ligament, (2) construct a scaphoid tether dorsally from the radius to the distal scaphoid, (3) construct a lunate tether dorsally from the dorsal horn of the lunate to the base of the third metacarpal, and (4) 8 weeks' fixation. If unstable but joint surfaces are satisfactory, treat as discussed under intermediate.

Intermediate: if same conditions are met as in "early", treat the same way. If not easily reduced or quite unstable post reduction but joint surfaces are satisfactory, reduce scaphoid, then treat with a stabilizing intercarpal fusion (STT or SC) plus construction of a dorsal lunate tether, as described in "early". If as just described but with significant damage to the radioscaphoid joint surfaces, reduce scaphoid and fuse to radius; if lunate is reducible, construct dorsal lunate tether; fix in position for 8 weeks.

Other: if none of the above conditions are met, treat with one of the salvage procedures, e.g., SLAC wrist procedure, PRC, RC, or RMC fusion, etc.

N Triquetrolunate (luno- or lunatotriquetral) dissociation

C Perilunate instability: ulnar component

T Early: if easily reducible and minimally unstable, repair TL interosseous ligament and construct dorsal tethers, one from the dorsal lunate horn to the radius, the other from the dorsum of the triquetrum to the base of the third metacarpal. Stabilize position with percutaneous fixation for 8 weeks. If unstable but major joint surfaces are satisfactory, reduce and perform lunotriquetral fusion.

Other: (1) ulnocarpal impingement and other distal ulna instability problems are common associates of LTD and may be the only conditions requiring treatment. (2) It is not easy, but it is very important to distinguish between LTD (a CID diagnosis) and CIND-VISI or CIC-VISI. If the latter diagnoses are the correct ones, the usual LTD treatment will not improve the deformity and may make it worse. (3) Fixed deformity, uncontrollable instability, or significant arthritis require salvage procedures such as PRC, fusion, etc.

N Proximal carpal row instability (PCRI)

C Carpal instability non-dissociative (CIND)

T Early: an occasional episode of acute deformity, VISI, DISI or both in alternating fashion will be seen after a single episode of trauma with definite localizing findings, i.e., avulsion of the insertion of the radiolunotriquetral dorsal ligament, rupture of the ulnar arm of the arcuate ligament or of the STT ligaments palmarly, etc. Such rare episodes can be treated satisfactorily with direct repair. However, most PCRI deformities are insidious in development and a

large number occur in higher-risk CIP individuals with lax wrist joints. When identified early (i.e., when still reducible) when only mildly unstable and with good joint surfaces, these can be treated satisfactorily by reducing the deformity and fixing the position with percutaneous fixation for 8–10 weeks after tightening the lax ligamentous areas dorsally and palmarly, and augmenting them with ligament or tendon graft reinforcement where necessary. The areas of capsuloligamentous reconstruction depend upon the presenting deformity, i.e., DISI or VISI. With a DISI deformity, one tightens/augments at the radiocarpal level palmarly, and dorsally at the midcarpal level or from the PCR to the MC bases. With a VISI deformity, it is preferable to tighten/augment the "space of Poirier", the ulnar arm of the arcuate ligament, and the STT palmar ligaments palmarly and the radiocarpal area dorsally. An occasional PCRI, usually presenting in negative ulnar variance, can clinically be controlled by direct pressure at the ulnar side of the triquetrum; such wrists may respond to ulnar lengthening to produce a slight positive ulnar variance, although even these may also benefit from capsuloligamentous tightening.

Late: markedly unstable PCRI is best treated by fusion, but the appropriate level of fusion may be difficult to determine, i.e., RC or M-C. If in doubt, temporary fixation of one joint system followed by passive stressing of the other often helps. If still in doubt, it is probably best to fuse the radiocarpal joint after aligning the PCR with both the radius and the DCR. RC fusion will not only control the VISI or DISI instability, but will stabilize any tendency toward UD, a problem which presents after many midcarpal fusions. With fixed deformity, significant joint damage, or other complicating factors, salvage with the usual procedures is indicated.

Addenda: (1) dislocations or fracture-dislocations are not included in this discussion of treatment for instability since their treatment is fairly well understood and outlined in many texts, including [1, 10, 11]. (2) Other categorizing systems are in use in the literature and alternate names are used for the conditions discussed above. The more common of these terms are: proximal carpal instability for radiocarpal instability, lateral carpal instability or rotary subluxation of the scaphoid for SLD, medial carpal instability for TLD, midcarpal instability, capitolunate instability, or mid-carpal anteromedial instability (MAMI) for PCRI or CIND. If the midcarpal instability is thought to be due to problems of the ulnar and palmar arcuate ligament, it may be called medial midcarpal instability; if the problem is felt to be at the palmar STT area, it may be called lateral midcarpal instability.

Conclusion

The motion requirements of the wrist in support of the most adaptable terminal effector in biology have resulted in a precariously balanced system of bones, joints, and control elements. The stability of the joint systems, particularly the closely inter-related carpal joint systems, is altered subtly as well as dramatically by many different lesions. Recognition of the individual clinical conditions has developed slowly over the last 40 years. A gradual understanding of the stages of these conditions and their inter-relationships is currently underway. Such understanding is altering the therapeutic techniques in the usual manner, i.e., by making it clear that no one technique is applicable to all stages of any of the instability problems. It is also becoming apparent that the instabilities overlap or combine more often than was previously thought. The instability factor is so important in the prognosis of all carpal injuries that it appears reasonable to include all of the common mechanical injuries in the instability categories.

References

1. Cooney WP, Linscheid RL, Dobyns JH (1991) Fractures and dislocations of the wrist. In: Rockwood CA Jr, Green DP, Bucholz RW (eds) Fractures in adults. Lippincott, Philadelphia, pp 563–678
2. Destot E (1926) Traumatismes du poignet et rayons X. Masson, Paris
3. Dobyns JH, Linscheid RL, Chao EYS, Weber ER, Swanson GE (1975) Traumatic instability of the wrist. In: Instructional course lectures, American Academy of Orthopedic Surgeons (Vol 24). Mosby, St. Louis pp 182–199
4. Fisk GR (1970) Carpal instability and the fractured scaphoid Ann R Coll Surg Engl 46:63–76
5. Gilford WW, Bolton RH, Lambrinudi C (1943) The mechanism of the wrist joint: With special reference to fractures of the scaphoid. Guys Hosp Rep 92:52–59
6. Gilula LA, Weeks PM (1978) Posttraumatic ligamentous instabilities of the wrist. Radiology 129:645–651
7. Linscheid RL, Dobyns JH, Beabout JW, Bryan RS (1972) Traumatic instability of the wrist. J Bone Joint Surg [Am] 54:1612–1632
8. Linscheid RL, Dobyns JH (1984) The unified concept of carpal injuries. Ann Chir Main 3:35–39
9. McConaill MA (1941) The mechanical anatomy of the carpus and its bearings on some surgical problems. J Anat 75:166–175
10. Sennwald G (1987) The wrist. Anatomical and pathophysiological approach to diagnosis and treatment. Churchill Livingstone, New York
11. Taleisnik J (1985) The wrist. Churchill Livingstone, New York
12. Taleisnik J (1988) Carpal instability: Current concepts review. J Bone Joint Surg [Am] 70:1262–1268
13. Cooney WP, Dobyns JH, Linscheid RL (1980) Fractures of the scaphoid: A rational approach to management. Clin Orthop 149:90–97
14. Cooney WP, Garcia-Elias M, Dobyns JH, Linscheid RL (1989) Anatomy and mechanics of carpal instability. Surg Rounds Orthop 1:15–24
15. Horii E, Garcia-Elias M, An KN, Bishop AT, Cooney WP, Linscheid RL, Chao EYS (1991) A kinematic study of lunotriquetral dissociation. J Hand Surg [Am] 16 355:355–362
16. Mayfield JK (1988) Pathogenesis of wrist ligament instability In: Lichtman DM (ed) The wrist and its disorders. Saunders, Philadelphia, pp 53–73
17. Berger RA, Landsmeer JMF (1991) The palmar radiocarpal ligaments: A study of adult and fetal human wrist joints. J Hand Surg [Am] 15:847–854
18. Drewniany JJ, Palmer AK, Flatt AE (1985) The scaphotrapezial ligament complex: An anatomic and biomechanical study. J Hand Surg [Am] 10:492–498
19. Johnston HM (1907) Varying positions of the carpal bones in the different movements at the wrist. J Anat 41:9–122
20. Kapandji A (1987) Biomécanique du carpe et du poignet. Ann Chir Main 6:147–169
21. Kauer JMG (1974) The interdependence of carpal articulation chains. Acta Anat 88:481–501
22. Kauer JMG (1986) The mechanism of the carpal joint. Clin Orthop 202:16 26
23. Kuhlman JN, Tubiana R (1988) Mechanism of the normal wrist. In: Razemon JP, Fisk GR (eds) The wrist. Churchill Livingstone, New York
24. Landsmeer JMF (1961) Studies in the anatomy of the articulation. The equilibrium of the "inter-

calated" bone. Acta Morphol Neerl Scand 3: 287–303

25. Lewis OJ, Hamshere R, Bucknill TM (1963) The anatomy of the wrist joint. J Anat 106:539–552

26. Linscheid RL (1986) Kinematic considerations of the wrist. Clin Orthop 202:27–39

27. McMurtry RY, Youm Y, Flatt AE, Gillespie TE (1978) Kinematics of the wrist. II. Clinical applications. J Bone Joint Surg [Am] 60:955–961

28. Mayfield JK, Johnson RP, Kilcoyne RF (1976) The ligaments of the human wrist and their functional significance. Anat Rec 186:417–428

29. Navarro A (1937) Anatomia y fisiologia del carpo. An Inst Clin Quir Exp 1:162–250

30. Razemon JP (1983) La maladie de Kienbock. Etude radiologique et therapeutique a propos de 22 cas de raccourcissement du radius. In: Razemon JP, Fisk GR (eds) Le Poignet. Expansion Scientifique Francaise, Paris. pp 204–209

31. Ruby LK, Cooney WP, An KN, Linscheid RL, Chao EYS (1988) Relative motion of selected carpal bones: A kinematic analysis of the normal wrist. J Hand Surg [Am] 13:1–10

32. Sarrafian SK, Melamed JL, Goshgarian GM (1977) Study of wrist motion in flexion and extension. Clin Orthop 126:153–159

33. Schernberg F (1984) Static and dynamic radio-anatomy of the wrist. Ann Chir Main 3:301–312

34. Taleisnik J (1976) The ligaments of the wrist. J Hand Surg 1:110–118

35. Viegas SF, Tencer AF, Cantrell J, Chang M, Clegg P, Hicks C, O'Meara C, Williamson JB (1987) Load transfer characteristics of the wrist. Part I. The normal joint. J Hand Surg [Am] 12: 971–980

36. Weber ER (1984) Concepts governing the rotational shift of the intercalated segment of the carpus. Orthop Clin North Am 15:193–207

37. Wright RD (1935) A detailed study of movement of the wrist joint. J Anat 70:137–142

38. Youm Y, McMurtry RY, Flatt AE, Gillespie TE (1978) Kinematics of the wrist. I. An experimental study of radio-ulnar deviation and flexion-extension. J Bone Joint Surg [Am] 60:423–431

39. Lichtman DM, Schneider JR, Swafford AR, Mack GR (1981) Ulnar midcarpal instability: Clinical and laboratory analysis. J Hand Surg 6:515–523

40. Sutro CJ (1946) Bilateral recurrent intercarpal subluxation Am J Surg 72:110–112

41. Vaughan-Jackson OJ (1949) A case of recurrent subluxation of the carpal scaphoid. J Bone Joint Surg [Br] 31:532–533

42. Obletz BE, Halbstein BM (1938) Non-union of fractures of the carpal navicular. J Bone Joint Surg 20:424–428

43. Howard FM, Fahey TH, Wojcik E (1974) Rotatory subluxation of the navicular. Clin Orthop 104: 134–139

44. Weber ER, Chao EYS (1978) An experimental approach to the mechanism of scaphoid waist fractures. J Hand Surg 3:142–148

45. Smith DK, Cooney WP, An KN, Linscheid RL, Chao EYS (1989) The effects of simulated unstable scaphoid fractures on carpal motion. J Hand Surg [Am] 14:283–289

46. Palmer A, Dobyns JH, Linscheid RL (1978) Management of post-traumatic instability of the wrist secondary to ligament rupture. J Hand Surg 6:507–532

47. Dobyns JH, Linscheid RL, Macksoud WS (1985) Proximal carpal row instability, nondissociative. Orthop Trans 9:574

48. Garcia-Elias M, Dobyns JH, Cooney WP, Linscheid RL (1989) Traumatic axial dislocations of the carpus. J Hand Surg [Am] 14:446–451

49. Johnson RP, Carrera GF (1986) Chronic capitolunate instability J Bone Joint Surg [Am] 68:1164–1176

50. Schernberg F (1984) Midcarpal instability. Ann Chir Main 3:344–348

51. Watson HK, Hempton RF (1980) Limited wrist arthrodeses. I. The triscaphoid joint. J Hand Surg 5:320–327

52. Watson HK, Goodman ML, Johnson TR (1981) Limited wrist arthrodesis. II. Intercarpal and radiocarpal combinations. J Hand Surg 6:223–233

Overuse Syndrome: A Common Soft Tissue Cause of Wrist Pain

VAUGHAN BOWEN[1] and MICHAEL WEINBERG[2]

Abstract. Twenty cases of overuse syndrome have been seen in our clinic. Overuse syndrome is a form of chronic repetitive strain injury in the upper extremity and frequently presents as undiagnosed wrist pain. The condition is characterized by a history of diffuse pain which is remarkably consistent from one patient to the next. Physical examination often reveals no positive features although muscle pain may occasionally be detected. Clinical investigative results are normal.

A psychological study of similar patients indicated that these patients did not differ from those in a control group.

Management of overuse syndrome consists of avoidance of aggravating factors, rest, splinting, and a gradual resumption of activity when symptoms have settled. Surgery should not be recommended.

Keywords: Overuse — Soft tissue — Wrist pain — Repetitive strain — Extraskeletal pain

Introduction

At present, there is considerable interest in the diagnosis and management of the painful wrist. The medical literature has recently tended to emphasize the skeletal causes of wrist pain and much less has been written about extraskeletal soft tissue causes. In our practice, soft tissue problems account for a high proportion of patients who present with wrist pain. Soft tissue causes of wrist pain can arise in any of the anatomical structures between the skin and the skeleton: the skin and subcutaneous layers, the peripheral nerves, the blood vessels, and the musculotendinous units. Our diagnostic philosophy is to initially determine the layer in which the pain originates and then to define the compartment, radial or ulnar, proximal or distal, in which the pain arises.

Musculotendinous causes of pain are common, especially among manual workers, and may occur in the form of acute injury or chronic repetitive strain injury.

Overuse syndrome is a form of chronic repetitive strain injury. Lockwood [1] described overuse syndrome as "an injury caused by the cumulative effect on tissues of repetitive physical stress that exceeds physiological limits". Fry [2] described overuse syndrome as "a painful condition of the hand and arm produced by hand-use-intense activity over long periods and use which is excessive for the individuals affected". He later described the confusing terminology that has arisen concerning tenosynovitis, overuse syndrome, and repetition strain injury [3]. It is important that overuse syndrome is differentiated from tenosynovitis which, by definition, is an inflammation of the tenosynovium.

Overuse syndrome is well known among musicians and athletes, but its association with activities in the workplace has not been emphasized [4]. Among the general public, there is a growing awareness of repetitive-motion injury in the workplace, and the number of cumulative trauma cases reported by workers increased nearly fourfold from 1985 to 1989 [5]. A number of our patients who presented with wrist pain were diagnosed as having overuse syndrome. In the majority of cases, this was related to work activity. This paper describes the etiology, management, and results in these patients.

[1] Divisions of Plastic and Orthopaedic Surgery and [2] Division of Plastic Surgery, University of Toronto. EN 10-243, Toronto General Hospital, 200 Elizabeth Street, Toronto, Ontario, M5G 2C4, Canada

Patients and Methods

A data registry was kept of all patients that presented to a busy, urban, tertiary referral, hand surgery practice. All patients who presented with wrist pain in a 34-month period between April, 1988 and February, 1991 were reviewed, and those that were diagnosed as having overuse syndrome were studied in detail. Demographic data were tabulated, and the etiological circumstances, presenting symptoms, clinical signs, management, and results of treatment were analyzed.

Results

In the 34-month period studied, a total of 332 new patients presented with the complaint of wrist pain. A wide spectrum of diagnoses was encountered. Skeletal diagnoses (bone and joint) were made in 197/332 patients and extraskeletal diagnoses (soft tissue) were made in 114/332 patients. There was one patient who was thought to have a non-organic cause of pain. There were twenty patients without a diagnosis; these were people whose diagnosis was uncertain after the initial clinical and radiological evaluation but who did not maintain follow-up throughout the process of investigation. It is known that some had only come for a second opinion and others had moved away from our city.

Among the extraskeletal diagnosis of wrist pain, there were 20 cases that had been labelled as overuse syndrome. Seventeen of the twenty were female and one other was a male-to-female transformation. In eighteen of the cases, the dominant right upper extremity was involved. The condition was almost always seen in light industry, blue collar workers. Fifteen were engaged in occupations that involved hours of highly repetitive activity on production lines, assembly lines, or in data processing. Three others took part in recreational activities that involved repetitive activity.

The presenting symptoms were remarkably consistent, both from patient to patient and from visit to visit in the same patient. The patients' pain appeared to be very real but its description was always rather unclear. Pain usually started insidiously and was dull and vaguely described as being variable in intensity and diffuse in location. Symptoms had almost invariably been present for months, were exacerbated by activity, and

tended to deteriorate with time. Patients characteristically used their uninvolved hand to demonstrate the direction of the pain's radiation to be dorsally and/or volarly. Some complained of weakness, a sensation of swelling, or sensory changes. Five thought they may have had an initial minor injury. Three had other predisposing factors: in two cases there was a disabling clinical problem in the contralateral wrist and, in the third, surgical exploration of the affected side revealed an anatomical abnormality in the flexor carpi ulnaris muscle.

The physical examination was usually unrewarding. None of the patients had visible soft tissue or bony abnormalities. None had any localizing signs, such as point tenderness or crepitus. Detailed examination of the wrists did not reveal any instability patterns and none of the patients were positive to any of the specific prevocative tests for instability in individual carpal articulations. The wrist range of motion and the neurovascular status were normal in all patients. Grip strength and rapid exchange grip tests tended to give rather inconsistent readings.

The patients were all investigated with plain radiographs, a blood test screen for the various forms of arthritis, electrodiagnostic studies, and technetium bone scintigraphy. None of the wrists demonstrated abnormalities. Some patients had been investigated by other additional tests, such as ultrasound, CT scan, MRI scan, and wrist arthroscopy. These never indicated a cause for the patients' symptoms.

Rest and splinting may have slightly alleviated symptoms in some of the cases, but, in general, physiotherapy, analgesics, nonsteroidal anti-inflammatory medications, and steroid injections were consistently unsuccessful. Five patients had undergone operations with no clinical improvement. All the patients had taken time away from work because of their pain, although ten were working at the time of review. Only one patient claimed to have recovered. The ability to continue working was closely related to the individual patient's ability to alter the working environment. Eight of the ten working patients had not only kept their jobs but had also diminished their symptoms by work modification. Only one working patient had a Workers' Compensation Board claim. Eight of the ten non-working patients had Workers' Compensation Board claims, and seven were in occupations where they could not control their work environment.

Table 1. A comparison of the clinical features of tenosynovitis and overuse syndrome

	Tenosynovitis	Overuse syndrome
Etiology	Repetitive use	Repetitive use
	Trauma	Unusual positioning
Symptoms	Pain — localized	Pain — vague, general
	Weakness from pain	General weakness
		Swelling in muscle
		Subjective sensory change
Signs	Tendon sheath swelling	Vague general tenderness
	Localized tenderness	
Management	Splint	Rest
	NSAID	
	Steroid injection	
	Tendon decompression	

NSAID, Nonsteroid anti-inflammatory drugs

Discussion

It is important to differentiate overuse syndrome from tenosynovitis. The two conditions are compared in Table 1. Patients with tenosynovitis tend to be more specific about etiology and have localized symptoms with positive clinical signs. They frequently respond well to management with anti-inflammatory medications. Patients with overuse syndrome tend to be much more vague about the etiology and localization of their symptoms, have few or no clinical signs, and do not respond to anti-inflammatory medications. Their clinical features, however, are consistent and appear to be very real.

There are many forms of tenosynovitis that cause pain in the region of the wrist. These and other extra-articular causes of pain in this region have been described by Wood and Dobyns [6].

Fry classified overuse syndrome according to severity [3]. He described convincing and reproducible tenderness in the overused structures of patients with this syndrome [7]. Tenderness was uncommon in our series, but this may be because our patients were seen late after the onset of the problem.

The medical literature contains a number of papers describing overuse problems in musicians and athletes [8, 9]. The recent surge of interest in competitive and recreational sports has been associated with a growing interest among physi-

cians and surgeons in the problems associated with sports-related injuries [10]. There has been a parallel development of interest in similar medical problems that are encountered in the performing artists [11].

Little has been written about overuse syndrome in the workplace and yet a number of factors, both historic and individual, allow the condition to develop in the work environment. In our city, many workers are employed in highly repetitive manual jobs in light-industrial factories. It is not surprising, therefore, that both tenosynovitis and overuse syndrome are responsible for so much of the chronic wrist pain that is seen.

A number of causative factors can be implicated in the etiology of both tenosynovitis [12] and overuse syndrome. These can be divided into general, local, and individual. General etiological factors are historic in nature and include events such as the invention of the assembly line and the advent of workers compensation legislation. Local etiological factors are found in the place of employment and may be related to 1 environment, such as the rate of work activity, number of hours worked per day, time between rest breaks, recent change in occupation, resumption of work after absence or other external work pressures, 2 equipment, such as its ergonomic design or weight, and 3 job training, such as technique, efficiency, or experience. Individual etiological factors may be physical, such as the presence of pre-existing musculoskeletal abnormality or injury, an imbalance of strength and flexibility or a lack of general fitness, or they may be mental, such as a desire to compete or a lack of understanding concerning the development of overuse conditions.

It seems likely that for a specific individual to develop overuse syndrome there must be a blend of extrinsic factors related to the work environment, equipment, and training, and intrinsic factors related to the patient's own pre-existing physical and mental state.

The pathophysiology of overuse syndrome is not entirely clear. Pitner [13] described injuries to the musculotendinous unit as the most frequent sports-related cause of wrist pain requiring medical attention. He noted that musculotendinous problems were implicated in up to 65% of all overuse injuries, while bone problems were implicated in 15% and nerve problems in only 2%. Herring [14] also described the pathogenesis of overuse problems in athletes.

The classic overuse injury to bone is a stress fracture and, although these may not always be obvious on a plain radiograph, the periosteal healing response can be demonstrated with a technetium bone scan. Overuse injury to nerves is not well understood but usually presents as an acute or chronic peripheral nerve compression. In view of the absence of localizing clinical or investigatory features in our patients, it is unlikely that either of these were pathophysiologically related to our cases of overuse syndrome. It would seem more likely that mild repetitive injury to the musculotendinous units was involved.

The current theories concerning the etiology of overuse syndrome have recently been summarized by Pitner [13]. These theories describe the relationship of the musculotendinous units to overuse injuries. In some cases, the tenosynovial coverings may become inflamed secondary to friction. In other cases, repetitive stress injury may cause damage to the tendons themselves. In theory, it is possible that if sustained loads in the physiological range are applied without sufficient recovery time, viscoelastic creep and a cumulative loss of molecular cross-linkages may occur. The amount, rate, and frequency of the stress have all been implicated in the microtrauma of repetitive stress injury. Other theories have implicated muscular factors. Metabolic theories center on the inability of the affected muscle to maintain sufficient aerobic production of ATP, possible due to ischemia. One theory places the fault on a lack of ATP and the subsequent derangement of calcium regulation in the cell, while another theory places the fault on an accumulation of metabolites, such as lactic acid. Mechanical theories relate muscle damage to direct disruption of muscle fibers and connective tissue from the process of contraction.

The patients in our study had no positive clinical features and there was no pathological evidence of disease. Are we correct in diagnosing them as having overuse syndrome? We believe we are partly justified because their case histories were so remarkably consistent and partly because of their similarity with descriptions in the medical literature. The alternative suggestion, that these patients might have had a psychological component to their symptoms, has been addressed by Langstaff et al. [15] in a long-term psychological study of young females with undiagnosed wrist pain. The results indicated that, although symptoms often did not settle with time, psychological morbidity was no greater among these patients than in a control group.

The management of overuse syndrome consists of avoidance of precipitating and aggravating factors [16]. The patient will have to stop work and should rest until the pain subsides. Splinting and physiotherapy, general conditioning, and strengthening to correct muscular imbalance (if present) may be useful at this stage. When the patient is ready to return to work, modification of technique and a gentle resumption of activity is appropriate. Surgery has nothing to offer and should not be recommended. In patients with chronic symptoms of overuse injury, it is unusual for a "cure" to be achieved; but, if it is possible to alter the work environment, individual patients may be successful in learning to live with the problem. Patients in occupations where they do not control their own work environment, especially if they are receiving workers' compensation, are unlikely to return to the causative occupation and will need to change their jobs.

References

1. Lockwood AH (1989) Medical problems of musicians. N Engl J Med 320:221–227
2. Fry HJH (1986) Overuse syndrome of the upper limb in musicians. Med J Aust 144:182–185
3. Fry HJH (1986) Overuse syndrome, alias tenosynovitis/tendinitis: The terminology hoax. Plast Reconstr Surg 78:414–417
4. Browne CD, Nolan BM, Faithfull DK (1984) Occupational repetition strain injuries. Med J Aust 140:329–332
5. Stix G (1991) Handful of pain. Pressure mounts to alleviate repetitive-motion injuries. Sci Am May: 118–119
6. Wood MB, Dobyns JH (1986) Sports related extra-articular wrist syndromes. Clin Orthop 202:93–102
7. Fry HJH (1986) Physical signs in the hand and wrist seen in the overuse injury syndrome of the upper limb. Aust NZ J Surg 56:47–49
8. Amadio PC, Russotti GM (1990) Evaluation and treatment of hand and wrist disorders in musicians. Hand Clin 6:405–416
9. Stern PJ (1990) Tendinitis, overuse syndromes, and tendon injuries. Hand Clin 6:467–476
10. Hunter — Griffin LY (ed) (1987) Overuse injury. Clin Sports Med 6 (2)
11. Amadio PC (ed) (1990) Hand injuries in sports and performing arts. Hand Clin N Am 6 (3)
12. Thompson AR, Plewes LW, Shaw EG (1951)

Peritendinitis crepitans and simple tenosynovitis: A clinical study of 544 cases in industry. Br J Ind Med 8:150–160

13. Pitner MA (1990) Pathophysiology of overuse injuries in the hand and wrist. Hand Clin 6:355–364

14. Herring SA, Nilson KL (1987) Introduction to overuse injuries. Clin Sports Med 6:225–239

15. Langstaff RJ, Ryley P, Barton NJ (1991) The natural history of undiagnosed wrist pain in young women. Presented at the International Symposium on the Wrist, Nagoya, Japan

16. Stone WE (1983) Repetitive strain injuries. Med J Aust 2:616–618

Dorsal Wrist Pain and Occult Ganglion

Toshihiko Ogino[1]

Abstract. The clinical features and prognosis of 15 patients with dorsal occult ganglion of the wrist are reported. Their ages ranged from 14 to 61 years. All complained of wrist pain which was aggravated by exercise. The pain had been present for periods ranging from 1 week to 5 years (mean 19.5 months). The range of motion of the wrist joint was restricted due to pain in 10 cases. There was tenderness on the dorsal surface around the lunate in all cases. X-ray findings were entirely normal. Ultrasonography was performed in 13 cases and all showed a small low-echogenic area in the subcutaneous tissue just dorsal to the lunate. Puncture was performed in 13 cases. In no case was it possible to sufficiently aspirate the jelly-like mucin into the syringe by puncture. Surgery was performed in 4 cases and occult ganglion was removed with its attachment to the scapholunate ligament; there was no recurrence of the ganglion postoperatively. In 7 cases in which puncture was performed, three patients continued to have pain and four were relieved of pain. The usefulness of ultrasonography for detecting dorsal occult ganglion was discussed on the basis of these results.

Keywords: Wrist — Ganglion — Ultrasonography — Magnetic resonance imaging — Pain

Introduction

There are many causes of chronic wrist pain, such as Kienböck's disease, carpal instability, disorders of the triangular fibrocartilaginous complex, arthritis, distal posterior interosseous nerve syndrome, and others. Occult ganglion, which is difficult to detect by palpation, is an additional cause of wrist pain [1, 2]. Although dorsal wrist ganglion is a very common disease, and is usually diagnosed easily, dorsal occult ganglion is considered to be relatively rare and its diagnosis by routine methods is difficult. The authors used ultrasonography to detect occult ganglion of the dorsal wrist and discovered that it is not a rare disease [3]. In this paper, the clinical features of dorsal occult ganglion are reported, and the usefulness of ultrasonography in detecting it is discussed.

Patients and Methods

During the past 7 years, I have examined 15 patients with dorsal occult ganglion of the wrist. Three of these patients were males and 12 were females. A history of dorsal wrist ganglion was positive in 2 cases. Sonographic examination was performed in 11 cases. The present study was carried out using a real-time 3.5, 5, or 7.5 MHz high-resolution scanner. For standardized sonographic examinations, the area to be examined was covered with polymer-gel conduction medium; longitudinal and transverse scans were performed.

Results (Table 1)

The age of the patients at their first visit to our clinic ranged from 21 to 51 years (mean 33.9 years). The right hand was affected in 7 cases and the left one in 8 cases. All the patients complained of pain in the wrist which was aggravated by exercise. The pain had been present for periods ranging from 1 week to 5 years (mean 19.5 months). The range of motion of the wrist joint was normal in 10 cases and was slightly limited

[1] Department of Physical Therapy, School of Allied Health Professions, Sapporo Medical College, Chuo-ku, Minami-3-jo, Nishi-17-chome, Sapporo 060, Japan

Table 1. Cases of occult ganglion of the dorsal wrist and results at follow-up

Case no.	Sex	Age (years)	Affected side	Period of wrist pain	Number of punctures[a]	Treatment	Follow-up period (years)	Tumor at follow-up	Pain at follow-up
1	Male	42	Left	2 Years	2	Surgery	4	Negative	Negative
2	Female	24	Right	2 Months	2	Surgery	4	Negative	Negative
3	Female	21	Left	2 Years	2		3	Negative	Positive
4	Female	26	Left	8 Months	2				
5	Female	22	Right	4 Years	1				
6	Female	31	Left	5 Years	3		3	Negative	Positive
7	Male	51	Right	2 Months	1[b]	Surgery	3	Negative	Negative
8	Male	58	Right	4 Years	0		1.5	Negative	Negative
9	Female	19	Left	1 Week	1		1.5	Positive	Positive
10	Female	50	Right	2 Years	1[b]	Surgery	1	Negative	Positive
11	Female	14	Right	1 Month	1		2	Positive	Negative
12	Female	61	Left	4 Years	1		0.5	Negative	Negative
13	Female	20	Left	1 Month	0				
14	Female	35	Right	1 Month	2				
15	Female	34	Left	1 Month	1		0.25	Positive	Negative

[a] The number which was needed to detect jelly-like mucin
[b] Puncture was performed only once and mucin was not detected

due to pain in 5 cases. Extreme dorsiflexion of the wrist induced pain in 10 cases, palmar flexion induced it in 2 cases, and extreme palmar and dorsal flexion in 3 cases. There was tenderness over the dorsal surface of the lunate bone in 10 cases, in the space between the lunate and scaphoid bones in 3 cases, and between the lunate and capitate bones in 1 case. No wrist tenderness was present in 1 case. X-ray findings were entirely normal in all cases but 1, in which roentgenograms revealed a small cystic shadow in the lunate. ^{99m}Tc scintigrams were performed in 2 cases and the results were normal.

Ultrasonography was performed in 13 cases and all except 1 showed a small low-echogenic area in the subcutaneous tissue just dorsal to the lunate bone. Because of its homogeneous echogenicity and the striking difference between the echogenicity of this area and the surrounding tissue, a dorsal occult ganglion was strongly suspected in all cases except 1. Puncture was performed in 13 cases. In no case was it possible to aspirate any thick jelly-like colorless mucin into the syringe, but a very small amount of mucin was found at the tip of the needle at the initial puncture in 5 cases, at the time of the second puncture in 5 cases, and at the third puncture in 1 case. In 2 cases, puncture was performed but no mucin was detected. Surgery was performed in 4 cases because of increasing pain. A dorsal occult ganglion was found at surgery and removed together with its attachment to the scapholunate ligament. The posterior interosseous nerve was resected at the wrist to denervate the dorsal wrist in 2 cases.

Eleven cases were followed up for periods ranging from 3 months to 3 years (mean 2.3 years). In the 4 cases in which surgery was performed, there was no recurrence of the ganglion; three of these patients had no pain, and one had only slight pain. In the 7 cases in which puncture was performed, three patients continued to have pain, and four were relieved of pain.

Case Report

The patient was a 61-year-old housewife who had been complaining of pain on the back of her non-dominant left wrist for 4 years. The pain increased after work, and she had some disability with respect to activities of daily living. There was a full range of motion and no deformity, but extreme extension of the wrist elicited pain. There was tenderness on the dorsal surface of the lunate. The findings on the roentgenograms were normal. An occult dorsal ganglion was suspected, and ultrasonography revealed a small homogeneous hypoechogenic area consistent with an occult ganglion (Fig. 1). Puncture was then performed, and although no sufficient amount of jelly-like mucin could be aspirated, some was found at the

Fig. 1. Ultrasonography in case 12 of Table 1. **a** Longitudinal scan. **b** Transverse scan. Ultrasonography revealed a small homogeneous hypoechogenic area adjacent to the carpal bones (*arrows*)

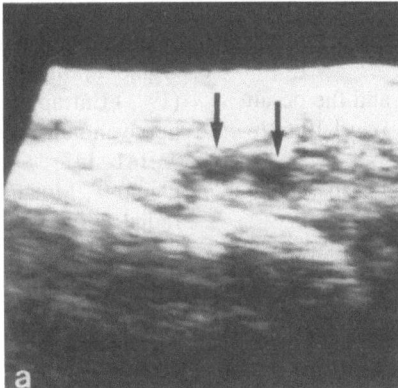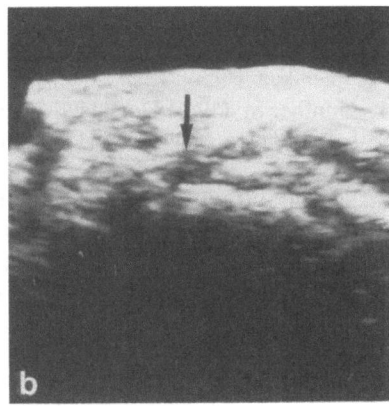

tip of the needle. The pain decreased gradually, and was absent 6 months after aspiration.

Discussion

From my experience, the chief complaint of all the patients with dorsal occult ganglion of the wrist was dorsal wrist pain. The duration of the pain varied, and there were some cases in which the correct diagnosis had not been made previously. It is not clear why small ganglions are painful. There is a relationship between ganglion size and severity of pain in the case of dorsal ganglion of the wrist. In this series, it was interesting to note that dorsal wrist pain disappeared in 2 cases when the ganglion grew to a size which was detectable by palpation. When a small ganglion occurs close to the attachment of the scapholunate ligament, it may cause pain but may be difficult to detect by palpation [4]. In such circumstances, differential diagnosis of the wrist pain becomes very important if treatment is to be effective.

The sensory branch of the posterior interosseous nerve is distributed to the dorsal wrist, and dorsal wrist pain is conducted through this nerve. Carr and Davis reported mechanical impingement of the sensory branch of the posterior interosseous nerve at the wrist as being a distal posterior interosseous nerve syndrome in 1985 [5]. This syndrome is also one of the causes of dorsal wrist pain which shows no abnormal roentgenographic findings. When no evidence of occult ganglion can be detected by diagnostic imaging techniques in patients with chronic dorsal wrist pain, there is the possibility of a false-negative diagnosis of dorsal occult ganglion. One of other possibilities is the distal posterior interosseous nerve syn-

drome. While a differential diagnosis between dorsal occult ganglion and distal posterior interosseous nerve syndrome is necessary, it is sometimes not possible. When this is the case, and the wrist pain is severe, surgical exploration of the dorsal wrist is recommended. During surgery, a meticulous attempt is made to detect dorsal occult ganglion and entrapment of the posterior interosseous nerve. If there is no occult ganglion on the dorsal wrist, the posterior interosseous nerve should be resected just proximal to the radiocarpal joint in order to relieve pain. In this series, denervation was combined with excision of the dorsal occult ganglion in 2 cases in which complete relief of pain was achieved. Denervation is one of the choices in the treatment of chronic wrist pain due to dorsal occult ganglion of the wrist.

In dorsal occult ganglion, plain roentgenograms usually reveal no abnormalities and the results of scintigrams are negative. Computed tomography, MRI, and ultrasonography are diagnostic methods which permit the imaging of tumors and tumor-like conditions. Computed tomography, however, sometimes fails to outline ganglions clearly [6], and does not have enough resolving power to detect small ganglions. MRI, on the other hand, has been reported to be useful in detecting small occult ganglions [7, 8]. On the basis of the present study, ultrasonography has been found to be useful in detecting dorsal occult ganglions. The procedure is easy and inexpensive. It provides higher resolving power and makes real-time imaging possible. Ultrasonography is non-invasive and is a valuable screening examination for dorsal occult ganglion.

References

1. Gunther SF (1985) Dorsal wrist pain and the occult scapholunate ganglion. J Hand Surg [Am] 10:697–703

2. Sanders WE (1985) The occult dorsal carpal ganglion. J Hand Surg [Br] 10:257–260

3. Ogino T, Minami A, Kato H, Itoga H, Takahata S (1988) The dorsal occult ganglion of the wrist and ultrasonography. J Hand Surg [Br] 13:181–183

4. Dellon AL, Seif SS (1978) Anatomic dissections relating the posterior interosseous nerve to the carpus, and the etiology of dorsal wrist ganglion pain. J Hand Surg [Am] 3:326–332

5. Carr D, Davis P (1985) Distal posterior interosseous syndrome. J Hand Surg [Am] 10:873–878.

6. Ogino T, Minami A, Kato H, Itoga H, Takahata S (1991) Entrapment neuropathy of the suprascapular nerve and ultrasonography. J Bone Joint Surg [Am] 73:141–147

7. Ogino T, Minami A, Kato, H (1991) Diagnosis of radial nerve palsy caused by ganglion with use of different imaging techniques. J Hand Surg [Am] 16:230–235.

8. Itoh Y, Uzawa M, Matsu K, Kuboi J, Nishiyama K, Yoshida K, Nemoto K (1991) Magnetic resonance imaging for painful wrist. 5th Annual Meeting of the Eastern Japan Society for Surgery of the Hand. February 9th, 1991. Sapporo

Carpal Bone Cyst

Satoshi Takahata, Toshihiko Ogino, Akio Minami, and Hiroyuki Kato[1]

Abstract. Roentgenograms of 1273 wrists of 877 outpatients and 156 wrists of 79 patients with vibration disease were reviewed in order to analyze the clinical and radiographic features of carpal bone cysts. The evaluation included the incidence, location, and size of the cysts. Correlations between incidence and age, sex, laterality, and ulnar variance were also evaluated. Another 10 wrists of ten patients with carpal bone cysts which had been treated surgically were also reviewed.

Among the outpatients, carpal bone cysts were found in 8.1% of the wrists, and in 18.6% of the patients with vibration disease. The incidence of cysts was higher in elderly patients, in those with vibration disease, and on the right side. Cysts tended to be located in the proximal carpal row. This suggests that exposure of the carpal bones to mechanical stress might cause carpal bone cysts.

The 10 patients who underwent surgical treatment were young, and their cysts were large and symptomatic. None of the patients had any symptoms after surgery. The histological findings of the operated cysts varied but most of them revealed some abnormality, such as intraosseous ganglions. Surgery should be considered in the treatment of symptomatic carpal bone cysts.

Keywords: Carpal bone — Bone cyst — Cystic lesion — Intraosseous ganglion — Ulnar variance

Introduction

We often find cystic lesions on roentgenograms of the carpal bones. Most cysts are asymptomatic, but sometimes they require surgical treatment. The purpose of this study was to analyze the

clinical and radiographic features of carpal bone cysts.

Patients and Methods

Non-Operated Cysts

Roentgenograms of 1273 wrists of 877 individuals among the general outpatient population of Hokkaido University Hospital and 156 wrists of 79 patients with vibration disease were reviewed. The evaluation included the incidence, location, and size of the cysts. Correlations between incidence and age, sex, laterality, and ulnar variance were also evaluated.

In this study, we defined carpal bone cysts as well-demarcated radiolucencies with or without marginal sclerosis and 2 mm or more in diameter (Fig. 1).

Operated Cysts

Another ten wrists of ten patients with carpal bone cysts treated surgically were also reviewed. The evaluation included pre- and postoperative symptoms and the histological diagnoses of the cysts.

Results

Non-Operated Cysts

Incidence. Carpal bone cysts were found in 103 out of 1273 wrists among the outpatients, an overall incidence of 8.1%. Among the patients with vibration disease, carpal bone cysts were found in 29 out of 156 wrists, for an overall incidence of 18.6%.

Location. Among the outpatients, 112 cysts were found in 103 wrists, with 42% in the lunate and

[1] Department of Orthopaedic Surgery, Hokkaido University School of Medicine, Kita 15-jo, Nishi 7-chome, Kita-ku, Sapporo 060, Japan

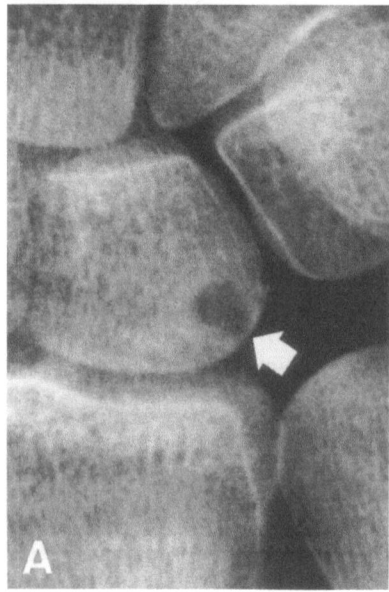 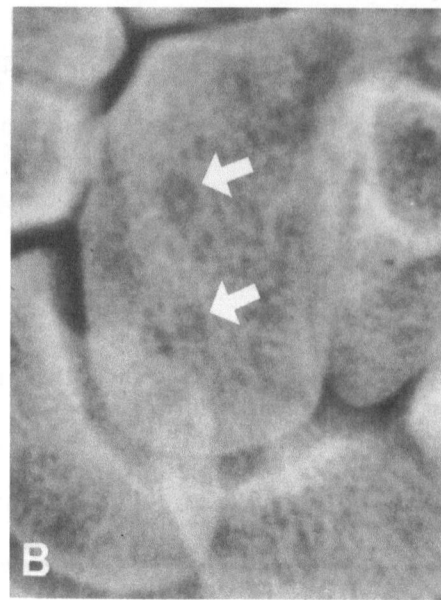

Fig. 1. A A carpal bone cyst is present in the lunate (*arrow*). **B** Cystic shadows in the capitate (*arrows*) did not meet the criteria of this diagnosis

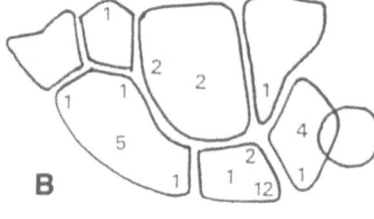

Fig. 2. Schematic representation of location and frequency of carpal bone cysts in **A** the general population of outpatients and **B** the patients with vibration disease

24% in the scaphoid. Among the patients with vibration disease, 34 cysts were found in 29 wrists, with 44% in the lunate and 23% in the scaphoid. Cysts tended to be found in the proximal carpal row and in proximity to the subchondral bone (Fig. 2).

Size. The diameters of 83% of the cysts in the outpatients and 94% of those in the patients with vibration disease were less than 7 mm (Table 1).

Age. The subjects were divided into 4 age groups. The patients with vibration disease ranged in age from 30 to 69 years. Among the outpatients, the incidence of cysts was higher in the older groups. This was also true of the patients with vibration disease. In each age group, the incidence in the patients with vibration disease was higher than among the outpatients (Table 2).

Sex. Among the outpatients, the incidence in both males and females was the same in the older

Table 1. Distribution of the cysts by size (%)

Diameter (mm)	2–3	4–6	7–9	>10
Outpatients	40	43	12	5
Patients with vibration disease	37	57	3	3
Operated cysts	0	50	25	25

Table 2. Incidence of carpal bone cyst (%)

	Overall	Male	Female	Right	Left
Outpatients (age range in years)					
0–29	1.0	0.3	3.0	1.4	0.5
30–49	6.8	4.3	9.0	7.7	5.8
50–69	13.0	13.8	12.7	16.2	9.9
>70	15.8	15.0	15.6	19.7	10.6
Overall	8.1	5.5	10.7	9.9	6.2
Patients with vibration disease					
30–49	10.7	10.7		14.3	7.1
50–69	21.3	21.3		23.0	19.7
Overall	18.6	18.6		20.5	16.7

groups (50 years of age or older), whereas the incidence was higher in females than males in the younger groups (under 50 years old). Thus, the overall incidence of carpal bone cysts was higher in females than in males. On the other hand, all the patients with vibration disease were male, and the incidences in each age group were higher than among the outpatients (Table 2).

Laterality. The incidence of carpal bone cysts was higher in the right wrist than in the left in all the outpatient age groups. The same was true for patients with vibration disease (Table 2).

Ulnar Variance. Among the outpatients, the incidence of carpal bone cysts was 10.4% in wrists with positive ulnar variance and 7.2% in wrists with zero ulnar variance. The incidence of carpal bone cysts was 26.9% in wrists with positive ulnar variance and 12.5% in wrists with zero ulnar variance in the patients with vibration disease. Wrists with negative ulnar variance were rare among both the outpatients and the patients with vibration disease.

Since many cysts were found at the proximal ulnar border of the lunate (Fig. 1.A), we reviewed the ulnar variance of wrists with cysts at the proximal ulnar border of the lunate. Thirty-one wrists of the outpatients had cysts at this location. There were 10 wrists with positive ulnar variance, 17 with zero ulnar variance, and 1 with negative ulnar variance. Information on the type of ulnar variance of the remaining three wrists is unavailable. Among the patients with vibration disease, 12 wrists had cysts in this location. There were seven wrists with positive ulnar variance, four with zero ulnar variance, and none with negative ulnar variance. Information on the type of ulnar variance of the remaining wrist is unavailable.

Operated Cysts

Another ten wrists (ten patients) with carpal bone cysts which were treated surgically were also reviewed. There were five patients under 30 years of age, four patients in the 30- to 49-year-old range, and one patient aged between 50–69 years. Five patients were males and five were females. Right and left wrists were equally affected.

Six cysts were located in the scaphoid, three in the capitate, two in the triquetrum, two in the hamate, and one each in the lunate, trapezium, and trapezoid. None of the cysts was less than 4 mm in diameter. One-half of the cysts were from 4 to 6 mm in diameter, and the other half had diameters greater than 6 mm (Table 1).

Preoperative symptoms consisted of pain in eight patients and swelling of the wrist in one patient. The remaining patient without any symptoms was treated with curettage and bone graft in order to prevent pathological fracture. Surgery included curettage and bone grafting in seven wrists, curettage alone in two, and resection of the affected bone in one. None of the patients had any symptoms after surgery with the exception of one who had subsequent wrist pain due to osteoarthritis.

Intraosseous ganglion was diagnosed histologically in the cysts of three patients, and one each of benign hemangioendothelioma, giant cell tumor of the tendon sheath, bone necrosis, bone cyst, and invagination of the synovium were revealed in five patients. The histological diagnosis of the cysts of the remaining two patients is unknown.

Discussion

Bugnion reported cyst-like lesions in 34.7%–50.8% (depending on the observer) of 600 cadaver wrists [1]. In the present study, carpal bone cysts were found in 8.1% of a general population of hospital outpatients and in 18.6% of the patients with vibration disease. The incidence of carpal bone cysts reported, however, may be influenced by the radiographic definition of "bone cyst". In fact, many cyst-like carpal bone shadows, especially in the capitate, were not diagnosed as carpal bone cysts in this study (Fig. 1.B).

The nature and pathogenesis of carpal bone cysts is obscure [1–4]. Schajowicz et al. thought that mechanical stress and repeated minor trauma near the surface of the bone might lead to intramedullary vascular disturbance with consequent foci of aseptic bone necrosis followed by intramedullary mucoid degeneration [2]. Eiken and Jonsson believed the cysts to be caused by intramedullary vascular disturbances, followed by bone resorption and fibroblastic proliferation [3].

In the present study, the incidence of cysts was higher in elderly patients, those with vibration disease, and on the right side. The cysts tended to be located in the proximal carpal row. This suggests that exposure of the carpal bones to mechanical stress might cause carpal bone cysts. The histological diagnosis of the operated cysts varied, and included intraosseous ganglion, bone necrosis, and bone cyst. The term "intraosseous ganglion" appears to have added to the confusion in terminology [3].

There is also the matter of whether the radiographically detected cystic lesion is the cause of pain and should be resected. In one series, 85% of the carpal bone cysts were asymptomatic [3]. The ten patients who underwent surgical treatment were young, their cysts were large and symptomatic and, in most, the histological findings were abnormal. Surgery should be considered in the treatment of symptomatic carpal bone cysts.

References

1. Bugnion JP (1951) Lesions nouvelles du poignet. Pseudokystes necrobiotiques. Kystes par herniations capsulaires. Arthrite chronique degenerative par osteochondrose marginale. Acta Radiol [Diagn] (Stockh) Suppl 90
2. Schajowicz F, Sainz MC, Slullitel JA (1979) Juxta-articular bone cysts (intra-osseous ganglia). J Bone Joint Surg [Br] 61:107–116
3. Eiken O, Jonsson K (1980) Carpal bone cysts. A clinical and radiographic study. Scand J Plast Reconstr Surg 14:285–290
4. Poznanski AK (1984) The hand in radiologic diagnosis, 2nd edn. Saunders, Philadelphia, pp 183–185

Congenital Deformities of the Carposcaphoid and Styloid Processes of the Radius in Mother and Son

Takatoshi Ohno,[1] Yasushi Suzuki,[1] Masahiro Asai,[1] Hideki Ando,[1] Takanobu Matsunaga,[1] and Takuji Tanaka[2]

Abstract. Congenital dysplasia of the radiocarpal and talocrural joints is extremely rare except in certain severe congenital disorders. We report on 2 cases of a congenital deformity involving a hyperplastic carpal scaphoid and a hypoplastic styloid process of the radius resulting in limitation of wrist extension in both wrists in a female and her son. The son also had an abnormal accessory bone on the distal end of the medial malleolus in both ankles. This is the first case report of such deformities in these anatomical regions.

Keywords: Familial congenital deformity — Radiocarpal joint — Wrist — Radial styloid process — Carpal scaphoid — Ankle — Accessory bone

Case Reports

Case 1

A 15-year-old male was treated in our hospital with fractures of the left ulna and radius due to a fall from a horizontal bar. Although his past medical history was otherwise unremarkable, he had been unable to extend his wrists since birth. When he supported himself with his hands, he always used the dorsal sides of the middle phalanx of all his fingers with the posterior and distal interphalangeal joints in the flexed position. There was no abnormal appearance of the wrists, but the extension of each measured approximately 0°, flexion 70°, radial deviation 10°, and ulnar deviation 25°. In addition, he could not fully extend his ankles. Ankle extension was measured at 5° and 0° in the left and right ankles,

respectively, and flexion was 30° bilaterally. X-ray films of the wrists in the anteroposterior plane showed bilateral hypoplasia of the styloid process of the radius and hyperplasia of the carpal scaphoid, (Fig. 1.a). The scaphoid was enlarged and projected into the position normally occupied by the radiostyloid process. Furthermore, radiograms of the ankles in the anteroposterior plane revealed a huge accessory bone distal to the medial malleolus bilaterally (Fig. 1.b). The accessory bone on the left side was larger than that on the right, and the left one near the subtalar joint space was partially joined to the medial malleolus. However, the remaining region was separated from the malleolus and showed irregular sclerotic changes. The accessory bone on the right ankle was slightly smaller and had no bony union with the malleolus.

Case 2

This 48-year-old female, the mother of the subject in case 1, also had bilateral limitation of wrist extension since birth, although the external appearance of the wrists was normal. There was no pain or swelling, the medical history was unremarkable, and ankle mobility was normal. Wrist extension was 35° on the right side and 30° on the left side, with flexion being approximately 70° bilaterally. The X-rays showed bilateral deformity of the carpal scaphoid and styloid processes of the radius and were similar to those of her son (Fig. 2).

Discussion

Familial congenital dysplasia of the radiocarpal joint is very rare except for certain congenital disorders associated with hypoplastic changes in the distal radius, the distal forearm muscles,

[1] The Department of Orthopaedic Surgery and [2] the First Department of Pathology, Gifu University School of Medicine, 40 Tsukasa-machi, Gifu 500, Japan

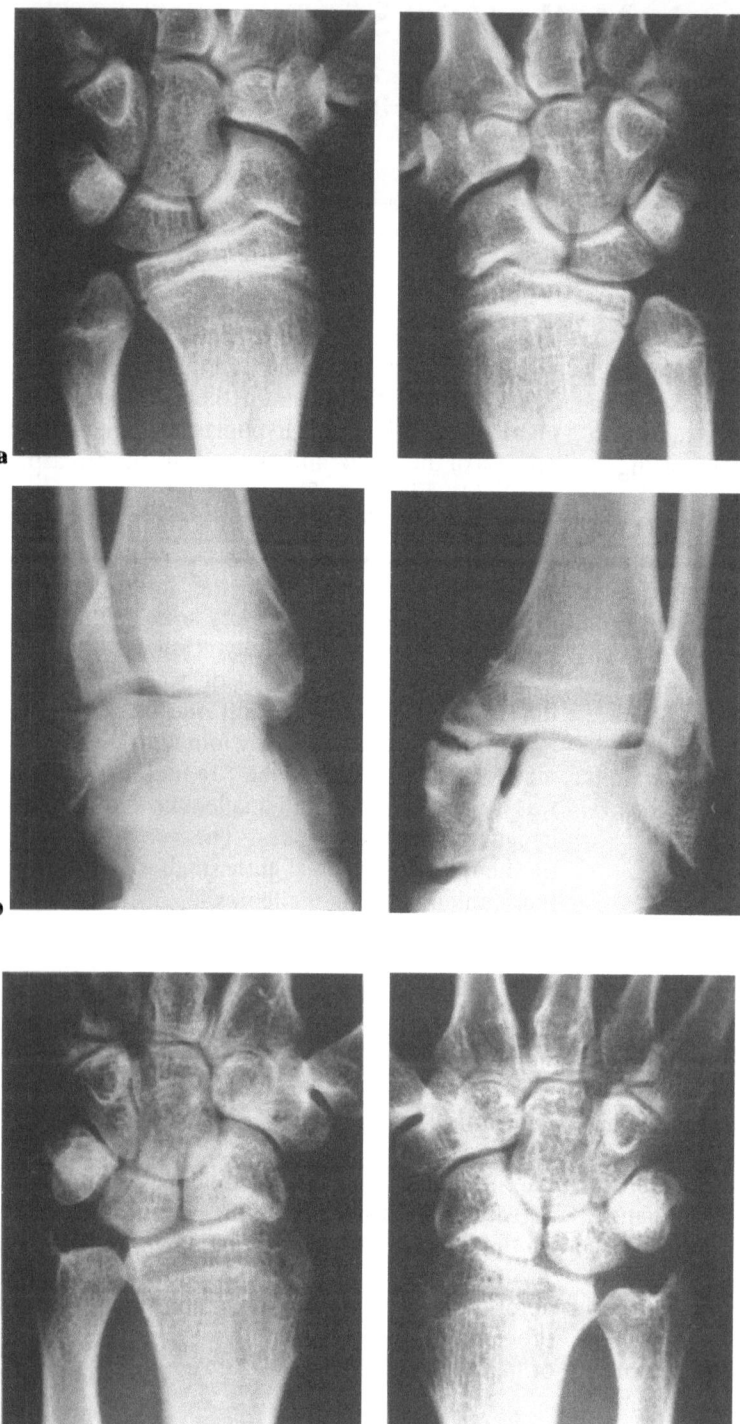

Fig. 1. Case 1. **a** Anteroposterior radiographs of the wrists demonstrating enlarged scaphoid and hypoplasia of radial styloid process. **b** Anteroposterior radiographs of the ankles demonstrating the accessory bone distal to the medial malleolus

Fig. 2. Case 2. Anteroposterior radiographs of the wrists showing a deformity similar to case 1

and the radial side of the hand [1, 2]. Several anomalies of the carpal scaphoid have been reported to date [3–10]. However, all involved hypoplasia or absence. In contrast, our cases showed hyperplasia of the scaphoid, which was enlarged and projected into the position normally occupied by the radial styloid process with no other deformity in the radial ray. It is difficult to speculate about the mechanism behind these unusual cases; however, two possibilities can be derived from previous reports (Fig. 3): fusion occurring between os radiostyloideum and the

Fig. 3. Possible causative mechanisms in case 1. *C*, Os centrale; *R*, Os radiale; *E*, OS radiale externum

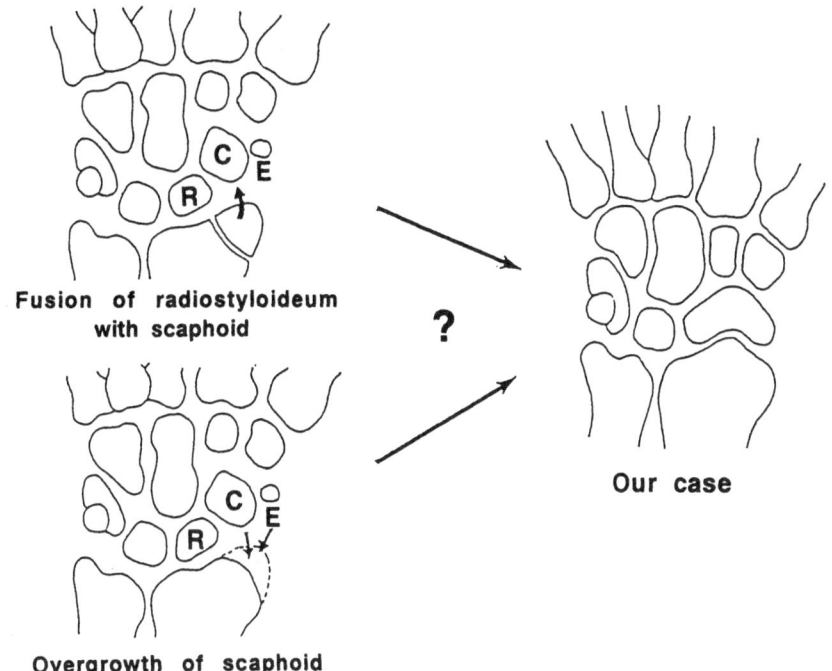

Fusion of radiostyloideum
with scaphoid

?

Our case

Overgrowth of scaphoid

carpal scaphoid, and hyperplastic growth of the carpal scaphoid occurring during the prenatal period.

O'Rahilly [11] categorized carpal and tarsal anomalies into 4 groups: (1) extensive anomalies (long bone deficiencies), (2) fusions, (3) accessory bones, and (4) bipartition. The following discussion relates to the latter 3 points of O'Rahilly's classification. The styloid process of the ulna and radius sometimes develops from a separate ossification center, and this occasionally fails to unite with the main bone, resulting in a disunited fragment called ulnostyloideum [11, 12] and radiostyloideum, respectively [13, 14]. On the other hand, several cases of fusion between the radius and carpal scaphoid have been reported [15–17]. These reports support our first speculation, that the second ossification center, the radiostyloideum, fuses with the carpal scaphoid.

In the embryo, the human carpal scaphoid is composed of two or three parts [18]: os centrale, os radiale, and (unusually) os radiale externum [19] which normally fuses to os centrale to form the tuberosity of the scaphoid. Some authors have described that hypoplasia, absence, or bipartition of the scaphoid are anomalies in the forming stage [5]. Similarly, overgrowth of the scaphoid might cause hypoplasia of the radiostyloid process during the fetal period. In addition, we could not find any prior case reports

mentioning the ankle deformity as that discovered in case 1. It most likely belongs to category 4 in O'Rahilly's classification, i.e., enlarged accessory bone, called os subtibiale [11]. In a roentgenographic study of 100 healthy children aged 6–12 years, Powell [20] found an accessory ossification center distal to the medial malleolus at a rate of 20%. Furthermore, in 50 adults without any history of injury, os subtibiale was observed in 4%. However, there were no submalleolar ossicles as large as those in our patient who may have the anomaly of the accessory ossification centers in both wrists and ankles — radiostyloideum in the wrists and subtibiale in the ankles — whose pathogenesis is uncertain.

It is interesting to note that these anomalies of both wrists and ankles (both are on the medial side when the human is viewed as a quadruped animal) are demonstrated together in the same individual. This might indicate that the genes which code the radial styloid process and medial maleollus are situated closely and express a similar phenotype in each region.

References

1. Radford PJ, Matthewson MH (1987) Hypoplastic scaphoid: An unusual cause of carpal tunnel syndrome. J Hand Surg [Br] 12:236–238

2. Treble NJ (1985) Congenital absence of the scaphoid in the "VATER" association. J Hand Surg [Br] 10:251–252

3. Davison EP (1962) Congenital hypoplasia of the carpal scaphoid bone. J Bone Joint Surg [Br] 44:816–827

4. Eaves J, Campiche P (1922) Note on a malformation of the carpus. J Bone Joint Surg [Am] 4:78–80

5. Hall RF, Keuhn D, Prieto J (1986) Congenital hypoplasia of the thumb ray with absent carpal navicular and hypertrophic styloid process of the radius: A case report. J Hand Surg [Am] 11:32–35

6. Hanley T, Conlon PC (1957) Congenital deformity of the carpus associated with maldevelopment of certain thenar muscles. J Bone Joint Surg [Br] 39:458–462

7. Hodgson AR (1943) Congenital retardation in development of the carpal navicular, first metacarpal, and styloid process of the radius. Br J Surg 31:95–96

8. Krauss CM, Herman TE, Holmes LB (1987) Unilateral carpal bone deformity in mother and son. Am J Med Genet 26:557–563

9. O'Rahilly R (1951) Morphological patterns in limb deficiencies and duplications. Am J Anat 89:135–193

10. Srivastava KK, Kochhar VL (1972) Congenital absence of the carpal scaphoid. J Bone Joint Surg [Am] 54:1782

11. O'Rahilly R (1953) A survey of carpal and tarsal anomalies. J Bone Joint Surg [Am] 35:626–642

12. Kelikian H (1974) Congenital deformity of the hand and forearm. Saunders, Philadelphia

13. Hauch PP (1946) The fate of an accessory ossicle. Br J Radiol 19:518–519

14. Marti T (1944) Ein interessanter Fall von Naviculare Bipartitum und akzessorischen Handwurzelknochen. Schweiz Med Wochenschr 74:960–962

15. Bunnell S (1956) Surgery of the hand, 3rd edn. Lippincott, Philadelphia, pp 932–935

16. Rauterberg E (1968) Beitrag zur Arbeit "Angeborene Synostose von Radius, Naviculare und Lunatum mit benachbarter Arthrose" von G. Reisinger und D. V. Torklus. Arch Orthop Unfall-Chir 63:133–134

17. Tognolo P, Poggi U (1963) Un raro caso di sinostosi congenita scaforadiale. Arch Putti Chir Organi Mov 18:418–421

18. Wood-Jones F (1942) Principles of anatomy as seen in the hand. Williams and Wilkins, Baltimore

19. Hardman TG, Wigoder SB (1928) An unusual development of the carpal scaphoid. Br J Radiol 1:155–158

20. Powell HDW (1961) Extra center of ossification for the medial malleolus in children. J Bone Joint Surg [Br] 43:107–113

Carpal Instabilities in Patients After Reduction of Lunate and Perilunar Dislocations

AKIO MINAMI, HIDEYA ITOGA, and MASATOSHI TAKAHARA[1]

Abstract. Twenty-five patients with lunate and perilunar dislocations were treated in our department during the past 10 years. Twenty-three of these patients were followed-up for more than 1 year (average 5 years 2 months), with two failing to obtain normal anatomical carpal architecture: one underwent arthrodesis of the wrist and the other had proximal row carpectomy. The remaining 21 patients were evaluated for this study. They were classified into 3 groups according to the existence of carpal instabilities after reduction, as determined by roentgenograms. Patients with a residual gap between the scaphoid and lunate of more than 3 mm after reduction of their dislocations were considered to have poor clinical results. These clinical analyses in patients after reduction of lunate and perilunar dislocation suggest a significant correlation between clinical results and carpal instabilities.

Keywords: Carpal instability — Dorsiflexed intercalated segment instability — Lunate dislocation — Perilunate dislocation

Introduction

Lunate and perilunar dislocations are comparatively uncommon and constitute only about 10% of all carpal injuries [1]. While many different forms of treatment have been advocated, the long-term results have not always been well documented [2–7]. There have been several reports detailing the carpal instabilities that occur in patients after reduction of lunate or perilunar dislocations with or without fracture of the scaphoid [8–13]. However, there have been few reports describing the correlation between clinical results and carpal instabilities in patients with these dislocations [8, 10, 13].

Within the past 10 years, 25 patients with lunate and perilunar dislocations were treated at the Hokkaido University Hospital and its affiliated hospitals. The following is a report of our findings on the relationship between the clinical results and carpal instabilities in these patients.

Patients and Methods

Twenty-five patients with lunate and perilunar dislocations were treated during the past 10 years. The ages of the patients at the first visit ranged from 18 to 53 years (average 28.4 years). Of these 25 patients, 23 were followed more than 1 year (average 5 years 2 months).

Four patients had palmar lunate dislocations and two had palmar perilunar dislocations. The remaining 17 patients had dorsal perilunar dislocations [14].

The interval between the dislocation and the initial visit ranged from 0 days to 8 months. Two patients were seen within 1 month of the time of injury and the remaining 21 patients were seen and treated more than 1 month after the dislocation. This suggests the propensity for perilunar dislocations to be neglected or misdiagnosed.

The injury occurred after a fall in 12 patients and was due to an automobile or industrial accident in 11 patients. The position of the injured wrist at the instant of trauma was with the forearm in pronation and the wrist in extension, as reported by all patients who could recall this detail.

[1] Surgery of the Hand, Department of Orthopaedic Surgery, Hokkaido University School of Medicine, Kita-15-Jo, Nishi-7-Chome, Kita-Ku, Sapporo 060, Japan

Treatment

Closed reduction was indicated and attempted in the two patients seen within 1 month of the time of injury. This procedure succeeded in only one of them and the other plus 19 of the 21 patients who had been seen later than 1 month from the time of injury, were treated by open reduction. Normal anatomical carpal architecture was obtained. Of the remaining two patients who were seen for relatively late treatment, one was treated by pan-arthrodesis of the wrist and the other by proximal row carpectomy. These two patients were excluded and the remaining 21 patients were evaluated for this study.

Fracture of the scaphoid was present in 15 of the 21 patients, and of these 15, 7 developed pseudoarthrosis. Five of them were treated by bone grafting using the Matti-Russe technique or the Herbert screw. The two remaining patients were not treated. Three patients had an associated fracture of the triquetrum for which no specific treatment was given. Median nerve paresis was observed in 12 patients after injury, all of whom recovered completely after reduction with no specific neutral decompression having been performed.

The external cast or splint support was used from 4 to 12 weeks (average 6.3 weeks). The dislocations of twelve patients, in whom open reduction was unsuccessful, were fixed internally with Kirschner wires.

Evaluation of Clinical Results

The clinical results were estimated according to a modification of the method of Green and O'Brien [14]. We employed 3 of their 5 criteria: pain in the wrist, range of motion of the wrist, and grasping power. We excluded the effect of the patient's returning to his original job because all our patients succeeded in doing so. The X-ray evaluation criterion was also excluded in order to analyze the correlation between the later clinical results and the roentgenographic findings after reduction of the dislocation. The distribution of points in each criterion in our clinical evaluation is shown in Table 1, with the clinical results being expressed as points.

X-Ray Findings

At the last follow-up examination, a series of lateral radiographs was obtained in all patients with the wrist in a neutral position, fully ex-

Table 1. Clinical evaluation. (From [13] with permission)

Pain:	None	50 Points
(50 points)	Cold weather symptoms	40
	Mild, no effect on activity	25
	Moderate, affects activity	10
	Severe	0
Range of motion:	140° or more	35 Points
(35 points)	100°–100°	25
	70°–100°	15
	40°–70°	10
	Less than 40°	0
Grip strength:	Normal	15 Points
(15 points)	Greater than 70% of normal	10
	Greater than 50% of normal	5
	Less than 50% of normal	0

tended, and fully flexed. Posteroanterior views were taken with the wrist in a neutral position, radially deviated, and ulnarly deviated. The roentgenograms of the affected wrist were compared with those of the unaffected wrist.

The 21 patients were classified into 3 groups according to X-ray findings in the posteroanterior view of the affected wrist after reduction of the dislocation. Group I consisted of eight patients with a gap between the scaphoid and lunate of more than three mm (Fig. 1). In group II there were three patients with incongruity between the lunate and triquetrum (Fig. 2). The ten patients in group III had an apparently normal anatomical carpal architecture.

The scapholunate angles were measured in the lateral X-rays with the wrist in a neutral position [8, 12]. In most of the patients who developed scaphoid non-union and in some in whom the scaphoids were united, there was often an angle between the proximal pole of the scaphoid and the distal pole. We did not measure the angle between these poles because the proximal poles of the scaphoid were too short to be measured in most cases. The longitudinal axis of the scaphoid was drawn through the midpoints of its proximal and distal poles. Accurate scapholunate angle measurements were obtained by correcting the angles in lateral X-rays with the wrist in 3 positions. The radiolunate and capitolunate angles were also measured in the lateral X-rays with the wrist in 3 positions. The changes of the radiolunate and capitolunate angles during the arc of motion from flexion to extension in the affected wrist were compared with these angles in the unaffected wrist.

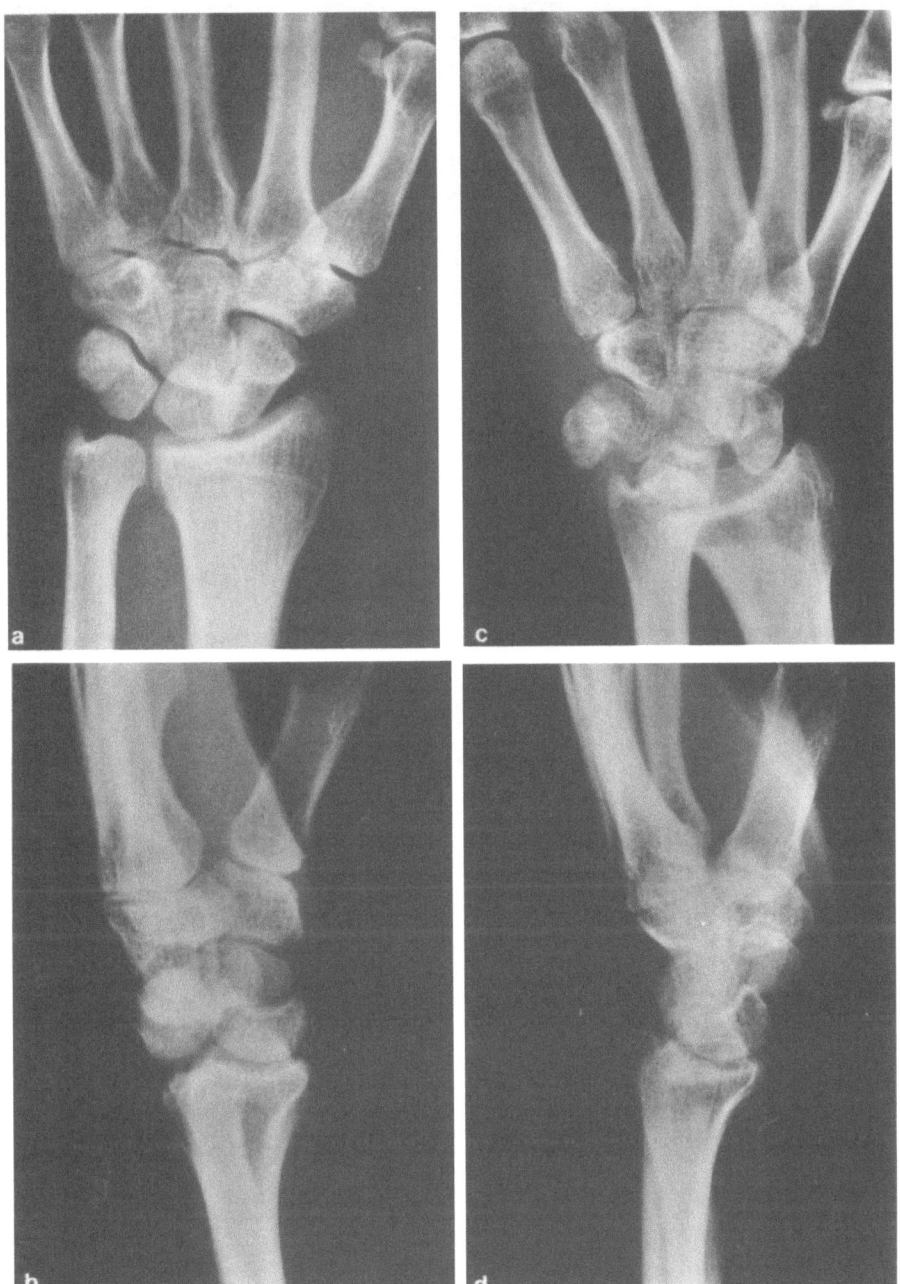

Fig. 1. Left perilunar dislocation in a 37-year-old male who was seen immediately after the trauma. **a, b** X-rays showed dorsal perilunar dislocation. Closed reduction was performed and reduction was obtained. **c, d** X-rays taken 12 months after closed reduction showed a 7.5 mm gap between the scaphoid and lunate and a scapholunate angle of 90°. The clinical result was 30 points. (From [13] with permission)

Results

Clinical Findings

The clinical results for the 21 patients after reduction of lunate and perilunar dislocations ranged from 30 to 90 points (average 62.3 points). Eight out of the twenty-one patients had less than 60 points (group I), with the range being from 30 to 55 points (average 38 points). In group II (three patients), clinical results showed 60–80

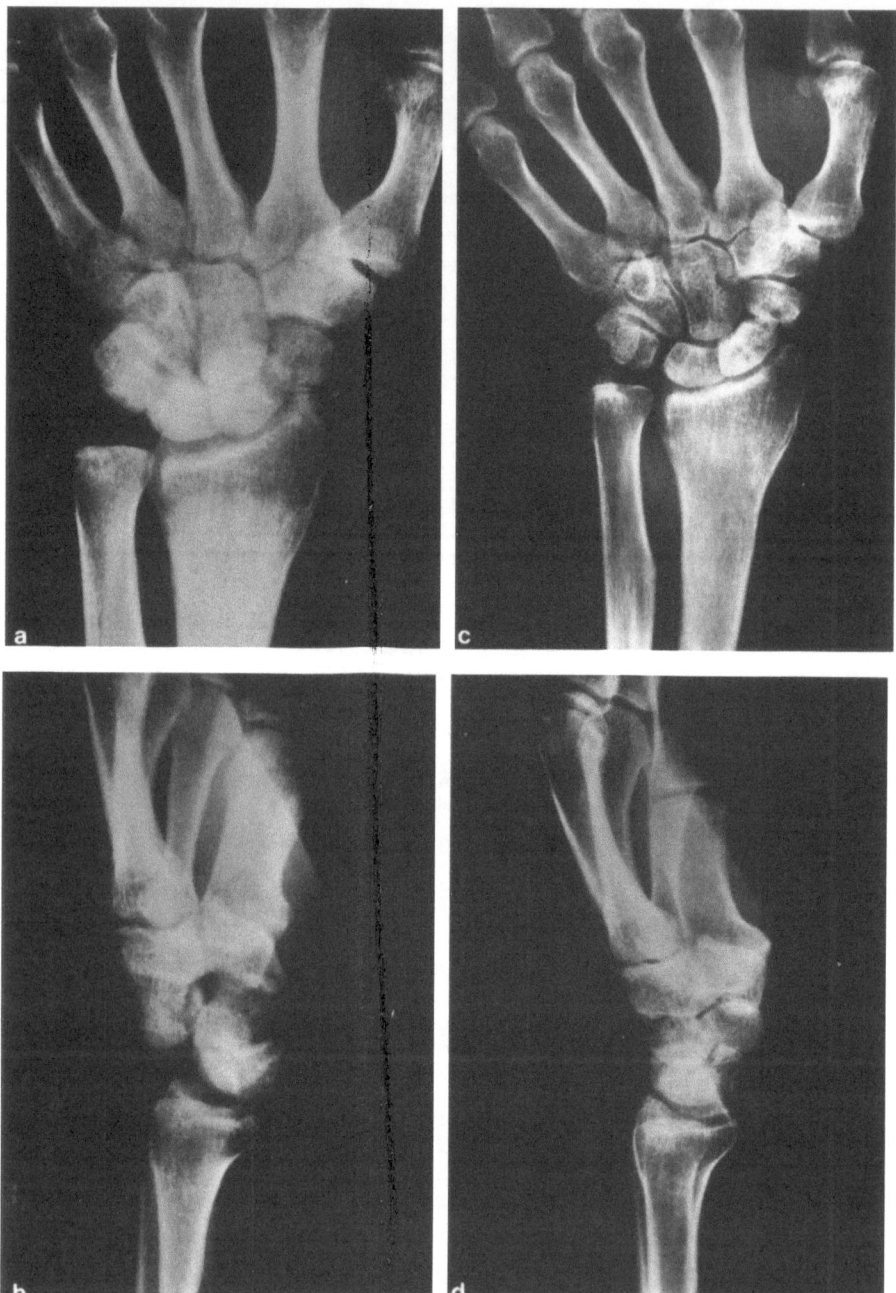

Fig. 2. Left perilunar dislocation with fracture of the scaphoid in a 36-year-old male who was seen 6 weeks after the trauma. **a, b** X-rays showed dorsal perilunar dislocation with fracture of the scaphoid. Open reduction was performed and reduction was obtained. **c, d** X-rays taken 3 years 8 months after open reduction showed incongruity between the lunate and triquetrum with a scapholunate angle of 80°. The clinical result were 80 points. (From [13] with permission)

points (average 70 points), and in group III (ten patients), the range was from 65 to 90 points (average 78 points). These results suggest that the existence of a gap between the scaphoid and lunate in the wrists of patients after reduction of the dislocation correlated significantly with poor clinical results.

There was no significant correlation between the clinical results of patients treated earlier or later from the time of injury. There also were no

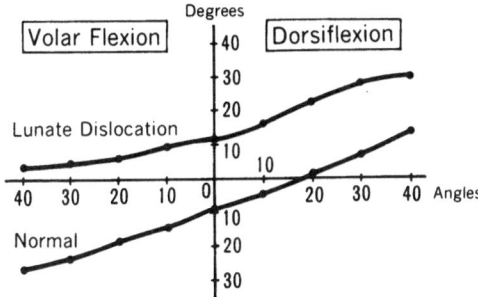

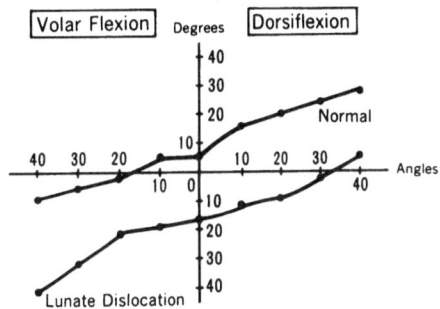

Fig. 3. Changes of radiolunate angles during the arc of motion from flexion to extension in affected and normal wrists. (From [13] with permission)

Fig. 4. Changes of capitolunate angles during the arc of motion from flexion to extension in affected and normal wrists. (From [13] with permission)

significant correlations between the periods of immobilization and the clinical results, and between the clinical results in patients with and without internal fixation after open reduction.

Fracture of the scaphoid was present in 15 of the 21 patients, and osteosynthesis was performed in 5 of them. Their clinical results averaged 72 points while the remaining ten patients showed an average of 60 points. However, there was no statistically significant difference between them. In three patients who had associated fracture of the triquetrum the clinical results averaged 72 points. Median nerve compression was associated with the injury in 12 patients whose clinical results averaged 56 points, while those of the remaining 9 patients averaged 65 points.

Roentgenographic Analyses

The scapholunate angle was measured in lateral X-rays with the wrist in a neutral position. The scapholunate angles ranged from 72° to 102° (average 90°) in the eight patients in group I. The scapholunate angles ranged from 65° to 80° (average 72°) in group II (three patients) and from 55° to 75° (average 64°) in group III (ten patients). On the other hand, the scapholunate angles ranged from 43° to 62° (average 46°) in normal control wrists (12 cases). Thus, the scapholunate angles in most patients after reduction of the wrist dislocation were greater than 60° in comparison to normal wrists which were equal to or less than 60°. This result suggests that X-rays of most of the wrists after reduction show dorsiflexed intercalated segment instability (DISI) [8–10, 12, 13] even though apparently normal carpal architecture was seen on the posteroanterior views, as in group III.

The position of the lunate and the motion in the radiocarpal and midcarpal joints were investigated by measuring the changes of radiolunate and capitolunate angles on flexion-extension lateral X-rays. These changes are shown in Fig. 3. The radiolunate angles were more than 0° (positive) during the arc of motion from flexion to extension in the affected wrist. This result shows that the lunate remains dorsiflexed throughout this motion rather than being flexed during palmar flexion. The range of radiolunate angles in the affected wrists during flexion-extension of the wrist were slightly smaller than those in normal wrists.

Changes of capitolunate angles during the arc of motion from flexion to extension in the wrist are shown in Fig. 4. Capitolunate angles remained below 0° (negative) relative to the dorsiflexed position of the lunate. However, the range of the capitolunate angles in the affected wrists during flexion-extension of the wrist was the same as that in the normal wrist.

Discussion

Linscheid et al. [8] reported on several patients with carpal instabilities occurring after reduction of lunate and perilunar dislocations. In this paper, we have attempted to correlate the clinical results with a measurement of the degree of carpal instability in patients following reduction of lunate dislocations.

In our series, patients with a gap between the scaphoid and lunate (group I) showed significantly poor clinical results. Patients with incongruity between the lunate and triquetrum (group II) and those with apparently normal

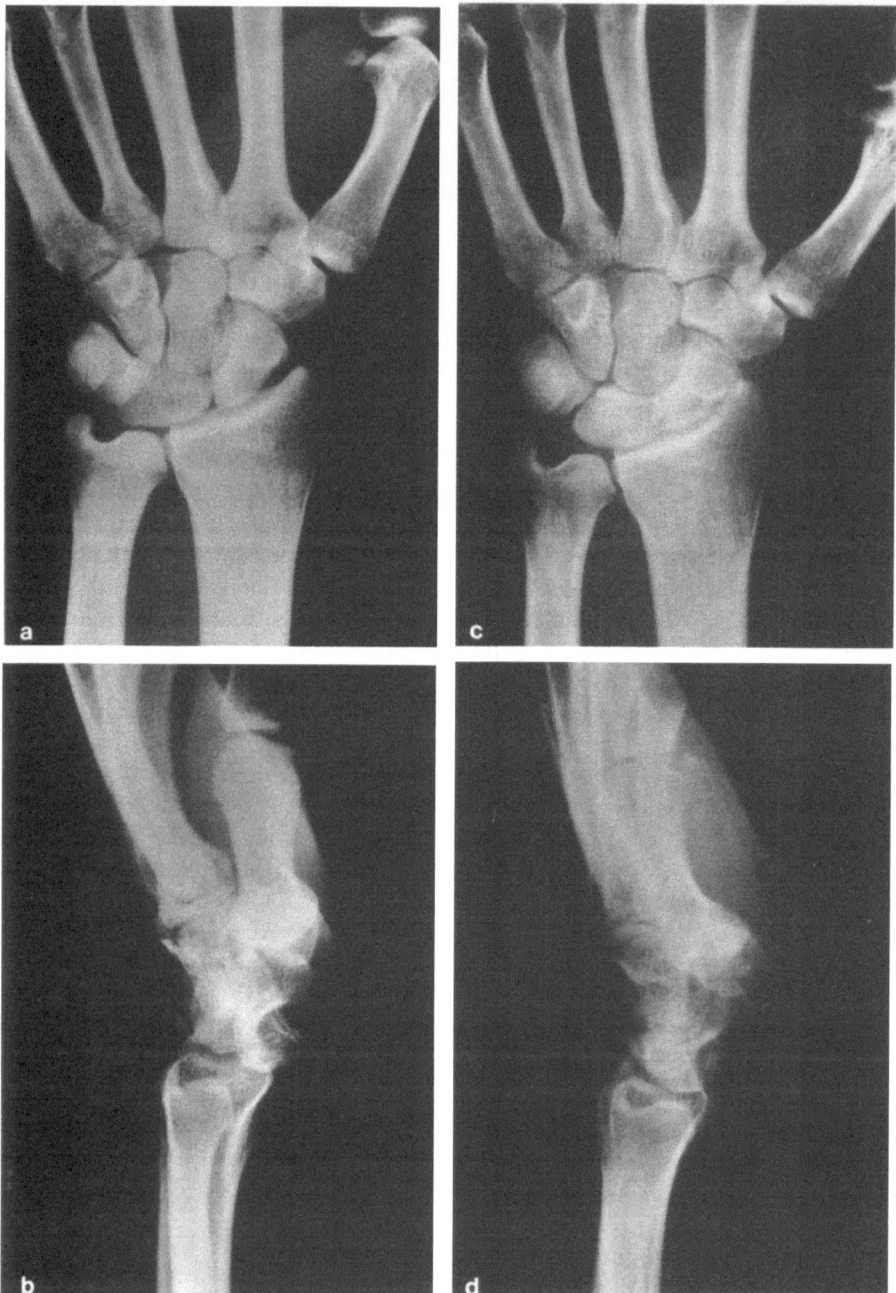

Fig. 5. Left lunate dislocation in a 22-year-old male who was seen 8 months after the trauma. **a, b** X-rays showed a palmar lunate dislocation. Open reduction with ligament reconstruction was performed. **c, d** X-rays taken 2 years and 1 month after open reduction showed normal anatomical carpal architecture with a scapholunate angle of 60°. The clinical result was 70 points. (From [13] with permission)

anatomical carpal architecture (group III) showed comparatively satisfactory clinical results. This suggests that the existence of a scapholunate gap significantly affects clinical results. On the other hand, the existence of lunotriquetral incongruity does not seem to affect clinical results. However, these patients may develop disabilities in the affected wrist after a longer-term follow-up [15].

Most of the patients showed a slight to severe DISI pattern [7–10, 12, 13]. Scapholunate angles averaged 90° in group I, 72° in group II, and 64°

in group III, compared with 46° in the normal control group. It is surprising that even patients in group III, who had normal anatomical carpal architecture in the posteroanterior X-rays, showed a slight DISI pattern.

In our study, there was no significant correlation between the clinical results in patients with and without internal fixation of the wrist after open reduction. After open reduction, two or three Kirschner wires were used in 12 patients, being introduced into the non-union site of the scaphoid and between the scaphoid and lunate in most cases. No Kirschner wire was introduced between the radius and proximal carpal row. Dobyns et al. [9] described that a minimum of two Kirschner wires should be introduced to stabilize the position of the radius, lunate, and the distal carpal row, and the position of the radius, scaphoid, and the distal carpal row. Introduction of Kirschner wires between the radius, lunate, scaphoid, and the distal carpal row is essential for maintaining the reduced position.

The clinical results in the 15 patients with fracture of the scaphoid and in the 3 patients with fracture of the triquetrum all averaged 72 points. From these results, it was difficult to determine whether or not fracture of the scaphoid and of the triquetrum actually affected the clinical results. However, the clinical results were not affected by any association with median nerve compression at the initial visit.

X-ray evaluation in this study indicated that the anatomical relationship between the lunate and scaphoid and the triquetrum and capitate should be accurately maintained in order to provide synergistic motion between the lunate and scaphoid during wrist movement. An anatomical carpal relationship appears necessary to achieve a satisfactory clinical result.

Palmer et al. [10] reported that if the rupture of the radioscapholunate ligament was seen within 4 weeks of injury, an antomical reduction maintained in plaster for 8 weeks led to good results. Ligament ruptures that could not be held in reduction or which were diagnosed after 4 weeks did poorly with immobilization only. Results after ligament reconstruction for late instabilities ranged from good to fair in 66% of their patients. Other surgical options include inter-carpal arthrodeses, proximal row carpectomy, or similar reconstructive procedures. In our series, three patients were treated by open reduction associated with ligament repair and three patients were treated by ligament reconstruction using the extensor carpi radialis longus tendon as described by Dobyns et al. [9]. Clinical results in these patients showed an average of 82 points with scapholunate angles of 54° (Fig. 5).

We agree with the suggestion of Palmer et al.: if a normal anatomical carpal relationship and synergistic motion between the lunate and scaphoid are not obtained, ligament repair is possible and ligament reconstruction between the lunate and scaphoid should be performed at the earliest opportunity.

Acknowledgments. We are grateful to Kiyoshi Kaneda, MD, Department of Orthopaedic Surgery, Hokkaido University School of Medicine, Sapporo, Japan, and to Ronald L. Linscheid, MD, Hand Section, Department of Orthopaedics, Mayo Clinic, Rochester, Minnesota, USA for their constant interest and guidance in this investigation.

References

1. Dobyns JH, Linscheid RL (1975a) Carpal injuries. In: Rockwood CA Jr, Green DP (eds) Fractures. Lippincott, Philadelphia, pp 385–440
2. Russell TB (1949) Inter-carpal dislocations and fracture-dislocations: A review of fifty-nine cases. J Bone Joint Surg [Br] 31:524–531
3. Aitken AP, Nalebuff EA (1960) Volar trans-navicular perilunar dislocation of the carpus. J Bone Joint Surg [Am] 42:1050–1057
4. Campbell RD, Lance EM, Yeoh CB (1964) Lunate and perilunar dislocations. J Bone Joint Surg [Br] 46:55–72
5. Stewart M, Cross H (1968) The management of injuries of the carpal lunate with a review of sixty cases. J Bone Joint Surg [Am] 50:1489
6. Fountain SS, Chapman MW, Bovill EG (1973) Fracture-dislocations of the wrist. J Bone Joint Surg [Am] 55:1319
7. Panting AL, Lamb DW, Noble J, Haw CS (1984) Dislocations of the lunate with and without fracture of the scaphoid. J Bone Joint Surg [Br] 66:391–395
8. Linscheid RL, Dobyns JH, Beabout JW, Bryan RS (1972) Traumatic instability of the wrist. Diagnosis, classification and pathomechanics. J Bone Joint Surg [Am] 54:1612–1632
9. Dobyns JH, Linscheid RL, Chao EYS, Weber ER, Swanson GE (1975b) Traumatic instability of the wrist. American Academy of Orthopedic Surgeries. Instructional Course Lecture 24:182–199

10. Palmer AK, Dobyns JH, Linscheid RL (1978) Management of post-traumatic instability of the wrist secondary to ligament rupture. J Hand Surg 3:507–532

11. Mayfield JK (1980) Mechanism of carpal injuries. Clin Orthop 149:45–54

12. Taleisnik J (1980) Post-traumatic carpal instability. Clin Orthop 149:73–82

13. Minami A, Ogino T, Ohshio I, Minami M (1986) Correlation between clinical results and carpal instabilities in patients after reduction of lunate and perilunar dislocations. J Hand Surg [Br] 11:213–220

14. Green DP, O'Brien ET (1980) Classification and management of carpal dislocations. Clin Orthop 149:55–72

15. Reagan DS, Linsheid RL, Dobyns JH (1984) Luno-triquetral sprains. J Hand Surg [Am] 9:502–514

Part VI. Wrist Arthroplasty

Technique and Indications of the Kapandji-Sauvé Procedure in Non-Rheumatoid Diseases of the Wrist

ADALBERT I. KAPANDJI[1]

Abstract. The Kapandji-Sauvé operation consists of arthrodesis of the distal radioulnar joint associated with a short segmentary resection of the lower ulnar shaft just above it. The original (1936) and two contemporary techniques of this operation are described.

History

As Buck-Gramcko showed recently [1], this technique was not invented by Lauenstein, whose publication in 1887 discussed the subperiostal resection of the distal end of the ulna after a distal fracture of the forearm [2], and again in 1890 when he described the "resection of the *medial meniscus of the knee*" [3]. The mistake came from Steindler in his book [4] in 1946. Gonçalves in 1974 was the first to clarify this question [5]. Taleisnik [6] in his book "*The Wrist*" (1985) recognized the paternity of Sauvé and Kapandji [2], but continued to name this procedure "Lauenstein's", as sanctioned for use in English-speaking countries.

Other procedures may be used in disorders of the distal radioulnar joint (DRUJ). One of the most commonly performed is the Moore-Darrach procedure which involves the excision of the ulnar head, first proposed by Moore in 1880 [7] and then by Darrach in 1912 [8] and in 1913 [9]. Taleisnik [6] states, however, that the French surgeon Desault [10] was the first to mention the resection of the ulnar head. Buck-Gramcko [1] who read Desault's paper did not find this to be mentioned, but discovered in another French surgeon's book, written in 1855 by Malgaigne [11], the mention of a resection of the ulnar head

after an irreducible dislocation of the DRUJ. The resection procedure of the ulnar head was recently modified by Bowers [12] who proposed hemi-resection with interposition of fibrous tissues.

In 1918, two French surgeons, Le Fort and Cololian [13] proposed a procedure of intentional pseudarthrosis of the lower ulnar shaft leaving the DRUJ undisturbed, thus the limitations of this joint's range of motion would be compensated by the pseudarthrosis. The same procedure was described and used in 1921 by Baldwin [14].

The ulnar shortening method was described by Darrach in 1913 [9], and elaborated upon by Milch [15] in 1941 with an improved osteosynthesis using a screw-fixed plate.

Ligamentous surgery in the treatment of a common luxation of the lower ulna was proposed in 1935 by Bazy and Galtier [16], but after observing the frequent failure of this procedure [17], two French authors, Sauvé and Kapandji [18], proposed an original one, combining the definitive fusion of the DRUJ with an intentional pseudarthrosis of the ulnar shaft above and close to the fusion, so as to compensate for the blocking of the DRUJ. In 1986, Kapandji [19] published an improvement of the original procedure which included an automatic lifting-up of the ulnar head in cases of positive ulnar variance.

Keywords: Distal radioulnar joint — Radius malunion — DRUJ instability — Ulnar head resection — Ulnar head fusion — Pronation-supination troubles

Techniques

Technique I

This is designed for chronic instabilities secondary to sprains and distal radioulnar dislocations. In this case, the ulnar head is in its proper location

[1] Clinique de l'Yvette, 43, Route de Corbeil, 91160, Long-jumeau, France

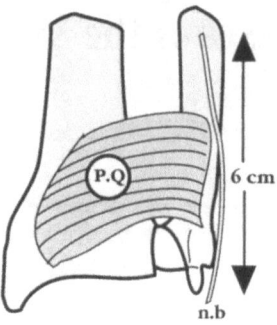

Fig. 1. Procedure I. The approach. A longitudinal skin incision, 6 cm-long, is made at the medial aspect of the wrist from the ulnar styloid process. Care must be taken to protect the subcutaneous branches of the ulnar nerve (*n.b.*). *P.Q.*, Pronator quadratus

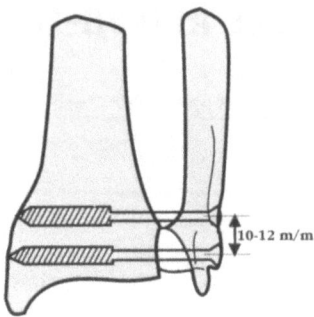

Fig. 3. Procedure I. The second screw is drilled, precisely parallel to the first one, at a level located 10 or 12 mm above it

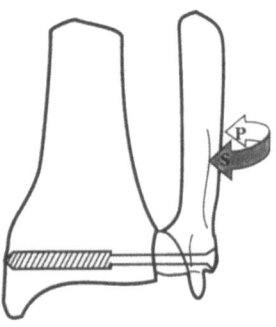

Fig. 2. Procedure I. The first screw. The lower ulnar shaft is exposed in an *extra-periosteal* way. With the wrist in the mid-position of pronation/supination (*PS*), the first screw is set transversally through the ulnar head. This is a temporary fixation

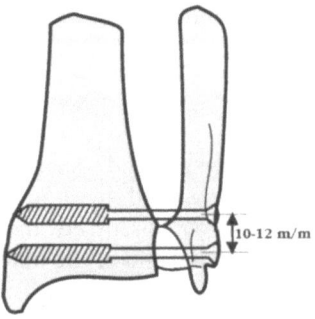

Fig. 4. Procedure I. The segmental resection of the ulnar shaft. The lower transversal cut of the ulnar shaft may be done at a level located 3–5 mm above the second screw, using an oscillating saw. The second cut, precisely parallel to the first one, is done 10–12 mm above it

at the sigmoid notch level and may be blocked in place. Following are the steps taken in this technique:

1. The approach is done through a 6 cm-long medial incision at the ulnar side of the wrist, beginning at the level of the ulnar styloid process and prolonged proximally (Fig. 1). It is of the utmost importance *not to wound the subcutaneous branches of the ulnar nerve*.
2. The lower ulnar shaft is exposed in an *extra-periosteal mode*.
3. Setting the wrist in mid-position of pronation/supination, a temporary fixation is done with a transversal screw passing through the DRUJ in the location of the definitive lower screw (Fig. 2).
4. In the same way, a second screw is drilled, precisely parallel to the first one, at a level

located 10 or 12 mm above it (Fig. 3). Note that this second screw was not mentioned in the original procedure: its role is to avoid the tilting of the distal ulnar fragment around the first screw. If there is not enough room, it can be replaced by a Kirschner wire and then put in later when the arthrodesis has been completed.
5. Then, the lower transversal cut of the ulnar shaft may be carried out at a level located 3–5 mm above the second screw, using an oscillating saw (Fig. 4).
6. The second cut (Fig. 4), precisely parallel to the first one, is done 10–12 mm above the first cut, and the segment of the ulnar shaft is brought away with its periosteum (Fig. 5), but keeping the fibers of the pronator quadratus in place; before liberating the bone segment from the pronator quadratus, this

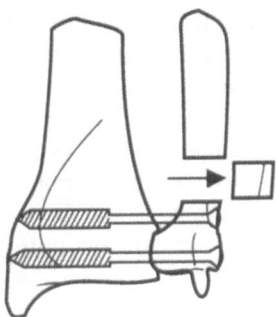

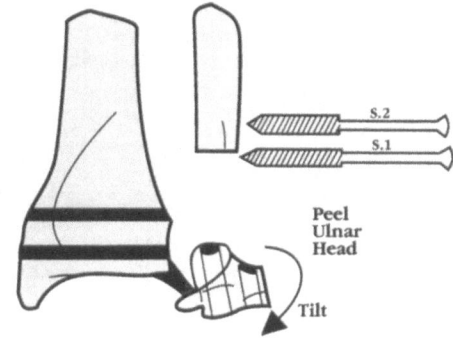

Fig. 5. Procedure I. The avulsion of the ulnar segment. The ulnar segment is brought away with its periosteum, but leaving the fibers of the pronator quadratus in place; the pronator quadratus is prepared in order to enter easily into the bony gap

Fig. 7. Procedure I. The preparation for arthrodesis. The cartilage of the ulnar head is also carefully peeled off: this is the indispensable condition of the joint fusion

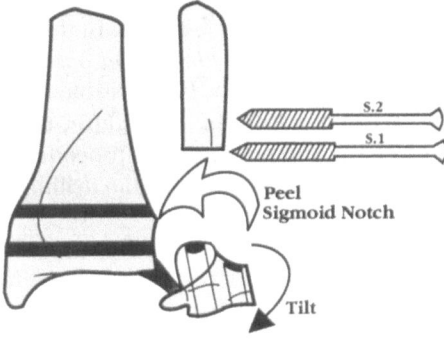

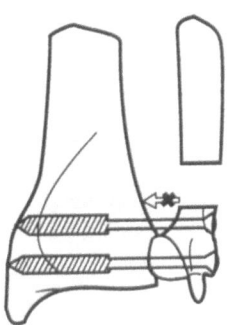

Fig. 6. Procedure I. The preparation for arthrodesis. After taking off the two temporary screws (*S.1*, *S.2*), the distal ulnar fragment is tilted medially around the "hinge" of the triangular fibrous cartilaginous complex (TFCC). The DRUJ can thus be open at its upper part, its capsula removed, but the TFCC is saved. The cartilage of the sigmoid notch of the radius is carefully peeled off: this is the indispensable condition of the fusion

Fig. 8. Procedure I. The DRUJ arthrodesis. The ulnar head is reset in its correct position and the two cancellous bone screws are again inserted into their holes. The length of these screws must be exactly calculated so that they contact the opposite wall of the radius. The lower screw must be tightened strongly, but not the upper one (*crossed arrow*): the axis of the distal part of the ulna must stay parallel to the axis of the radius

muscle is gently separated from the anterior aspect of the radius, so as to enter easily into the bony gap.

7. The two temporary screws are removed (Fig. 6) and the distal ulnar fragment is tilted medially around the "hinge" of the triangular fibrous cartilaginous complex (TFCC).

8. It is thus possible to open the DRUJ at its upper part, to remove its capsula, and evaluate the status of the TFCC which must not be resected except if it is already destroyed.

9. The cartilage of the sigmoid notch of the radius (Fig. 6) and of the ulnar head (Fig. 7) is carefully peeled off: this is the indispensable condition of the fusion.

10. The ulnar head is reset in its correct position and the two cancellous bone screws are again inserted in the two prepared holes (Fig. 8). The length of these screws must be exactly calculated so that they contact the opposite wall of the radius. The lower screw must be tightened strongly, but not the upper one: the axis of the distal part of the ulna must stay parallel to the axis of the radius. We do not put a cancellous graft between the radius and the ulna as Gonçalves does.

11. The gap between the two extremities of the ulna is filled by the already liberated pronator quadratus to avoid bony reconstruction (Fig. 9); the muscle fibers are fixed medially on

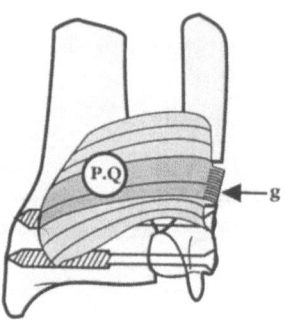

Fig. 9. Procedure I. The pronator quadratus interposition. The ulnar gap is filled by the already liberated pronator quadratus (*P.Q*) to avoid bony reconstruction; the muscle fibers are fixed medially on the fibrous tissues so as to maintain them in the gap (*g*)

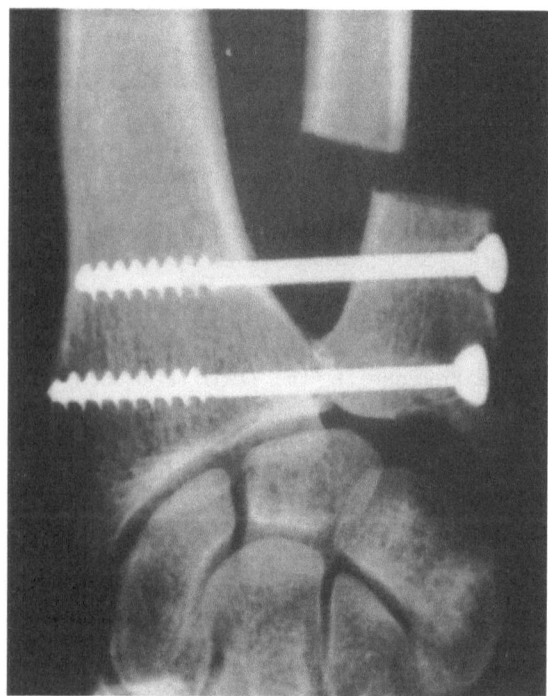

Fig. 10. Procedure I. The frontal radiograph. This radiograph shows all the characteristics of a good technique: tight coaptation between the ulnar head and the radial sigmoid notch, correct position and good length of the two screws, a lower cut adequately distal, and a not too-wide gap

the fibrous tissues so as to maintain them in the gap.

12. The skin is carefully closed without disturbing the subcutaneous nervous branches; a suction drain is put under the skin closure and taken off after 3 or 4 days.

13. Lateral and frontal radiographs are taken (Fig. 10) and show all the characteristics of a good technique: tight coaptation between the ulnar head and the radial sigmoid notch, good position and length of the two screws, a lower cut sufficiently distal, and not too wide a gap.

14. No cast is applied; rehabilitation must be undertaken as soon as the postoperative pain begins to diminish.

Technique II

The second procedure, described by Kapandji [19], is especially designed for the limitations of the prono-supination range of motion after Colles' fractures, when a shortening of the radius causes an incongruency of the distal radioulnar joint with a *positive ulnar variance*. In this cases, *it is necessary to lift up the ulnar head before blocking it* in the sigmoid notch. It is possible to do that by guesswork, but with this procedure, the lifting up is automatic and precise. This procedure is the same as the first one, except for the drilling of the screw holes.

Before beginning the operation, the *excessive length of the ulna* must be calculated on the frontal radiograph (Fig. 11). Normally, the ulnar variance is *negative*: the inferior aspect of the ulnar head is located 2mm above the inferior edge of the radial sigmoid notch. If the ulnar head level is located *e* m/m under the level of the sigmoid notch, *excess of the ulnar length A* is evaluated: $A = e + 2$. For example, if $= 3$mm, then $A = 5$. The steps involved in this technique are as follows:

1. The hole of the lower screw is drilled at its usual place (Fig. 12), but *only in the ulnar head* and at its center.

2. The hole of the second screw is drilled parallel to the first one, 10–12mm above it, and also *only through the ulna*.

3. The third hole is drilled, the wrist being in mid-position of pronation/supination, parallel to the others holes, *both in the ulna and the radius*, at a level located at the distance A (Fig. 12) from the second one.

4. The length of the segmental shaft resection B is calculated according to the desired wideness G of the gap (Fig. 12):

$$B = A + G$$

so that after the lifting-up of the ulnar head A, a gap (G) remains.

5. The lower cut is done in a transversal plane,

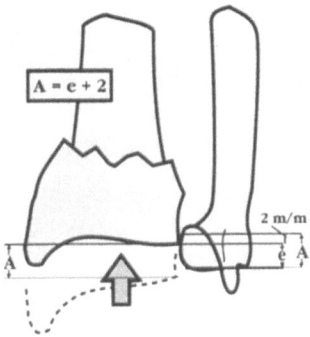

Fig. 11. Procedure II. The pre-operative calculations. With the normal ulnar variance being quoted *negative* at −2 mm and in the other hand the excess of the ulnar length being *e*, the lifting value *A* is the sum of *e + 2*

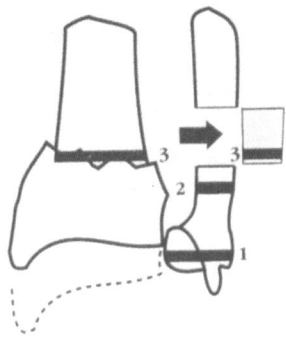

Fig. 13. Procedure II. The ulnar segmental resection. Removal of ulnar shaft segment between the two cuts and the management of the pronator quadratus are the same as in technique I

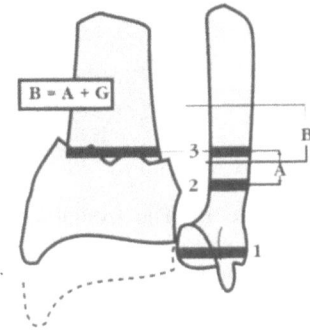

Fig. 12. Procedure II. The three holes. The first hole (*1*) is drilled horizontally in the middle of the ulnar head and *only in it*. The second hole (*2*), which is parallel to the first one, is drilled at a level located 10–12 mm above it, *only in the ulna*. The third hole (*3*) is also parallel, and the wrist, being in mid-pronation/supination position, is drilled at a distance *A* above the second one, both in the ulna and the radius. Then, the cuts may be done. The lower cut is made on the ulna just under the third hole (*3*). The lower cut, parallel to the first one, is made at a distance *B* equal to *A + G* (the desired wideness of the gap)

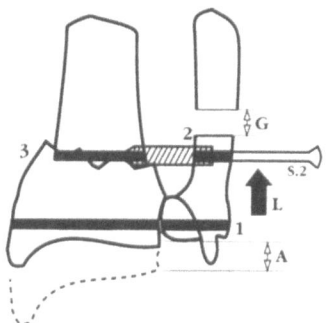

Fig. 14. Procedure II. The lifting-up of the ulnar head. The upper screw (*S.2*) is first set into the hole (*2*) of the ulna, and, after lifting it up in order to make it coincident with the hole (*3*) in the radius, it is screwed into this radial hole: the gap is at its pre-calculated value *G*, and the ulnar variance is now normal at −2 mm

parallel to the screw holes, at a level located just *under the upper hole*.

6. The upper cut, parallel to the first one, is done at a level located at a distance *B* from the first one. The upper hole in the ulna is thus included in the resected shaft segment, which is removed in the same way as in the procedure I, after liberating the pronator quadratus from the anterior aspect of the radius (Fig. 13).
7. Then, the automatic lifting-up of the ulnar head is done (Fig. 14) by inserting the upper screw in the second hole of the ulna and lifting

it to the level of the only hole in the radius, into which it is screwed.

8. Drilling of the lower ulnar hole is completed in the radius (Fig. 15) and the lower screw is set into it: a frontal radiograph shows the lifting-up of the distal ulna, the *normalization of the ulnar variance*, and the good positioning of the two screws.
9. The last part of this procedure is then performed under the same conditions as in technique I: the two screws are removed, the DRUJ is opened, the cartilages are peeled off, and the two screws are set definitively. They must make contact exactly with the opposite wall of the radius. The lower screw must be tightened strongly, but not the upper one (Fig. 16). The pronator quadratus is gently driven and fixed into the gap and the skin is closed.

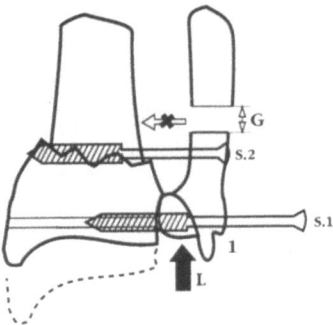

Fig. 15. Procedure II. The setting of the two screws. With the upper screw (*S.2*) being half-tightened, the hole (*1*) in the ulnar head is completed in the radius and the lower screw (*S.1*) is inserted into it

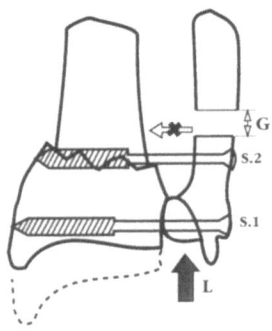

Fig. 16. Procedure II. Tightening the screws. The lower screw (*S.1*) is completely tightened; contrarily, the upper screw (*S.2*) is not tightened too much because the axis of the radius and the ulna must stay parallel

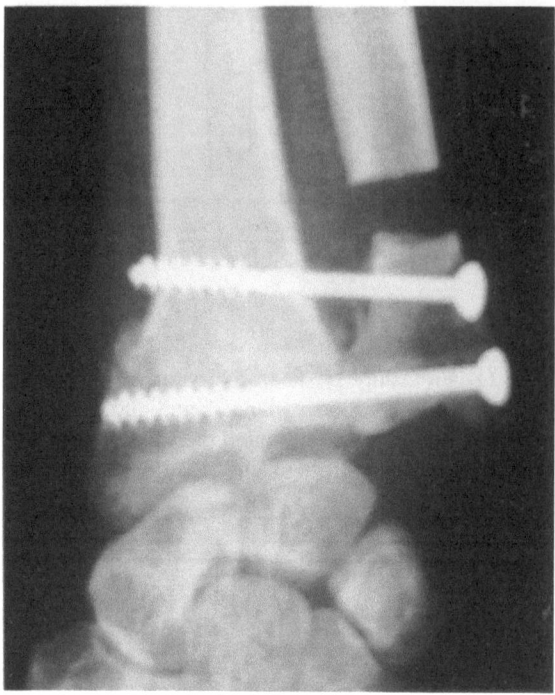

Fig. 17. Procedure II. The frontal radiograph. This view shows the good positioning and length of the two screws as well as the firm fixation of the ulnar head

The gap must be as narrow as possible, only 7 or 8 mm, and as low as possible, in order to avoid ulnar stump instability. The gap can be narrower in rheumatoid indications, where secondary ossifications are not frequent, than in post-traumatic indications where postoperative calcifications are possible. The interposition of pronator quadratus fibers is of the utmost importance to avoid these complications.

A frontal radiograph (Fig. 17) will show the satisfactory positioning and length of the two screws as well as the firm fixation of the ulnar head. A lateral radiograph (Fig. 18) will show the correct orientation of the radial glena.

Post-Operative Care

A cast is not necessary, because passive and active rehabilitation must begin as soon as possible to

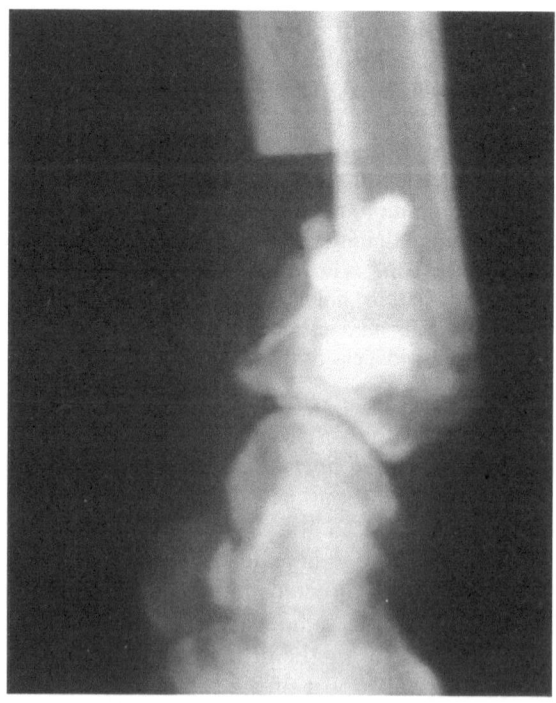

Fig. 18. Procedure II. The lateral radiograph showing the correct orientation of the radial glena

Fig. 19. The "waiter's test". In the first position (*I*), this test evaluates the wrist capability for complete extension and pronation. In the second position (*II*), it evaluates the wrist strength in rectitude and complete supination. Test II is positive when a tray bearing a filled glass can be held on the supinated hand without spilling the water. In the third position (*III*), the firmness of the rectitude and supination is evaluated

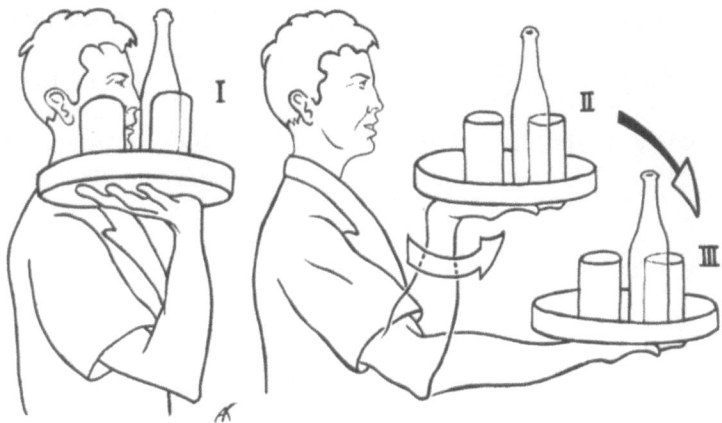

the time when the postoperative pain begins to diminish.

It is not mandatory to remove the screws, because the achievement fusion is very difficult to confirm. If their heads are correctly embedded, they do not cause problems. With time, it is expected that the bony extremities become smoother, especially the upper one.

Results

The range of pronation-supination becomes normal within 3 weeks to 2 months. The supination may be considered as normal when the "waiter's test" is normal (Fig. 19): a tray bearing a filled glass can be held on the supinated hand without spilling the water. Sometimes, this test is positive, but may be painful at first.

The range of flexion-extension of the wrist is not modified in comparison to the previous ROM. The pain disappears in 3–6 months. The previously poor wrist stability is improved, allowing the person to unwind screws and caps and to turn doorknobs.

With early rehabilitation, the grasp becomes the same as it was before the operation, and even stronger within 3–6 months.

The cosmetic appearance is good because the axis of the hand is normal: there is neither ulnar deviation nor medial shifting. It is better than that in ulnar head avulsion. Rarely, there is a slight depression at the medial side of the wrist, but this is not visible because the scar is normally hidden under the wrist.

Complications

There are sometimes *paresthesias* distally to the scar on the medial border of the wrist and dorsally to the fourth and fifth fingers. When the subcutaneous branch of the ulnar nerve is simply bruised, these disappear in a few weeks. However, when the nerve is damaged, the complications are definitive and very troublesome, making it very important to be careful in protecting every neural branch.

The most significant complication is *painful instability of the ulnar stump*: the lower extremity of the upper segment of the ulna is hyper-mobile, especially when the pronated hand bears the body's weight. This mobility is accompanied by pain, especially in the extreme range of pronation or supination or in supporting a weight with the supinated hand. This complication is due to the hyper-mobility of the ulnar stump, because the gap has been left too large and the ulnar upper cut was too proximal. It is for this reason that the cut must be as low as possible and the gap not too wide. If these conditions are met, the painful instability of the ulnar stump does not occur. Note that this complication is also possible in other ulna-resecting procedures, such as the Moore-Darrach or Baldwin.

Indications

This procedure may be used not only instead of the resection of the distal end of the ulna (Moore-Darrach) in rheumatoid dislocations of the distal radioulnar joint, where it is associated with synovectomy and re-alignment of the dorsal tendons, but also in *traumatic complications* such

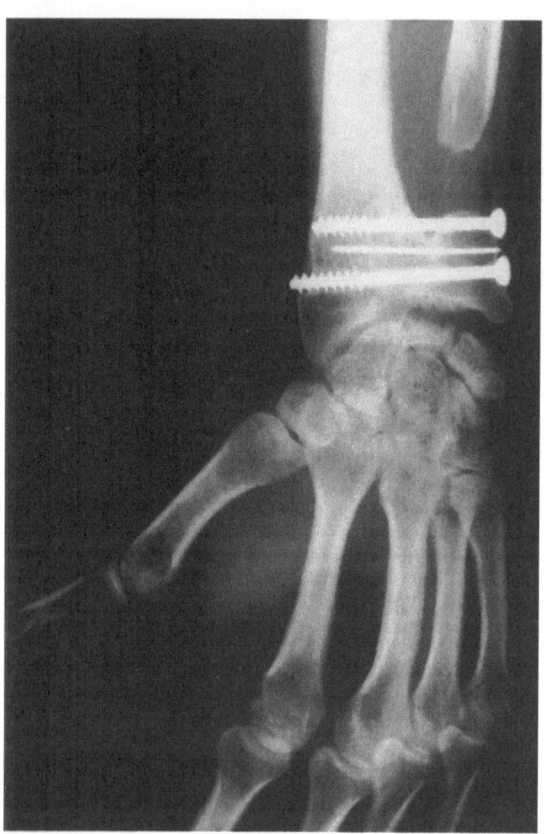

Fig. 20. Radiograph of a case of Madelung's dislocation treated with a combined procedure. The Kapandji-Sauvé procedure may be used in combination with a graft interposed between the radius and ulna in Madelung's dislocation and in cases of chronic instability. The result seen here are excellent

as dislocations, sprains, chronic instabilities, and stiffness of the DRUJ secondary to Colles' fractures, Galeazzi's fractures, lower ulnar and ulnar-head fractures, and even in certain two-bone fractures. It is of great value in malunion after fractures of the lower radial extremity [20, 21] and some surgeons venture to combine it with a radial osteotomy, firmly fixing it with a screwed plate. I once used this procedure, combined with a graft set between the radius and ulna, in a case of chronic instability in Madelung's deformity (Fig. 20) and the results were excellent.

The important criterion for the indication of this procedure is the loss of the linking system between the two bones of the lower extremities. At the present time, the ligamentous procedures are not reliable enough and a simple shortening of the ulna cannot be a good solution because instability will persist.

Summary

The Kapandji-Sauvé operation consists of an arthrodesis of the distal radioulnar joint associated with a short segmentary resection of the lower ulnar shaft located just above it.

As Buck-Gramcko showed recently, this original technique was not devised by Lauenstein, but by Sauvé and Kapandji. Two techniques are described, following the original one which had been proposed in 1936.

The first technique is designed for chronic instabilities following sprains and distal radioulnar dislocations. It is also used in rheumatoid diseases. In these indications, the ulnar head is in its proper location at the sigmoid notch level and may be blocked in place. The original procedure I is described with some small modifications: the extra-periostal approach of the lower ulnar shaft, the temporary fixation of the ulnar head with two screws in mid-position of pronation-supination, the segmental resection of the ulnar shaft above the screws, the opening of the distal radioulnar joint (DRUJ) after removing the screws, the peeling of the radial sigmoid notch and of the ulnar head in order to achieve an arthrodesis, and, finally, the definitive resetting of the two screws in the prepared holes. An important technical point is the filling of the ulnar shaft gap with the fibers of the mobilized pronator quadratus, in order to avoid the uniting of ossifications in the gap. It is also important to begin rehabilitation as soon as the postoperative pain begins to wane.

The second procedure is especially designed for the limitations of the pronosupination motion after Colles' fractures, with an incongruency of the distal radioulnar joint due to a *positive ulnar variance*. In this cases, it is *necessary to lift up the ulnar head before blocking it in the sigmoid notch*. This procedure does this automatically and precisely. It is essentially the same as the first one except for the drilling of the holes. Before the beginning of the operation, the excess of ulnar length must be calculated on the frontal radiograph, measuring the ulnar head level (located e m/m) under the level of the sigmoid notch. Thus, *excess of the ulnar length* (A) is evaluated: $A = e + 2$ (2 = the normal ulnar variance). Then, three transversal and parallel holes are drilled in the ulna: the first one in the center of its head, the second one 10–12 mm above, and the third at a distance (A) from the second one, also drilling the radius as the wrist is set in a mid-pronation/supination position. The length of the segmental shaft resection (B) is calculated according to the desired width (G) of the gap: $B = A + G$, so that after the lifting-up of the ulnar head (A), a gap (G) remains. The lower transversal cut is done parallel to the screw holes at a level located just under the upper hole. The upper cut, parallel to the first one, is done at a level located at a specific distance (B) from the first one. The upper hole in the ulna is thereby included in the resected shaft segment, which is removed (Fig. 13) in the same way as in procedure I, after liberating the pronator quadratus from the anterior aspect of the radius. Then, the final steps of this procedure are performed in the same manner as in technique I: the two screws are removed, the DRUJ is opened, the cartilages are peeled off, and the two screws are set definitively, taking the same precautions. The pronator quadratus is gently moved to and fixed in the gap, and the skin is closed. Note that the screws may be left in place.

The pronation-supination range of motion becomes normal within 3 weeks to 3 months. The flexion-extension ROM is not modified, but the grasp strength may increase within 3–6 months.

There are two types of complications: paresthesias that may be avoided by using a careful approach, and, most important, the *painful instability of the ulnar stump*. The latter results from hyper-mobility of the distal extremity of the upper ulnar segment when the pronated hand supports the body weight, accompanied by pain, especially in an extreme range of pronation or supination or in supporting a weight by the supinated hand. This complication is due to the too-large width of the gap and the too-proximal location of the ulnar's upper segment. Consequently, the cut must be as low as possible and the gap not excessively wide. Note that this painful instability of the ulnar stump is also possible in other procedures which involve resecting the ulna, as the Moore-Darrach or Baldwin.

The indication of this procedure is not only in rheumatoid dislocations of the DRUJ, where it is associated with synovectomy and re-alignment of the dorsal tendons, in place of resection of the distal end of the ulna (Moore-Darrach), but also in *traumatic complications* such as dislocations, sprains, chronic instabilities and stiffness of the DRUJ, secondary to Colles' fractures, Galeazzi's fractures, lower ulnar and ulnar head fractures, and even in certain two-bone fractures. It is of great value in mal-union after fractures of the lower radial extremity. This procedure, combined with a graft set between the radius and ulna, may also be used in chronic instability from Madelung's dislocation.

The important criterion for selecting this procedure is the loss of the linking system between the two bones of the lower extremities. At the present time, ligamentous surgery is not reliable enough, and a simple shortening of the ulna cannot be a good solution because of the possibility that instability will persist.

References

1. Buck-Gramcko D (1990) On the priorities of publication on some operative procedures on the distal end of the ulna. J Hand Surg [Br] 15:416–420
2. Lauenstein C (1887) Zur Behandlung der nach karpaler Vorederarmfraktur zurükbleibenden Störung der Pro- and Supinationbewegung. Centralblattfür Chirurgie 14:433–435
3. Lauenstein C (1890) Zur Frager der Derangement internedes Khiegelenks. Deutsche Medizinisch Wochenschrift 16:169–170
4. Steindler A (1946) The traumatic deformities and disabilities of the upper extremity. Chartes Thomas, Springfield, Illinois
5. Gonçalves D (1974) Correction of disorders of the distal radio-ulnar joint by artificial pseudarthrosis of the ulna. J Bone Joint Surg [Br] 56:462–464
6. Taleisnik J (1985) The wrist. Churchill Livingston, New York, p 423
7. Moore EM (1880) Three cases illustrating luxation of the ulna in connection with Colles' fracture. Medical Record 17:305–308
8. Darrach W (1912) Anterior dislocation of the head of the ulna. Ann Surg 56:802–803
9. Darrach W (1913) Partial excision of the lower shaft of the ulna for deformity following the Colles' fracture. Ann Surg 57:764–765
10. Desault P (1791) Mémoire sur les luxations de l'extrémité inférieure du cubitus. J Chir 1:78
11. Malgaigne J-F (1855) Traité des fractures et luxations, vol II. JB Baillère (ed) Paris
12. Bowers WH (1985) Distal radio-ulnar joint arthroplasty: The hemi-resection-interposition technique. J Hand Surg [Am] 10(2):169–178
13. Le Fort R, Cololian P (1918) Les pseudarthroses et pertes de substances de la diaphyse du cubitus et en particulier de sa moitié inférieure. Considérations thérapeutiques. Rev Orthop 3° série, 6:117–150
14. Baldwin WI (1921) Orthopaedic surgery of the hand and wrist. In: Jones Sir R (ed) Orthopaedic surgery of injuries. Henry Frowde, Hodder and Stroughton, London, pp 241–282

15. Milch W (1941) Cuff resection of the ulna for malunited Colles' fracture. J Bone Joint Surg [Am] 23:311–313

16. Bazy L, Galtier M (1935) Traitement sanglant de la luxation isolée de l'extrémité inférieure du cubitus en avant. J Chir 45:868–876

17. Sauvé L, Kapandji M (1933) Constitution d'un ligament péri-cubital inférieur. Bull Mem Soc Nat Chir Paris 59:237–239

18. Sauvé L, Kapandji M (1936) Nouvelle technique de traitement chirurgical des luxations récidivantes isolées de l'extrémité inférieure du cubitus. J Chir 47:589–594

19. Kapandji AI (1986) Opération de Kapandji. M et Sauvé. L. Techniques et indications dans les affections non rhumatismales (in French and English) Ann Chir Main 5:181–193

20. Baciu C (1976) L'opération de Kapandji-Sauvé dans le traitement des cals vicieux de l'extrémité inférieure du radius. Ann Chir 31:323–329

21. Baciu C, Zgabura I, Roventa N, Chicu EI (1965) Résultats éloignés après l'opération de Sauvé-Kapandji pour le traitement des fractures de Pouteau-Colles vicieusement consolidées. Acta Orthop Belgica 31:920–935

Tendon Ball Grafting in Wrist Surgery

Katsumi Suzuki, Toshitaka Nakamura, Hideki Furukawa, Yoshiki Minami, and Motonori Yamaura[1]

Abstract. Our tendon ball grafting technique, described herein, is recommended in partial replacement surgery of the wrist.

Out of 13 cases, nine were followed-up, including 7 cases with Kienböck's disease which were studied clinically and radiologically. One case each of Kienböck's disease, malunited scaphoid, and unstable ulnar head are summarized.

Keywords: Wrist surgery — Tendon ball graft — Kienböck's disease — Biological spacer

Introduction

The following is a description of our surgical technique of autogenous tendon ball grafting as well as of our methods of treatment.

Since 1970, many authors have reported success in tendon ball grafting in cases of Kienböck's disease [1, 2]. As of 1967, we have grafted the pedicled tendon ball as a biological spacer in place of the bone that was excised due to Kienböck's disease, excising both the proximal part of the malunited scaphoid and the radial half of the degenerated unstable ulnar head.

Surgical Technique for Kienböck's Disease

The merits and disadvantages of replacement procedures for Kienböck's disease are summarized in Table 1.

Recently, we began to prefer pedicled tendon ball grafting because it works as a harmless and biological spacer of the excised bone. In addition, the autogenous graft of the tendon ball may change into a cartilage one after several years postoperatively [2].

Under general anesthesia or axillar block anesthesia, the patient's arm which is affected from Kienböck's disease (stage 3 or 4) is lifted and a fixed pneumatic tourniquet is inflated at 250 mmHg for about 90 minutes.

Through a proximal volar skin incision, the palmaris longus tendon is cut at the musculotendonous junction and pulled out into the distal wound atraumatically (Fig. 1).

The tendon is stretched transversely 1.5–3.5 cm proximal to the proximal carpal crease to both sides, in order to create a thin tendon sheet. The proximal part of the tendon is then rolled up into a ball and enclosed in the tendon sheet by using several 6-0 nylon sutures (Fig. 2).

We also approach the volar carpal capsule between the median nerve and the flexor tendons in distal wounds. A rectangular capsular incision is made and the flap is retracted distally. All the necrotic lunate fragments are excised through the capsular slit.

After washing the operative area with saline, we insert the tendon ball in place of the bone. The edges of the capsular ligament are sutured tightly after confirmation that the pedicle does not disturb local functions. Oozing or bleeding points are coagulated bipolarly following release of the tourniquet. The edges of the skin are then sutured and the wrist is fixed into a functional position for about 3 weeks.

Case Presentations

Case 1

S.K., a 37-year-old male carpenter, had suffered from right wrist pain due to Kienböck's disease unassociated with trauma since June, 1984. On

[1] Department of Orthopaedic Surgery, School of Medicine, University of Occupational and Environmental Health, Yahatanishiku, Kitakyushu City 807, Japan

Table 1. Replacement surgery for Kienböck's disease

	Simple excision	Silastic implant	Dorsal flap	Tendon ball grafting
Indication: Stage	3 or 4	3 or 4	3 or 4	3 or 4
Strenuous activity	Unable	Able	Unable	Unable
Approach	Dorsal	Dorsal	Dorsal	Volar
Technique	Facile	Facile	Facile	Complex
Postoperative fixation	3 Weeks	3 Weeks	3 Weeks	3 Weeks
Foreign body reaction	No	Yes	No	No
Cartilagenous transformation	No	No	No	Possibly
Carpal displacement	Yes	No	Slight	Moderate
Devised by	F Stahl 1947 [3]	AB Swanson 1970 [4]	SH Nahigian 1970 [5]	RE Carroll 1970 [1]

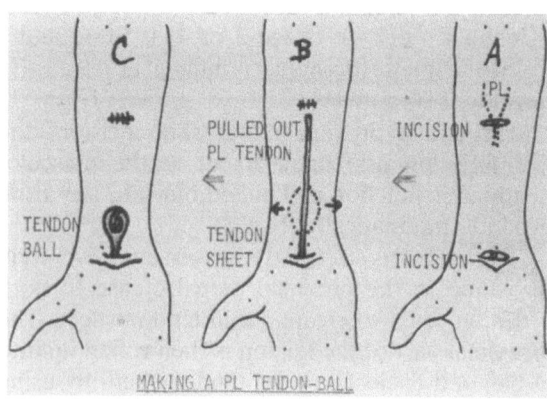

Fig. 1. Schematic representation of devising a palmaris longus tendon ball on the right forearm

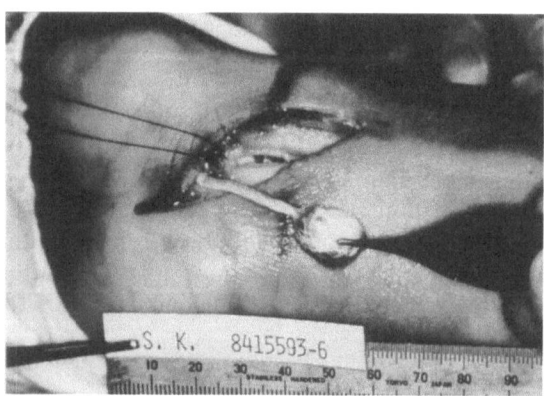

Fig. 2. Palmaris longus tendon ball graft of the right hand

January 14, 1985, a pedicled graft of the palmaris longus tendon ball was performed on the affected wrist (stage 3). Preoperative active flexion/extension was 25°/32° and postoperative active flexion/extension increased to 50°/50°. Preoperative active radial/ulnar deviation was 10°/10°, but the postoperative deviation increased to 15°/20°. Grip power increased from 18 to 42 kg postoperatively. As of August 24, 1989, he was still working and was free of pain (Fig. 3).

Case 2

K.O., a 29-year-old male water supply worker, broke his right ulnar styloid process in a fall from his motorcycle on July 10, 1985. The wrist was set in a plaster cast at another clinic. On February 23, 1987, the modified Bower's procedure with an extensor carpi ulnaris tendon ball graft was performed on his unstable distal radioulnar joint. Preoperative active flexion/extension increased from 45°/60° to 60°/65° following surgery. Preoperative active radial/ulnar deviation changed from 10°/45° to 16°/40° degrees postoperatively, and postoperative grip power was 51 kg. As of February 5, 1991, he is working without any complaints (Fig. 4).

Case 3

H.N., a 23-year-old male florist, fell from a ladder on October 20, 1984 and broke his right scaphoid bone. On April 15, 1985, the proximal half of his right scaphoid was excised, an extensor carpi radialis longus tendon ball was grafted, and a part of the radial styloid was excised. Preoperative active flexion/extension increased from 13°/40° to 33°/58° postoperatively. Preoperative active radial/ulnar deviation increased postoperatively from 18°/21° to 25°/25° and grip power increased from 13 to 46 kg. As of August 30, 1987, he was working but still suffered from slight carpal pain after heavy work (Fig. 5).

Fig. 3. Wrist X-rays of case 1.
a Before surgery and **b** 4 years
and 7 months after surgery

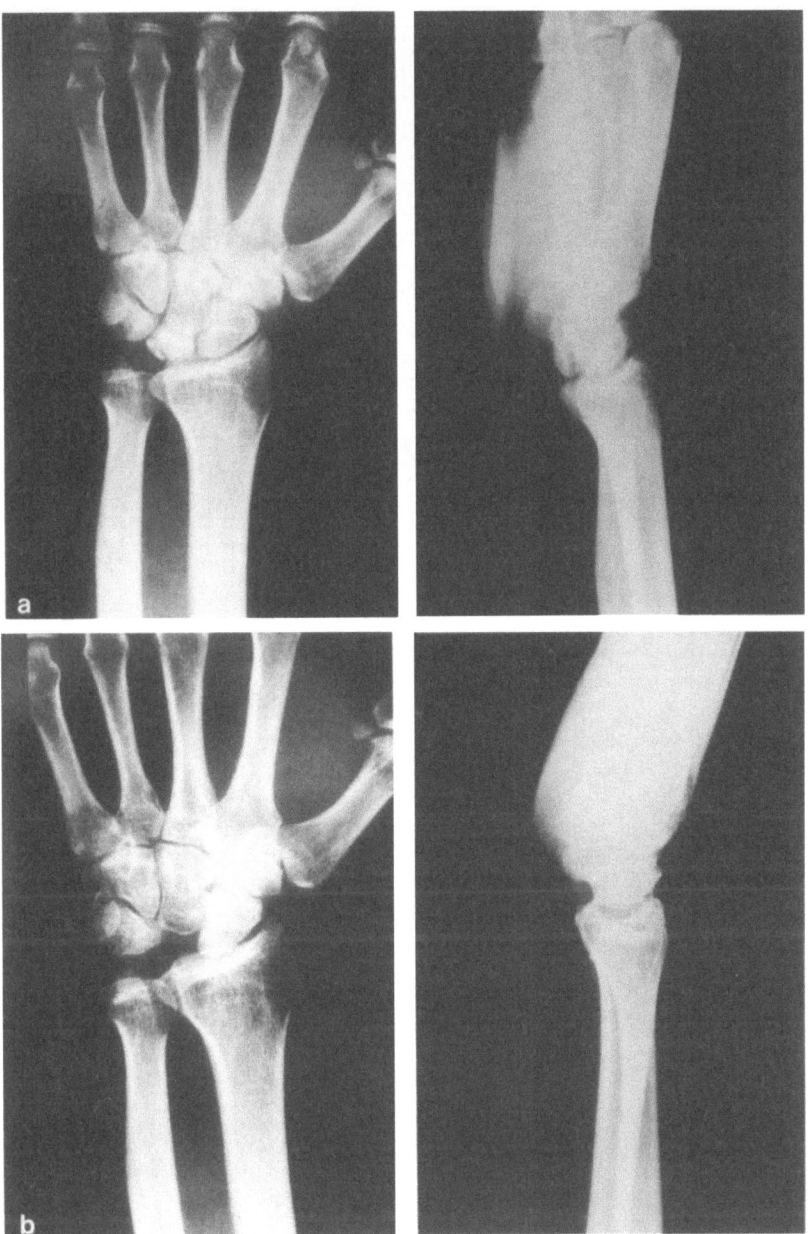

Results of Tendon Ball Grafting

Out of 13 patients who had undergone a tendon ball grafting operation, 9 were followed up postoperatively from 11 months to 28 years and 8 months (average 5 years and 9 months). Among these nine patients, there were 7 cases of Kienböck's disease (stage 3 or 4), 1 malunited scaphoid, and 1 unstable distal radioulnar joint. After

convalescence, they were all able to engage in their former occupations.

In the cases of Kienböck's disease, the preoperative range of carpal flexion-extension was 57° to 113° (average 80°), which increased to 80° to 125° postoperatively (average 108°; $P < 0.05$ by the paired t-test). The range of the preoperative carpal radial-ulnar deviation was 20° to 65° (average 45°) and increased to 40° to 60° (average 54°) postoperatively (not significant).

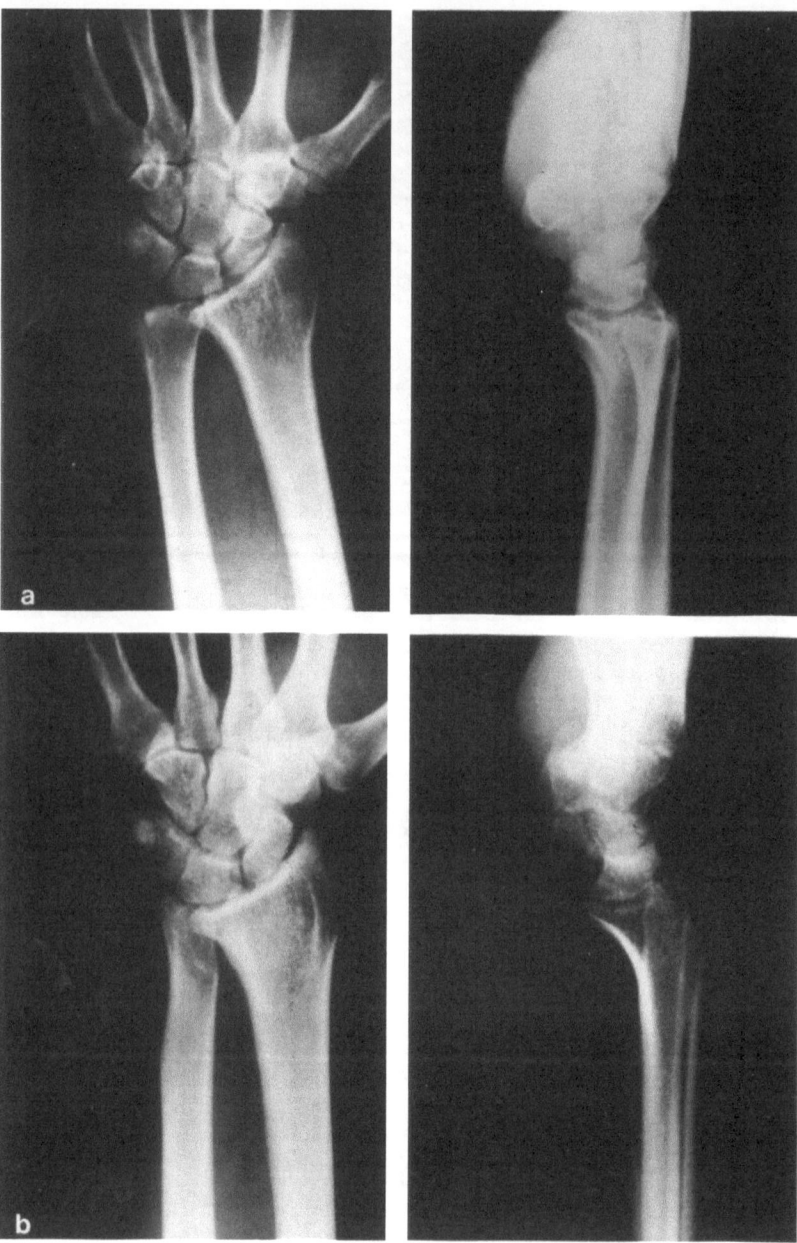

Fig. 4. Wrist X-rays of case 2. **a** Before surgery and **b** 4 years after surgery

Preoperative grip power was from 18 to 25 kg (average 20 kg) in the affected hand, which increased to 23–44 kg (average 33 kg) postoperatively ($P < 0.05$ by the paired t-test).

The carpal/height ratio changed from an average of 0.49 to 0.47 postoperatively (not significant). The carpal/ulnar distance ratio was reduced from an average of 0.28 to 0.23 postoperatively (not significant). The radioscaphoid angle also decreased from an average of 63° to 52° (not significant).

By postoperative magnetic resonance imaging examinations of 3 grafted wrists, we were able to detect slightly reduced joint spaces with no evidence of any ossifications.

Conclusions

Because it is soft elastic and is able to completely fit the space, the pedicled tendon ball graft works as a biological and harmless replacement of the

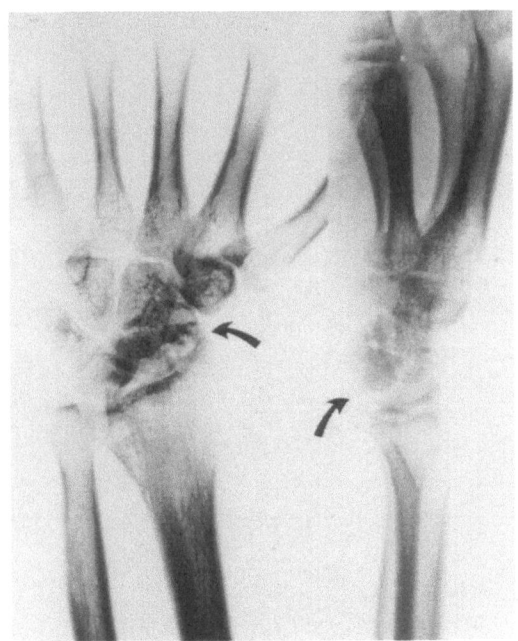

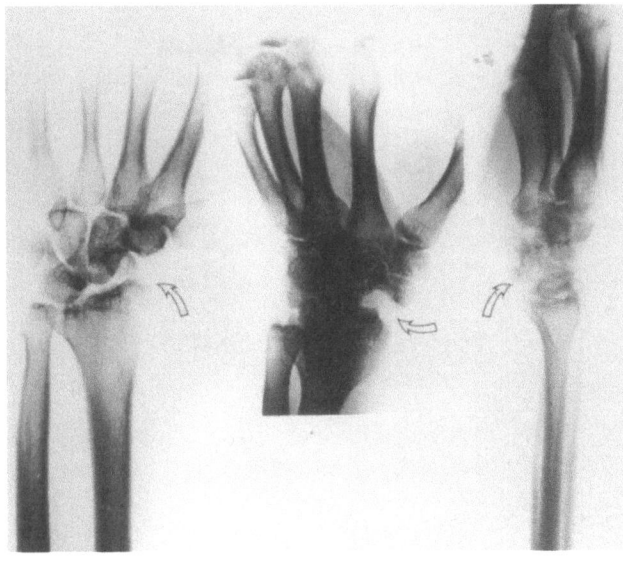

a

b

Fig. 5. Wrist X-rays of case 3. **a** Before surgery and **b** after surgery. *Black arrows*, destroyed scaphoid; *white arrows*, tendon ball grafted space

excised bone. Technically, the procedure of creating and fixing this graft in the joint is relatively uncomplicated, and its being prepared in the operated arm at the time of surgery makes it more convenient. According to Horita et al. [2], this ball may change to cartilage due to synovial circulation after several years postoperatively. For these reasons we recommend the pedicled tendon ball graft technique in partial replacement surgery of the wrist.

However, the graft has in sufficient resistance to mechanical stress and does not show distinct vascular supplies angiographically.

References

1. Ishiguro T (1984) Experimental and clinical studies of Kienböck's disease. J Jpn Orthop Assoc 58:509–522
2. Horita K, Ikuta Y, Murakami K, Ochi M, Mochizuki Y (1990) An experimental study on the bone-core tendon ball replacement for the treatment of Kienböck's disease. J Jpn Soc Surg Hand 7:767–771
3. Stahl F (1947) On lunatomalacia. Acta Chir Scand 95(Suppl 126):3–133
4. Swanson AB (1970) Silicone rubber implants for the replacement of the carpal scaphoid and lunate bones. Orthop Clin North Am 1:299–309
5. Nahigian SH, Li CS, Richey DG, Shaw DT (1970) The dorsal flap arthroplasty in the treatment of Kienböck's disease. J Bone Joint Surg [Am] 52:245–252

Silicone Rubber Sheet Interpositional Arthroplasty for Rheumatoid Arthritis of the Wrist

HIROSHI ONO, SUSUMU TAMAI, and HIROSHI YAJIMA[1]

Abstract. Although several procedures of inter-positional arthroplasty are available, silicone rubber sheet interpositional arthroplasty seems to be particularly suitable for the rheumatoid wrist. In our clinic, we have performed 21 operations in 19 patients using this procedure, and 19 wrists in the 17 of the patients who were followed-up for more than 1 year were evaluated. The patients' age ranged from 8 to 66 years (average 41 years). There were 18 females and 1 male. The right wrist was affected in 10 cases, the left in 5, and both in 2. According to Steinbrocker's classification, 1 case was stage II, 14 stage III, and 4 stage IV. The follow-up period ranged from 1 year to 4 years 8 months (average 3 years).

Postoperatively, pain was relieved in all and the swelling subsided. Roentgenologically, the radio-carpal joint space was preserved in all. However, the inserted sheet migrated dorsoradially in 4 cases; the sheet was removed in two of these patients and it was replaced with a new sheet 39 months later in one patient.

The average ROM of the 19 wrists pre- and postoperatively was as follows: dorsiflexion increased from $27.1°$ to $29.7°$, palmar flexion decreased from $27.1°$ to $18.2°$, supination increased from $66.4°$ to $76.4°$, and pronation increased from $70.8°$ to $75°$. The grip strength was increased from 10 to 16 kg.

The advantages of this operation include (1) ease of performing the procedure, (2) preserved joint mobility, (3) replaceability, and (4) salvageability.

Keywords: Rheumatoid arthritis — Wrist joint — Synovectomy — Silicone rubber sheet — Arthroplasty

Introduction

The treatment of rheumatoid arthritis of the wrist is divided into two major therapeutic approaches, conservative and operative. The former includes systemic rheumatoid medication, i.e., non-steroid anti-inflammatory drugs (NSAIDs), disease-modifying anti-rheumatoid drugs (DMARDs) and steroids, and splinting in proper alignment as the treatment of first choice. Operative therapy consists of synovectomy, arthroplasty, and arthrodesis.

Synovectomy is widely used for the treatment of rheumatoid arthritis of the wrist joint [1]. However, a number of cases have developed joint contracture or bony ankylosis after this procedure, and most patients do not want to undergo arthrodesis for the wrist. Silicone rubber sheet interpositional arthroplasty for maintaining wrist joint motion [2], developed by Jackson and Simpson in 1979 [3], seems to be a reliable substitutive procedure for total wrist replacement.

In this study, we introduce our operative technique of silicone rubber sheet arthroplasty and report our results from using this procedure.

Operative Technique

Under regional block or general anesthesia, a longitudinal straight incision is made over the dorsum of the wrist. The extensor retinaculum is raised from the ulnar to the radial side in a single continuous sheet, 2.5 cm in width, from the distal margin. If extensor tenosynovitis is severe, tenosynovectomy should be performed. The dorsal capsule of the wrist joint is opened transversally, and synovectomy of the radiocarpal, intercarpal, and distal radioulnar joints is performed as completely as possible. If the lower end of the ulna is unstable, eroded, or causing pain,

[1] Department of Orthopaedic Surgery, Nara Medical University, 840 Shijo-cho, Kashihara, Nara 634, Japan

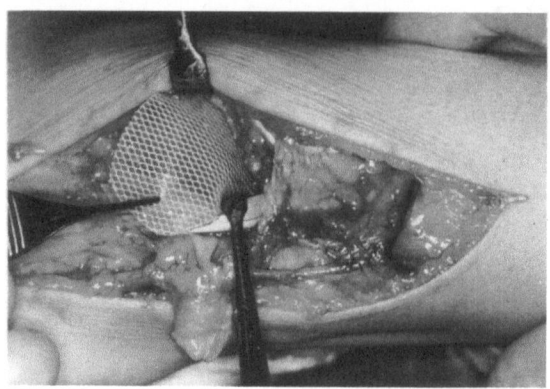

Fig. 1. Operative method. A silicone rubber sheet (*arrow*) is inserted into the radiocarpal joint.

it is resected according to Darrach's method. If pannus or bony destruction is present on the radiocarpal joint surface, it is curretted and smoothed. A 1 mm-thick Dacron meshed silicone rubber sheet (Dow Corning Corporation, Michigan, USA,) is trimmed to fit the distal joint surface of the radius, and is inserted gently with smooth forceps into the radiocarpal joint space (Fig. 1). To prevent later displacement of the sheet, it is fixed to the radiodorsal side of the joint capsule with 5–6 interrupted stitches using 4-0 braided nylon (Surgilon). The dorsal wrist joint capsule is carefully closed, and the extensor retinaculum is passed under the extensor tendons and sutured to the dorsal wrist joint capsule for reinforcement. An ulnar strip of retinaculum can be used to hold the extensor carpi ulnaris in its anatomical position when necessary. The skin is closed and the hand is placed in a plaster cast in the neutral position for 3 weeks. The cast is then removed and active motion exercise using a dynamic splint is commenced.

Patients and Methods

In our clinic, 21 operations on 19 patients with silicone rubber sheet interpositional arthroplasty have been performed from April, 1984 to December, 1990. In this study, we evaluated 19 wrists in 17 of the patients who were followed-up for more than 1 year postoperatively (Table 1). The patients' age at operation ranged from 8 to 66 years, (average 41 years). There were 18 females and 1 male. The right wrist was affected in 10 cases, the left in 5, and both in 2. Five cases had

the monoarthritic type of rheumatoid arthritis and 12 had the polyarthritic.

According to Steinbrocker's classification [4], 1 case was stage II, 14 were stage III, and 4 were stage IV. Before surgery, 11 cases were treated with NSAIDs alone, 14 cases with DMARDs, and 2 cases with steroid therapy. The duration of disease prior to surgery ranged from 3 months to 10 years 6 months (average 3 years 11 months). Subjective and objective evaluation was performed before and after the operation, as detailed below.

Subjective Evaluation

The patients were questioned as to degree of pain, tenderness, local sensation of heat and swelling, restriction of activities of daily living (ADL), and wrist stability.

Objective Evaluation

The grip strength and active range of motion (ROM) of the wrist were measured. The carpal height ratio was calculated roentgenographically in the posteroanterior plane by Youm's method [5]. The radiolunate joint space was measured by the distance between the distal radial joint surface for the lunate and proximal lunate joint surface for the radius in the posteroanterior plane (Fig. 2).

Results

The follow-up postoperative period ranged from 1 year to 4 years 8 months (average 3 years).

Subjective Evaluation

Pain and tenderness of the wrist joint were relieved in all patients. Local sensation of heat also disappeared in all, and swelling around the wrist joint was improved in all but one patient. None of the 19 wrists showed clinical evidence of recurrence of synovitis. All patients retained wrist joint stability and had no complaints of severe restriction in activities of daily living. All patients but two were satisfied with this procedure. The two exceptions were dissatisfied because of the poor range of wrist motion that had been achieved.

Objective Evaluation

The average grip strength was increased from 10 kg preoperatively to 16 kg postoperatively

Table 1. Clinical characteristics

Case	Sex	Age (years)	RA Type	Stage[a] Pre-op	Stage[a] Post-op	Duration of disease (months)	Follow-up Period (months)	Grip power (kg) Pre-op	Grip power (kg) Post-op	TAM Pre-op	TAM Post-op	CHR Pre-op	CHR Post-op
T.O.	F	19	Poly	III	III	24	36	13	20	325°	300°	52.7	50.0
T.S.	F	71	Poly	III	III	120	18	1	4	195°	220°	47.2	48.1
T.M.	F	30	Poly	III	IV	28	56	20	22	205°	170°	52.5	45.6
K.K.	F	49	Poly	IV	IV	80	15	8	11	175°	160°	45.6	47.4
S.I.	M	46	Poly	III	IV	98	39	15	32	240°	245°	41.5	45.7
S.M.	F	53	Mono	III	III	25	40	9	17	140°	245°	55.2	58.6
K.S.	F	32	Poly	III	IV	13	45	12	15	220°	150°	59.3	54.2
M.U.	F	18	Poly	III	III	24	47	13	25	270°	285°	55.3	56.1
				III	III	28	43	25	25	280°	250°	52.6	50.0
H.M.	F	66	Poly	IV	IV	3	18	17	15			48.4	49.2
				III	IV	7	14	14	16			51.7	46.8
T.K.	F	44	Mono	III	III	37	35	1	10	295°	335°	56.9	55.0
A.S.	F	11	Mono	III	III	46	32	5	15	230°	225°	48.9	50.0
M.F.	F	27	Poly	III	III	36	32	4	20	215°	215°	36.4	39.4
Y.N.	F	49	Poly	IV	IV	126	34	10	4	240°	205°	46.4	46.4
M.A.	F	56	Mono	III	IV	14	54	5	6	225°	200°	50.9	52.8
E.T.	F	49	Poly	IV	IV	120	22	13	14			47.5	37.3
E.O.	F	58	Poly	III	III	60	49	1	9				
K.O.	F	52	Mono	II	II	10	53	15	23				

RA, Rheumatoid arthritis; Poly, polyarthritic; Mono, monoarthritic; TAM, total active motion; CHR, carpal height ratio; Pre-op, preoperatively; Post-op, postoperatively
[a] Steinbrocker's classification

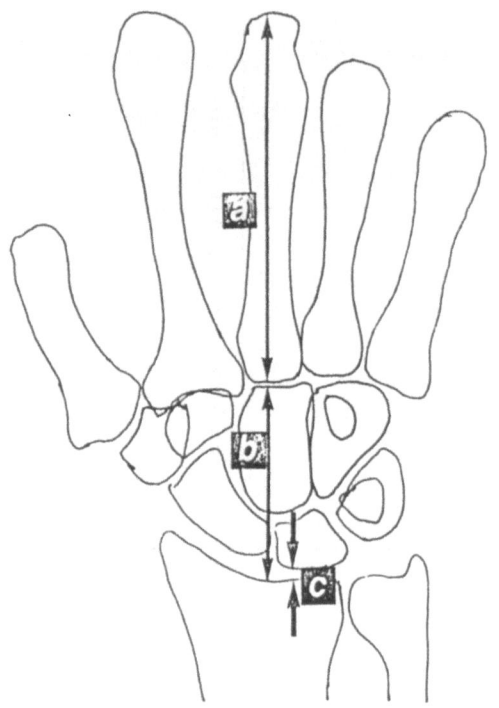

Fig. 2. Roentgenographical evaluation. Carpal height ratio (CHR) = b/a × 100 (%). Radiolunate joint space = c mm

(Table 1). Only three patients had decreased grip strength postoperatively, all of whom had stage IV according to Steinbrocker's classification in addition to severely affected elbows and fingers.

Range of Motion (ROM)

The average ROM of the 19 wrists pre- and post-operatively was as follows: dorsiflexion increased slightly from 27.1° to 29.7° (12 cases increased and 7 decreased postoperatively), palmar flexion decreased from 27.1° to 18.2° (6 cases increased, 3 were unchanged, and 10 decreased), pronation increased from 70.8° to 75° (8 cases increased, 6 were unchanged, and 4 decreased), supination increased from 66.4° to 76.4° (9 cases increased, 9 were unchanged), radial flexion decreased from 6° to 2.9° (3 cases increased, 4 were unchanged, 7 decreased, 5 were not measured), and ulnar flexion increased from 18.7° to 20.4° (7 cases increased, 4 were unchanged, 3 decreased, 5 were not measured). The average total active motion of the wrist, i.e., the sum of dorsiflexion, palmar flexion, pronation, supination, radial flexion and ulnar flexion, was 232° preoperatively and 230° postoperatively.

Radiological Evaluation

According to Steinbrocker's classification at the time of review, there was 1 case in stage II, 9 in stage III, and 9 in stage IV. Five cases progressed from stage III to stage IV, with no change in status seen in the remaining cases.

Roentgenologically, the radiocarpal joint space was preserved without fusion in all cases. The average radiolunate joint space increased from 1.28 mm preoperatively to 2.22 mm postoperatively, while the average carpal height ratio was slightly decreased, from 49.4% preoperatively to 48.6% postoperatively (Table 1). In 6 cases, intercarpal joint destruction and fusion progressed, resulting in a decreased carpal height ratio despite preservation of maintaining the radiolunate joint space.

The inserted sheet migrated dorsoradially in 4 cases; the sheet was removed after 16 months in 1 and after 2 years in the other. In one patient, the sheet was replaced at the time of a second operation 39 months later. One of the three removed sheets was found to be perforated centrally, while the others were intact. At 1 year after removal of the silicone rubber sheet, the radiocarpal joint space in 1 case was seen to be preserved on roentgenological examination.

Case Reports

Case 1

S.M., a 53-year-old female, was initially seen at our hospital in April, 1985 presenting with pain in her right wrist. She received gold therapy for 2 years but the wrist pain worsened. Roentgenologically, the wrist was in stage III of Steinbrocker's classification (Fig. 3). Silicone rubber sheet arthroplasty was performed on April 23, 1987. At follow-up 46 months after the operation, she felt no wrist pain and her grip strength increased from 9 kg preoperatively to 17 kg postoperatively. The ROM of her right wrist was as follows: dorsiflexion which was 25° preoperatively increased to 40° postoperatively, palmar flexion from 25° to 35°, radial flexion from 5° to 15°, ulnar flexion from 20° to 35°, pronation from 30° to 70°, and supination from 35° to 50°. Roentgenologically, the silicone rubber sheet was in a good position, and the radiolunate joint space remained 2 mm wide (Fig. 4). She has been very satisfied with the results of this procedure.

Fig. 3. Case 1, a 53-year-old female. Preoperative X-ray shows a stage III wrist

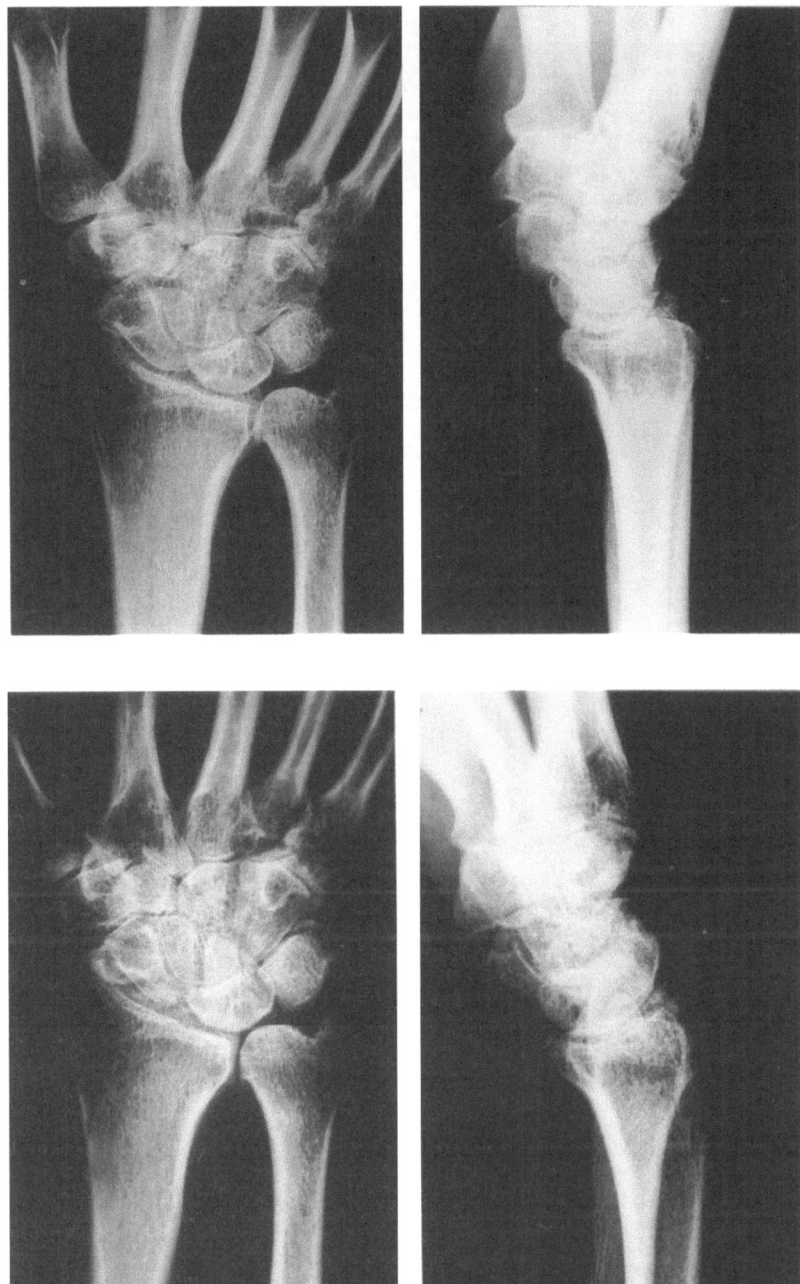

Fig. 4. Case 1. At follow-up 46 months postoperatively, the wrist was still in stage III. The silicone rubber sheet was in a good position

Case 2

S.I., a 46-year-old male, had been treated for rheumatoid arthritis at another hospital for 8 years. On June 26, 1984, he consulted our hospital and underwent a silicone rubber sheet arthroplasty on August 2, 1984. At that time, his left wrist was classified as Steinbrocker's stage III (Fig. 5.a). Two years after the operation, the silicone rubber sheet was displaced dorsally (without accompanying pain) and upon removal (Fig. 5.b) was found to be intact. At follow-up 1 year after removal of the sheet, he felt no wrist pain and the postoperative ROM of his wrist was not decreased. Radiological examination revealed that his left wrist was still in stage III,

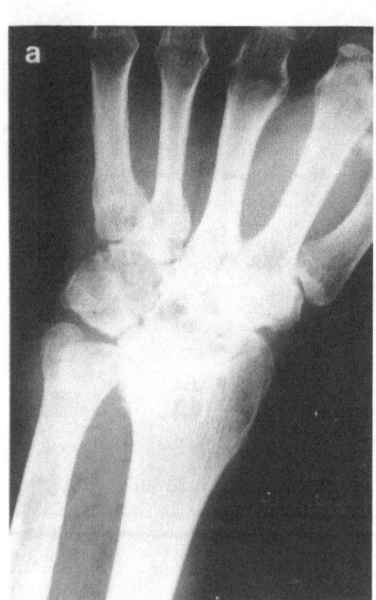
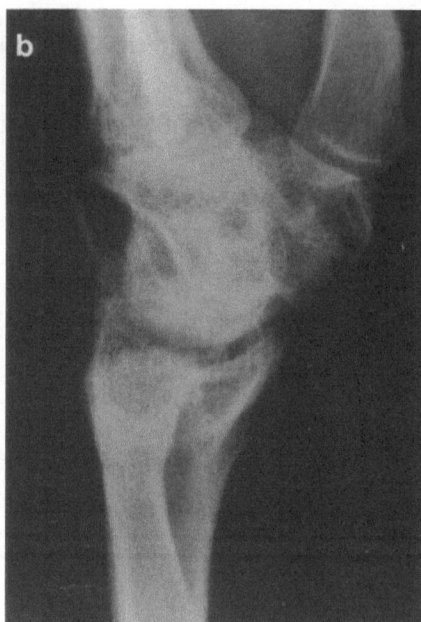

Fig. 5. Case 2, a 46-year-old
male. **a** Preoperative X-ray
shows a stage III wrist. **b** The
silicone rubber sheet was displaced dorsally 2 years postoperatively

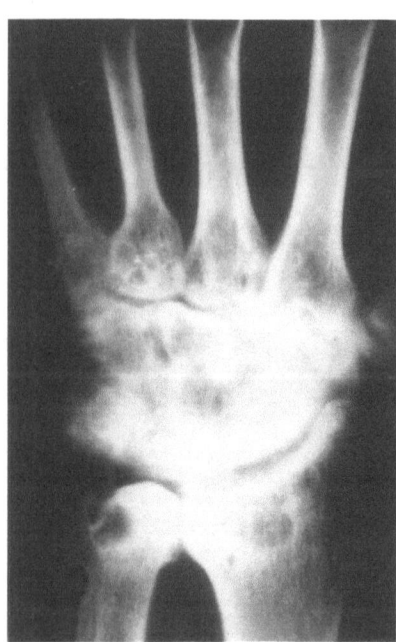
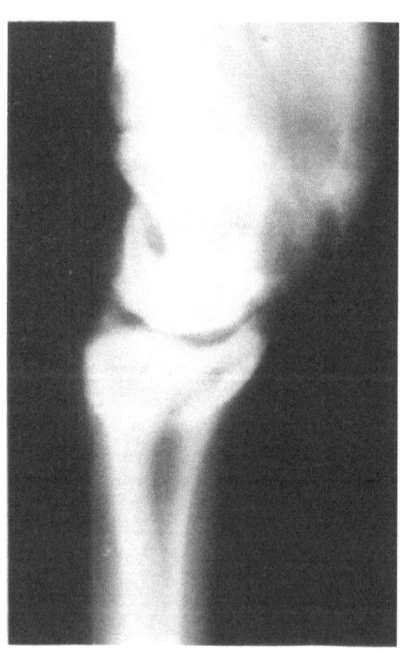

Fig. 6. Case 2. The wrist was
still in stage III and the radiolunate space was maintained 1
year after removal of the sheet

while the radiolunate distance remained 2 mm
even at 1 year after removal of the sheet (Fig. 6).

Case 3

A.S., an 8-year-old female, was initially seen
at our hospital on May 9, 1986 with pain and
limitation of ROM in her right wrist and digits.
Roentgenological examination revealed that the

radiocarpal joint was destroyed and that the
carpal bones were eroded at multiple sites (Fig.
7.a). The rheumatoid factor was positive. She was
diagnosed as having juvenile rheumatoid arthritis
and was treated conservatively in the beginning,
but the pain and limitation of ROM worsened.
She underwent synovectomy and silicone rubber
sheet arthroplasty on February 5, 1987. At follow-
up 32 months after the operation, she felt no wrist

Fig. 7. Case 3, an 8-year-old female. **a** Preoperative X-ray shows destruction of the radio-carpal joint. **b** At follow-up 32 months after surgery, the radiolunate joint surface was seen to be preserved and the sheet was in a good position

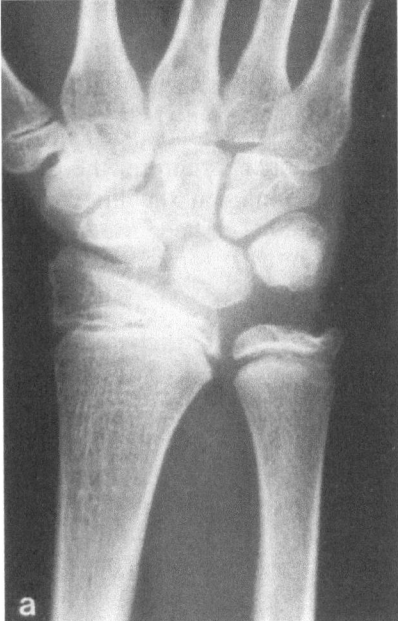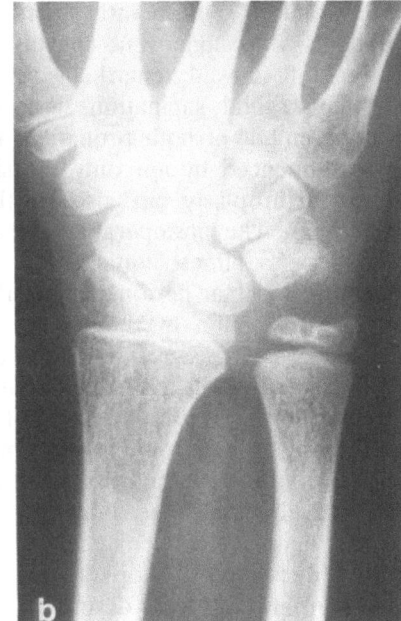

pain and her grip strength and ROM of the wrist increased remarkably. Roentgenologically, the radiolunate joint space was found to be preserved and the sheet was in a good position. Her daily lifestyle was unrestricted (Fig. 7.b).

Discussion

The wrist is the keystone to the rheumatoid hand. The importance of stability, absence of pain, and mobility are crucial for the continued optimal use of the entire hand in the patient with rheumatoid arthritis. In spite of early management, including systemic medications and splints, increasing soft tissue damage and bone and joint destruction in some patients necessitate surgical intervention, such as synovectomy, arthrodesis, or arthroplasty. In 1979, Jackson and Simpson [3] classified the rheumatoid wrist into 3 groups. In the acute group, the joint shows synovitis but no evidence of cartilage destruction, and synovectomy can be carried out. Synovectomy undoubtedly achieves good pain relief, but numerous cases have been found to develop joint destruction, contracture, or ankylosis on long-term follow-up. Thus, some surgeons have concluded that synovectomy is indicated only for the relief of wrist pain. In the chronic group, the joint shows destruction, dislocation, and instability or ankylosis in a poor functional position, requiring arthrodesis or total joint replacement [6, 7]. Total joint replacement of the wrist is not popular, thus arthrodesis is performed for this stage in most cases. The choice of treatment is most difficult in the intermediate group in which the wrist shows synovitis and destruction of cartilage and bones but with retention of stability. In such patients, we perform silicone rubber sheet arthroplasty [8], as developed by Jackson and Simpson in 1979, in order to maintain wrist motion. Therefore, the major indications for silicone rubber sheet arthroplasty are joints which are erosive or ulcerous with synovitis but stable, joints without subluxation or dislocation, and joints with contracture or ankylosis.

Silicone rubber sheet arthroplasty has the great advantage of preservation of wrist joint motion without instability [9]. In our study, palmar flexion of the wrist joint decreased from 27.1° preoperatively to 18.2° postoperatively, because the dorsal capsule of the wrist joint was reinforced by the extensor retinaculum. On the other hand, dorsiflexion of the wrist joint increased postoperatively. Thus, the total active motion of flexion-extension of the wrist joint slightly decreased postoperatively, with good dorsiflexion of the wrist joint, which is more important for the activities of daily living. Almost all the patients felt that the wrist was more useful postoperatively. Both pronation and supination increased from a mean of 66.4° and 70.8° preoperatively to

76.4° and 75° postoperatively, respectively. The patients who underwent concurrent distal ulna resection showed remarkable improvement of pronation and supination, indicating that the improvement of both pronation and supination was influenced by not only the silicone rubber sheet arthroplasty but also by the distal ulna resection. The postoperative decrease in radial flexion was almost equal to the postoperative increase in ulnar flexion, and so the total active range of motion of the wrist at the time of review was the same as before the operation. Consequently, silicone rubber sheet arthroplasy maintains the ROM of the wrist which is lost when only synovectomy is performed.

The radiolunate joint space increased postoperatively, which accounts for the increased carpal height ratio. Conversely, the carpal height ratio decreased postoperatively, because the intercarpal joints were destroyed and fused.

In case 2, we confirmed that the distal radial joint surface was covered with a material resembling cartilage at the time the sheet was removed. In addition, the radiolunate joint space was maintained without fusion even 1 year after removal of the sheet. Therefore, it was concluded that the silicone rubber sheet induces joint repair with tissue resembling fibrous cartilage. Other advantages of silicone rubber sheet interpositional arthroplasty include (1) ease of performing the procedure, (2) low cost, (3) replaceability, and (4) salvageability.

One of the drawbacks of this procedure is the possibility of displacement of the sheet. Four implants were displaced dorsoradially and fifteen remained in place. To prevent dislocation of the sheet, it was fixed to the radiodorsal or palmar capsule of the wrist joint with 5–6 interrupted stitches using 4-0 braided nylon (Surgilon), and the dorsal capsule of the wrist joint was reinforced by the extensor retinaculum under the extensor tendons. Another problem with this procedure is fracture and fragmentation of the sheet. A silicone rubber sheet reinforced with Dacron mesh should be used to prevent early fragmentation. The silicone rubber sheet with Dacron mesh can be fixed with sutures to the capsule without causing microfractures; two of the three sheets which were removed in this series were found to be intact.

Another drawback is associated with concomitant extensor tendon repair in cases with subcutaneous rupture of the extensor tendons. In some of our cases undergoing silicone rubber sheet arthroplasty, extensor tendon repair (i.e., tendon grafts or tendon transfers) was performed simultaneously. The results in these cases were very poor because of adhesion of the extensor tendons. Thus, in cases with extensor tendon rupture, the extensor tendon should be repaired at the first operation, with the silicone rubber sheet interpositional arthroplasty being performed at a second operation.

Conclusions

Silicone rubber sheet interpositional arthroplasty with synovectomy was evaluated in a total of 19 wrists in 17 patients. This surgical procedure maintained the range of the rheumatoid wrist joint motion. The advantages of silicone rubber sheet arthroplasty include ease of the procedure, preserved joint mobility, induction of joint repair, replaceability, and salvageability. The problems associated with this procedure include displacement, fracture and fragmentation of the sheet, and management of extensor tendon rupture.

References

1. Straub LR (1956) The rheumatoid hand. Clin Orthop 15:127–139
2. Tillman K, Thabe H (1981) Technique and results of resection and interposition arthroplasty of the wrist in rheumatoid arthritis. Reconstr Surg Traumatol 18:84–91
3. Jackson IT, Simpson RG (1979) Interpositional arthroplasty of the wrist in rheumatoid arthritis. Hand 2:169–175
4. Steinbrocker T, Traeger CH, Batterman RC (1949) Therapeutic criteria in rheumatoid arthritis. JAMA 140:659–662
5. Youm Y (1978) Kinematics of the wrist. I. An experimental study of radial-ulnar deviation and flexion-extension. J Bone Joint Surg [Am] 60:423–431
6. Vicar AJ, Burton RI (1986) Surgical management of the rheumatoid wrist — Fusion or arthroplasty. J Hand Surg [Am] 11:790–797
7. Volz RG (1977) Total wrist arthroplasty. Clin Orthop 128:180–189
8. Tamai S, Mizumoto S, Yajima H (1987) Silastic sheet arthroplasty for rheumatoid wrists. J Jpn Soc Surg Hand 4:633–638
9. Robertson GA, Bailey BN (1985) Silicone rubber sheet interposition arthroplasty for the painful rheumatoid wrist: A long-term review Br J. Plast Surg 38:190–196

Radial Styloid Wedge Osteotomy for Early SLAC Wrist, Nonunion of the Scaphoid and for Painful Radial Styloid Impingement Syndrome: A Preliminary Report

Minoru Shibata,[1] Hidehiko Saito,[1] Junichi Hasegawa,[1] Toshiaki Hara,[2] Kazuhiko Sasagawa,[2] and Noburu Nakabe[2]

Abstract. Painful arthritis around the radial styloid is induced in scapholunate advanced collapse of the wrist (SLAC). This change also occurs in non-union of the scaphoid and in triscaphe arthrodesis.

We devised a closing wedge osteotomy of the radial styloid as a treatment for this problem. We removed a radially based wedge of bone with an angle of 8° from the subchondral bone of the inter-articular ridge separating the lunate and scaphoid fossae. The articular surface of the inter-articular ridge was kept intact. The defect was closed and fixed by using staples. A short arm cast was applied for 4 weeks.

We performed these procedures in 5 wrists of four patients (2 females and 2 males). The patients' ages ranged from 47 to 55 years (average 51.5 years). This series included two cases of scapholunate advanced collapse, two with both radial styloid impingement and ulnar abutment syndrome, and one with aseptic necrosis of the scaphoid bone (Preiser's disease).

The radioscaphoid space was opened immediately after surgery suggesting decompression in that joint. All patients regained a pain-free wrist, with the follow-up period ranging from 6 to 30 months except for the most recent case. The space in the radioscaphoid remained open after the operation in each patient. All the patients were relieved from pain, tenderness, and swelling in the radiocarpal joint shortly after surgery and soon returned to their original jobs. There has been no sign of progressing arthritis or collapse of carpal bones noted thus far. The preoperative range of the operated wrist was maintained postoperatively.

Intraoperative measurement of contact pressure of the radiocarpal joint was carried out in one of the patients. Manual compression or simultaneous contraction of flexor and extensor tendons using electric stimulation clearly demonstrated shifting of the contact pressure from the radial to the ulnar side. Similar results were obtained regardless of the wrist position.

Closing wedge osteotomy of the radial styloid effectively unloads contact pressure at the radial side of the radiocarpal joint without inducing instability or contracture of the wrist joint. This new operative procedure may be a useful treatment for SLAC wrist, especially in the early stage.

Keywords: Radial styloid — Wedge osteotomy — SLAC wrist — Non-union of the scaphoid — Radial styloid — Impingement syndrome

Introduction

Arthritis at the most radial portion of the radioscaphoid joint occurs in the early stage of scapholunate advanced collapse (SLAC) wrist. Non-union of the scaphoid induces a similar type of arthritic change and triscaphe arthrodesis frequently causes a painful radial styloid impingement syndrome. This arthritic change eventually involves the entire radioscaphoid joint and requires a salvage operation, such as the so-called SLAC procedure [1]. To avoid progression to this advanced stage, we devised a new type of osteotomy that relieves the load on the radioscaphoid joint. The aim of this paper is to introduce this new operative treatment and present its results.

[1] Orthopedics Department, Niigata University School of Medicine, Asahimachidori-1 Niigata City 951, Japan
[2] Engineering Department, Niigata University, Ikarashicho-1, Niigata City, 950-21 Japan

Operative Procedures

A dorsoradial approach is used. An oblique incision is made over the dorsal lateral side of the radial styloid and deepened to the extensor retinaculum, which is divided between the second and the third dorsal compartment. Tendons are retracted radially and ulnarly. The radial part of the distal radius is exposed subperiosteally. Two lines are marked using a pair of Kirschner wires with an intervening angle of 8°, placing its apex just ulnar to the dorsal radial tubercle, which is the dorsal end of the scapholunate inter-articular ridge. An osteotomy is carried out using a power saw along these K-wires to the level of the subchondral bone of the inter-articular ridge. The articular surface of the inter-articular ridge must be kept intact. The defect can be easily closed by manipulating the K-wire inserted into the radial styloid. The extensor pollicis longus tendon and the radial sensory nerve must be carefully protected from injury during the procedure. Bone fixation is obtained using staples (Fig. 1). A short arm cast is applied for 4 weeks and finger motion exercises are started soon after the operation.

Patients

These procedures were applied clinically to 5 wrists of four patients (2 females and 2 males). The patients' ages ranged from 47 to 55 years (average 51.5 years). Two of them had advanced scapholunate collapse associated with scaphoid fracture, two had both radial styloid impingement and ulnocarpal abutment syndrome, and one had Preiser's disease. The follow-up period ranged from 6 to 20 months (average 17 months) except for the most recent case which was followed-up for 2 months.

In one of these patients, contact pressure at the radiocarpal joint was measured using pressure-sensitive conductive silicone rubber (Yokohama Rubber Co., CS-577-RSC) connected to a personal computer (Epson 386LS) equipped with an analogue digital converter (Contec AD-12-16T-98, 25 ms sampling speed).

Case Presentation

Case 1

The patient was a 55-year-old male gymnastic teacher who was seen in January, 1989 with pain

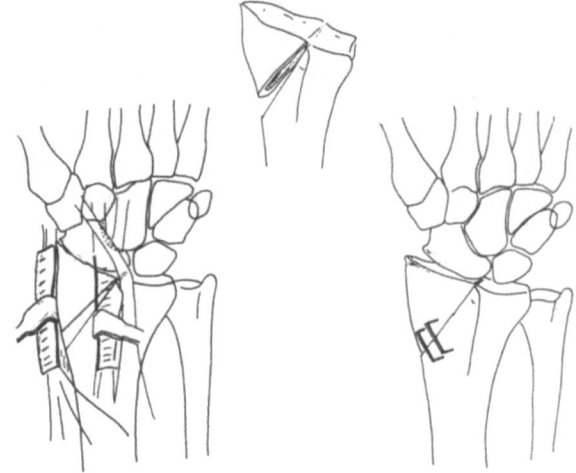

Fig. 1. Operative procedures. The entrance is between the second and third compartments and the radial styloid is exposed. A radially based wedge with an 8° intervening angle at subchondral bone of the inter-articular ridge is made. The articular surface is maintained intact and the defect is closed. Staples are used for bone fixation, and a short arm cast is applied for 4 weeks

and swelling in the radial side of his right wrist joint. His past history revealed a fracture around his right wrist which occurred when he fell down from a horizontal bar about 20 years before the operation.

Radiography and tomography of the right wrist joint showed non-union of the proximal pole of the scaphoid and osteoarthritis of the radio-scaphoid joint (Figs. 2a, b). Active range of motion of the right wrist joint measured 40° of dorsiflexion, 50° palmar flexion, 25° ulnar deviation, and 15° radial deviation. Arthrography demonstrated immediate contrast-medium leakage into the midcarpal joint (Figs. 3a, b). Radial styloid osteotomy was indicated for decompression of the radioscaphoid joint. Care was taken to protect the radial sensory nerve and the second dorsal compartment was identified and opened. A proximally and radially based wedge with a 10° apex angle was removed and closed. Temporary bone immobilization using Kirschner wires was followed by fixation using staples. Immediate postoperative X-rays demonstrated opening of the space of the radioscaphoid joint, indicating the release of contact pressure in the joint (Figs. 4a, b).

Thirty months postoperatively, union of the osteotomy site was attained and the opening

Fig. 2. a Preoperative non-treated scaphoid fracture with degenerative arthritis of the radioscaphoid joint. **b** Preoperative tomography. An osteophyte in the radial styloid and a narrowed radioscaphoid joint are shown

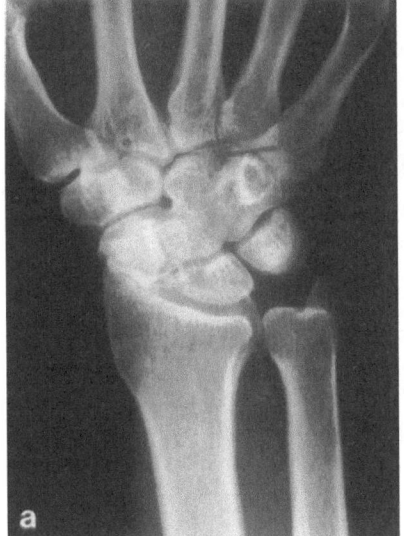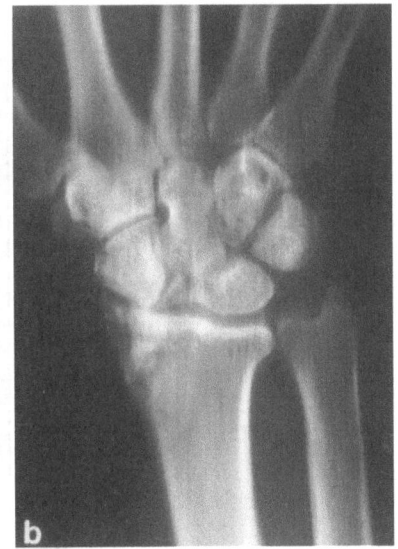

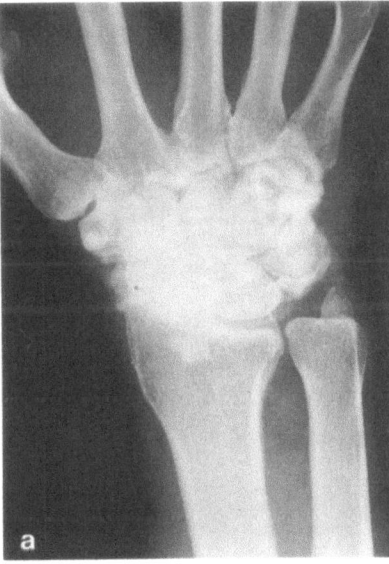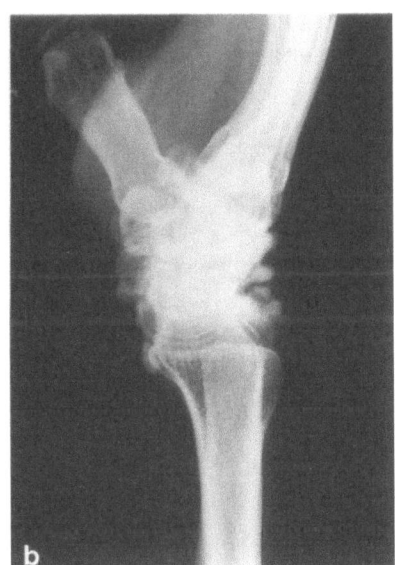

Fig. 3a, b Arthrography. Injection of medium into the radioscaphoid joint immediately showed leakage into the midcarpal joint

of the radioscaphoid joint was maintained (Fig. 4.c). The patient could not perform gymnastic exercises such as using the horizontal bar and hand-standing nor bat a ball before the operation. Postoperatively, the patient can do all these activities without pain.

Case 2

This 39-year-old male cook was seen with a 2-month history of right wrist pain. Tenderness was noted on the radial styloid and ulnocarpal areas of his right wrist joint. Physical examination elicited pain in the radiocarpal and ulnocarpal joints by forearm rotation and radial deviation of the affected wrist joint. Radiography showed minimal spur formation at the radial styloid (Fig. 5.a). An arthrogram showed leakage of contrast medium into the midcarpal and intercarpal joints and also at the distal radioulnar joint by injection into the radiocarpal joint (Fig. 5.b). We suspected both radial styloid impingement and ulnocarpal abutment syndrome. Arthroscopic examination was done followed by radial styloid wedge osteotomy and ulnar bone shortening. We used a plate and screws for the immobilization of the ulna. An

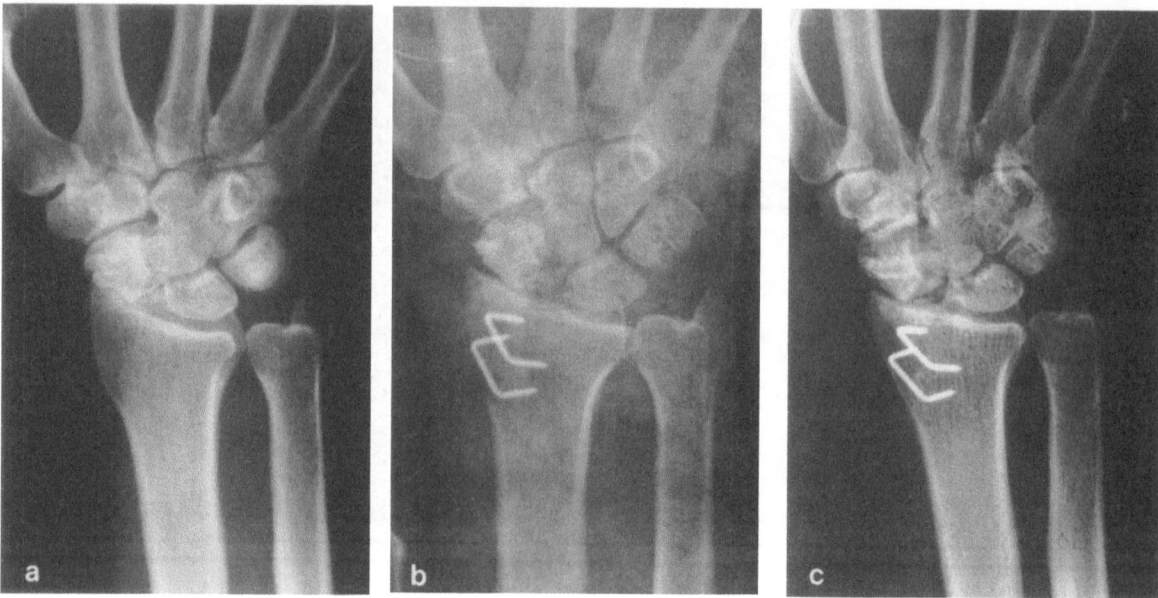

Fig. 4. **a** Before osteotomy. **b** Immediately after the closing radial styloid wedge osteotomy. The radioscaphoid joint is opened. **c** At 30 months postoperatively the radioscaphoid joint remains open

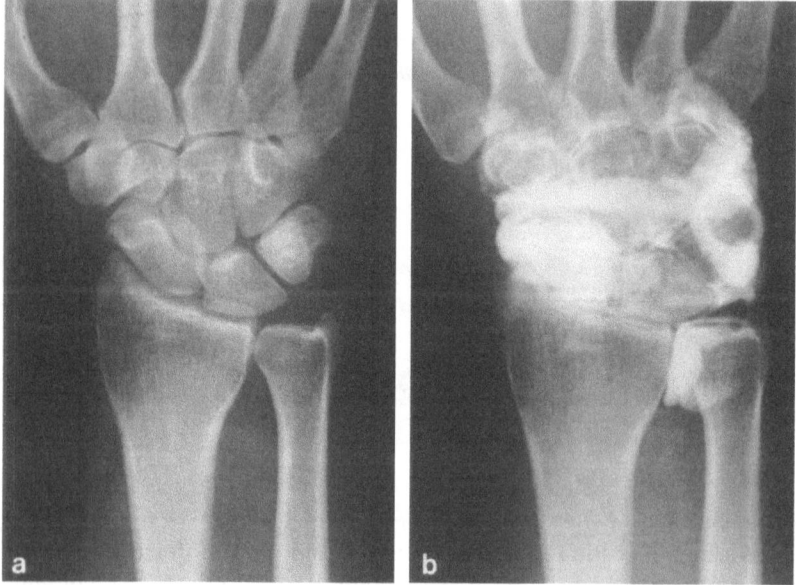

Fig. 5. **a** Before the operation. **b** Arthrogram showing contrast-medium leakage into both midcarpal and ulnocarpal joints

intraoperative radiograph confirmed 7° of closing of the radial styloid angle and 2 mm of shortening of the ulnar bone (Figs. 6.a, b). The radioscaphoid joint space remained opened and wrist joint pain was relieved soon after the operation. The patient was free from pain 2 years postoperatively (Fig. 6.c).

Case 3

The patient was 47-year-old female who suffered from pain at the radial side of her left wrist joint. Radiography and tomography proved to be similar to advanced scapholunate collapse with fracture of the proximal scaphoid (Figs. 7.a, b).

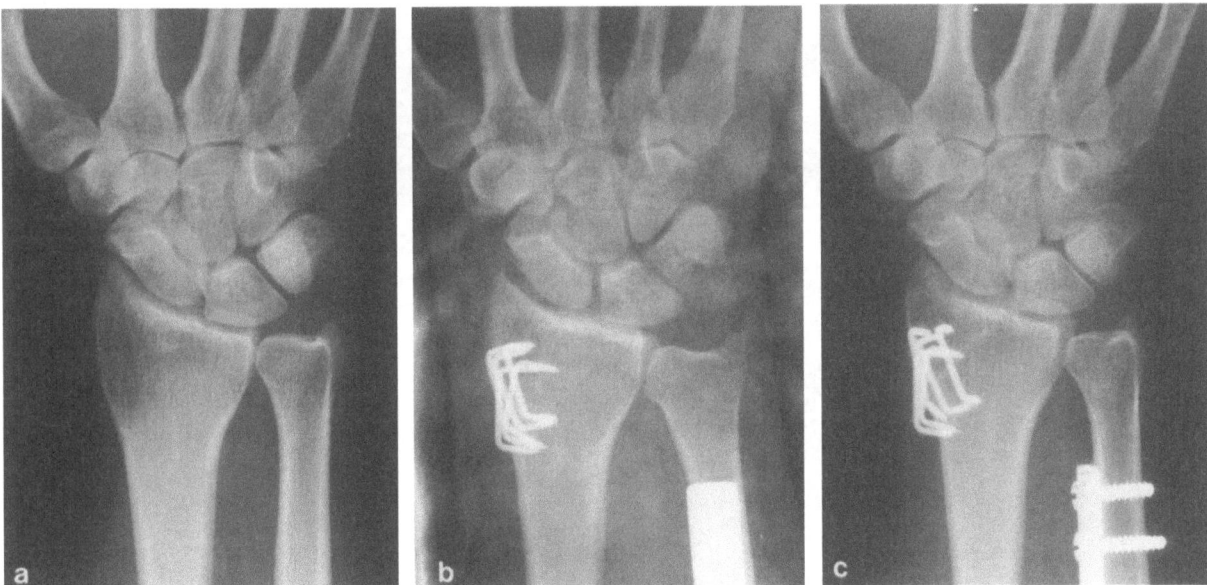

Fig. 6. a Before osteotomy. **b** Immediately after the closing radial styloid and ulnar shortening osteotomy. **c** At 24 months postoperatively the radioscaphoid joint space remains open

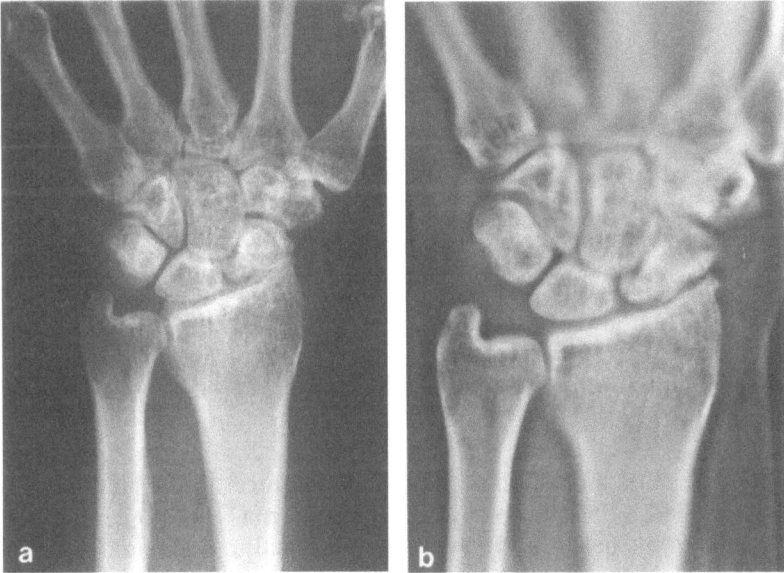

Fig. 7. a Preoperative plain X-ray and **b** tomography showing a non-united scaphoid fracture and degenerative arthritis in the radioscaphoid joint

A closing radial styloid wedge osteotomy was indicated. A wedge with a 6° angle was resected and arthrotomy was then done. The fracture site of the scaphoid was exposed, but the fragment was too small for reduction and internal fixation. We left it in place. We then introduced a sensor using pressure-sensitive conductive silicone rubber into the wrist joint to measure the contact pressure in the radiocarpal and ulnocarpal joints. The sensor has 5 measuring points aligned in the frontal plane with its central point sitting on the scapholunate inter-articular ridge. The thickness of the sensor is 0.8 mm and its maximal measurable pressure is 1.5 MPa. We confirmed the sitting position of the sensor with direct vision and with X-rays before and after measurement

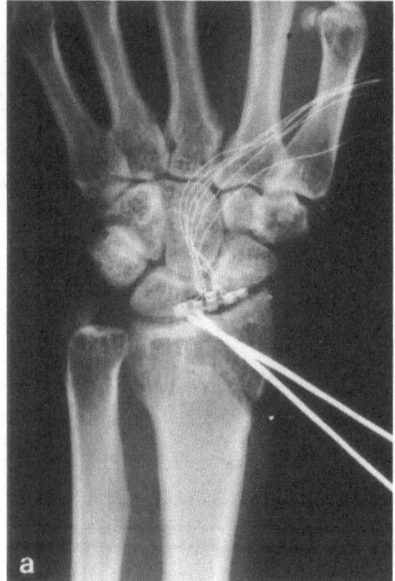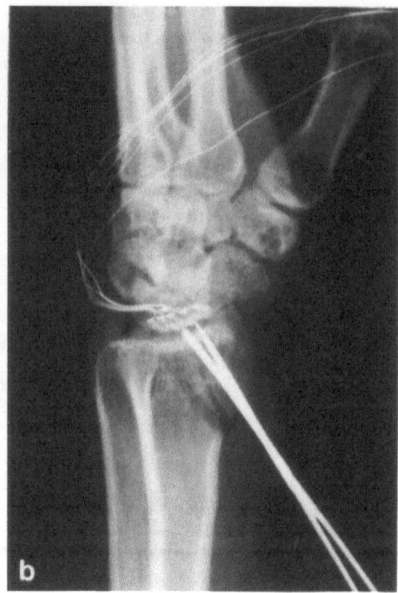

Fig. 8. a, b After resection of the wedge and insertion of the sensor. The Position of the sensor was confirmed. We measured contact pressure before and after closing the defect by manipulating the K-wires inserted into the radial styloid

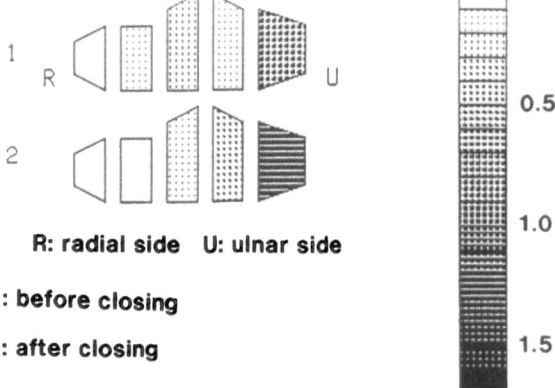

flexor:6v extensor:6v wrist in neutral position   (Kgf/cm²)

R: radial side   U: ulnar side

1: before closing

2: after closing

Fig. 9. Measurement of contact pressure by muscle contraction using electric stimulation. The contact pressure shifts from the ulnar to the radial side after closure of the defect

(Figs. 8a, b). Longitudinal compression force was applied by manual or by simultaneous contraction of the flexors and extensors using electric stimulation.

Six volts was given simultaneously through needles inserted into the flexors and extensors before and after closing the defect created by the osteotomy. The distribution of the contact pressure shifted to the ulnar side and the pressure on the radial side was markedly decreased by closure of the defect (Fig. 9). Longitudinal compression was then applied manually with the wrist joint in a neutral position and in radial and ulnar deviations. Shifting of the contact pressure to the ulnar side and decompression at the radioscaphoid joint were consistently noted in the wrist joint at each position (Fig. 10). An immediate postoperative X-ray showed opening of the radioscaphoid joint (Fig. 11b). Nine months postoperatively, the joint space remained open (Fig. 11c) and the patient was free from pain. The preoperative range of motion of her left wrist joint was preserved.

Results

X-Ray Findings

Widening at the radial part of the radioscaphoid joint space was demonstrated with an intraoperative X-ray in each case.

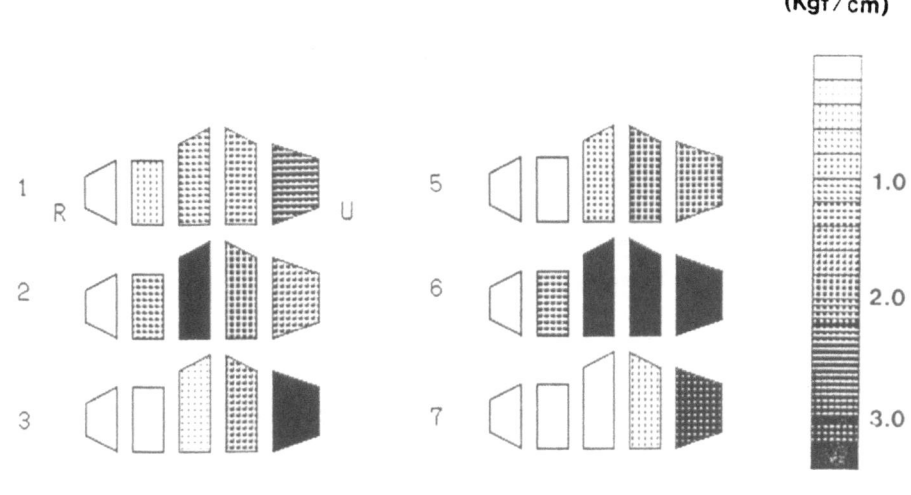

1: before closing   wrist in neutral   5: after closing   wrist in neutral

2: before closing   wrist in radial deviation 6: after closing   wrist in radial deviation

3: before closing   wrist in ulnar deviation   7: after closing   wrist in ulnar deviation

Fig. 10. Measurement of contact pressure in the radiocarpal joint using manual compression. Note the similar shift of the contact pressure from the ulnar to the radial side after closing the wedge despite changing the position of the wrist

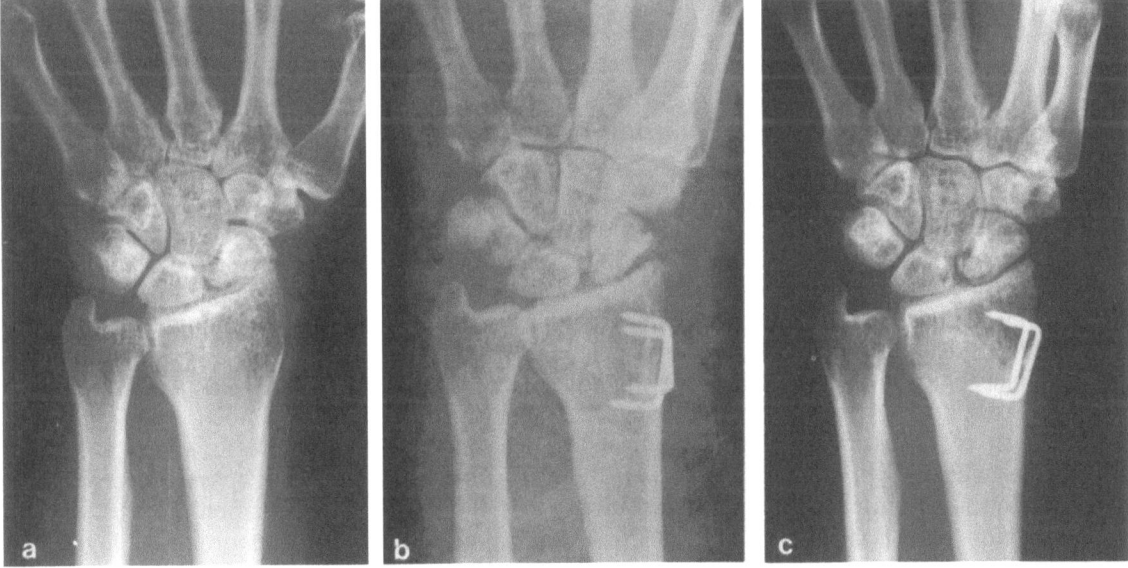

Fig. 11. a Preoperative. **b** Immediately postoperative. **c** The space in the radioscaphoid joint is maintained in an open position

There has been no sign of progressing arthritis or collapse of carpal bones noted at a maximal follow-up period of 24 months.

All cases showed relief from pain, tenderness, and swelling soon after surgery, and most of the patients soon returned to their original jobs. This operation was done extra-articularly and the preoperative range of motion of the operated wrist was maintained postoperatively.

An intraoperative measurement of contact pressure of the radiocarpal joint was done. Manual compression or simultaneous contraction

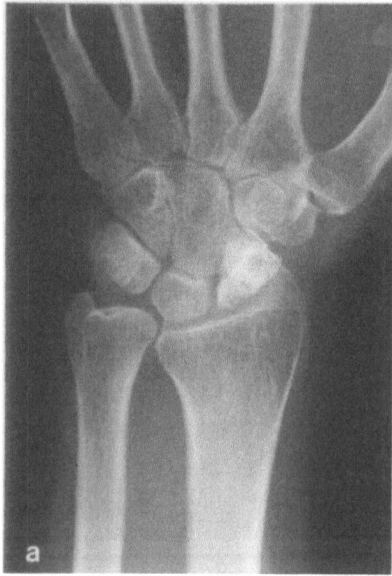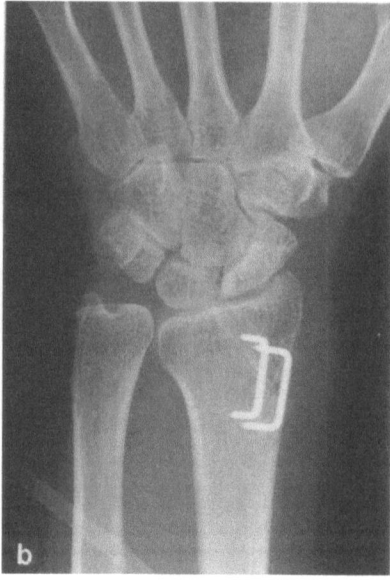

Fig. 12. a Before osteotomy. Rotatory instability and sclerosis of the scaphoid are seen. **b** Postoperatively (1.5 months). The radioscaphoid joint is widened and rotation of the scaphoid is improved

of the flexors and extensors using electric stimulation clearly demonstrated ulnar shifting of the contact pressure with decompression in the radio-scaphoid joint after closing osteotomy. Similar results were obtained regardless of the position of the wrist joint (Figs. 9, 10)

Discussion

The distal radius has an elliptical fossa for articulation with the scaphoid and a spherical fossa for the lunate. Periscaphoid articular malalignment associated with rotation of the scaphoid brings about a specific pattern of arthritis or impingement, while the radiolunate joint is significantly resistive to degenerative change [2]. This degenerative change initially involves the radioscaphoid joint and eventually the capitolunate joint as the rotation of the scaphoid develops. In this advanced stage, the capitate migrates proximally and radially on the capitolunate joint, resulting in destruction of the capitolunate articulation. Further carpal collapse associated with capitate migration involves the hamate-lunate joint. Untreated scaphoid non-union produces a similar arthritic pattern.

Watson recommended capitate-lunate-hamate-triquetrum arthrodesis and replacement of the scaphoid with a Silastic prosthesis [1]. Recently, he has been using a slightly smaller-sized silicone prosthesis for better fitting. However, it is widely known that repeated load to the silicone prosthesis

often induces serious synovitis. Experimental study [3] revealed that the silicone scaphoid implant is a load-bearing implant even when undersized or combined with a limited carpal fusion. For this reason, silicone synovitis should still be a concern in a reconstruction using the SLAC procedure. Currently, he removes the scaphoid and retains the space empty in order to circumvent silicone synovitis [2, 4]. This procedure seems to be a reasonable choice as the salvage procedure for the advanced stage of SLAC wrists. However, this extensive procedure sacrifices motion and may not be necessary for those patients in the early stage whose arthritis is limited to the radioscaphoid joint. The radiolunate becomes the only joint that receives the total load to the wrist after reconstruction by the SLAC procedure. If the styloid wedge osteotomy is performed, the closed radial styloid still shares some longitudinal compression force in extreme situations, such as lifting heavy objects with the wrist joint in radial deviation. In this way, the styloid osteotomy can be more physiological than the SLAC procedure.

Triscaphe arthrodesis has been widely used in the treatment of triscaphe degenerative arthritis [1, 2, 5], rotatory subluxation of the scaphoid [6, 7], and Kienböck's disease [8]. However, triscaphe arthrodesis produces radiocarpal impingement syndrome. Painful radial styloid impingement arises in 33% of successful triscaphe arthrodesis [4]. Roger and Watson [4] recommend radial styloidectomy for radiocarpal impingement and this is now routinely incorporated as the first step in the triscaphe arthrodesis procedure. However, an effective radial styloidectomy for radial styloid impingement syndrome may require release of the radiocapitate or radial collateral ligaments, and result in instability or ulnar translation of the carpus. One anatomical study revealed that a short oblique osteotomy, generally used in conjunction with triscaphe arthrodesis, disrupts 92% of radial collateral ligaments and 9% of radioscaphocapitate ligaments [9].

This series includes a case with Preiser's disease that was treated by a closing radial styloid osteotomy. This procedure should unload the contact pressure to the scaphoid but it is too early for evaluation of the results at the present time (Figs. 12a, b).

Conclusion

Closing wedge osteotomy of the radial styloid effectively unloads contact pressure at the radial side of the radiocarpal joint while maintaining stability and range of motion of the wrist joint through the radiolunate joint. Although further accumulation of clinical experience is needed, closing radial styloid osteotomy may be a useful procedure for SLAC wrist, especially in the early stage.

References

1. Watson HK, Ryu J (1984) Degenerative disorders of the carpus. Orthop Clin North Am 15:337–353
2. Watson HK, Vender MI (1988) Operative hand surgery, 2nd edn. Churchill Livingstone, New York, pp 135–154
3. Viegas SF, Patterson RM, Peterson PD, Crossley M, Foster R (1991) The silicone scaphoid: A biomechanical study. J Hand Surg [Am] 16:91–97
4. Roger WD, Watson HK (1989) Radial styloid impingement after triscaphe arthrodesis. J Hand Surg [Am] 14:297–301
5. Bertheussen K (1981) Partial carpal arthrodesis as treatment of local degenerative changes in the wrist joint. Acta Orthop Scand 52:629–631
6. Watson HK (1981) Limited wrist arthrodesis. I. The triscaphoid joint. J Hand Surg [Am] 5:629–631
7. Watson HK, Ryu J (1986) Limited triscaphoid intercarpal arthrodesis for rotatory subluxation of the scaphoid. J Bone Joint Surg [Am] 68:345–349
8. Watson HK, Ryu J, DiBella A (1985) An approach to Kienböck's disease: Triscaphe arthrodesis. J Hand Surg [Am] 10:179–187
9. Siegel DB, Gelberman RH (1991) Radial styloidectomy: An anatomical study with special reference to radiocarpal intercapsular ligamentous morphology. J Hand Surg [Am] 16:40–44

Surgical Treatment of Rheumatoid Wrists

In Kim, Jung-Man Kim, Seung-Koo Rhee, Yong-Sik Kim, and Sung-Tae Kim[1]

Abstract. Surgical procedures on rheumatoid wrists are often recommended for the alleviation of various associated problems. For example, early synovectomy is strongly indicated, and partial wrist fusion has proven to be effective in patients with moderate destruction of articular cartilage, deformities, and pain. However the use of total arthrodesis and arthroplasty is still in controversy. The proper surgery for rheumatoid wrist should be determined by the clinical severity of disease and radiological findings.

Keywords: Rheumatoid wrist — Surgical treatment — Synovectomy — Partial wrist fusion — Arthroplasty

Introduction

The treatment principle of rheumatoid arthritis (RA) is to achieve painless, normal-ranged joints through surgical or medical means before the occurrence of permanent joint deformities. With the wrist being essential for fine motions of the fingers, the rheumatoid wrist will induce loss of digital dexterity, weakened grasping power, and finally the loss of use of the hand. It is well known that the wrist is the initial site of synovitis in only 2.7% of the rheumatic patients — almost six times less frequently than hand involvement — but is eventually involved in close to 95% of all rheumatic patients in later stages [1]. Therefore, various surgical approaches should be considered for the rheumatoid wrist when the painful swelling, limited motion, and deformation of the wrist have not improved despite adequate medical treatment over a period of several months; the method of surgery will be usually chosen by the severity of the wrist joint involvement as seen radiologically.

Traditionally, the surgical options are open synovectomy or other soft tissue realignment procedures in the initial stage of the disease and wrist arthrodesis in the advanced cases. Recently, however, arthroscopic surgery in the wrist has been developed, reducing the duration of hospitalization and convalescence period. In addition, the distinctly improving techniques of arthrodesis or total wrist arthroplasty (TWA) with remarkably advanced wrist biomechanics makes the postoperative results better, even in the rheumatoid wrist.

The purposes of this study are to determine the optimal time and surgical procedure, and to evaluate the efficacy of arthrodesis or TWA in the rheumatoid wrist.

Patients

A retrospective study was done on 42 rheumatoid wrists in 28 rheumatic patients who underwent various types of surgery at the Department of Orthopaedic Surgery, St. Mary's Hospital (Seoul) from November, 1980 to May, 1990. They were operated upon because of exacerbation of the disease process in spite of receiving physiotherapy and various medications, including gold therapy, for more than 7 months, each having been followed-up for a minimum of 1 year.

Case Analysis

Most of the patients were females (23/28, 84%) with an average age of 43 years. According to the American Rheumatoid Association (ARA) criteria, 25 of the total 28 patients were classified as having classic rheumatoid arthritis (RA) and 3

[1]Department of Orthopaedic Surgery, St. Mary's Hospital Catholic University Medical College, 62, Yoido, Young Deung Po-Ku, Seoul, 150-010 Korea

Table 1. Classification and case analysis

Classification by ARA criteria	No. of patients	No. of wrists	Range of age (years)	Sex M : F
Classic RA	25	38	47	2 : 15
Definite RA	3	4	40	3 : 8
Probable RA	0	0		
Total	28	42	(Mean: 43)	5 : 23

Table 2. ARA Functional classes. (From [19])

Class	Definition	No. of cases
I	Completely able to carry out all usual duties without handicaps	0
II	Adequate for normal activities despite handicaps of limited motion at one or more joint	0
III	Limited only to few or none of the duties of usual occupation or self-care	25
IV	Incapacitated largely or wholly: bed-ridden or confined to wheelchair; little or no self-care	3

Table 3. Classification of rheumatoid wrist preoperatively according to the ARA radiological stages. (From [3])

Stage	X-ray Findings	No. of wrists
Early	No X-ray changes Soft tissue swelling[+]	17
Moderate	Osteoporosis[+] Slight caritilage destruction[+] No joint deformities	8
Severe	Cartilage and bone destruction[+] Osteoporosis[++] Joint deformity[+]	12
Terminal	Fibrous or bony ankylosis	5
Total		42

[+] Slight or mild
[++] Moderate

Table 4. Indications for synovectomy

Indications	No. of complaints
Progressive pain and LOM	12
No effects of medication for more than 6 weeks	11
Recurrent synovitis	1
Progressive deformity	1
	25 CCs (13 wrists)
Radiological ARA findings	
Early	7
Moderate	5
Severe	1

LOM, Limitation of motion; *CCs*, chief complaints

had definite RA (Table 1). Bilateral involvement was present in 28 wrists of 14 patients and unilateral involvement in 14. According to the ARA functional classes by Steinbrocker et al. [2], 25 patients were classified as being in class III (severely disabled) and the remaining 3 patients in class IV (wholly incapacitated) (Table 2).

We tried to analyze all the patients according to the ARA radiological stage by Barren [3] because the method of surgical treatment would be chosen by the radiological findings on the severity of the condition. The classifications of the stages were "early", the most common (17 wrists), "moderate" (8), "severe" (12), and "terminal" with joint ankylosis (5) (Table 3).

Surgical Indications

Synovectomy was done in 13 wrists in patients with 25 complaints. Persistent progressive pain and limited wrist motion that continued for more than 6 weeks despite various medical measures were the operative indications of synovectomy. Radiologically, the lesions were in the early stage in 7 wrists, moderate in 5, and severe in 1. Arthroscopy was performed on 11 wrists, while open synovectomy was carried out in 2 cases because of

painful postero-lateral subluxation, articular erosion, and snapping. A padded splint was applied for 2 weeks postoperatively, after which gradual wrist motion was allowed (Table 4).

Wrist arthrodesis was performed in 24 rhumatoid wrists of patients with 52 complaints which included severe pain, progressive fibrous or bony ankylosis, and wrist deformites or instabilites due to carpal bone destruction. There was no case of unstable wrist associated with the extensor tendon rupture. There were 11 wrists in the severe stage and 13 wrists in the terminal stage according to the ARA radiological criteria (Table 5). Six wrists in 3 patients were fused bilaterally and 18 wrists had unilateral fusion. The fusion angle of the wrist was 10°–20° of dorsiflexion for unilateral or dominant wrists (bilateral involvement) but 10°–20° of palmar flexion for non-dominant wrists in cases of bilateral involvement. Autogen-

Table 5. Indications for wrist arthrodesis

Indication	No. of complaints
Marked pain when using crutches	21
Fibrous or bony ankylosis	17
Marked instability as the result of carpal destruction	14
Rupture of wrist extensors (ECRL and ECRB)	0
	52 CCs (24 wrists)
Radiological ARA findings	
Severe	11
Terminal	13

ECRL, Extensor carpi radialis longus; *ECRB*, extensor carpi radialis brevis

Table 6. Surgery of the rheumatoid wrist

Operation	No. of wrists	Subtotal
Synovectomy		13
Arthroscopic	11	
Open	2	
Arthrodesis		24
Unilateral	18	
Bilateral	6	
Total (involving 2nd and 3rd CMC joint)	19(4)	
Partial wrist arthrodesis	5	
Total wrist arthroplasty (Protek)	5	5
Total	42	42

CMC, Carpometacarpal

Table 7. Indications for total wrist arthroplasty

Indications	No. of complaints
Bilateral involvement with fibrous or bony ankylosis	5 wrists
Radiological ARA findings	
Severe	1
Terminal	4

Table 8. Results of synovectomy. (From [4])

Criteria		Wrists (*n*)
Excellent	Swelling (−)	9
	Free motion	
	Strength preserved or increased	
	No X-ray changes	
	No complaints	
Good	Minimal swelling at op. site	2
	Occ. slight pain usually after exertion	
	No loss of strength	
	No progression of X-ray changes	
Fair	Significant recurrence of synovial thickening	2
	Persistent pain	
	Some progression of X-ray changes	
Poor	Recurrence of synovitis	0
	Severe progressive destructive changes in X-ray	

Op., Operation; *Occ.*, occasional

ous iliac chip bone grafts were put into the fused wrist, fixed with two Kirschner wires, and immobilized with a sugar-tong cast for 6–10 weeks (average 7.2 weeks). In 5 wrists (24 cases), partial wrist arthrodesis was carried out, e.g., radioscapholunate fusion, because the mid-carpal joints were preserved relatively well. The second and third carpometacarpal joints were fused simultaneously because of extensive cartilaginous erosion of the whole wrist (Table 6).

The Protek TWA was performed in 5 cases of radiologic severe or terminal stages and only in cases of bilateral involvement. The ulnar head was not excised in 3 wrists out of 5 TWA cases as part of the hemi-resection interpositional technique (HIT), but was excised in 2 cases as part of the standard technique for TWA (Table 7). Postoperative immobilization with a short arm splint was kept with the wrist in a neutral position for 3 weeks, and gradual active wrist motion was then allowed but with the splint in place at night for another 8 weeks.

Results

All of the patients were followed-up for a minimum of 12 months (average 17 months) after the operation with no evidence of immediate postoperative complications.

The radiological results of synovectomy in the early and moderate stages were analyzed by four grades according to the criteria of Kessler and Vainio [4], and were excellent and good in 11 cases (11/13, 84.6%) but only fair in 2 cases (2/11, 15.4%) because of tenosynovitis of the fingers and involvement of the distal radioulnar joint 4 months after arthroscopic synovectomy (Table 8).

The results of a total of 24 cases with wrist arthrodesis were analyzed according to the criteria of Dupont and Vainio [5] and were good in all of them. Partial wrist fusion involving the radio-

Table 9. Results of arthrodesis. (From [5])

Analysis		Wrists (n)
Good	Bone fusion	24
	Subjective feeling of an increase of power on grasping	
	Subjective feeling and generally more functional	
Poor	Absence of any one or more of the above three conditions	0

scapholunate joint in 5 cases also obtained good results and more than 50% of the wrist motion could be preserved after partial wrist fusion. In conclusion, partial wrist arthrodesis was very effective in moderate degrees of involvement (Table 9).

The final results in 5 cases with TWA were relatively good, but they were totally dependent upon the severity of rheumatoid involvement in the adjacent joints and tendons. The preservation of the ulnar head in TWA was effective in preventing pathological ulnar deviation of the wrist joint in which the ulnar head is excised as in the ordinary technique of TWA (cases 1, 3). The initial wrist range of motion (ROM) after TWA was good but tended to decrease gradually. The overall results of TWA showed that the flexion-extension ROM of the wrist was improved markedly, but neither the radioulnar deviation nor the pronation-supination ROM were increased postoperatively (Table 10).

In conclusion, wrist arthrodesis was the most effective technique for relieving the wrist pain but was not effective in the TWA group (Table 11).

Case Illustration

Case 1 (Fig. 1)

This 17-year-old female high-school student had been suffering from progressive classical RA for 1 year. The condition for both wrists was classified as class III by ARA functional criteria and in the terminal stage by ARA radiological staging (Fig. 1.A). The dominant right wrist was fused to 20° of dorsiflexion. The second and third carpometacarpal (CMC) joints were not included in the fusion area, but the distal radioulnar joint was because of severe pain due to dislocation and cartilageinous erosion (Fig. 1.B). Complete bony union was obtained 3 months later, and finger motion and power were relatively good as of the last follow-up at 18 months. The left wrist (Fig. 1.C) was treated by the Meuli TWA, and this type provided her with better function for the past 27 months postoperatively (Fig. 1.D) with 15° of volar flexion and 65° of dorsiflexion (Fig. 1.E). The distal ulna head was resected by the original techniques for TWA.

Case 2 (Fig. 2)

A partial right wrist fusion including the radioscapholunate bones was performed on this 48-year-old housewife who had definite RA for the previous 6 years. The condition was classified as class III by ARA functional classification and in the severe stage by ARA radiological staging (Fig. 2.A). The distal radioulnar joint was not included in the fusion area, and solid bony union was obtained by 3 months after fusion. At present, 25 months later, 40° of dorsiflexion and 30° of palmar flexion are possible, with remission of the disease (Fig. 2.B).

Case 3 (Fig. 3)

This 32-year-old housewife had previously undergone an arthroscopic wrist synovectomy because of progressive classical RA for the last 7 years. The condition was classified radiologically as being in the severe stage (Fig. 3.A). The distal ulna head was resected in the original TWA procedure, and we thought this could be one of the causes of ulna deviation of the hand in RA postoperatively. Therefore, TWA was done with hemi-resection arthroplasty in order to preserve the distal ulnar stability (Fig. 3.B) and the final results 1 year postoperatively were adequate, with

Table 10. Results of total wrist arthroplasty

Range of motion	Preoperative	Postoperative	% Changes
Flexion-extension	20°	85°	+325%
Radioulnar deviation	10°	10°	0
Pronation and supination	130°	130°	0

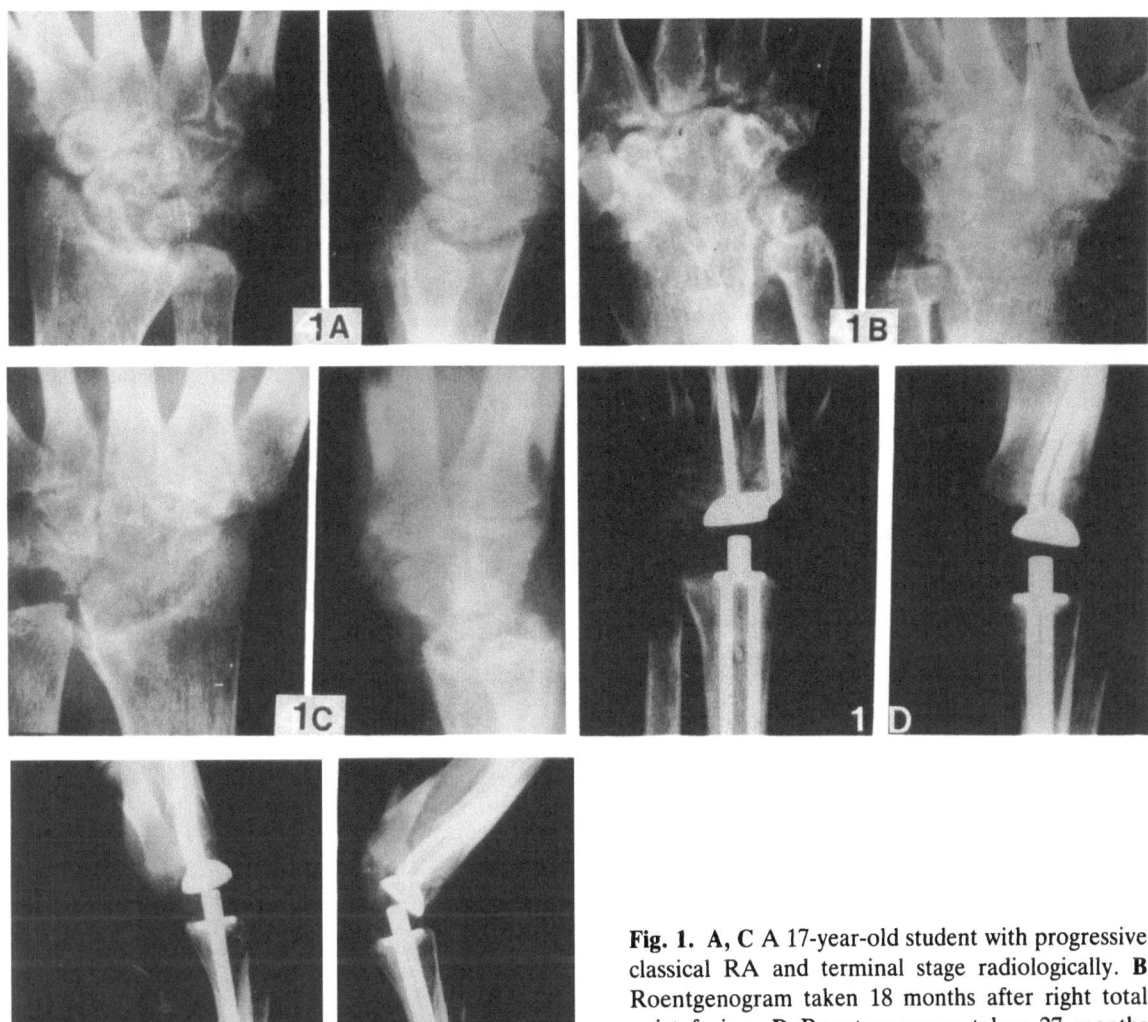

Fig. 1. A, C A 17-year-old student with progressive classical RA and terminal stage radiologically. **B** Roentgenogram taken 18 months after right total wrist fusion. **D** Roentgenogram taken 27 months after left total wrist arthroplasty (TWA). **E** showing maximal wrist motions with 15° of volar flexion and 65° of dorsiflexion

Table 11. Comparison of severity of pre- and postoperative pain

Surgical procedure	Preoperative	Postoperative
Synovectomy	3.6	2.3
Arthrodesis	4.7	1.2
Total wrist arthroplasty	4.2	1.8

Pain	Points
None	1
Mild, occasionally	2
Moderate	3
Marked, serious	4
Severe, disabling	5

20° of palmar flexion and 40° of dorsiflexion, although mild persistent pain on exercise was still present.

Discussion

Rheumatoid arthritis can be classified as monocyclic, polycyclic, and progressive types according to the severity of clinical symptoms. Statistically, only about 35% of the monocyclic, 50% of the polycyclic, and 15% of the progressive types recover after various forms of medications and surgeries [6]. In addition, 15%–47% of RA patients will require various surgical interventions due to

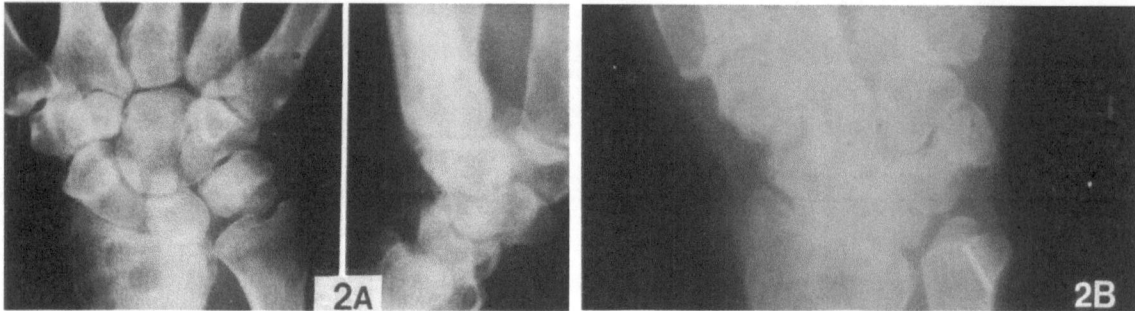

Fig. 2. A A 48-year-old housewife with definite RA and severe radiological stage. **B** Roentgenogram taken 25 months after partial wrist fusion including the radioscapholunate joint

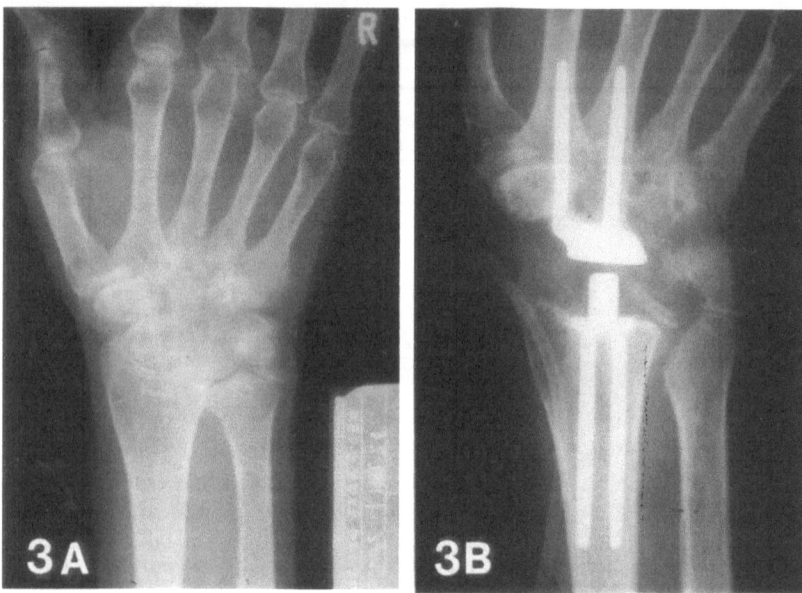

Fig. 3. A A 32-year-old female with classical RA and severe radiological stage. **B** Roentgenogram taken immediate after TWA showing preserved ulnar head

progression of the disease [2, 3, 7, 8]. However, with regard to the surgical results, in 1974, Allander [7] reported that only 80% of major operations and 30% of minor operations were effective for 293 RA patients, and that these results are dependent upon selection of the patient, the patient's knowledge about the surgery and expected results, and the surgical methods.

It is well known that the wrist is the key joint in the upper extremity, and that wrist stability is very important to normal function and strength of the hand. The wrist is also commonly involved in most cases of RA [1]. Consequently, we analyzed the patients with rheumatic wrists in order to select the optimal treatment for the various stages of rheumatoid involvement and to examine the role of the distal radioulnar joint as well as the

efficacy and indications for wrist arthrodesis and TWA.

Surgery, when indicated in RA, should not be delayed. The deformity of one joint will cause secondary changes in adjacent joints and eventually develop a severe fixed deformity. Early preventive treatment should be initiated before this occurs [9–12]. Generally, it is wise to perform the operations during a stabilized period of the disease progression and when the erythrocyte sedimentation rate (ESR) is low. Aspirin may cause a bleeding tendency and so must be replaced by other anti-inflammatory drugs at least 1 week before surgery. The ARA radiological findings provided the best guidelines for selecting the method of surgery. In this study, most of the patients were housewives and had long-term bilateral involvement. For cases in less than the moderate radiological stage, synovectomy or other soft tissue surgery was preferred. On the other hand, for those in the severe stage with extensive bony destruction and osteoporosis, arthrodesis or TWA was preferred but the choice depened upon other factors, such as the patient's general condition, the presence of multiple joint involvement, age, and occupation.

The results of synovectomy are known to differ according to the joints involved. For example, hip synovectomy is effective only in cases with early radiological changes, but good results in the knee joint can be expected even in cases past the moderate stage. The wrist joint is a complex organ, having eight carpal bones, and becomes much more complicated in combination with the second and third CMC joints and the distal radioulnar joint in transmitting force. Consequently, wrist synovectomy was recommended only in cases in less than the moderate stage of joint destructions as seen on X-rays. Open dorsal wrist synovectomy had the disadvantages of prolonging the initiation of rehabilitation and the difficulty in excising the volar synovium. Recently, arthroscopic volar and dorsal synovectomy, which had been relatively uncommon, have been widely attempted. However, unlike other joints, the main pathology of the rheumatoid wrist is not limited to synovitis but also extends to tenosynovitis of extensor tendons. In particular, we did not expect good results with arthroscopic surgery alone in cases with subluxation of the distal radioulnar joint associated with the involvement of the second and third CMC joint.

Dorsolateral subluxation of the distal radioulnar joint and painful snapping are common in advanced RA [13]. In these conditions, the Darrach operation has been used conventionally [14], but the resection of the distal ulna, especially in an active young male, the TFCC (triangular fibrocartilage complex) will be injured and result in radiocarpal instability associated with excessive volar and ulnar translation of the carpals. This is because the distal ulna is the attachment site of the TFCC which prevents the excessive anteroposterior and ulnar translation of carpal bones during wrist motion [15]. The rupture of extensor tendons at the distal end of the resected ulna has also been reported [16]. We have performed the Darrach operation for painful subluxation of the radioulnar joint on three rheumatoid wrists which showed progressive ulnar deviation of the hand and pathological translation of the carpal bones in

long-term follow-up. In order to minimize these complications, we have sometimes chosen the hemiresection interpositional arthroplasty procedure [17], Sauvé-Kapandji operation [18], or silastic ulnar head replacement, rather than excise the ulnar head, and have obtained good results.

Partial wrist arthrodesis in severe or terminal radiological stages was preferred before performing total wrist arthrodesis or TWA [19]. The results of all 5 cases of partial wrist fusion for the radioscapholunate bones were relatively good and more than 50% of the wrist motion could be preserved. As for simultaneous fusion of the second and third CMC joints, we have confined it to cases with abnormal physical and X-ray changes because these joints are normally immobile, although Carrol and Dick [8] stated that it was desirable to include these joints to accomplish a large grafted bone for total wrist joint fusion.

Another controversy concerns the position of wrist fusion, with 10°-20° of dorsiflexion in unilateral cases being more widely accepted for maximal daily activities. In light of the possibility of bilateral wrist involvement in RA being high [1, 10], consideration of wrist fusion on each side is needed. We fused the dominant wrist in 10°-20° of dorsiflexion and the non-dominant wrist in 0°-20° of volar flexion, an essentially neutral position of less then 10°, because of the patient's preference on a cosmetic basis rather than for convienence in daily activities and possible compensation for the limited wrist motion by finger motions. To preserve the thumb function and grip strength of the fingers, we took care not to damage the first, fourth, and fifth CMC joints which have 15°-30° of motion in flexion.

The use of the TWA procedure is still controversial because there are no effective ways to fix the artificial joint into the medullary canal of the second and third metacarpals and radius, and the volar and dorsal carpal ligaments, wrist flexors and extensors are the active stabilizers in the wrist joint. If we consider that the wrist joint space will need to be released up to a maximal 5/8 inches for lifting a weight of 40 lbs [20], we can understand the difficulty of achieving a successful TWA. We have performed five TWAs of the Meuli type, and have followed each patient for more than 25 months. Although the complications and revision rates of TWA are reported in the literature as being high [20], all of our patients are reasonably satisfied with the remarkable relief of pain and the return of functional abilites of their wrist. We believe that for the dominant wrist in patients with bilateral wrist involvement and the other involved wrist in those who underwent arthrodesis on one wrist, TWA could be carried out to reconstruct the disabled wrist.

References

1. Millender LH, Nalebuff EA (1973) Arthrodesis of the rheumatoid wrist. J Bone Joint Surg [Am] 55:1026–1034

2. Steinbrocker O, Traeger CH, Batterman RD (1944) Therapeutic criteria in rheumatoid arthritis. JAMA 140:659–662

3. Barron JN (1969) The assessment of suitability for surgery in general timing of operation. Ann Rheum Dis 28(Suppl):74–76

4. Kessler I, Vainio K (1966) Posterior (dorsal) synovectomy for rheumatoid involvement of the hand and wrist. A follow-up study of sixty-six procedures. J Bone Joint Surg [Am] 48:1085–1095

5. Dupont M, Vainio K (1986) Arthrodesis of the wrist in rheumatoid arthritis. Study of 140 cases. Ann Chir Gynaecol 57:513–519

6. Feric DC, Smyth CY, Clayton ML (1983) Medical considerations and management of rheumatoid arthritis. J Hand Surg [Am] 8:662–666

7. Allander E (1974) Need for reconstruction surgery for rheumatoid arthritis. Scand J Rheumatol 3:183

8. Carrol RE, Dick HM (1971) Arthrodesis of the wrist for rheumatoid arthritis. J Bone Joint Surg [Am] 53:1365

9. Findley TW, Halpern D, Easton JKM (1983) Wrist subluxation in juvenile rheumatoid arthritis: Pathophysiology and management. Arch Phys Med Rehab 64:6

10. Granberry WM, Mangum GL (1980) The hand in the child with juvenile rheumatoid arthritis. J Hand Surg [Br] 5:105

11. Maldonade-Cocco JA, Garcia-Morteo O, Spindler AJ (1980) Carpal ankylosis in juvenile rheumatoid arthritis. Arthritis Rheum 23:1251

12. Sones DA (1968) Surgery for rheumatoid arthritis. Timing and techniques: General and medical aspects. J Bone Joint Surg [Am] 50:576

13. Bell MJ, Hill RJ, McMurty RY (1985) Ulnar impingement syndrome. J Bone Joint Surg [Br] 67:126–129

14. Darrow JC Jr, Linscheid RL, Dobyns JH, Mann JM III, Wood MB, Beckenbaugh RD (1985) Distal ulnar resection for disorder of the distal radio-ulnar joint. J Hand Surg [Am] 10:482–491

15. Palmer AK, Werner FW, Murphy D, Glisson R (1985) Functional wrist motion: A biomechanical study. J Hand Surg [Am] 10:39–46

16. A.A.O.S (American Academy of Orthopedic Surgery) (1987) Orthopedic knowledge, update 2. Home study syllabus, pp 250–251

17. Bowers WH (1985) Distal radio-ulnar joint arthroplasty: The hemiresection-interposition technique. J Hand Surg [Am] 10:169–178

18. Sauvé I, Kapandji IA (1936) Nouvelle technique pour le traitement chirurgical des lexations recidivantes isolees de lextremite inferieure du cubitus. J Chir 47:589–594

19. Rozing PM, Kauer JMG (1984) Partial arthrodesis of the wrist. An investgation in cadavers. Acta Orthop Scand 55:66–68

20. Volz RG (1977) Total wrist arthroplasty. A new approach to wrist stability. Clin Orthop 128:180–189

Treatment of Chronic Dislocation of the Distal Radioulnar Joint: Comparative Studies Between Reconstruction and Resection of the Distal Ulna

Seung-Koo Rhee, Soon-Yong Kwon, Hee-Dai Lee, Jong-Hoon Park, and Jin-Young Kim[1]

Abstract. From January 1981 until March 1990, a total of 32 cases of chronic dislocation of the distal radioulnar joint was treated surgically, and the follow-up results were compared between the group which underwent reconstruction and those who had resection of the distal ulna (the Darrach operation). The results obtained were as follows: (1) there was marked postoperative improvement in pain, range of motion, and grip strength in all 32 cases, and (2) in comparing the long-term follow-up results between the reconstruction (13 cases) and Darrach operation groups (19 cases), relief from pain was marked in the former, while the range of motion and grip strength scores were similar in both groups. It was concluded that the distal ulnar head and distal radioulnar joint were singularly important in preservation of normal wrist function. While various methods of treatment of distal radioulnar derangement are available, the results of reconstruction surgery are more favorable than those of the Darrach operation.

Keywords: Chronic dislocation — Distal radioulnar joint — Reconstruction — Resection of distal ulna — Darrach operation

Introduction

Dislocations or subluxations of the distal radioulnar (DRU) joint are not uncommon, but they are often neglected to be treated. In 1984, Palmer and Werner reported that approximately 81.6% of the load applied on a wrist model was borne by the distal radius and 18.4% by the distal ulna [1]. Thus, ulnar variance will change the load borne by the distal ulna, with the DRU joint playing an important role in the integrated forearm-wrist-hand function biomechanically, as does the lateral malleolus in the ankle joint [2]. Recently, reconstruction of the dislocated DRU joint to normal anatomic proportions began to be performed more commonly than the resection or Darrach operation [3].

The purpose of this study was to find out the biomechanical significance of the DRU joint by analysis of long-term follow-up results, comparing those of 19 reconstructed cases and 13 cases of the Darrach operation group, all treated for a dislocated DRU joint.

Patients

Thirty-two patients with deranged DRU joints, who were treated at the Department of Orthopaedic Surgery, St. Mary's Hospital (Seoul, Korea) from January, 1981 until March 1990, were chosen as the subjects of this research. In all the cases, it was impossible to immediately close reduction because the patients presented more than 3 weeks after the initial injury. Surgery was considered for all. Their ages ranged from 18 to 56 years (average 31 years). There were 19 males and 13 females, and 24 of them had right wrist injuries (Table 1).

Causes of Dislocation

The most common cause of dislocation was fracture of the forearm bones (22 cases), and among them, Colles' fracture (18 cases) was the most frequent followed by Kienböck's disease and rheumatoid arthritis. Only one case involved an anterior dislocation, and the others had posterolateral dislocations (Table 1).

[1] Department of Orthopaedic Surgery, St. Mary's Hospital, Catholic University Medical College, 62, Yoido, Youngdeungpo-ku, Seoul, 150-010, Korea

317

Table 1. Analysis of chronic distal radioulnar dislocation in 32 patients

Cause (*n* cases)	Treatment (*n* cases)
Colles' fracture (18)	Radioulnar tenodesis (1)
Kienböck's disease with	Arthroplasty
negative ulnar variance (4)	Darrach operation (13)
Rheumatiod arthritis (4)	HIT (2)
Galeazzi's fracture (2)	Osteotomy
Fracture of both forearms (2)	Ulnar shortening (6)
Positive ulnar variance (1)	Ulnar lengthening (1)
Unknown (1)	Radial lengthening (4)
	Radial shortening (1)
	Angular osteotomy of the
	distal radius (1)
	Sauvé-Kapandji
	operation (3)

HIT, Hemi-resection interpositional technique

Physical Findings and Diagnosis

Dull pain around the DRU joint on wrist motion and bony prominance due to a dislocated distal ulnar head were the most common complaints. Limitation of motion and snapping were also seen but not to a severe degree (Table 2).

The preoperative grip strength, measured in only 8 cases, was maximally decreased up to 50% than that of the normal adult.

The ulnar head and the triquetrum were not in a straight line in wrist AP X-rays, and the long axis of the ulna was located posteriorly in the posterior dislocations and anteriorly in the anterior dislocations in relation to that of the radius in lateral wrist films.

Treatment

Reconstruction of a dislocated DRU joint was done in 19 cases using tenodesis with dorsal retinacular ligaments, osteotomy at the distal radius or ulna, hemiresection interpositional arthroplasty (HIT) and the Sauvé-Kapandji operation, especially in younger or hard laborers without injuries to the articular cartilage of the DRU joint. The patients were monitored for an average of 5.5 months (from 7 weeks to 27 months) postoperatively.

The Darrach operation was performed in 13 patients, with 4 cases of rheumatoid arthritis and 9 cases of severe comminuted fracture of the ulnar head with marked destructive changes of the articular cartilage. They were followed-up for an average of 26 months (from 12 weeks to 9 years) postoperatively (Tables 1, 2).

Results

Radiological Changes

Three cases out of a total of thirteen (23.1%), which had been followed-up for more than 26 months after the Darrach procedure, radiologically showed the typical complications as

Table 2. Comparison between the Darrach operation and the reconstruction groups

	Darrach (13 cases)	Reconstruction (19 cases)
Age (years)	27–46 (average, 32)	18–56 (average, 30)
Sex (M/F)	8/5	11/8
Etiology Rheumatoid arthritis	2	2
Trauma	9	13
Ulnar variance	1	4
Unknown	1	0
Chief complaint		
Pain	12	10
Limitation of motion	9	4
Clicking	6	2
Deformity	14	8
Follow-up period	12 weeks-9 years (average 26 months)	7 weeks-27 months (average 5.5 months)

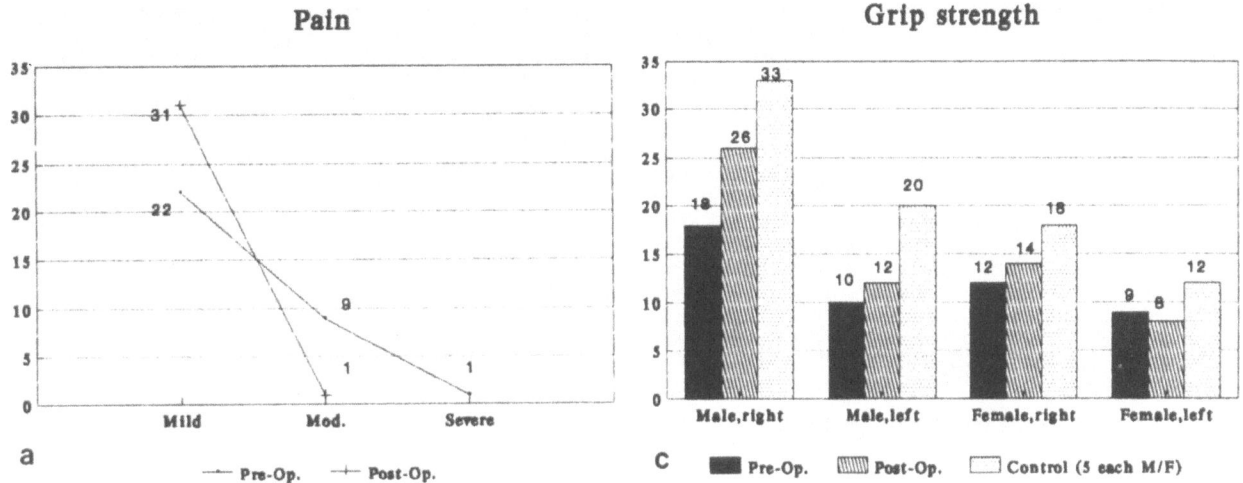

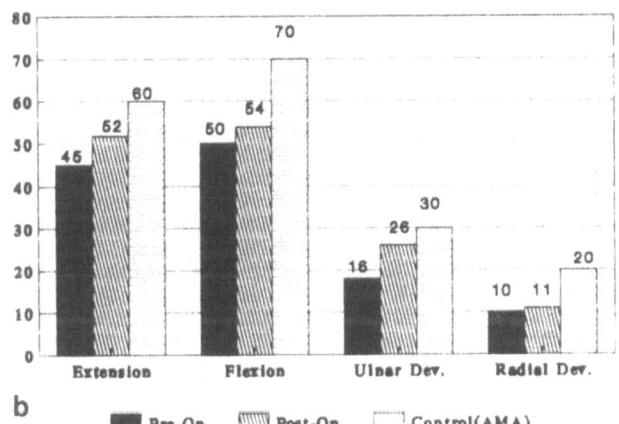

Fig. 1. Pre- and postoperative functional results in all cases

described below in case 1, among them ulnocarpal translation, scapholunate dissociation, and osteoarthritic changes on the radiolunate joint. However, in none of the reconstruction cases, which had been followed-up for more than 5.5 months postoperatively, were any radiological changes detected.

Pre- and Postoperative Functional Results

Pain, range of wrist motion, and grip strength of the fingers were evaluated. Preoperatively, 22 patients suffered from mild wrist pain which was moderate in 9 patients. Postoperatively, however, 31 out of 32 patients complained only of mild, occasional pain (Fig. 1.a).

The range of wrist motion as measured by AMA criteria was improved postoperatively in all patients, there was a large increase in the amount of wrist extension, but the degree of radial deviation increased slightly (Fig. 1.b).

Grip strength was compared with the mean strength of the wrists of five normal males and females (age range 20–40 years) as measured by a Preston dynamometer. Postoperatively, it was markedly increased in the right hand of the male patients but diminished in the left hand of the female patients (Fig. 1.c).

Comparative Clinical Results

Pain, range of motion, and grip strength at the last follow-up were also compared in both groups. Grip strength was measured in only 4 cases in each group. Pain relief was remarkable in the reconstruction group (Fig. 2.a), but the extent of

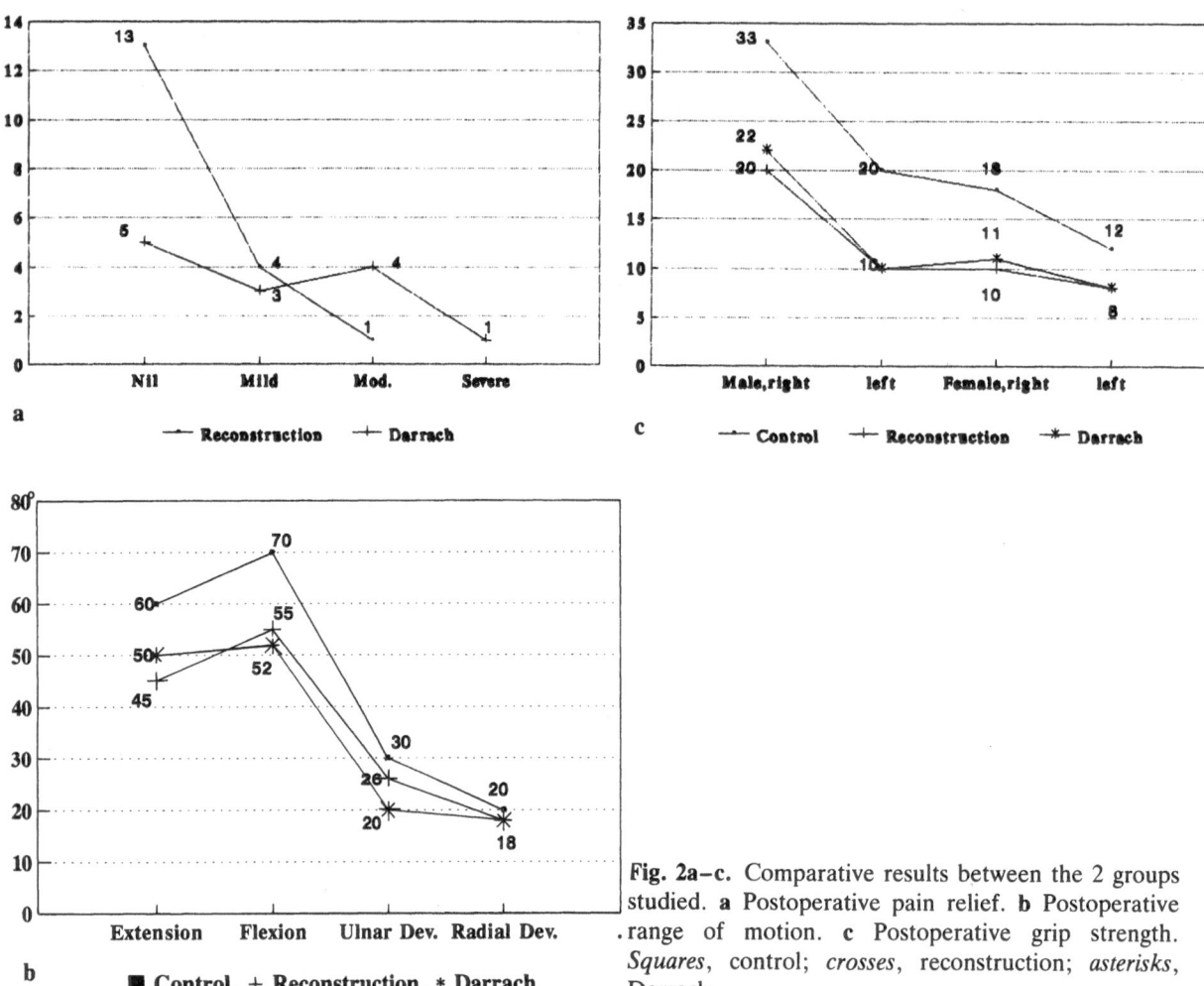

Fig. 2a–c. Comparative results between the 2 groups studied. **a** Postoperative pain relief. **b** Postoperative range of motion. **c** Postoperative grip strength. *Squares*, control; *crosses*, reconstruction; *asterisks*, Darrach

restoration of wrist motion and grip strength was similar in both groups (Figs. 2b, c).

Case Illustrations

Case 1. O-G Kim, 46/M: the Darrach Operation

This patient had been treated conservatively for a comminuted fracture of the distal radius 12 years ago. Three years after the fracture, he underwent the Darrach operation because of persistent pain and limited wrist motion in all directions and radiologically evidenced radial shortening and disruption of the DRU joint (Fig. 3.A). Nine years after the Darrach operation, ulnocarpal sliding of carpal bones and severe osteoarthritic changes between the RU joint on X-rays were shown (Fig. 3.B); he complained of persistent, painful and limited wrist motion. Partial wrist fusion including the radiolunate was done.

Case 2. O-S Kim, 49/F: the Hemi-resection Interpositional Technique (HIT)

In this comminuted Galeazzi's fracture dislocation (Fig. 4.A), the HIT was done with resection of only the bony fragments of the distal ulnar head, but repair of the triangular fibrocartilage complex (TFCC) and the ulnar collateral ligament was carried out simultaneously. No definite bony changes were found 7 years after the operation, but a slight widening of the DRU joint was noted (Fig. 4.B). Clinically, good results were obtained.

Case 3. O-S Nam, 31/F: the Sauvé-Kapandji Operation

This patient had complained of bony prominance of the ulnar head, painful snapping, and limited wrist motion for 2 years after a right forearm bone fracture (Fig. 5.A). Sauvé-Kapandji pro-

Fig. 3. A 46-year-old male laborer with radial shortening and disruption of the distal radioulnar joint. **A** Roentgenogram taken before the Darrach operation. **B** Roentgenogram taken 9 years after the operation showing marked ulnar translation of carpal bones and osteoarthritis on the radiolunate joint

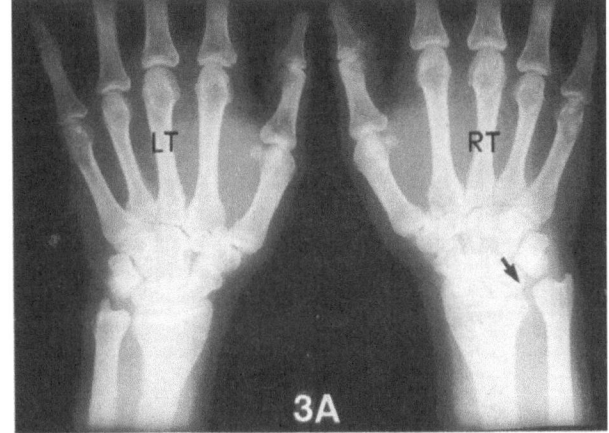

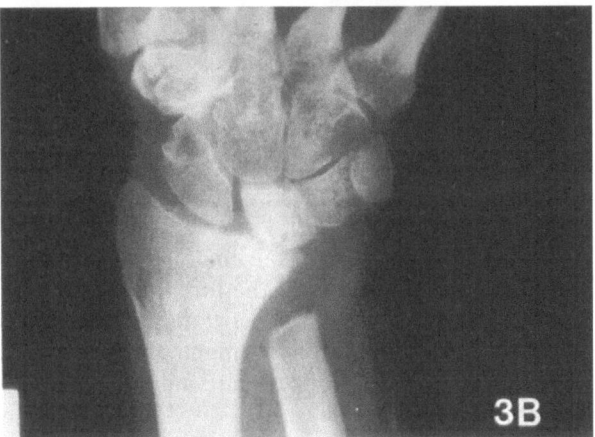

Fig. 4. A 49-year-old female with comminuted Galeazzi's fracture-dislocation. **a** Initial roentgenograms. **b** Roentgenogram taken 7 years after the hemi-resection interpositional technique (HIT)

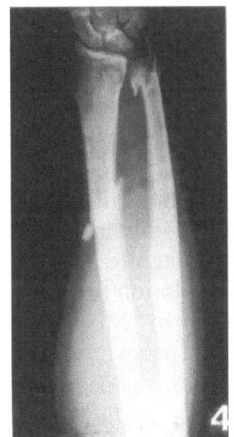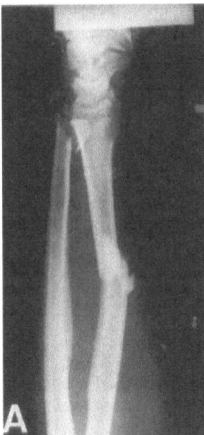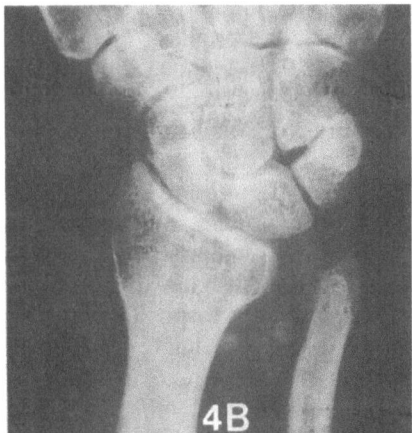

cedures were carried out, and the fascia and periosteum around the osteotomy site were carefully repaired to prevent painful friction between the distal end of the osteotomized ulna and the adjacent muscle during rotation of the forearm (Fig. 5.B). The follow-up at 9 months revealed good clinical results.

Discussion

We examined the anatomic characteristics of the DRU joint using two wrists from cadavers. The ulnar head articulated with the sigmoid notch of the distal radius which was angled distally and ulnarly to the surface of the ulnar

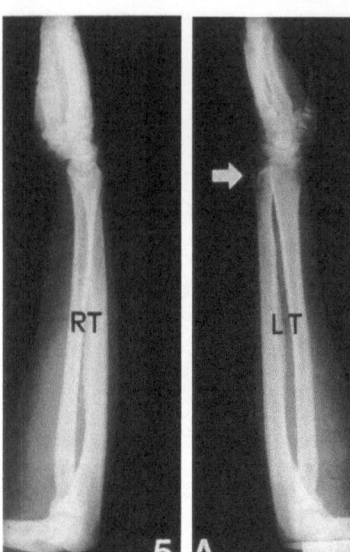
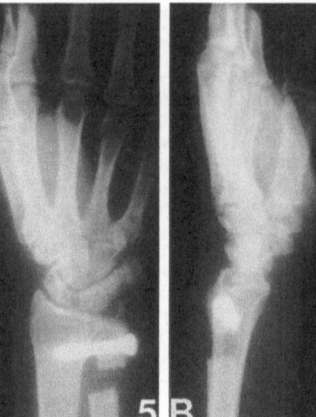

Fig. 5. A 31-year-old female with posterior dislocation of the distal ulnar head. **a** Both forearms, lateral views. **b** Roentgenograms taken 9 months after the Sauvé-Kapandji operation

head by approximately 20°. Biomechanically, it is well known that the distal ulnar head is not immobile during rotation of the forearm, having 8°–9° of lateral sliding during wrist motion, a few degrees of posterodistal movement in forearm pronation, and anteroproximal migration in forearm supination [4–6].

In 1987, Crenshaw [7] stated that the stabilizers of the DRU joint were the ulnar collateral ligament, articular disc, anterior and posterior RU ligaments, and pronator quadratus muscle. However, in 1981, Palmer and Werner [8] stressed that the TFCC contained the most important structures for stabilizing the DRU joint, with this complex consisting of the articular disc and the anterior and posterior DRU ligaments. Through our cadaver studies, we have also confirmed that the TFCC is comprised of the ligamentous and cartilagenous structures that suspend the distal radius and ulnar carpus from the distal ulna.

According to Palmer and Werner [1], approximately 81.6% of the axial loads in the wrist are known to be borne by the distal radius and 18.4% by the distal ulna. They also reported that removal of the TFCC could decrease the loads borne by the distal ulna by approximately 6.2% and result in 93.8% of the loads being borne by the distal radius, and, of course, 100% of the axial loads would be borne by the distal radius in resections of the ulnar head. They also revealed that the distribution of the load on the wrist varied according to the length of the ulna. For example, negative ulnar variance with 2.5 mm of shortening resulted in an increase of the force borne by the distal radius to 95.7% of the total axial loading to the wrist. On the other hand positive ulnar variance with 2.5 mm of lengthening might result in a decrease of the force borne by the distal radius to 58.1%. Brand et al. [9] also reported the average daily axial loading of the normal adult wrist to be more than 500 kg. All of these biomechanical obervations on the DRU joint suggest how important are the normal anatomical relationships of the this joint. Therefore, there has been a recent trend to maintain the normal anatomical relations of a disrupted DRU joint caused by various injuries or diseases.

Dislocation of the DRU joint may be frequently combined with Galeazzi's, Colles', or Smith's fracture and rarely result independently and in isolation from external torsional force over the forearm. Mechanically, a posterior dislocation will be caused by excessive pronation but an anterior dislocation will result from excessive supination of the forearm. Most dislocations are posterior ones in this study, only 1 out of 31 cases was anterior. The dislocation of the DRU joint caused by a forearm bone fracture could be easily missed by physicians because the clinical symptoms are relatively mild. Therefore, it was not uncommon to discover that there had been a dislocation after the fracture had healed. Radiologically, it is difficult to diagnose a posterior subluxation, but the diagnosis can be easily made in dislocations if the ulnar head and triquetrum do not lie on a straight line in AP wrist X-rays.

Acute posterior dislocation could be reduced by pushing the distal ulna head anteriorly in a position of 90° of elbow flexion and full supination of the forearm. Afterwards, long arm cast immobilization or cross-pinning with Kirschner wires for 6 weeks is necessary. All of ours were chronic cases; we performed distal ulnar resection for 13 cases and 6 various kinds of reconstructions for 19 cases to preserve the normal anatomic relations of the DRU joint. There were no specific indications for each operation, but we have tried to reconstruct the DRU joint rather than perform excisions in younger patients without arthritic changes detected in X-ray films and in heavy laborers. Among the 19 reconstruction cases, osteotomy at the distal radius or ulna was performed in 13 cases, Sauvé-Kapandji procedures [10] in 3 cases, HIT in 2 cases, and tenodesis in 1 case.

In the Sauvé-Kapandji operation, the pronation-supination motion did not occur on the DRU joint but rather on the site of the osteotomy. Consequently, the cut end of the distal ulna should be well covered with fascia or surrounding muscle to prevent pain and snapping at the osteotomy site. Interposition with fatty or other soft tissue was also necessary to prevent reunion of the osteotomy site [11]. HIT, which was reputed initially performed in 1952 by Dingman [12], is a modification of the Darrach operation for an intraarticular fracture of the ulnar head, and is commonly used in rheumatoid arthritis or ulnocarpal impingement syndromes. We have performed HIT for 2 cases with rheumatoid arthritis and obtained good results: diminution of pain and prevention of recurrent subluxation, osteoarthritic changes, and ulnar deviation. Many operative methods of tenodesis using flexor carpi ulnaris (FCU) [4], fascia lata, and free tendon graft [13] for dislocation of the DRU joint have been advocated [14]. We have performed FCU stabilization in 1 case using the extensor retinacular flap created initially by Spinner and Kaplan [15]. It was simple to execute, needing only a single skin incision, and good range of motion was obtained postoperatively.

Accordingly, the results of the long-term follow-up of 10 out of 13 patients (76.9%) who underwent the Darrach operation were found to be good, with no serious abnormal changes occurring to the biomechanics of the wrist. These results did not mean that the Darrach procedure is a totally reliable operation, even in the light of the long-term follow-up, since many authors [16, 17] reported on complications, such as painful snapping or rupture of the extensor tendon at the ulnar stump, or osteoarthritic changes on the radiolunate joint. To prevent these complications, Tsai and Stillwell [18] reported a way of stabilizing the ulnar stump by tying the FCU to the ulnar stump, ECU, and around the distal radius. Furthermore, as shown in case 1, serious complications after a Darrach operation, such as ulnar-carpal sliding, osteoarthritis of the radiolunate joint, and painful limitation of motion, are so critical to the patient that there is no other treatment option except partial arthrodesis of the wrist joint. Therefore, the indication of the Darrach procedure should be carefully selected, although generally, in cases with ulnocarpal impingement syndrome, posttraumatic osteoarthritis, or instability of the DRU joint, rupture of the TFCC, and advanced rheumatoid arthritis, it would still be the treatment of choice. The likelihood of these complications could increase in the elderly or those with heavy labor occupations, and if the cases were followed up for much longer periods, but we nevertheless believe that these complications can be minimized by careful reconstruction of the periosteal sleeve and preservation of the interosseous and distal ligamentous support after minimal resection of the distal ulna.

References

1. Palmer AK, Werner FW (1984) Biomechanics of the distal radioulnar joint. Clin Orthop 187:26
2. Palmer AK (1988) The distal radioulnar joint. In: Bowers WH (ed) Surgical procedures for the distal radioulnar joint. The wrist and its disorders. Saunders, Philadelphia, pp 220–231
3. Darrach W (1942) Colles' fracture. N Engl J Med 226:594–596
4. Bunnel S (1956) Surgery of the hand, 3rd ed. Lippincott, Philadelphia
5. Ekenstam FW (1984) The distal radioulnar joint. Doctoral thesis. Acta Universitatis Up Salvensis Uppsala Universitet, Uppsala
6. Ray RD, Johnson RJ, Jameson RM (1951) Rotation of the forearm — an experimental study of pronation and supination, J Bone Joint Surg [Am] 33:993
7. Crenshaw AH (1987) Campbell's operative orthopaedics, 7th ed. Mosby, St. Louis

8. Palmer AK, Werner FW (1981) The triangular fibrocartilage complex of the wrist — anatomy and function. J Hand Surg [Am] 6:153

9. Brand PW, Beach RB, Thompson DE (1981) Relative tension and potential excursion of muscles in the forearm and hand. J Hand Surg 3:209

10. Sauvé I, Kapandji AI (1936) Nouvelle technique pour le traitement chirurgical des luxations recidivantes isolees de lextremite inferieure du cubitus. J Chir 47:589–594

11. Bowers WH (1982) The distal radioulnar joint. Operative hand book. Churchill Livingstone, New York, pp 743–769

12. Dingman PVC (1952) Resection of the distal end of the ulna (Darrach Op.). J Bone Joint Surg [Am] 34:893–900

13. Fulkerson A, Watson DH (1988) Surgical procedures for the distal radioulnar joint. In: Bowers WH (ed) The wrist and its disorders. Saunders, Philadelphia, pp 232–243

14. Hui FC, Linscheid RL (1982) Ulnotriquetral augmentation tenodesis. J Hand Surg [Am] 7:230

15. Spinner M, Kaplan EB (1970) Extensor carpi ulnaris: Its relationship to stability of the distal radio-ulnar joint. Clin Orthop 68:124–129

16. Kesslu I, Hecht O (1970) Present application of the Darrach procedure. Clin Orthop 72:254–260

17. Newmeyer WL, Green DP (1982) Rupture of extensor tendons following resection of the distal ulna. J Bone Joint Surg [Am] 64:178–182

18. Tsai T, Stillwell JH (1984) Stabilization of the ulnar stump using the FCU — a modification of the Darrach procedure. J Bone Joint Surg [Br] 9:289–294

An Original Prosthesis of the Distal Radioulnar Joint

Adalbert I. Kapandji[1]

Abstracts. Pronation-supination is one of the most important motions of the upper limb, indispensable to the orientation of the hand. It is often problematic, particularly in distal radio-ulnar joint (DRUJ) dislocations after Colles fracture and in other circumstances, isolated ulnar fractures, two-bone fractures, Galeazzi fractures, and also in rheumatoid arthritis. Many procedures are proposed for the treatment of pronation-supination troubles or traumatic painful instabilities of the DRUJ but in all these procedures except that by Milch, the risk of painful instability of the ulnar stump is real, such as after a Kapandji-Sauvé or a Moore-Darrach operation. When this occurs, ulnar stump stabilization is very difficult to obtain. Ligamentoplasties have been proposed but their results are hazardous. Then the idea of a mechanical fixation by mean of a DRUJ prosthesis emerged. After considering the characteristics of this joint, it appears that a "ball and socket" joint prothesis is convenient with little losseness. The original principles of the DRUJ prothesis are: cementless fixation but with screws, composition of the articular pieces and a metal spherical head fitting with an HD polythylene cup. The articular surfaces are supported by two pieces: the proximal part, set on the ulnar stump, bearing a hollow hemisphere, coated with an HD polyethylene cup and fixed with a transversal screw on an intra-medullary stem; and the distal part, holding a sphere, the ball, fitting with the cup and fixed on the radius lower extremity by two special screws. Two models with the same proximal part were designed depending on whether or not the ulnar head was to be saved. The indication of this DRUJ prothesis is painful instability of the ulnar stump when the ulnar resection is too large, after a Kapandji-Sauvé procedure or after a Moore-Darrach procedure. The DRUJ arthroplasty technique is also described, that needs a few additional ancillary tools. Until now, these protheses have been used in 2 cases, with or without a saved ulnar head. The results seem to have been favourable, with a total range of pronation-supination, stability, and painlessness. Obviously, it is too early to know their final value; we know that with clinical experience, the techniques will evolve, mainly the in fixation system. However, it seems important to make it known as an additional possibility in the treatment of DRUJ problems.

Keywords: Distal radio-ulnar joint — Wrist prosthesis — Instability of the distal radioulnar joint — Ulnar stump instability — Dislocation of the distal radio-ulnar joint — Stiffness of the distal radio-ulnar joint — Pronation supination of the forcarm

Introduction

The pronation-supination motion is problematic in many cases because the two bones of the forearm are linked for that function [1]: the shape of each one is congruent to that of the other, and the two radioulnar joints work simultaneously [2]. A simple modification of the length or shape of one or both bones is sufficient to seriously impair this motion. The distal radioulnar joint (DRUJ) may be dislocated in five circumstances (Fig. 1).

The most frequent is *Colles' fracture* in which it is possible to see a widening of the joint, a rotation of the radial sigmoid notch in two planes, and a relative lengthening of the ulna due to compression of the distal radius. As it is very

[1] Clinique de l'Yvette, 43, Route de Corbeil, 91160 Longjumeau, France

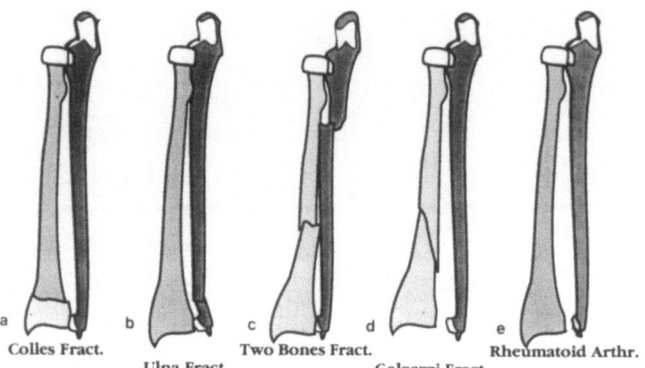

Fig. 1. The five causes of pronation-supination problems. **a** Colles' fracture. **b** Ulna fractures. **c** Two forearm bones fractures. **d** Galéazzi's fracture. **e** Rheumatoid arthritis

Colles Fract.

Ulna Fract.

Two Bones Fract.

Galeazzi Fract.

Rheumatoid Arthr.

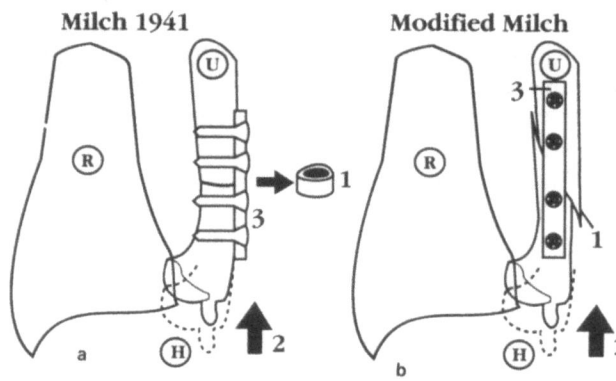

Milch 1941

Modified Milch

Fig. 2. Milch's procedures. **a** The original (1941) [6] and **b** the current one using an oblique section and sliding it before fixing it to a plate [7]

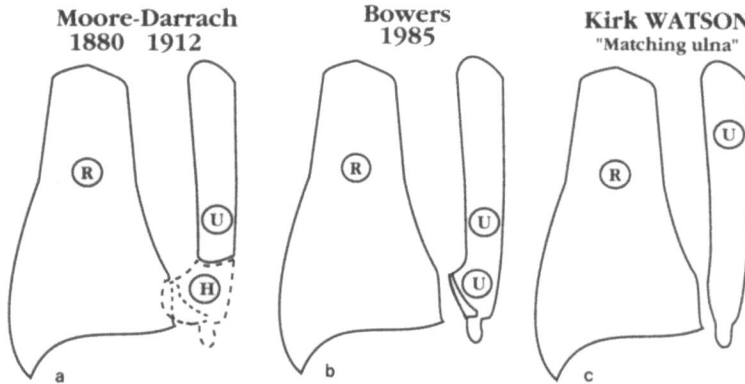

Moore-Darrach 1880   1912

Bowers 1985

Kirk WATSON "Matching ulna"

Fig. 3. The resection of the ulnar head. **a** Total excision according to Moore [8] and Darrach [9], **b** partial resection, according to Bowers [10] with or without fibrous interposition [5], **c** the "matching ulna" according to Kirk Watson

difficult to precisely reduce this type of fracture, mal-union often occurs and the problems are not so much those of flexion-extension than of pronation and, especially, supination [3].

Other circumstances produce pronation-supination impairments, such as isolated *ulnar fractures*, especially at its distal extremity, *two-bone fractures* which are difficult to reduce without osteosynthesis, a radial fracture combined with a DRUJ luxation [4], the so-called *Galeazzi's*

fracture and, finally, the destruction of the ulnar head in *rheumatoid arthritis*.

There are many procedures for treating problems of pronation-supination or for traumatic painful instabilities of the distal radioulnar joint. The Milch procedure (1941) [5, 6] consists of shortening the ulna (Fig. 2) with a shaft segmental resection of the ulna combined with a plate osteosynthesis (Fig. 2.a), so that the ulnar head will be exactly at the level of the radial

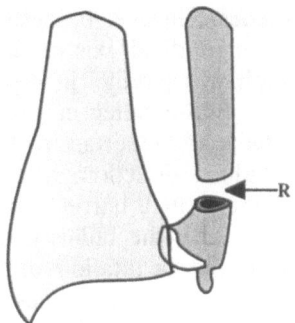

Fig. 4. The isolated resection (R) of the ulnar shaft first proposed in 1917 by Le Fort and Cololian [12] then in 1924 by Baldwin [11]

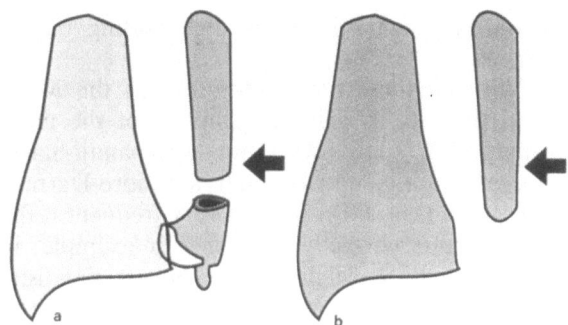

Fig. 6. The instability of the ulnar stump (*arrow*) may occur **a** after a Kapandji-Sauvé procedure or **b** after a Moore-Darrach procedure

The Kapandji-Sauvé Procedure 1936

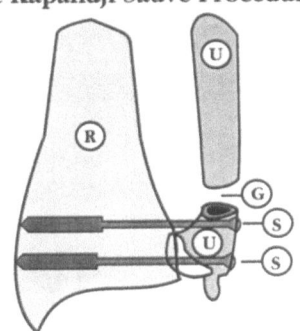

Fig. 5. The Kapandji-Sauvé procedure [13] proposed in 1986. It consists of a fusion of the DRUJ, the ulnar head being fixed with one or two screws (S) combined with a segmental resection of the ulnar shaft, creating a pseudarthrosis (G) just above the DRUJ fusion

The Kapandji-Sauvé Procedure 1936

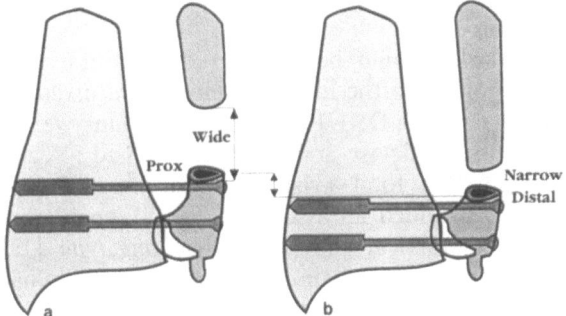

Fig. 7. How to prevent an ulnar stump instability **a** In the Kapandji-Sauvé procedure, the stump instability may be avoided **b** by a lower cut as distal as possible and a resection as limited as possible so as to not risk ossifications between the two bony extremities

sigmoid notch [7]. At this time, it is preferable to making an oblique osteotomy (Fig. 2.b) and fix the two extremities after sliding them together. It is a good procedure if there is no dislocation of the DRUJ, which is not always the case.

The Moore (1888) [8] — Darrach (1912) [9] procedure (Fig. 3.a) consists of an excision of the ulnar head which improves the pronation-supination range of motion, but may favor an ulnarly shifting of the carpus. Moreover, if the ulnar resection is too vast, an instability of the ulnar stump may occur.

The Bowers (1985) [10] partial resection of the ulnar head (Fig. 3.b) is a better solution for carpus stability, but the pronation-supination motion does not always work perfectly. It is the reason why this partial resection has evolved to a

"custom-made" resection or "matched ulna" (Kirk Watson) — a resection along 4–5 cm from the ulnar styloid process (Fig. 3.c) — which does work better than the other ones, if the ulna has kept its normal length.

The Baldwin procedure (1924) [11], following the work of two French surgeons Le Fort and Cololian (1917) [12], makes only a segmental shaft resection of the ulna (Fig. 4), closely above the DRUJ, which is not touched. In this way, the pronation-supination motion becomes free.

The Kapandji and Sauvé (1936) [13, 14] procedure — wrongly attributed to Lauenstein [15–19] — consists of a fusion of the DRUJ combined with the above-mentioned ulnar segmental resection (Fig. 5). The results for the pronation-supination range of motion are mostly good, and there is no medial shifting of the carpus.

With all these procedures, except the Milch one, the risk of painful instability of the ulnar stump (Fig. 6) is real (after a Kapandji-Sauvé operation (Fig. 6.a) or after a Moore-Darrach operation (Fig. 6.b)) but not very frequent if the technique is correctly applied. For example, in the Kapandji-Sauvé procedure (Fig. 7), the distal section must be as low as possible, and the gap as narrow as possible (Fig. 7.b) without risking ossification between the bony extremities. In the Moore-Darrach procedure, the resection of the ulnar head must be as short as possible. When this complication occurs, ulnar stump stabilization is very difficult to obtain: some investigators have proposed a looping technique using the flexor carpi ulnaris tendon and others a lengthening of the ulnar stump, but the results are inconsistent.

In what could be considered a natural progression came the idea of a *mechanical fixation*, by means of a DRUJ prosthesis. We think we are the first to devise and build it. We had already proposed a total wrist prosthesis in 1982 [20] which included an associated DRUJ prosthesis. The anatomical joint is a *trochoid type* [13, 21–23], with a cylindrical solid surface, the ulnar head fitting with a cylindrical hollow surface, the radial sigmoid notch. However, *this is not*

a very cylindrical surface, because, during the motion, the longitudinal axis of the two bones (Fig. 8), which was parallel in supination (Fig. 8.a), becomes non-parallel in pronation (Fig. 8.b). Thus, the articular surface is slightly convex in the longitudinal direction, and the cylinder looks rather like a small barrel. Furthermore, in pronation (Fig. 9.b), the radius is crossing over the ulna, with the facilitation of the anterior concave curvature of the two bones in supination (Fig. 9.a) becoming opposed in pronation. The radius thereby becomes shorter relative to the ulna. If we consider the radius (Fig. 10) as being

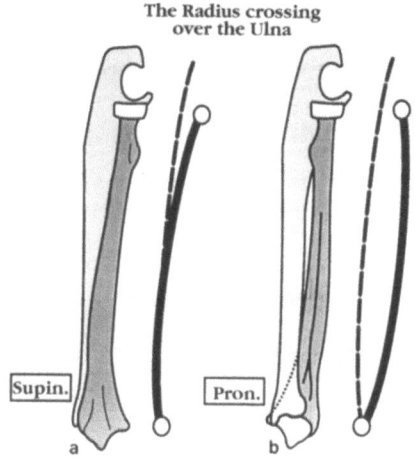

Fig. 9. **a** In supination, the curvatures of the two bones are facing anteriorly, **b** while in pronation they are opposite to each other so as to match up and make possible a complete range of motion

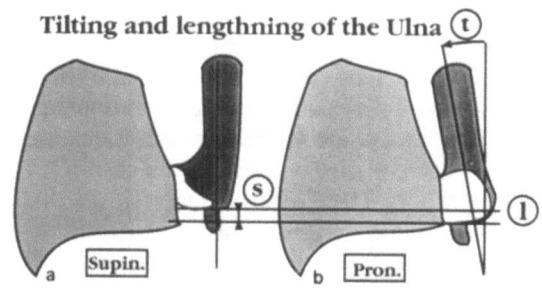

Fig. 10. The modifications in the DRUJ during pronation. **a** In supination, the axis of the ulna and the radius are parallel, and the ulna is slightly shorter than the radius (s): this is the ulnar variance. **b** In pronation, the two axes are not parallel and the ulna is tilting (t) with regard to the radius, which becomes shorter in reference to the ulna which seems to be longer (l). The ulnar variance diminishes by 2–3 mm

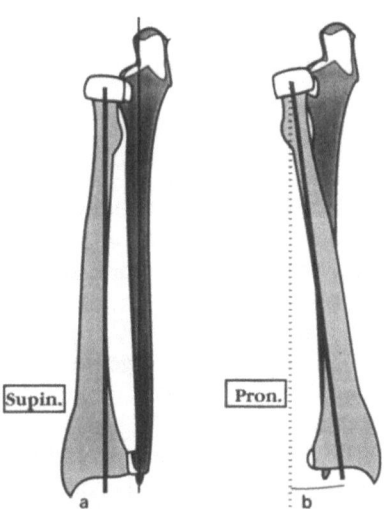

Fig. 8. The obliquity of the radius in pronation. **a** As in supination, the longitudinal axis of the radius is parallel to that of the ulna, **b** In pronation, the radial axis crosses that of the ulna, being is located in front of it

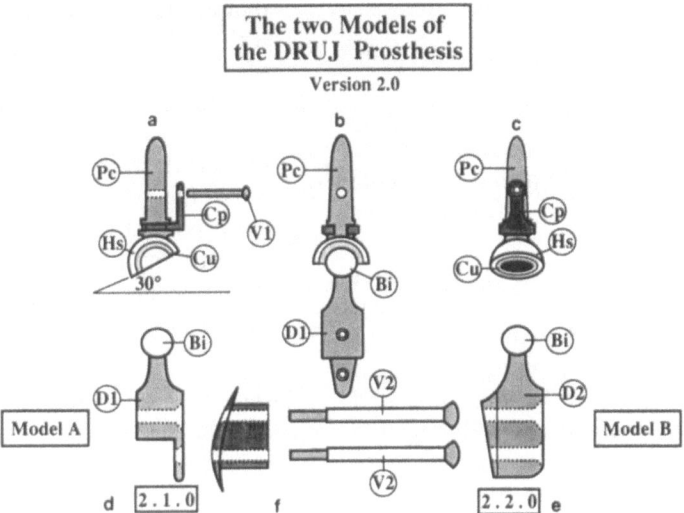

Fig. 11. The DRUJ prosthesis. The proximal part is common to the two models. **a** A cut view with the stem (*Pc*), the ulnar counter-plate (*Cp*), the oblique (*30°*) hemispherical cup (*Hs*) coated with HD polyethylene, and the fixation screw (*V1*). **b** A lateral view wherein the counter-plate is seen by the end of its fork. **c** A medial view wherein the counter-plate is seen on the stem. The distal part is different for each model, but it supports the spherical surface (*Bi*) of the prosthesis which fits with the cup coated with HD polyethylene. **d** In Model A (2.1.0), the distal part (*D1*), with its special hollowing-out, is fixed with two screws both on the radius and on the intact ulnar head. In the center, the distal part's inferior plate which is fixed on the ulnar head can be seen. **e** In Model B (2.2.0), the distal part (*D2*) is complete and fixed directly in the radial sigmoid notch. **f** The system of fixation of the distal part is composed of two long screws (*V2*), threaded only at their extremities with the rest being coated with hydroxyapatite, and the radial counter-plate with a median partition set perpendicularly to the plate, and two threaded tubes into which the screws are tightened

immobile (Fig. 10.a), the lower ulna in pronation (Fig. 10.b) is tilting and lengthening. These movements are not very large, but need a ball and socket joint with a small amount of looseness.

The original principles of the DRUJ prothesis (Fig. 11) are: *cementless fixation* but with *screws* giving immediate and definitive firmness and the allowing of rapid rehabilitation. The articular pieces are composed of a metal spherical head (Bi) fitting with an HD polythylene cup (Cu). The articular surface is spherical so as to allow mobility of all the components of this complex joint. The two articular surfaces are supported by two pieces: the proximal part (A–B–C), holding a hollow hemisphere (Hs), coated with an HD polyethylene *cup* (Cu), fixed with a screw (V1) in the ulna, and a distal part (D–E), holding the sphere, *the ball* (Bi), fitting within the cup, and fixed on the radius by two screws (V2) tightening a radial counter-plate (F).

Two models of the prosthesis were designed depending on whether or not the ulnar head was to be saved, i.e., a prosthesis after a Kapandji-Sauvé procedure with the intact ulnar head or a prosthesis after a Moore Darrach procedure without ulnar head preservation. For both models, the proximal part is the same, with a stem (Pc) introduced into the prepared medullary ulnar canal and fixed with a screw on an ulnar counter-plate (Cp).

The distal part is different according to the type of the prosthesis: (1) for model A, the distal piece (D), with a special hollowing-out, is fixed with two screws both on the radius and on the intact ulnar head, and (2) for model B, the distal piece (E) is fixed with two screws directly on the radius onto the sigmoid notch. The indication of this DRUJ prothesis is *painful instability of the ulnar stump* which may occur after a Kapandji-Sauvé procedure when the ulnar resection was too wide and too proximal, and after a Moore-Darrach procedure when the ulnar head resection was too large.

The DRUJ arthroplasty technique is done as

follows:

1. A medial 10-cm approach, saving the sub-cutaneous nervous branches.
2. Dissection of the ulnar head region, keeping it in its proper place when it has been saved.
3. Dissection of the ulnar stump with a minimal stripping of the periosteum and only on its medial aspect.
4. Preparation of the prothesis bed, and, after good positioning, fixation with two screws and blocked on the radial counter-plate.
5. Preparation of the ulnar stump: (a) cutting it with an alternating saw at the level indicated with a special gauge, and (b) widening the medullary canal with a special reamer.
6. Introduction of the stem of the proximal piece into the medullary canal with the oblique cup facing laterally.
7. Using a special key, drawing down the cup (2 or 3 mm) so that it fits exactly with the ball to its contact point and turning it 180° so that it faces *medially*.
8. Putting the forked radial counter-plate on the distal piece, pushing it onto the ulnar medial wall, and fixing it with a screw after making the holes in the bone. The holes must be made at first with a thin drill and, after

temporarily taking out the proximal piece, with a slightly larger drill, all at the diameter of the screws.
9. At this point, the proximal piece may be returned to its proper position and firmly fixed with the screw.
10. Now, the prosthesis may be tested. It must work correctly with a 180° range of motion without any tendency of luxation of the ball from the cup. This is why the cup is positioned after a drawing down and a 180° rotation to make it face medially.

Used in 1 case with and 1 without a remaining ulnar head, the results of these 2 types of prosthesis seem to have been favorable, achieving a total range of pronation-supination, stability, and relief of pain. Obviously, it is too early to know the final value of this prosthesis, based on only 2 cases, but it seemed important to make it known as an additional possibility in the treatment of the DRUJ problems.

We knew that, in time and with clinical experience, some of its secondary characteristics would evolve, mainly for its fixation system. Two types of a new model is available, the Mark 2.1.0. (model A) and the Mark 2.2.0 (model B). The proximal and the distal parts are smaller and the

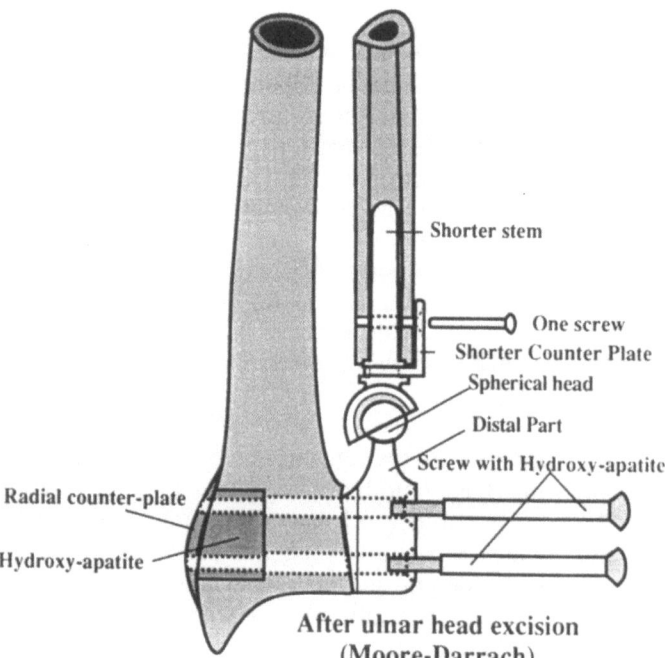

Shorter stem

One screw
Shorter Counter Plate
Spherical head

Distal Part
Screw with Hydroxy-apatite

Radial counter-plate

Hydroxy-apatite

After ulnar head excision
(Moore-Darrach)

Fig. 12. The DRUJ prosthesis 2.2.0 set in place. The proximal part is set in the prepared ulna: the stem is in the medullary canal, the ulnar counter-plate in position, there is lengthening of the stem and orienting of the cup medially, and it is fixed with the screw. The distal part is firmly fixed on the radial sigmoid notch with the two long screws, passing through the radial epiphysis and tightened on the radial counter-plate. This schema shows the main modifications to version 1.

fixation system has improved, particularly for the distal part which is firmly attached on the radial epiphysis with two screws tightened on a radial plate located on its lateral aspect. The screws, the plate, and the lateral side of the distal plate are coated with hydroxyapatite, in preparation for being glued to the adjacent bone.

The differences can be noted on the drawing of a Mark 2.2.0 set in place, (Fig. 12): there is a shorter stem and counter-plate in the ulnar stump, fixed with only one screw, and the distal part is smaller, with coated screws fitting with the lateral radial plate. Consequently, the ulnar resection is also smaller and its periosteum-stripped area more limited. Essentially, this prosthesis is indicated in two "second-look" situations: painful ulnar stump instability after Kapandji-Sauvé, and after a Moore-Darrach procedures. Perhaps it will be used in unstable stumps after a Bowers procedure. It is possible that, in the future, when its reliability will be definitively established, this prosthesis will be used primarily. We are working toward this end.

References

1. Kapandji AI (1975) Pourquoi l'avant-bras comporte-t-il deux os? Ann Chir 29(5):463–470
2. Kapandji AI (1986) Biomechanik des Carpus und des Hangelenkes. Orthopäde 15:60–73
3. Kapandji AI (1977) Le membre supérieur soutien logistique de la main. Ann Chir 31(12):1021–1030
4. Desault M (1791) Mémoire sur la luxation de l'extrémité inférieure du cubitus. J Chir 1:78
5. Milch H (1936) Dislocation of the inferior end of the ulan: Suggestion of a new operative procedure. [Am] J Surg 47:589–594
6. Milch H (1941) Shortening of the ulna with osteosynthesis in inferior luxation of the ulnar head. J Bone Joint Surg [Am] 23:311–313
7. Milch H (1942) So-called dislocation of the lower end of the ulna. [Am] Surg 116:282–292
8. Moore EM (1880) Three cases illustrating luxation of the ulna in connection with Colle's fracture. Med Rec 17:305
9. Darrach W (1912) Anterior dislocation of the head of the ulna. [Am] Surg 56:802–803
10. Bowers WH (1985) Distal radio-ulnar joint arthroplasty: The hemiresection-interposition technique. J Hand Surg [Am] 10:169–178
11. Baldwin WI (1921) Orthopaedic surgery of the hand and wrist. In: John Sir Robert (ed) Orthopædic surgery of injury. Henry Frowde and Hodder and Stroughton, London
12. Le Fort R, Cololian P (1917) La resection segmentaire isolée de la diaphyse cubitale inférieure. Rev Orthop 3(6):117–150
13. Kapandji AI (1986) Opération de Kapandji-Sauvé. Techniques et indications dans les affections non rhumatismales. Ann Chir Main 5:181–193
14. Sauvé L, Kapandji M (1936) Nouvelle technique de traitement chirurgical des luxations récidivantes isolées de l'extrémité inférieure du cubitus. J Chir 47:589
15. Gonçalves D (1974) Correction of the disorders of the distal radio-ulnar joint by artificial pseudo-arthrosis of the ulan. J Bone Joint Surg [Br] 56:462
16. Lauenstein C (1880) Zur Frage der derangement interne des kniegelenk. Dtsch Med Wochenschr 16:169–170
17. Lauenstein C (1887) Zur Behandlung der nach Karpaler Vorderarmfraktur zurükbleibenden Störung der Pro- und Supinations-Bewegung. Zentralbl Chir 23:433
18. Steindler A (1940) Orthopedic operations: Indications, techniques and results. Charles C. Thomas, Springfield, Illinois
19. Taleisnik J (1985) The wrist Vol 1. Churchill Livingston, New York
20. Kapandji AI (1982) Principes et expérimentation d'une nouvelle famille de prothèses de poignet de type cardan. Ann Chir Main 1(2):155–167
21. Kapandji AI (1977) La radio-cubitale inférieure vue sous l'angle de la prono-supination. Ann Chir 31(12):1031–1039
22. Kapandji AI (1980) Physiologie Articulaire — Schémas commentés de Mécanique Humaine Vol. I, le Membre Supérieur. 5 ème Edition Maloine Ed. Paris.
23. Kapandji AI (1987) Biomécanique du carpe et du poignet., Ann Chir Main 6:147–169

Keywords Index